Health Now: An Integrative Approach to Personal Health Version 1.0

By

Linda B. White

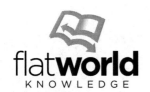
flatworld
KNOWLEDGE

Health Now: An Integrative Approach to Personal Health Version 1.0

Linda B. White

Published by:

Flat World Knowledge, Inc.
1111 19th St NW, Suite 1180
Washington, DC 20036

Brief Contents

Contents

About the Author

LINDA B. WHITE, MD

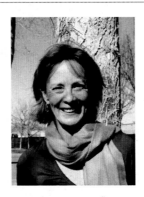

Source: Courtesy of Amber Paugh.

Linda B. White, MS, MD, has specialized training in radiology, pediatrics, and adolescent medicine. During the 1980s, she taught human physiology at Metropolitan State University of Denver before shifting to full-time freelance writing, editing, and consulting. In 2004, she returned to Metro State as faculty in the new Integrative Therapies Program. There she developed and taught a number of classes: personal health, medical terminology, physiology of aging, holistic pediatrics, botanical pharmacology, herbal medicine, stress physiology, and sleep science. She coauthored *Kids, Herbs, & Health*; *The Herbal Drugstore*; and *500 Time-Tested Home Remedies and the New Science Behind Them*, contributed to other books, and has published many magazine articles on health.

Acknowledgments

Special thanks go to the following people:

- Melissa Yu, my Flat World Knowledge project manager, for her efficiency, organizational skills, and gracious editorial guidance.
- Steve Rissman, ND, Metropolitan State University of Denver, for his contributions to the men's health sections.
- Christine Odell, PhD, Metropolitan State University of Denver, and Amy Terry, BA, CPT, for their contributions to the fitness chapter.
- Darcy White, MPH, Emory University; Sandra Stenmark, MD; and Mike Bizeau, PhD, Metropolitan University of Denver, for directing me toward timely research.

And thanks go to the following astute reviewers of this book:

- Liza Allen, MS, Mesa Community College
- Charkarra Anderson-Lewis, University of Southern Mississippi
- Lisa Bernardo, PhD, RN, MPH, Carlow University School of Nursing
- Mike Bizeau, PhD, Metropolitan State University of Denver
- Jewel Carter-McCummings, Montclair State University
- James Clark, University of Texas at San Antonio
- Christine Davis, University of North Carolina at Charlotte
- Jose Gonzales, MS, Plymouth State University
- Una Gordon, El Centro College
- Stephanie Huskey, Tennessee Wesleyan College
- Jeri Lloyd, Piedmont Virginia Community College
- Hal Marchand, Western Illinois University
- Janet Marquard, California State University Northridge
- Heidi Paquette, RN, MS, Marquette University
- James Pennington, Springfield College
- Ramin Radfar, Wofford College
- Rodney Ragsdale, M.A., West Hills Community College
- Linda J. Romaine, Raritan Valley Community College
- Tammy Schiek, M.A., Rockford College
- Heather Seitz, PhD, Johnson Community College
- Jennifer Spry-Knutson, Des Moines Area Community College
- Michelle Tollefson, MD, Metropolitan State University of Denver
- Jennifer Vickery, Winthrop University
- Charles B. White, JD
- Shari Willis, Rowan University

Dedication

Dedicated to Leonard Wisneski, MD, and Carol Jensen, RN, M.Ed., for their visionary work to transform health care and medical education.

Preface

Welcome to *Health Now: An Integrative Approach to Personal Health*, published by Flat World Knowledge, which is dedicated to high-quality textbooks at an affordable cost. Knowledge of personal health has a value that lasts a lifetime. This book will help students identify lifestyle changes that promote their health and wellness and prevent disease. Students will learn how personal habits ripple outward, affecting them, those they love and work with, and, ultimately, the local and global environment.

By book's end, students will possess what medical professionals call health literacy. Not only will they have a firm grasp of health basics, but when presented with unfamiliar medical information or dubious health claims, they'll be able to consult credible sources for answers. Students will know how to communicate with their health care practitioner and make informed decisions.

ORGANIZATION

The book's overall organization mirrors that of competing books. However, *Health Now* leads with information on the ways of practicing medicine: conventional, complementary, alternative, holistic, and integrative. The last, integrative medicine, represents the brave new world of health care. It shifts the focus from treating disease to keeping patients healthy, addresses all aspects of an individual's health (not just physical function), and considers all therapies with evidence of effectiveness and safety. Whereas competing texts relegate information about complementary medicine to the last chapter, *Health Now* provides information on relevant, evidence-based therapies throughout the book.

In keeping with the integrative model, the book emphasizes strategies to optimize health and avoid disease. Most Americans die of chronic and largely preventable diseases. The seeds of these illnesses are planted early. For that reason, the book repeatedly presents modifiable risk factors.

CHAPTER SUMMARIES

The book begins with an overview of health and wellness, proceeds through the pillars of good health, moves to the most common illnesses facing Americans, and concludes with the interrelationship between personal and environmental health.

Here are chapter overviews:

- Chapter 1 defines health and wellness, explores health trends and unmet challenges at home and abroad, and provides skills for positive behavior change.
- Chapter 2 examines the types of health care: conventional, alternative, complementary, holistic, and integrative.
- Chapter 3 explains the stress response, discusses the damaging effects of long-term stress, and reviews methods of managing stress.
- Chapter 4 reviews the stages of sleep, sleep needs through the life cycle, the perils of sleep deprivation, sleep disorders, and ways to improve sleep.
- Chapter 5 examines psychological health: factors that promote it, factors that erode it, signs of psychological disorders, and treatment options.
- Chapter 6 explores the value of healthy relationships, types of relationships, the effects of sex and gender on health, and skills for improving social health.
- Chapter 7 focuses on sexual and reproductive health with an emphasis on how to maximize the benefits and minimize the risks associated with intimate sexual relationships. It provides information on reproductive options, sexually transmitted infections, and common reproductive system conditions in men and women.
- Chapter 8 teaches nutrition basics, recommendations on healthy eating, dietary challenges, and contemporary trends in the food industry.
- Chapter 9 discusses the damaging effects of sedentary lifestyles, the benefits of regular exercise, government activity guidelines, types of exercise, tips for working physical activity into daily life, and sports safety.
- Chapter 10 reviews body weight and body composition, the current crisis in overweight and obesity in the United States and the world, causes and consequences of obesity, strategies for achieving and maintaining healthy body weight, and common eating disorders.
- Chapter 11 explores the reasons people use and abuse addictive substances, the health effects of commonly used substances, and the tools that help people quit.

- Chapter 12 covers unintentional injuries (accidents) and intentional injuries (violence), with emphasis on personal and community strategies to reduce accidents and violence.
- Chapter 13 explains basic immune system function, factors that undermine and bolster immune system health, disorders of this system, and strategies for preventing infection.
- Chapter 14 reviews the types of disease-causing microorganisms, the common infections affecting the major bodily systems, warning signs of serious infections, preventive strategies, and treatment options.
- Chapter 15 presents important facts about diabetes mellitus and the major cardiovascular diseases, including statistics, causes, signs and symptoms, risk factors, protective factors, and management.
- Chapter 16 explains cancer, common types of cancer, risk factors, protective factors, screening and diagnostic tests, and treatment approaches.
- Chapter 17 investigates the complex interrelationship between personal environmental health, pollution, water management, climate changes, and the ways individuals can promote planetary health.

FEATURES

While this book can serve as a resource for anyone interested in health, it has unique advantages for students and instructors. Its conversational style makes medical information accessible. Each chapter contains several staple and innovative features as follows:

- **Historical overview:** Many chapters begin with a summary of historical milestones culminating in our current understanding of health.
- **Learning objectives by section:** Instead of a long list of learning objectives at the beginning of the chapter, we divide the learning objectives by section and offer exercises and key terms for every section in the book. Students can make sure they understand key concepts before moving to the next section. Instructors can readily reorganize, delete, and modify sections within chapters to make the book their own.
- **Video and audio clips:** Book chapters contain videos from YouTube and health organizations that help cement or augment many of the concepts.
- **Tips on staying healthy:** Whenever appropriate, chapters contain self-assessments, skills for making positive behavioral changes, preventive measures, appropriate home management of minor illnesses, guidelines for contacting a medical professional, and information on research-backed treatments.
- **Additional resources:** Each chapter contains book and website suggestions to read more on certain topics.
- **Timely research:** Chapters contain highlights from cutting-edge studies.
- **Customizable features:** Flat World Knowledge's digital-first platform lets educators take control and personalize their textbooks to match their learning objectives and, ultimately, increase student success.

I hope you will enjoy this book as much as I enjoyed writing it for instructors, professors, and students.

Best wishes for a great semester or quarter!

Linda B. White, MD

This book seeks to increase your knowledge about personal health. To the best of our knowledge, the information provided is accurate, as of the time of publication. Please do not use this book to substitute for professional medical care or advice. If you have medical concerns or questions, always seek guidance from a health care professional. The author and publisher are not responsible for the accuracy of any content added by faculty.

CHAPTER 1
Health for Life

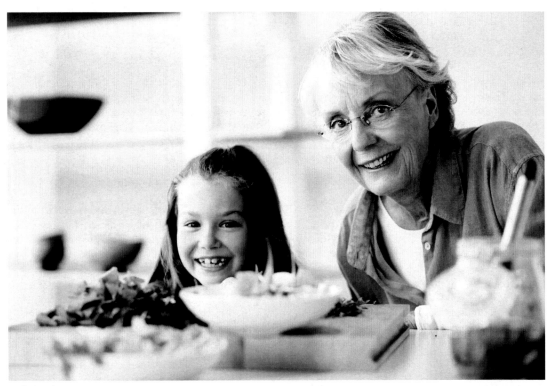

© *Thinkstock*

Around the world, people value physical health, as well as mental, emotional, social, and spiritual well-being. Despite the importance of health, our behaviors often compromise this precious resource. When suboptimal behaviors become habitual, we cease to connect them to ill health. We don't get enough sleep, neglect our relationships, eat junk food, stress out, sit too much, and exercise too little—yet can't figure out why we feel tired most of the time.

It doesn't have to be that way. Habits can change. Health should evolve naturally, pleasurably. Appreciating beauty, feeling joy and compassion, enjoying friends, engaging with work, having a sense of purpose, savoring delicious food, moving our bodies, spending time in nature, taking time to rest and sleep—all these things promote vitality. They also prevent illness and speed recovery when illness strikes.

This chapter will explore the elements of health and wellness, national and global health challenges, and the lifestyle patterns that promote vibrant health.

Health is the outcome of living well.

- Alice Waters, author, activist, and restaurateur

1. DEFINING HEALTH AND WELLNESS

LEARNING OBJECTIVES

1. Define health and wellness.
2. Analyze the relative contributions of medical care, genetics, personal behaviors, and environmental factors in determining health and longevity.
3. Describe the dimensions of wellness.

What do you mean when you say someone is healthy? That the person lacks the outward signs of disease? That he or she appears physically fit? That his or her skin glows and eyes shine? Health is not always an easy word to pin down. For many years, health referred to the absence of disease. Western physicians examined the body for signs of physical illness, with little acknowledgment of other components of health.

In the mid-1940s, the World Health Organization (WHO) defined **health** as "a state of complete physical, mental, and social well-being and not merely the absence of disease."[1] Optimal health allows people to enjoy long, productive lives.

Optimal health has become synonymous with **wellness**. The WHO defines wellness as "the optimal state of health." The organization further explains the two focal points of wellness: (1) "the realization of the fullest potential of an individual physically, psychologically, socially, spiritually and economically," and (2) "the fulfillment of one's role expectations in the family, community, place of worship, workplace, and other settings."[2] Optimum wellness is also termed "high-level wellness."

Health and wellness are neither static nor passive. You are a work in progress. Some agents beyond your control—genetics, environmental exposures, age—affect your health. However, your lifestyle choices hold great power to either promote or undermine health. Wellness is an active process, one in which individuals deliberately adopt lifestyle patterns that promote their health. Most of us desire high-level wellness. And having a disability or chronic illness doesn't prevent people from obtaining that goal.

No one lives forever. The maximum human lifespan is about 125 years.[3] Although people increasingly make it to age 100, precious few live much longer. The average life expectancy in the United States is 78.7 years.[4] Before death, many people have developed chronic (long-term) illnesses. In any given population of people, the gap between the actual and optimal state of health is known as the **burden of disease**.

health

According to the WHO, "A state of complete physical, mental and social well-being and not merely the absence of disease."

wellness

Optimal health achieved through an active process by which an individual makes healthy choices.

burden of disease

The gap between the actual and optimal state of health; often measured by resultant disability and premature mortality.

1.1 Determinants of Health

What makes one person healthy and another ill? Why do some people sustain long, vigorous lives while others suffer persistent illness and premature death? Research yields some surprising answers. For instance, only 10 percent of untimely deaths are caused by shortfalls in medical care.[5] Family history and genetics contribute to 30 percent of illness and death. On the other hand, personal behaviors and environmental and social factors carry far greater weight in determining health and longevity.

FIGURE 1.1 Drivers of Premature Death

Four domains drive premature death. As you can see, insufficient medical care is responsible for only 10 percent of these deaths. While genetics and family history more powerfully shape health, a person's behaviors are the most important. Furthermore, these domains interact.

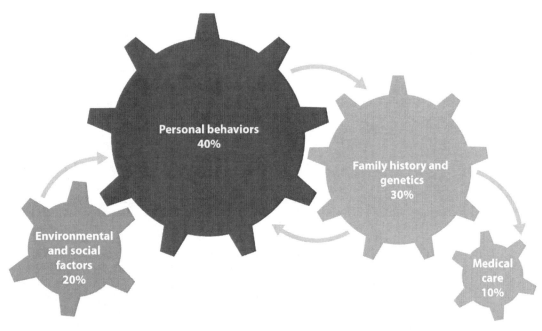

Source: Courtesy of Kaiser Permanente.

Another way to view health is from an ecological perspective. Ecology is a branch of biology that studies the complex relationships of organisms to one another and to their physical environments. In 1988, scientists began applying this model to human health.[6] The basic concept is that multiple levels of influence affect human health. Furthermore, these levels interact in complex ways.

FIGURE 1.2 Social-Ecological Model of Health

Health can be viewed in an ecological framework, starting with an individual's genetics and behaviors and expanding outward to social relationships, community resources, and greater societal influences.

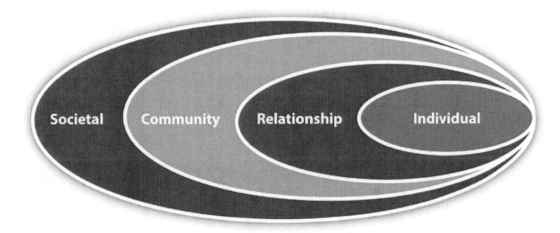

Source: Adapted from Centers for Disease Control and Prevention. The social-ecological model: a framework for prevention. 2009. Available at: http://www.cdc.gov/violenceprevention/overview/social-ecologicalmodel.html.

Figure 1.2 illustrates four levels: individual, relationship, community, and societal factors. You have the most control over your own health-related behaviors and the least over societal factors.

Individual Influences

Some of these factors are outside of your control: genetics, family history, age, gender, race, and sexual orientation. You have the power to modify other factors: beliefs and values, resiliency, coping skills, financial resources, education, health literacy, and health-related behaviors (diet, physical activity, sleep, substance use, sexual behaviors).

Relationships

Relationships include formal and informal social networks: family members, friends, roommates, classmates, coworkers, clubs, and support groups. Social support benefits health, particularly when friends and peers model and encourage health-promoting behaviors. In contrast, discord and violence undermine health; so does associating closely with people who abuse substances, engage in risky sexual behaviors, have consistently unhealthy diets, and disdain physical exercise.

Community Factors

Resources include the quality of neighborhoods, schools, religious institutions, housing, clinics and hospitals, parks and recreation centers, workplaces, air and water, and transportation. The cohesiveness of community members also figures in. In a pivotal examination of the health determinants published in online journal *Health Affairs* in 2002, J. Michael McGinnis and colleagues wrote, "Our genetic predispositions affect the health care we need, and our social circumstances affect the health care we receive."[7]

Greater Societal Influences

Society and culture establish norms and attitudes about health-related issues such as diet, physical activity levels, body weight, smoking, substance abuse, sexuality, and violence. Intolerance and inequality based on gender, age, race/ethnicity, and sexual preference socially and economically marginalize those groups. The country's overall economic health influences employment rates as well as the funding of social services, education, and health care. Environmental conditions directly impact health. Public health policies (public smoking bans, gun-control laws, seatbelt laws, universal vaccination, health insurance mandates) affect whole populations.

1.2   Family History and Genetics

In the past, discussions pitted genetics against environmental factors: nature versus nurture, genetic endowment as opposed to everything else—social environment, diet, activity levels, and environmental influences. However, we know nature and nurture interact intricately, engaging in a lifelong dance.

We inherit our genes from our parents. From there, ecology acts on those genes to affect our biology. Genetic traits can also color our responses to that ecology. So do the behaviors we learn from our parents, other role models, and the media. Multiple influences shape our physical, emotional, psychological, social, and financial health.

Within each of your cells (the basic working units in your body) is a nucleus, which contains your genetic information. The **genome** is the complete set of **deoxyribonucleic acid (DNA)**. DNA contains building blocks called nucleotides, which are arranged sequentially along chromosomes like beads on a necklace. The four nucleotide bases act like letters of the alphabet to spell out a code.

Chromosomes are threadlike structures containing DNA and protein. Humans have 23 chromosomes. Most cells contain a pair of each chromosome for a total of 46. (Sperm and egg cells contain 23 chromosomes.)

Each chromosome contains many genes. A **gene** is the basic unit of heredity. Each gene is made of a specific sequence of nucleotide bases and codes for a particular protein. In 2003, the US Human Genome Project identified and sequenced all 20,500 human genes. The genome forms a blueprint for the structure and function of the body.

Proteins perform your body's essential functions. They form structural components in your body (bones, ligaments, tendons, teeth, hair) and enzymes, which catalyze chemical reactions. The collection of proteins expressed by the genome is called the **proteome**.

genome

The complete set of genetic information in an organism.

deoxyribonucleic acid (DNA)

A molecule that encodes genetic instructions in the chromosomes; contains nucleotides.

chromosome

A structure containing DNA and protein.

gene

The basic unit of heredity; a sequence of nucleotides in DNA that codes for a protein.

Only about 2 percent of deaths in this country are purely genetic in nature.[8] Some diseases have a strong genetic component. A few are caused by a single mutated gene. Examples include sickle cell anemia (a mutation that distorts red blood cells), Tay Sachs disease (an enzyme deficiency that results in accumulations of fatty material in the brain), and cystic fibrosis (a defect that makes mucus sticky and difficult to clear in organs such as the lungs). Through advances in genomic medicine, scientists are learning to control, and perhaps someday cure, diseases caused by a single mutation.

However, the marked health disparities and major diseases burdening the United States are not caused by genetic variations. The common chronic diseases of modern life stem from a complex interaction of genes, lifestyle habits, and environmental exposures. These so-called **multifactorial diseases** include common chronic conditions such as cardiovascular disease, diabetes, cancer, obesity, and Alzheimer's disease. While these diseases may have genetic risks, they manifest from genetic vulnerability *plus* life experiences. As George Bray, MD, a renowned obesity researcher, famously put it, "Genetics loads the gun; the environment pulls the trigger."

Our experiences and exposures modify **gene expression**, the conversion of genetic information into a protein. Not all genes are "read" (transcribed into proteins). That's because, within the chromosomes, DNA is coiled around special proteins. In the chromosomes, the DNA winds around histones (a particular type of protein). Genes that are tucked within this coil can't be read. Substances can also bind to genes (and their associated proteins) to prevent or allow their expression. Some genes promote or suppress the expression of other genes.

Epigenetics is the study of the reactions that influence gene expression. *Epi* is Greek for "above." Epigenetics literally means above the genome. It explains why, despite sharing the same genes, a muscle cell looks different from a nerve cell and why the health of identical twins differs. Epigenetic changes can be inherited, even though the genes are not changed. Inherited traits, therefore, can be genetic or epigenetic.

FIGURE 1.3 The Chromosome

Inside the nucleus are the chromosomes, each of which contains many genes.

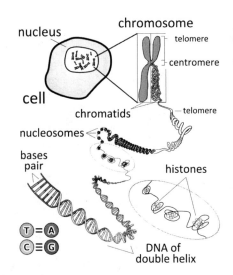

Source: KES47. 2010. Available at: http://commons.wikimedia.org/wiki/File:Chromosome_en.svg.

Video Clip 1.1

Epigenetics
Identical twins, by definition, share the exact same genes. However, environmental factors can alter the way our genes are expressed. That's why identical twins aren't really identical. Epigenetic changes can be passed along to the next generation. This Nova Science Now (PBS) video explains epigenetics, including the genetics and epigenetics of identical twins.

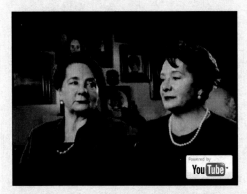

View the video online at: http://www.youtube.com/v/Xjq5eEslJhw
Source: PBS NOVA.

---

multifactorial diseases

Medical conditions caused by a complex interaction of genes, lifestyle habits, and environmental exposures.

gene expression

The process whereby the information encoded in a gene produces a protein.

epigenetics

The study of heritable changes caused by activation or deactivation of genes rather than alternations in the DNA sequence.

Prenatal and Early Childhood Experiences

Our experiences begin in the womb. Certain prenatal (before birth) exposures—malnutrition, toxins, infections—negatively affect the fetus's growth and development.

In the late 1980s, David Barker, MD, PhD, professor of clinical epidemiology at the University of Southampton, England, and his colleagues showed that babies small at birth were at risk for developing high blood pressure and heart disease later in life.[9] Provided with plenty of calories, low-birth-weight babies display catch-up growth and face a greater likelihood of becoming obese and developing diabetes.[10]

Barker's work sparked the "fetal origins of adult disease" hypothesis, which marked a radical departure from the belief in the 1950s that the fetus was largely protected from the mother's experiences with alcohol, cigarettes, drugs, and stress.[11] Instead, Barker and others posited that early life events can predispose people to chronic conditions that may not appear until middle age. Rather than changing the genes, these early experiences—good or bad—modify gene expression. Furthermore, epigenetic alterations can be passed to the next generation.

In addition to prenatal influences, negative experiences in childhood shape brain development, potentially leading to learning impairments, anxiety, depression, increased reactivity to stress, and substance abuse.[12] Adverse childhood experiences have social, cultural, economic, and environmental roots. They contribute to and perpetuate disparities in health and socioeconomic status. The fetal origins hypothesis suggests that the best way to safeguard the health of the next generation is to optimize the health of their parents.

 Video Clip 1.2

A Biologist's Mother's Day Song
This music video explains genetics and epigenetic influences such as the prenatal environment.

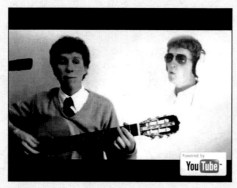

View the video online at: http://www.youtube.com/v/osWuWjbeO-Y
Source: Adam Cole, musician and biologist.

1.3 Environmental Determinants of Health

People exercising in Haikou People's Park, Haikou City, Hainan Province, China.

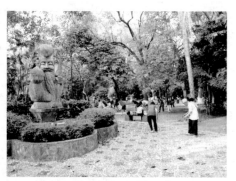

Source: Anna Frodesiak. 2012. Available at:

http://commons.wikimedia.org/wiki/

File:Haikou_People%27s_Park_-

_people_exercising_-_01.jpg.

Environmental determinants are those physical elements that affect health. The natural environment includes plants, animals, natural resources, weather, and climate change. Access to natural landscapes ("green spaces") positively influences human health.

The manmade environment gives us buildings (housing, workplaces, recreation centers, cultural events centers, industrial operations) and transportation. Our activities can both create aesthetically pleasing works and give rise to damaging pollutants.

As discussed, environmental influences begin before birth. Exposures to various chemicals can affect the eggs and sperm that combine to form an individual. The mother's nutritional status, stress level, and overall health determine the environment in which a fetus develops. Early childhood experiences—some infectious diseases, abuse, neglect, family discord, and malnutrition—can have profound influences on health in adult life.

Throughout life, toxic exposures can increase the risk of cancer and other chronic diseases. Contaminants such as toxic chemicals and microorganisms in food, water, air, and soil pose health risks. Geographic location can determine exposure to noxious substances. Around the world, the poor are more likely than the rich to live near industrial operations and disposal sites for toxic waste. In developing countries, people often lack the luxury of clean drinking water. They may heat their homes by burning coal, which releases respiratory irritants.

The built environment shapes health. Buildings for residences and workplaces need to be safe. Communities designed for motor vehicle transportation promote inactivity and obesity. On the other hand, communities that create safe pedestrian and bicycle routes improve health by reducing pollution and encouraging physical activity. People with ready access to recreation centers and safe green spaces have better physical and mental health. Chapter 17 will discuss environmental health in more detail.

1.4   Socioeconomic Determinants of Health

Socioeconomic factors include your social experiences and economic realities. *Socioeconomic status (SES)* refers to one's position in society based on education, occupation, and income. SES factors encompass social support, access to educational and job opportunities, availability of healthy foods, exposure to actual and media violence and chaos, prevailing attitudes and norms that relate to tolerance and acceptance, economic disparities, and the safety of neighborhoods.[13] Included in this discussion are race (which is biologically based) and gender (which is biologically and culturally based) because they influence SES and contribute to health disparities.

Family

You inherit your genes from your biological parents. Your family also powerfully shapes your attitudes, values, eating habits, physical activity patterns, methods of managing stress, and social skills. Healthy families support and love one another, share responsibilities, eat together, enjoy leisure activities together, and don't abuse substances. Well-nurtured children have better health and survival rates.

Education

Educational level predicts health and longevity. Surveys show that college graduates are twice as likely as those who hadn't graduated from high school to be in excellent health.[14] Among people aged 45 to 64, the death rate for those with the highest level of education is 2.5 times lower than for people with the lowest education.[15]

Education helps to close the racial-disparity gap between whites and nonwhites. One study found that, compared with whites with less than 12 years of education, blacks and Hispanics with 16 years of education lived an additional 7.5 and 13.6 years, respectively.[16] Persistent racial discrimination and a two-tiered education system probably explain why most educated white men outlived the least educated black men by 14.2 years. The gap was 10.3 years for highly educated white women versus less educated black women.

Nevertheless, education promotes health for multiple reasons. Higher educational attainment correlates with better jobs, higher income, higher social status, health insurance coverage, less smoking, more physical activity, and less obesity. Taking a class in personal health gives you many tools and increases your *health literacy*, your ability to locate and understand health information, to obtain health services and to make informed health care decisions.[17] Greater health literacy is linked to a reduced risk of hospitalizations, emergency room visits, and deaths.

Financial Status

Poverty contributes to an estimated 6 percent of **mortality** (death).[18] Income inequality (the difference in income between the richest and the poorest citizens) has widened over recent decades. For every 1 percent increase in income inequality, mortality rates rise 0.4 for those at the bottom. Possibly more important than absolute income level is how poor you feel. Feeling poor is stressful, which is bad for your health. Relative to more affluent neighborhoods, poor neighborhoods tend to have higher crime, worse pollution, suboptimal schools, scarcer grocery stores, and fewer parks and other green spaces—all of which undermine health and well-being.

mortality

Death.

Race and Ethnicity

Race refers to categories of people based largely upon physical appearance: the color of skin, hair, and eyes and the shape of the nose, eyes, and jaw. Ancestry influences these appearances. Ancestry also shapes **ethnicity**, as do culture, nationality, language, traditions, and beliefs. While race is inherited, ethnicity is acquired. Any given race contains a host of ethnic groups. People who look white may identify with entirely different ethnic groups: Scandinavian, Australian, New Englanders, and so on. People with brown skin might fit into the pigeonhole for Hispanic yet be Dominican, Puerto Rican, Cuban, Spanish, or Brazilian.

The racial divisions used by the US Census Bureau are white, black (African American), American Indian or Alaskan Native (also called Native Americans), and Asian (also called Asian American) or Pacific Islander. Multiracial refers to a blend of two or more races.

Ethnicity affects health by influencing dietary patterns and attitudes toward education, substance use, physical activity, and health care. Only a few diseases fall along racial lines. For example, sickle cell disease mainly affects people of African and Mediterranean descent; cystic fibrosis tends to affect

race

Categories of humans based largely upon physical characteristics.

ethnicity

Refers to groups of people defined by their culture, traditions, nationality, or ancestry.

people of Northern European ancestry. Note that race is largely based on superficial biological characteristics. Of the genetic variation among humans, there's far more variation within a continental group (e.g., Africans, Asians, Europeans) than between one race and another.[19]

Nevertheless race contributes significantly to health disparities. A 2006 US study found a nearly 21-year life expectancy gap between Asian American females and urban black males.[20] In 2009, the death rate for blacks was 1.3 times higher than for whites.[21] In 2011, the infant mortality rate was more than twice as high for blacks as for whites.[22] On the other hand, Hispanics have made gains in life expectancy, which was 81.4 years in 2011.[23] Compare that to life expectancy for whites (79 years) and blacks (75.3 years).

Causes of death and disease prevalence vary by race. For instance, the number one cause of death in whites, blacks, American Indians, and Alaska Natives is heart disease.[24] For Hispanics, Asian Americans, and Pacific Islanders, cancer is the top killer and heart disease is second. Hispanics are more vulnerable to diabetes, blacks to stroke, and whites to Alzheimer's disease. Relatively more deaths from accidents, liver disease, and diabetes affect American Indians and Alaska Natives.

A number of factors contribute to race-related health disparities. At the top of the list is *racism*, a bias toward or against members of a particular race. The presumption is that one race is somehow better or worse than another. Ungrounded stereotypes take root. Discrimination based on race hinders upward mobility among social classes and undermines health.[25] Marginalization is stressful. Language barriers can further hamper the success of immigrants.

Underprivileged racial minorities more often live in poor neighborhoods marred by substance use, violence, substandard housing, and suboptimal schools. Green spaces, parks, recreation centers, and grocery stores (stocked with fresh produce) are often in short supply. Access to health care may be limited. Some experts believe that social conditions are the main causes of racial health disparities and far outweigh biological risk factors and access to medical technology.

Gender

Sex is biologically based. The WHO defines *gender* as "the socially constructed roles, behaviours, activities, and attributes that a given society considers appropriate for men and women."[26] American women outlive men by five years. In 2011, the life expectancy for men was 76.2 years versus 81.1 years for women.[27] A complex interplay of biological and cultural differences contributes to this difference. Hormonal differences affect vulnerabilities to certain illnesses. Women are more likely to suffer from depression and osteoporosis (brittle bones). Men are more likely to die from accidents and violence. Women more often consult with health professionals for preventive care and sick care. Chapter 6 will discuss theories about gender-based health disparities in more detail.

Medical Care

Conventional medical care has a limited effect on people's health. Insufficient medical care accounts for an estimated 10 percent of deaths.[28] Researchers and scientists predict that, as the population continues to age (and requires more medical care), that number will rise. Older people tend to have more diseases, many of which can be managed by medical treatment. No matter one's age, medical treatment can be lifesaving, particularly in the face of overwhelming infection or traumatic injury. Vaccinations prevent many infections that once cut life short. Medical technology helps diagnose and promptly treat many diseases.

On the other hand, medical care sometimes causes harm. A landmark 1999 study from the Institute of Medicine reported that as many as 98,000 people die each year from medical errors—more than deaths from car crashes, AIDS, and breast cancer.[29] A 2011 study revealed that the problem was perhaps even worse.[30] One out of three hospital patients in the United States experienced a medical error. Examples include hospital-acquired infections, adverse drug reactions, surgical injuries, and surgeries on the wrong site.

Personal Behaviors

Modifiable lifestyle patterns contribute to an estimated 40 percent of deaths.[31] Each day, you make important decisions about diet, physical activity, substance use, and sex. You decide how you'll handle life's curveballs, whether you stress out or view them as challenges to master. You budget how much time you make for sleep and socializing.

Four unhealthy behaviors—lack of physical activity, insufficient intake of fruits and vegetables, tobacco use, and excessive alcohol consumption—cause most of the illness and death related to chronic diseases. A British study tracked the impact on longevity of those four health behaviors over a span of 11 years. People with the lowest scores (smoked, didn't exercise, drank too much, and didn't consume at least five servings of fruit and vegetables a day) had four times the risk of dying relative to their peers who made the healthiest choices.[32]

1.5   The Dimensions of Wellness

In a move away from examining health on the physical plane alone, experts have defined wellness according to six to seven dimensions. While some sources omit environmental wellness, physical environments clearly influence people's health and well-being.

In Chapter 2, we'll discuss the holistic model, which holds that these dimensions interact and that optimal wellness requires that people mobilize their strengths and shore up weaknesses in all areas. For now, here are the seven dimensions and their attributes. In Section 3, you'll have a chance to assess your health in each area.

- **Physical** wellness takes into account a number of biological factors: level of physical fitness, presence or absence of disease or injury, and a person's ability to take care of himself or herself.

- **Emotional** wellness refers to the overall balance of a person's emotional state (happy, sad, angry, tranquil, etc.), awareness of emotions, and ability to express emotions freely and appropriately. People with positive emotional health are capable of trust, intimacy, and love. They are generally happy, optimistic, and self-confident and feel they accomplish what they set out to do.

- **Social** wellness springs from emotional wellness. Socially healthy people enjoy satisfying interpersonal relationships.

- **Intellectual** wellness refers to the ability to organize and express ideas; to think critically, rationally, and analytically; to maintain a sense of curiosity; and to solve problems using brainpower. Skills learned in the classroom can be used in life experiences. Creativity and zest for learning keep people vital and engaged throughout life.

- **Spiritual** wellness provides a sense of meaning and purpose in life. Spiritual people possess a set of beliefs, principles, and values that guide their decisions. They rise above intolerance, petty grievances, and grudges toward compassion, forgiveness, and altruism (a selfless concern for the well-being of others). They may have a sense of being part of a grander scheme. For many people, participation in organized religions forms the anchor of their spiritual life. Others may express their spirituality through creative arts, nature, meditation, and acts of service.

- **Occupational** wellness entails identifying passions and career goals, preparing to meet those goals (which is one purpose of college), and finding work that pays the bills and provides a sense of personal satisfaction. Work can be paid or unpaid, including volunteer activities and scholastic pursuits. Financial stability is important. Its opposite generates stress and reduces access to healthy food, safe living situations, and health care—all of which jeopardize health. It's also important to find a healthy balance between work and play. As a college student, you're working on achieving that balance now.

- **Environmental** wellness refers to the safety and cleanliness of your physical environment, as well as your attitude toward the environment and your commitment to improving it. Environmental toxins can make you sick. On the other hand, beauty in your environment enhances your well-being. Your contributions toward protecting the planet—recycling, conserving natural resources, reducing pollution, preserving wilderness areas—have an impact and provide a sense of personal engagement.

Video Clip 1.3

Wellness Dimensions

This video explains the connection between the wellness dimensions and the concept of wellness as a life journey.

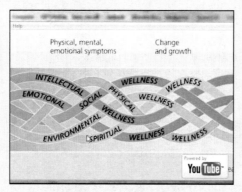

View the video online at: http://www.youtube.com/v/ZnMZ44RkE6k

Each of us moves along a continuum of health and wellness. Some days we feel under the weather; other days we're brimming with vitality. In Section 3, we'll discuss the dimensions of wellness and the keys to promoting your own health and wellness.

KEY TAKEAWAYS

- Health and wellness are more than the absence of disease.
- The most important determinant of health and longevity is personal behaviors. Genetic and family history, social factors, and environmental factors also influence health. Medical care, while critical, is the least important factor.
- Optimal wellness encompasses health in all the domains of a person's life. The dimensions of wellness include physical, emotional, social, intellectual, spiritual, occupational, and environmental.

DISCUSSION QUESTIONS

1. Medical care has a relatively small contribution toward preventing premature death. Does that surprise you? Why do you think personal behaviors have a greater impact? Provide an example from your own life to support or dispute that contention.

2. Some medical services do prevent illness and promote longevity. Provide two examples of services you've received from your health provider that kept you healthy.

3. Discuss the meaning of spirituality in your life. Consider what gives you a sense of meaning and purpose—the things you do that make you feel connected to something grander than yourself and the rituals you follow that make you at peace.

2.   GLOBAL AND NATIONAL HEALTH CONCERNS

LEARNING OBJECTIVES

1. Discuss trends in global health, including the top causes of disability and death.
2. Analyze health trends in the United States and list the top causes of death.
3. Compare and contrast the health of US citizens to the health of citizens in other affluent nations.
4. Describe the US government's Healthy People initiative.

2.1   Health around the World

Global health relates to populations around the world. Although it transcends national concerns, the well-being of people in far-flung countries affects us all. Human health and wellness, education, income, productivity, environmental health, and political stability all intertwine.

For many years, international organizations such as the United Nations and the World Health Organization have focused on reducing and eliminating **communicable diseases**, illnesses caused by infectious agents or their toxins that people can acquire from other humans, animals, and the environment (contaminated food, air, water, soil, etc.). Illnesses such as infectious diarrhea, malaria, tuberculosis, and AIDS prematurely end lives.

Some of these infections are **acute illnesses**, meaning they last a short time. Acute illnesses can be mild or life-threatening. Many cases of infectious diarrhea are acute, though they can be deadly, especially in infants and small children. On the other hand, tuberculosis and AIDS are **chronic illnesses**, meaning they last longer than three months.

Communicable diseases are rampant in the developing world. Their solutions lie in providing clean water and food, sanitation, vaccinations, and strategies to eradicate disease-causing agents from the environment. Antimicrobial drugs help treat those infections that elude prevention. These advances increase quality and quantity of life.

More recently, international experts have recognized the parallel threat of **noncommunicable diseases**, illnesses that are not infectious or readily transmissible. The top noncommunicable conditions are obesity, cardiovascular disease, type 2 diabetes, cancer, and chronic lung disease. These illnesses are chronic, sapping health for years before death occurs.

For decades, noncommunicable diseases have caused significant **morbidity** (illness) and mortality in the developed world. As the "Western lifestyle" of tobacco; inactivity; and salty, fatty, sugary foods has spread around the globe, these chronic diseases have likewise become common in developing countries. These risk factors contribute to disease **incidence** (the number of new cases of a condition occurring within a certain time frame) and **prevalence** (how many people have the condition at any point in time).

Recent analyses of changes in disease incidence and prevalence around the globe have yielded expected as well as startling findings. The Institute for Health Metrics and Evaluation periodically measures the world's most significant health problems and evaluates their possible solutions. Their 2010 Global Burden of Disease study analyzed health statistics from 50 countries and compared the data collected in 1990.[33] Here are some of the key findings:

- The world's inhabitants are living longer, mainly because fewer infants and children succumb to infectious diseases.
- In many developing countries, a number of positive changes have increased longevity: public health initiatives (clean water, proper disposal of sewage, vaccinations), improved nutrition, and family planning (which reduces the birth rate and increases the survival of those children who are born).
- Africa is the one continent that hasn't significantly improved conditions of extreme poverty: maternal and infant mortality, childhood infections, malnutrition, malaria, and AIDS.
- As cars become more available in developing countries, the incidence of roadway injuries has escalated.
- The incidence and prevalence of chronic, noncommunicable disease has increased substantially. People live long enough to develop these conditions, and medical advances have extended the life

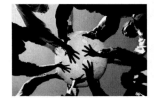
© Thinkstock

communicable diseases

Illnesses caused by infectious agents or their toxins that people can acquire from other humans, animals, and the environment (contaminated food, air, water, soil, etc.).

acute illnesses

Those illnesses that last a short period of time.

chronic illnesses

Those illnesses that last three months or longer.

noncommunicable diseases

Illnesses that are not infectious or readily transmissible.

morbidity

Illness.

incidence

When talking about diseases, the term refers to the rate at which new cases appear.

prevalence

When talking about diseases, the term refers to the proportion of the population affected with that condition at a particular period of time.

of those who have these illnesses. That means that those years gained aren't necessarily spent in good health.

- The biggest health risks for chronic illness and death are high blood pressure, tobacco use, physical inactivity, and overweight and obesity.
- The top two causes of death worldwide are now heart disease and stroke (brain injury due to interrupted blood flow).
- Other chronic, lifestyle-related conditions that have increased include diabetes and painful conditions such as arthritis and low back pain.
- The prevalence of substance abuse and mental illnesses rose. Untreated mental disorders now account for 13 percent of the global burden of disease, with depression alone ranking as the third leading cause of disease burden.[34]
- People are now living long enough to develop dementia, a group of conditions marked by progressive loss of intellectual and social function. Between 1990 and 2010, Alzheimer's disease (the most common type of dementia) tripled.

Other researchers found that, in 2008, of the 57 million people who died, 36 million succumbed to noncommunicable conditions.[35] While their ill effects may not be as dramatically apparent as symptoms of infectious illnesses, they do rob people and nations of health, productivity, prosperity, and years of life.

Noncommunicable, chronic diseases are also more expensive and complicated to prevent and treat than acute infectious illnesses. Antibiotics and vaccinations against infectious diseases are relatively cheap. Distributing mosquito nets and draining standing water where malaria-carrying mosquitoes breed dramatically reduce malaria. However, changing the factors that fuel most noncommunicable diseases is more difficult. Doing so requires a complete revamping of the food industry, eating habits, activity levels, sleep habits, and stress levels.

Top Causes of Death and Disability Worldwide

The Global Burden of Disease studies estimate disability-adjusted life years (DALYs), which are the sum of years lost due to premature mortality and years lived with a disability. Here are the leading causes of DALYs worldwide for 2010:[36]

1. heart disease (ranked 4th in 1990)
2. lower respiratory infections (ranked 1st in 1990)
3. stroke (ranked 5th in 1990)
4. diarrheal disease (ranked 2nd in 1990)
5. HIV/AIDS (ranked 33rd in 1990)

2.2 Health in the United States

Since the nation's founding, the trend has been that each generation of Americans enjoyed longer, healthier lives than the last. During the 20th century, US life expectancy rose an astounding 30 years.[37] In 1900, the life expectancy at birth was 47.3 years. The average American man lived 46.3 years; women lived 48.3 years.[38] The three leading causes of death were tuberculosis, pneumonia and influenza, and diarrheal illnesses.[39] By 1999, the longevity rates had climbed to 76.7 years (73.9 years for men and 79.4 years for women). The three leading causes of death were heart disease, cancer, and stroke.[40] Notice the change in the top killers from infectious diseases to chronic diseases associated primarily with personal habits.

Public health improvements paved the way for living longer. They included sanitation and hygiene, family planning, improvements in the food supply, and immunizations (vaccinations) against childhood infectious diseases. Better medical care for women during pregnancy and childbirth drove down maternal and infant deaths. Contraceptives allowed women to avoid teen pregnancies and to space births, which improved children's health. In addition to immunization programs, antibiotic treatment of bacterial infections also helped children and young adults survive to older ages. Improvements in medical technology played a much smaller role in extending life, though medical treatment increases the survival of those with chronic illnesses.

FIGURE 1.4 Population Pyramids

The figure on the top is the population pyramid for Angola, Africa. The figure on the bottom represents the population pyramid for the United States.

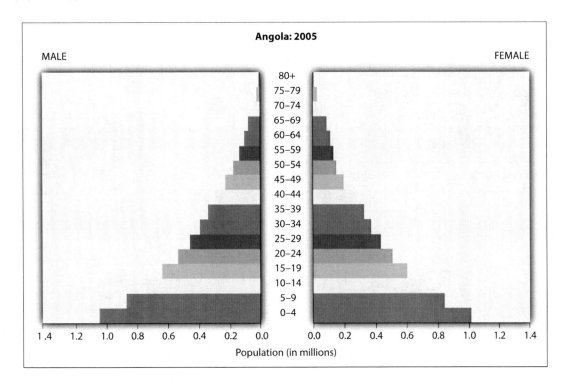

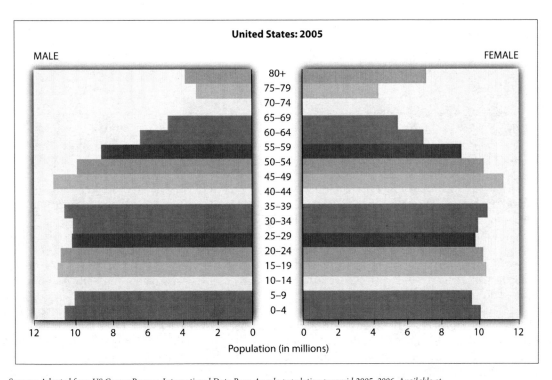

Sources: Adapted from US Census Bureau, International Data Base. Angola population pyramid 2005. 2006. Available at:

http://commons.wikimedia.org/wiki/File:Angola_population_pyramid_2005.png; US Census Bureau, International Data Base. US-2005. 2010.

Available at: http://commons.wikimedia.org/wiki/File:Us-2005.jpg.

Another trend has been a marked increase in the proportion of older adults in the population. In the past, the most populous age group was infants and children. As you can see in Figure 1.4, that situation still holds in Africa and other countries where infectious diseases and malnutrition continue to cut life short. In the United States and other developed countries, the graph has become more rectangular. In fact, organizations such as the World Health Organization note that populations around the world are rapidly aging.

Four factors explain that shift toward a population top-heavy in older adults:

1. Thanks to the public health measures listed, childhood death rates have fallen.

2. The period of increased prosperity following World War II led to the "baby boom," with high birth rates between 1946 and 1964.

3. Birth rates subsequently declined. That's because contraceptives became more available and parents no longer feared their children would die of infections.

4. Life expectancy increased.

Now older Americans (those 65 and up) are the fastest growing segment of the population. The proportion of people over age 85 has also increased dramatically. At the turn of the 20th century, 4.1 percent of Americans were over the age of 65.[41] By 2004, that percentage tripled to 12.4 percent. In 2010, 13 percent of Americans were 65 and up. Baby boomers have begun to enter their senior years. By 2030, an estimated 71 million older adults will make up 20 percent of the population.[42] After 2030, this growth is expected to slow once the last baby boomers blow out the candles on their 65th birthday cakes.

FIGURE 1.5 Rising Numbers of Older Americans

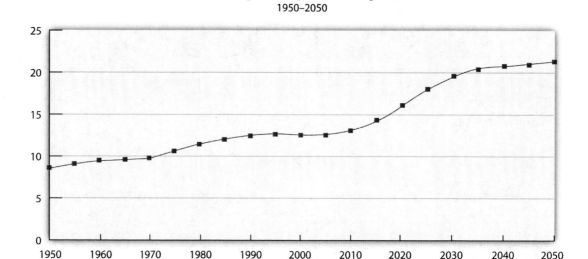

Percentage of US Population over Age 65, 1950–2050

Source: Adapted from Federal Interagency Forum on Aging-Related Statistics/US Census Bureau. Population age 65 and older and age 85 and older.

Available at: http://www.agingstats.gov/Main_Site/Data/2012_Documents/Population.aspx.

Unfortunately, increased longevity combined with the "Western lifestyle" has bred chronic diseases. About 80 percent of American elders live with at least one chronic condition.[43] Chronic illness accounts for 70 percent of deaths in the United States and 75 percent of health care expenditures.[44]

However, long-term medical conditions such as obesity, diabetes, and high blood pressure have become more common at all ages, even children. In 2010, at least one chronic illness plagued 147 million Americans—half the adult population.[45] Obesity, inactivity, poor nutrition (cheap, fast, widely available junk food), smoking, stress overload, sleep deprivation, social isolation, and other ills have increased the proportion of chronic diseases.

Two-thirds of American adults and one-third of children and teens are now overweight or obese.[46] ,[47] Since 1980, the prevalence of childhood obesity has tripled.[48] Over the past 30 years, childhood obesity has more than doubled and teen obesity has tripled.[49] Unfortunately, overweight and obesity in childhood often persists into adulthood, which raises the risk of associated chronic illnesses such as diabetes, heart disease, stroke, arthritis, and some cancers. Experts predict that, unless society halts this trend, this generation of children will be the first not to live longer than their parents.[50] In addition to the health burdens, the economic burden of lost productivity and increased health care costs will be staggering.[51]

What's perhaps most startling is our poor ranking compared to peer nations. In early 2013, researchers from the National Research Council and Institute of Medicine published an analysis of health and longevity called *U.S. Health in International Perspective: Shorter Lives, Poorer Health.*[52] The subtitle says it all. Here are the findings of this study and a follow-up analysis of the data.[53]

- Compared to 16 other affluent democracies, US life expectancy is shorter. The life expectancy at birth is now 78.7 years (76.3 for men, 81.1 for women).[54] Compare that to Japan (80 for men, 86 for women).[55]

- More Americans die before age 50 and are sicker by the time they reach that age. In fact, much of the gap in life expectancy had to do with higher mortality before age 50.

- The United States' ranking for key indicators of health is at the bottom. Recent immigrants to the United States have better health than the natives.

- The United States has higher rates of low-birth-weight babies (an indicator of poor maternal health), premature babies, and infant mortality.

- The United States has higher rates of teen pregnancies and sexually transmitted infections, including HIV (human immunodeficiency virus, which can cause acquired immunodeficiency syndrome, or AIDS).

- Higher rates of unintentional injuries (especially from motor vehicle collisions) and homicides (mainly from firearms) claim the lives of many American youths.

- Americans have a higher prevalence of anxiety, depression, impulse control, and substance abuse disorders.

- Alcohol and drugs sicken and kill more Americans. In fact, drug overdoses are a big contributor to deaths under age 50.

- Americans are more likely to develop obesity, heart disease, diabetes, and chronic lung disease, and general disability is higher.

- Americans smoke less and do better at controlling blood pressure and cholesterol levels (two heart disease risk factors) and detecting cancer and treating cancer.

- Americans who do survive to age 75 are more likely to hang on longer than do seniors in other countries.[56]

The big question is why, despite spending more on health care than any other country, has the health of US citizens steadily slipped?[57]

A number of factors probably contribute. As Chapter 2 discusses in more detail, our medical system focuses on treating rather than preventing disease.

The aforementioned 2013 comparison between the United States and other peer nations addressed underlying causes.[58] Compared to citizens of other affluent nations, the authors noted the following:

- Americans consume more calories (and often from food that's unhealthily prepared).

- US social welfare programs are less comprehensive and less generous.

- Americans are more likely to travel by car (and less likely to fasten their seatbelts), which decreases physical activity.

- Americans own more guns, which contributes mightily to homicides and suicides.

- When it comes to health policy changes, Americans resent government intrusion.

- Americans have higher rates of poverty, higher numbers of uninsured, and poorer education of youth.

- Curiously, even more advantaged US citizens have relatively worse health than those in peer countries.[59]

- Another factor is that, although Americans have the highest per capita income of the affluent countries, they have more income inequality.[60]

In addition to multicountry objective comparisons, surveys show Americans don't rate their own health very highly. One in five rates his or her health as fair or poor.[61] Many Americans admit to neglecting the personal behaviors that maintain health. Many say they suffer from too much stress, too little sleep, and not enough time for quality relationships.

Some people don't recognize the importance of lifestyle factors to health. Even when they do, there's a gap between knowing and doing. Over half of respondents in one survey agreed to the importance of regular physical activity, but only about one-quarter met that goal. Nearly 60 percent believed a healthy diet was important to health, yet only 31 percent said they actually ate well.[62]

The problem seems to be getting worse. Another national survey revealed that the proportion of Americans who adhered to four key elements of a healthy lifestyle—eating enough fruits and vegetables, exercising regularly, maintaining healthy weight, and moderating alcohol intake—fell from 15 percent to 8 percent between 1988 and 2006.[63] People primarily blame lack of time, money, and willpower as barriers to healthier living.

FIGURE 1.6 Per Capita Health Care Spending in Industrialized Countries

The United States spends more health care dollars per person than any other developed country but doesn't earn as much from its investment.

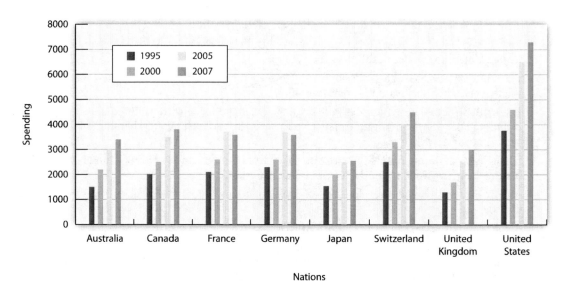

Nations

Source: Adapted from Sugar-Baby-Love. Total health expenditure per capita, US dollars PPP. Data source: OECD Health Data 2010. Available at: http://commons.wikimedia.org/wiki/File:Total_health_expenditure_per_capita,_US_Dollars_PPP.png.

On a brighter note, the 2011 National College Health Assessment found that 62 percent of college students (67 percent of men and 59 percent of women) rate their health as very good or excellent. Nearly 93 percent of students rate their health as good.[64]

Health Care Expenditures

Americans spend far more on medical care than any other country. In 2011, the United States spent an estimated $2.7 trillion on health care, which translates to nearly 18 percent of the gross domestic product.[65],[66] In 1960, the United States spent an average of $143 per person on health care.[67] By 2011, the per person cost had ballooned to $8,684 per person—about 2.4 times the per capita expenditure in the United Kingdom.[68],[69] If the maxim "You get what you pay for" held true, the United States would be the healthiest nation on earth. But as you've already seen, we're not.

Increased investment in expensive medical technology has been a driving force behind skyrocketing spending. Furthermore, doctors may order expensive diagnostic tests, but even the odds of identifying a treatable malady are low—a practice driven, in part, by physicians' fear of malpractice litigation. And indeed, malpractice cases directly and indirectly drive up costs.

If you're thinking you're not the recipient of those funds, you're probably right, particularly if you're young and relatively healthy. Three-quarters of US health care spending goes toward managing chronic illnesses, primarily cardiovascular disease, cancer, and diabetes.[70] Half of health care spending goes toward treating a mere 5 percent of Americans, particularly people over age 65, who have more chronic illness and who are also covered by Medicare. As the population continues to age, health care costs are expected to rise accordingly.

In order to manage the health care needs of the aged—without sacrificing the care of our youth—we need to get smarter about how we spend our medical dollars. According to the Institute of Medicine, of the $2.5 trillion in US health care spending in 2009, 30 percent of it ($765 billion) went toward unnecessary medical services, overpriced services, excessive administration costs, inefficient delivery, missed opportunities for prevention, and fraud.[71] To view an animated graphic of health care costs, go to http://iom.edu/Reports/2011/The-Healthcare-Imperative-Lowering-Costs-and-Improving-Outcomes.aspx.

Some physician groups have taken steps to stop wasteful spending. In 2012, nine medical societies, including the American College of Physicians and the American College of Cardiology, came together to reduce unnecessary medical treatments.[72] For instance, people with no evidence of heart or lung disease shouldn't need a routine chest X-ray before surgery or hospital admission. People with mild symptoms of sinus infection don't need expensive diagnostic tests or antibiotics. To find out more, go to choosingwisely.org.

2.3 Common Causes of Death in the United States

For over 85 years, heart disease has been the number one cause of death in the United States.[73] Cancer, stroke, chronic lung disease, and unintentional injuries (accidents) have ranked in the top 10 for many years, though they tend to shift positions. (See the sidebar "The 10 Leading Causes of Death in 2011 for Americans of All Ages".)

The 10 Leading Causes of Death in 2011 for Americans of All Ages

1. Heart disease
2. Cancer
3. Chronic lower respiratory diseases (asthma, chronic bronchitis, and emphysema)
4. Stroke and related diseases of the blood vessels supplying the brain
5. Unintentional injuries (accidents)
6. Alzheimer's disease (the most common type of dementia)
7. Diabetes mellitus
8. Influenza and pneumonia
9. Kidney diseases
10. Suicide

Source: Hoyert DL, Xu J. Deaths: preliminary data for 2011. Natl Vital Stat Rep. 2012;61(6):4. National Center for Health Statistics. Centers for Disease Control and Prevention. Available at: http://www.cdc.gov/nchs/data/nvsr61/nvsr61_06.pdf. Accessed January 25, 2013.

Patterns for causes of death shift depending on the age group considered. For instance, in people under age 44, unintentional injuries (accidents) top the list. Chronic diseases take time to develop and to become serious enough to cause death. The following list is for adolescents and young adults. Of the 12,032 deaths due to unintentional injuries, nearly 7,000 involved motor vehicle accidents. Driver inexperience and alcohol play huge roles in those accidents. In 2010, 10,228 people of all ages (one-third of all traffic-related deaths) died in alcohol-impaired motor vehicle accidents.[74]

The 10 Leading Causes of Death in 2011 for Americans 15 to 24 Years Old

1. Unintentional injuries (accidents)—of these 12,032 deaths, nearly 7,000 involved motor vehicle accidents
2. Suicide
3. Homicide
4. Cancer
5. Heart disease
6. Congenital disorders (those present from birth)
7. Influenza and pneumonia
8. Stroke and related diseases of the blood vessels supplying the brain
9. Pregnancy and childbirth
10. Chronic lower respiratory diseases

Source: Hoyert DL, Xu J. Deaths: preliminary data for 2011. Natl Vital Stat Rep. 2012;61(6):30. National Center for Health Statistics. Centers for Disease Control and Prevention. Available at: http://www.cdc.gov/nchs/data/nvsr61/nvsr61_06.pdf. Accessed January 25, 2013.

We all have to die at some point. However, most of the conditions that sicken and prematurely kill Americans could be avoided or postponed. In a study published in 2009 in *PLoS Medicine*, researchers analyzed data from the National Center for Health Statistics to determine the numbers of deaths attributable to 12 key risk factors for preventable causes of death.[75] The researchers found that, of the 2.5 million deaths in 2005, almost half a million stemmed from tobacco smoking and 400,000 could be pinned on high blood pressure. Other research shows that tobacco use shortens life expectancy by 10 years.[76] The sidebar "The 12 Leading Preventable Causes of Death" shows how researchers ranked the top risk factors.

The 12 Leading Preventable Causes of Death

1. Smoking
2. High blood pressure
3. Overweight and obesity
4. Physical inactivity
5. High blood glucose (sugar)
6. High LDL cholesterol
7. High dietary intake of sodium (salt)
8. Low dietary intake of omega-3 fatty acids (the kind found in seafood)
9. High dietary intake of trans fatty acids (largely man-made fatty acids created by adding hydrogen atoms to polyunsaturated fatty acids to make them more solid and stable at room temperature; found in many processed foods)
10. Alcohol use
11. Low intake of fruits and vegetables
12. Low intake of polyunsaturated fatty acids

Source: Danaei G, Ding EL, Mozaffarian D, et al. The preventable causes of death in the United States: comparative risk assessment of dietary, lifestyle, and metabolic risk factors. PLoS Med. 2009 Apr 28;6(4):e1000058. Available at: http://www.ncbi.nlm.nih.gov/pmc/articles/PMC2667673/?tool=pubmed.

2.4 Healthy People Initiatives

In 1979, the US Department of Health and Human Services established an initiative called Healthy People. The program established measurable targets for improving the nation's health at the end of each decade. For example, some of the goals for 1990 were to reduce infant mortality by 35 percent and childhood deaths by 20 percent. Most of the objectives were met.

Three decades later, the program continues. Healthy People 2020 established ambitious yet achievable goals for a number of areas.[77] Here are some examples of those goals.

- Increase health insurance coverage for 83 percent of people in 2008 to 100 percent.
- Adolescent health improvements include increasing school safety, increasing the proportion of teens who receive wellness checkups, increasing high school graduation rates, reducing the proportion involved in crimes (as perpetrators or victims).
- The following goals aim to lighten the burden of common chronic diseases:
  - reduce disability due to chronic illnesses such as arthritis and back pain;
  - reduce deaths caused by stroke and heart disease;
  - reduce the proportion of people with high blood pressure;
  - reduce cancer death rates, increase the proportion of Americans who receive recommended screening tests for cancer, and reduce the number of adolescents who visit tanning salons; and
  - reduce the number of cases of newly diagnosed diabetes and the death rate due to diabetes.
- Objectives for improving health behaviors include to
  - increase the proportion of people at all ages who meet federal guidelines for physical activity,
  - reduce tobacco use in people of all ages and increase smoking-cessation success, and
  - decrease the number of people of all ages who use addictive substances and increase treatment for people with substance abuse problems.

- Objectives for environmental health include to
    - increase work commutes made by bicycling and walking and taking mass transit,
    - reduce the risk of adverse health events caused by airborne toxins, and
    - reduce domestic water use.
- Objectives for eliminating health disparities include to improve availability and access to nutritious food, high-quality education, decent and safe housing, health insurance, and reliable and affordable public transportation.[78]
- An important addition to the 2010 goals is addressing sleep deprivation. Key goals in this area are to increase the proportion of Americans who get enough sleep and to reduce the motor vehicle crashes caused by drowsy drivers.

 Video Link 1.1

Determinants of Health: Reaching Healthy People 2020 Goals

This Healthy People 2020 video discusses how identifying weak links in health determinants paves a way toward solutions that improve health and well-being.

http://www.healthypeople.gov/2020/about/DOHAbout.aspx

KEY TAKEAWAYS

- Around the world, life expectancies and the burden of chronic disease have gone up.
- Infectious diseases have steadily come under control in the developing world. However, many people still lack access to safe drinking water, sanitation, and hygiene.
- The United States spends more on health care than any other nation.
- People in other affluent nations live longer and have generally better health than Americans.
- The leading causes of death in the United States could be prevented or postponed.

DISCUSSION QUESTIONS

1. Explain why the prevalence of chronic disease has increased around the world.
2. Discuss the major advances that have reduced the fatality rate for infectious diseases.
3. Examine the "The 10 Leading Causes of Death in 2011 for Americans 15 to 24 Years Old" sidebar. Compare the top three causes of death in that list with the top three causes of death in people 45–64 years old (cancer, heart disease, and unintentional injuries). What factors account for the differences in cause of death between these two age groups?

3. TAKE CHARGE OF YOUR HEALTH

LEARNING OBJECTIVES

1. Assess your current level of wellness.
2. Examine and apply theories about how people make behavioral changes.
3. Learn ways to improve your health behaviors.

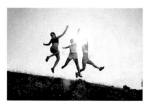
© Thinkstock

You've learned that genetics, heredity, socioeconomic factors, and environmental factors all contribute to health. It's time to address the personal habits—the elements you can control. Once you recognize the importance of lifestyle habits, you can exert a healthy measure of personal responsibility for your health.

Consider yourself the architect of your health and well-being. We're all works in process. Your lifestyle habits promote either construction or demolition. Take a hard look. Like the architect on any remodeling project, you first assess the raw materials, looking for strengths and weaknesses in the design. You do your homework, design a step-by-step plan, and, provided with the necessary tools, build on your assets to create a firm foundation for vitality now and for healthy aging.

If you want to live a long and robust life, follow the pillars of good health:

- Eat well. That means eating vegetables or fruit at every meal, enough to cover half your plate. Other food groups to include are seafood, meat, poultry, nuts, seeds, and whole grains. View foods with added sugar (most processed foods and beverages) as occasional treats. Eat only when you're hungry.
- Engage in physical activity every day. Try to get 30 minutes of aerobic exercise (the kind that's intense enough to let you talk but not sing) five days a week. Do strength training twice a week. To maintain flexibility, move your joints through their full range of motion.
- Make time for friends and family. Nurture those relationships that make you feel secure and happy. Let go of those that only hurt you. Choose friends whose attitudes, values, and habits you admire. Research increasingly shows elements of physical and mental health are "catching."[79]
- Stay away from tobacco smoke and other toxic substances. Other people's smoke harms your health too. Smokeless forms of tobacco also damage health.
- Get enough sleep. Most people need about eight hours of sleep a night. You know you're sleeping enough if you awaken refreshed and feel alert throughout the day.
- Learn to control stress. Stress is unavoidable and, in limited amounts, good for you. Excessive stress undermines health.
- Manage your weight. Overweight and obesity raise the risk for many illnesses. While proper diet and regular exercise help, additional strategies can improve success.
- Maintain hope, optimism, and a generally positive approach to life.
- Find your passion. People who feel a sense of meaning and purpose live longer.[80]
- Start living better now. Your lifestyle affects your well-being now and also sets the stage for your health in old age.

Assess Your Wellness

Earlier, you learned that wellness has at least six components. You'll feel at your best if you're satisfying needs in all domains. Many of these areas overlap. For instance, if you have a drinking problem, your health in all areas will decline.

Rather than focus on risk assessment, it can be more motivating to consider your score for preventing illness and promoting your overall well-being. Notice what you're already doing well.

Examine the following list, placing a check in front of each item that applies to you.

Physical

_____At each meal, half of my plate is fruits and vegetables.

_____I avoid highly processed foods (those high in refined grains and added sugar).

_____I engage in 30 minutes of moderate aerobic exercise (the kind that elevates your heart and breathing rate) most days of the week (for a weekly minimum of 150 minutes).

_____I do muscle-strengthening exercises two days a week (lift weights, work with resistance bands or against the resistance of my body weight, yoga, Pilates, heavy gardening).

_____I routinely get enough sleep (I awake feeling refreshed in the morning and feel alert throughout the day).

_____I rarely feel stressed out.

_____I don't smoke or use other tobacco products.

_____I drink no more than one (if you're a woman) or two (if you're a man) alcoholic beverages a day.

_____I never binge drink (consume five or more drinks at a time if you're a man, four if you're a woman).

_____I wear a seatbelt when I'm in a car and a helmet when cycling, skiing, and skating.

_____I never operate a car or motorcycle under the influence of alcohol or drugs.

_____I am not sexually active or practice safe sex (consistently use condoms and use contraceptives to prevent pregnancy).

_____I examine my breasts or testicles each month.

_____I am up to date on immunizations.

_____I get recommended screening tests (e.g., blood pressure, Papanicolaou ["Pap"] tests).

Emotional

_____I enjoy my life.

_____I recognize and accept my emotions.

_____I can express my emotions to other people in appropriate ways.

_____I usually feel optimistic.

_____I appreciate the good things in my life.

_____I am self-confident.

_____I have a healthy self-esteem (feel good about myself and believe in my value and worth).

_____I am able to trust myself and other people.

_____I take time to relax.

_____I (would) seek professional help for signs or symptoms of physical or mental illness.

Social

_____I make friends easily.

_____I generally get along with people.

_____I make time to socialize.

_____I feel supported by friends and family.

_____I am capable of establishing close bonds with people.

_____I enjoy giving as much as getting in my social relationships.

_____I am honest and trustworthy in my relationships.

_____I am able to ask for help.

Intellectual

_____I enjoy learning and mastering new skills.

_____I'm interested in what other people do and think.

_____I keep up on current affairs through credible news media.

_____I make decisions calmly.

_____I solve problems by examining my options and acting accordingly.

_____I view challenges as learning opportunities.

_____I learn from my mistakes.

_____I have a creative pursuit.

_____I can ask questions when I don't understand something.

_____I have a sense of humor.

Spiritual

_____I have a sense of purpose.

_____I believe my life has meaning.

_____I have a strong set of values that help me do right.

_____I am able to feel compassion for people different from me.

_____I am able to forgive.

_____I engage in community service projects or otherwise help others.

_____I have found an expression of my spirituality (attending religious services, meditating regularly, spending time in nature, playing music, and creating art).

_____I feel a part of something greater than myself.

Occupational/Financial

_____I have a career goal.

_____I am learning skills that will help me achieve my career goals.

_____I take academic pursuits seriously.

_____I am financially secure.

_____My work gives me a sense of personal satisfaction.

_____I am able to balance work and play.

_____I stick to my budget, keeping track of and prioritizing my expenditures.

_____I'm careful with credit cards, avoiding debt by not overspending and by paying off my monthly charges.

Environmental

_____I feel safe in my neighborhood.

_____My personal space makes me feel peaceful and secure.

_____I can usually sleep without loud noises (or other disturbances) awakening me.

_____I have ready access to green spaces (city parks, gardens, or natural environments).

_____My campus provides bins to recycle paper, glass, and plastic—and I use them.

_____I turn off lights, computers, monitors, and other electrical devices when I leave my room.

_____I use only as much water as I need.

_____I never litter.

_____I believe my efforts to protect the environment matter.

How did you do? No one's perfect. Most people will have a couple unchecked spaces in each category. Some things aren't entirely under your control, such as the serenity of your environment and your need to take on financial debt to attend college. In which area do you have the most work to do?

3.1 Making Positive Behavioral Changes

We make changes all the time. Many we embrace enthusiastically: learning to drive a car, going to college, adopting a pet, getting married, and becoming a parent. Some habits—those that you do almost reflexively—can be hard to change. That's especially true if undesirable habits provide immediate gratification or if their absence causes withdrawal symptoms.

Sometimes it's those automatic behaviors—the tendency to lapse into negative thinking, grab a cookie rather than an apple, down a beer at a party—that are hardest to change. Perhaps you decide to give up sodas. You go to lunch and see a cooler full of soda. Your intellect tells you, "Soda is full of sugar. If I keep drinking the stuff, I'm going to gain weight." The hedonist in you says, "Yes, but it tastes good." Commercials suggest that drinking this particular brand is fun. Everyone around you is drinking soda. If you've already paid for an unlimited meal plan, it won't cost you any additional money. Too many times, the pleasure seeker wins.

On the other hand, you've already broken habits. Presumably, you've long since given up pacifiers and cherished stuffed animals. You changed schools and learned to become more independent of your family. It just takes courage, perseverance, and a bit of sweat.

None of us experience success in all our ventures. When it comes to personal health, our approach can be irrational and inconsistent. Resolutions to exercise more, eat better, lose weight, or quit tobacco don't always stick.

Public health experts have long studied what it takes to change health behaviors. During the 20th century, they tried to understand why people weren't universally responding to informational campaigns about the risks of smoking, the ruinous effects of alcoholism, and the benefits of vaccinations. Clearly, knowledge alone wasn't sufficient. If it were, all doctors would be lean, physically fit, and lacking in vices like tobacco use.

Beginning in the 1940s, researchers learned how people made decisions affecting their health and what elements supported successful adoption of positive lifestyle modifications.[81] Since then, scientists have put forth several models to explain how people make behavioral changes. One prominent theory is the Health Belief Model.

Health Belief Model

Developed in the 1950s, the Health Belief Model remains a widely used framework for explaining health behaviors.[82] The model holds that motivation is key to making positive changes. In addition to knowledge, other motivating factors for giving up a bad habit and/or adopting a health behavior include the following:

1. **Perceived susceptibility.** You believe you're vulnerable to diseases or other adverse consequences associated with an undesirable behavior. The following is an example: "All sexually active people are at risk for human papillomavirus. Some strains of the virus cause cancer. A vaccine helps prevent it."

2. **Perceived severity.** You believe the consequences can be dire. Take the following example: "Alcoholism can wreck families and cause cirrhosis of the liver. My uncle was an alcoholic. He lost his job. His wife divorced him. Liver disease turned his skin and the whites of his eyes yellow. He died before he reached 60."

3. **Perceived benefits.** You believe that positive actions will avert and improve your risks. Here's an example: "My doctor says that even if I only lose seven pounds, my blood sugar may return to normal, and I won't need medication for diabetes."

4. **Perceived cost-to-benefit ratio.** You believe that the benefits of your action will outweigh any costs. For instance, a person might think, "If I quit smoking, I might gain weight. But with the money I'll save from not buying cigarettes, I could join a gym. If I'm not smoking, it will be easier to exercise. I won't catch as many colds."

   Four main factors influence the cost-to-benefit analysis:

   a. **Perceived barriers to action.** These are the things individuals think will make it difficult to adopt and maintain a new behavior. For instance, you want to quit smoking but believe you're too stressed to take that on right now. Or you would like to eat more fruits and vegetables but don't live near a grocery store and don't have a car.

   b. **Sense of self-efficacy.** Self-efficacy means you believe you have the power to achieve your goals. You also believe that your actions make a difference to your health. Positive self-efficacy furnishes the necessary motivation, confidence, problem-solving skills, determination, and tenacity for long-term lifestyle changes. Past experiences will shade that perception, which is why it helps to remember past successes. Probably years of avoiding sweets, flossing, tooth brushing, and routine dental hygiene have prevented you from having a mouthful of rotted teeth.

   c. **Subjective assessment of starting to take action.** If you perceive this adventure in a positive light, you're more likely to persist. Stay alert to encouraging signs. Perhaps you've incorporated exercise into your routine in order to lose weight. Even before the scales register lost pounds, you might feel more energetic by day, have better mental focus, and fall asleep more easily at night.

   d. **Social milieu.** Social influences establish norms. If many people around you disdain exercise, eat junk food, smoke, drink heavily, or express negative attitudes, those behaviors start to seem normal. Stepping outside the norm isn't easy. It helps to hang out with people who set the bar higher, who have already achieved (or are working toward) your goal. Having even one supportive friend can make a big difference. Better yet your living and work situations support, reinforce, and reward healthy lifestyles.

Transtheoretical Model: Stages for Behavior Change

The Transtheoretical Model describes the stages people pass through as they initiate positive behavioral changes. The model attempts to explain how people take action to improve health. Some of these stages' elements overlap those described in the Health Belief Model. Here are the five stages:[83]

1. **Precontemplation.** At this stage, an individual has no intention of changing. He or she may be ignorant of or in denial of a problem. Or past failures to change have led to a resigned hopelessness. He or she may react with resistance or defensiveness to others' attempts to help. If the individual is conscious of a health threat, he or she may feel changing isn't worth the effort ("Everyone in my family is overweight") or may feel that change may be offset by a disadvantage ("If I quit taking my roommate's Ritalin, I might not get the As I need to go to law school").

2. **Contemplation.** The individual gains awareness, believes he or she ought to make a change, and intends to take action within six months. He or she may gather information and weigh the pros and cons of the new behavior—without necessarily doing anything. The Southern expression, "I'm fixin' to do it," sums up that stage. Many people become stuck in this stage.

3. **Preparation.** The individual makes plans and intends to take action within a month. He or she has now decided that the pros of making a positive change (e.g., using a condom every time you have sex) outweigh any inconvenience (going to a store and buying the condoms). In addition, the negatives of not modifying the behavior (becoming infected with HIV) outweigh any reluctance to change. The person takes initial steps in the right direction. For instance, someone vowing to begin an exercise program may investigate gym memberships, shop for athletic shoes, or read a book about running.

4. **Action.** Behavior shifts. Positive actions continue for six months. The individual goes from smoking a pack to half a pack a day, eats an apple instead of a donut, drinks seltzer water rather than beer, or laces up his or her sneakers and heads out the door. The individual also overcomes barriers and accesses resources. Maybe the person moves to a substance-free dorm, gets a prescription for a nicotine patch, meets with a nutritionist, works with an athletic trainer, or joins a support group.

5. **Maintenance.** At this stage, the behavioral change has lasted over six months. The person figures out ways to resist temptation and otherwise prevent relapse.

6. **Termination.** The person has gained complete confidence in this new lifestyle and feels no temptation to relapse. The positive behavior now starts to feel routine and necessary. For instance, someone who has taken up jogging now feels out of sorts when she or he misses a day, someone who commits to eating more fruits and vegetables loses the desire to eat a bag of pork rinds, and someone who quit smoking now abhors the smell of burning tobacco. You're probably already at this stage for a number of behaviors—buckling your seatbelt, brushing your teeth, consistently using a condom.

The passage from stage to stage is neither linear nor irreversible. Some stages may be skipped, especially if there's a sudden sense of urgency. (For instance, a heart attack can belatedly motivate someone to quit cigarettes cold turkey.) And people may relapse, which moves them back a stage or two. Often people cycle back and forth between stages. They take two steps forward, one step back. Sometimes the pros of the positive behavior outweigh cons. Other times, the cons outweigh the pros. For instance, you might decide to give up baked goods for a while. You feel better. People start to notice improvements in your appearance. But it's your birthday and a friend has baked you a cake. That doesn't mean you can't get back on target the next day.

3.2 Changing for the Better: Skills for Success

A number of skills will make you successful in your goals of improving your health and well-being. Here are some specific tips.

- **Do it for you.** You're more likely to hang in there if you want to change than if you're trying to please someone else. Tell yourself you're worth the effort and capable of positive change. After all, these modifications should ultimately make you feel better.

- **Create precise goals.** For instance, wanting to become more muscular or lose weight is vague. More specific targets include being able to run a half marathon in three months or fitting into the jeans you wore freshman year. Specificity will motivate you and give you a yardstick by which to measure progress.

- **Decide where to set the bar.** If it's too high, you'll become frustrated. If it's too low, you may not feel inspired. Are you an overachiever or an underachiever? If you tend to be an overachiever, especially if that predisposition typically results in feeling burnout, you may want to start with more modest goals. If you're a self-identified slacker, why not aim higher? Maybe you'll surprise yourself.

■ **Post your goals.** Put them on your screensaver, write them on bookmarks, or put a note on your refrigerator. Make sure you see them often.

■ **Take it one day at a time.** Divide your long-term goal into doable chunks. Go one day without a cigarette. Exercise for 30 minutes today. Eat one breakfast of fruit and yogurt, skipping the baked good. Wake up each day, ready to recommit to your goal.

■ **Find enjoyable substitutions.** Giving something up is harder if something good doesn't take its place. Find a healthier (more rewarding, more fun) alternative for the behavior you want to quit. If you focus on the new thing (rather than the old habit), you shift from the problem to the solution. For instance, if you want to reduce the time you spend watching videos, you might instead join an intramural sports team, learn to play the harmonica, or help out at a food bank.

■ **Use your strengths and skills.** Those assets enable you to scale perceived barriers and resist temptations. Humans too often focus on problems and negative emotions. Instead, make a list of your talents. Perhaps you're kind, steady, independent, social, resourceful, creative, generous, patient, intellectual, witty, and tenacious. All these skills can help you adopt and maintain a new health habit.

■ **Surmount barriers.** Tangible roadblocks (not yet having a pair of running shoes) can be relatively easy to identify and solve. Don't forget about the intangibles—your own attitudes and beliefs. Is your identity tangled up with the behavior you want to switch? Perhaps you have prided yourself on being a "party animal" but now realize drinking and carousing into the wee hours isn't working out well. In order to change, you will need to convince yourself that this new lifestyle suits you better and makes you feel proud. You're now the kind of person who gets up at 7 a.m., clear-eyed and ready for a jog.

■ **Dodge temptations.** Look for the cues with which you associate undesirable habits (coffee and cigarettes, parties and alcohol, television and junk food). Break those associations. Willpower is a finite resource. Eventually, the part of you that wants immediate gratification or relief from cravings will outmuscle your better self. If you're trying to reduce calories, use a smaller plate, stock your living quarters with healthy but low-calorie foods, and get rid of junk food.

■ **Create contingency plans for battling temptations and cravings.** Will you write in a journal or play music? Take 10 slow, deep breaths? Call your support buddy? Go for a walk?

■ **Identify outside resources.** The list depends on the goal. Resources might include friends, family members, informal support groups, and professionals (registered dietitians, certified athletic trainers, physical therapists, doctors, nurses, health educators, coaches, and counselors). Ask for help. You deserve it.

■ **Pick a role model.** This admirable person could be someone you know, a celebrity, a scholar, or even a fictional character (but not one with super powers). The main thing is that your hero worked hard to achieve his or her goals—goals you share. If the person is a celebrity, tape a photo to your wall. Be inspired.

■ **Inform close friends of your goal.** Solicit their support. It can help you persist and feel proud of your achievements. Also, "coming out" with your goals may act as insurance against backsliding.

■ **Team up.** Find a buddy with the same objective. If your friend is dedicated to the cause, you'll feel more committed too. Meet for workouts. Cook a healthy meal together. Call each other when the urge to relapse seems overwhelming.

■ **Track your progress.** Find a way to document small, progressive changes: weekly photographs (weight, waist circumference), a food diary, a record of weights lifted or miles run, a log of the hours you sleep each night, a journal of stress symptoms, and a tally of cigarettes or alcoholic drinks consumed each day. A written record helps you appreciate that, with many small steps, you've scaled a mountain.

■ **Pay attention to positive signs and symptoms.** Maybe you notice that you feel more cheerful and focused after you get a good night's sleep, more energetic after moderate exercise, more joyous after doing something nice for a friend, and more confident when you make ample time to study for an exam. These are signs of more vitality and success in your life.

■ **Reward success.** Establish milestones that deserve a prize. Take care that the treat doesn't undermine your long-range objective. In other words, if you're working to improve your diet and lose weight, a slice of chocolate cake may only engender guilt, but a new pair of (slimmer) jeans will strengthen your resolve. Treasure compliments from friends.

■ **Be flexible.** Not every day turns out as planned. Relapses happen. If you judge yourself harshly, you may become too consumed with guilt, shame, and hopelessness to get back on track. Turn those negative feelings into motivations. Forgive yourself, but don't give up on the prize. It's perseverance that counts, not perfection.

■ **Remember, you are enough—as you are right now.** If anyone has told you otherwise, disregard that erroneous opinion. No one's perfect. Everyone has room for improvement. Just because someone makes straight As, boasts a well-defined musculature, eats homegrown fruits and vegetables, has a flock of adoring friends, or carries a yoga mat around campus—none of these things make him or her better than you.

Behavioral Change Contract

Go back to your assessment of wellness in the eight dimensions. Pick one thing you feel ready to change now.

1. Describe the change you want to make. Be as specific as possible. Vague: "I want to eat healthier meals." Specific: "I will eat a vegetable or fruit with every meal." Or, "I will eat raw carrots instead of French fries."

   _____

   _____

2. Write down the date you start to adopt this behavior. _____

3. Write down the date by which you hope to achieve that goal. _____

4. List short-term goals. For instance, if you plan to run a half marathon in three months, map out exercise targets for each week. If you plan to eat more fruits and vegetables, write out a sample menu. (Note: Some goals can't be "chunked." Buckle your seatbelt each time you get into a car. Use a condom every time you have sex.)

   a. _____

   b. _____

   c. _____

5. List perceived barriers to this change.   List your strategies for surmounting each barrier.

   a. _____   a. _____

   b. _____   b. _____

   c. _____   c. _____

6. List outside resources that will promote your success (books, websites, recreation centers, health center, family, friends, coaches, doctors, therapists, clergy, etc.).

   a. _____

   b. _____

   c. _____

7. List possible temptations.   Describe a contingency plan for resisting.

   a. _____   a. _____

   b. _____   b. _____

   c. _____   c. _____

8. Write down your reward for completing your long-term goal.

   _____

9. Provide the name of a buddy to whom you'll report your progress and call upon when you feel tempted to revert to old habits. _____

10. Sign the contract to indicate your commitment to   Ask a witness or behavior-change buddy to
    your goals.   sign as well.

    Date   Date

    _____   _____

    Your signature   Witness

    _____   _____

KEY TAKEAWAYS

- Researchers have generated theories to explain how people make health-related decisions. The most prominent theory in health education is the Health Belief Model.
- The Transtheoretical Model describes the stages people pass through as they initiate positive behavioral changes.
- A number of skills help individuals successfully change their behaviors for the better.

DISCUSSION QUESTIONS

1. You can learn a lot about your own health risks by creating a family health tree. Completing a pedigree that goes back a few generations can require research. The National Human Genome Research Institute provides some tools: http://www.genome.gov/Pages/Education/Modules/YourFamilyHealthHistory.pdf. See if you can at least go back to your grandparents. If you're not able to contact any blood relatives, write whatever you know about your family health history.

   Once you finish, note any illnesses or deaths that occurred before age 50. The earlier the onset, the greater the chance that it has a genetic component, though usually behaviors still play a role. Illnesses arising later in life probably have strong lifestyle and environmental components. How might your awareness of possible disease vulnerabilities affect your lifestyle choices?

2. Go to this Healthy People 2020 website: http://healthfinder.gov/myhealthfinder/Default.aspx. Make the appropriate selections in the widget. You'll then receive health recommendations for someone your age and sex. Click on one of them and write down three things that you learned.

3. Choose an unhealthy behavior you or your peers commonly engage in. Using the Health Belief Model, analyze this behavior according to possible perceptions of susceptibility, severity, benefits, and barriers to change. Examples include not wearing helmets while cycling, binge drinking, smoking, and not using condoms.

4. Identify a health behavior you'd like to change. Examine the stages of the Transtheoretical Model. Note which stage you're in now and explain why. What will it take to push you to the next stage?

5. Around the world, tobacco is a leading preventable cause of death. It contributes to the top killers: heart disease, chronic lung disease, stroke, and many cancers. Why do you think so many people continue to smoke?

4. RECOMMENDED RESOURCES

4.1 Books

Glanz K, Rimer BK, Viswanath K, eds. *Health Behavior and Health Education: Theory, Research, and Practice*. 4th ed. San Francisco, CA: Jossey-Bass; 2008. Available at: http://www.ihepsa.ir/files/h1.pdf.

Heat C, Heath D. *Switch: How to Change Things When Change Is Hard*. New York, NY: Broadway Books; 2010.

4.2 Organizations and Websites

Centers for Disease Control and Prevention. http://www.cdc.gov.

Healthy People 2020. http://www.healthypeople.gov.

Human Genome Project Information. http://www.ornl.gov/sci/techresources/Human_Genome/home.shtml.

National Center for Health Statistics. http://www.cdc.gov/nchs.

National Human Genome Research Institute. http://www.genome.gov.

World Health Organization. http://www.who.int.

4.3 Video

Chromatin, Histones and Epigenetics. All Things Science. http://www.allthingsscience.com/video/732/Chromatin-Histones-and-Epigenetics.

ENDNOTES

1. WHO definition of health. World Health Organization. Available at: http://www.who.int/about/definition/en/print.html. Accessed January 27, 2013.

2. Smith BJ, Tang KC, Nutbeam D. WHO health promotion glossary: new terms. *Health Promotion International Advance Access.* 2006. doi:10.1093/heapro/dal033. Available at: http://www.who.int/healthpromotion.../HP%20Glossay%20in%20HPI.pdf. Accessed December 29, 2011.

3. Weon BM, Je JH. Theoretical estimation of maximum human lifespan. *Biogerontology.* 2009 Feb;10(1):65–71. doi:10.1007/s10522-008-9156-4.

4. Hoyert DL, Xu J. Deaths: preliminary data for 2011. *Natl Vital Stat Rep.* 2012;61(6):2. National Center for Health Statistics. Centers for Disease Control and Prevention. Available at: http://www.cdc.gov/nchs/data/nvsr/nvsr61/nvsr61_06.pdf. Accessed January 25, 2013.

5. McGinnis JM, Williams-Russo P, Knickman JR. The case for more active policy attention to health promotion. *Health Aff (Millwood).* 2002 Mar–Apr;21(2):78–93. Available at: http://content.healthaffairs.org/content/21/2/78.long. Accessed December 8, 2012.

6. McLeroy KR, Bibeau D, Steckler A, Glanz K. An ecological perspective on health promotion programs. *Health Educ Q.* 1988;15(4):351–377.

7. McGinnis JM, Williams-Russo P, Knickman JR. The case for more active policy attention to health promotion. *Health Aff (Millwood).* 2002 Mar–Apr;21(2):83. Available at: http://content.healthaffairs.org/content/21/2/78.long. Accessed January 30, 2013.

8. McGinnis JM, Williams-Russo P, Knickman JR. The case for more active policy attention to health promotion. *Health Aff (Millwood).* 2002 Mar–Apr;21(2):78–93. Available at: http://content.healthaffairs.org/content/21/2/78.long. Accessed January 30, 2013.

9. Barker DJP, Osmond C, Winter PD, Margetts B, Simmonds SJ. Weight in infancy and death from ischaemic heart disease. *Lancet.* 1989 Oct 21;2(8669):984–985.

10. Forsén T, Eriksson J, Tuomilehto J, Reunanen A, Osmond C, Barker D. The fetal and childhood growth of persons who develop type 2 diabetes. *Ann Intern Med.* 2000 Aug 1;133(3):176–182.

11. Almond D, Currie J. Killing me softly: the fetal origins hypothesis. *Int J Epidemiol.* 2002;31:1235–1239. Available at: http://www.princeton.edu/~jcurrie/publications/Killing_Me_Softly.pdf. Accessed December 30, 2011.

12. Shonkoff JP, Garner S; the Committee on Psychosocial Aspects of Child and Family Health. From the American Academy of Pediatrics technical report: the lifelong effects of early childhood adversity and toxic stress. *Pediatrics.* 2012;129:1 e232–e246. [Published ahead of print.] doi:10.1542/peds.2011-2663.

13. Determinants of health. Health People 2020. HealthyPeople.gov. Available at: http://www.healthypeople.gov/2020/about/DOHAbout.aspx. Accessed February 25, 2013.

14. Summary health statistics for the U.S. population: National Health Interview Survey, 2011. Vital and Health Statistics, Series 10, No. 255. National Center for Health Statistics. Available at: http://www.cdc.gov/nchs/data/series/sr_10/sr10_255.pdf. Accessed January 27, 2013.

15. McGinnis JM, Williams-Russo P, Knickman JR. The case for more active policy attention to health promotion. *Health Aff (Millwood).* 2002 Mar–Apr;21(2):78–93. Available at: http://content.healthaffairs.org/content/21/2/78.long Accessed January 30, 2013.

16. Olshansky SJ, Antonucci T, Berkman L, et al. Differences in life expectancy due to race and educational differences are widening, and many may not catch up. *Health Aff (Millwood).* 2012;31(8):1803–1813. Available at: http://content.healthaffairs.org/content/21/2/78.long. Accessed January 30, 2013.

17. Board on Neuroscience and Behavioral Health. Institute of Medicine. Health Literacy: A Prescription to End Confusion. National Academies Press. 2004, p. 31. Available at: http://www.nap.edu/openbook.php?record_id=10883&page=31. Accessed February 6, 2013.

18. McGinnis JM, Williams-Russo P, Knickman JR. The case for more active policy attention to health promotion. *Health Aff (Millwood).* 2002 Mar–Apr;21(2):78–93. Available at: http://content.healthaffairs.org/content/21/2/78.long. Accessed January 30, 2013.

19. Jorde LB, Wooding SP. Genetic variation, classification and "race." *Nat Genet.* 2004;36: S28–S33. doi:10.1038/ng1435.

20. Murray CJ, Kulkarni SC, Michaud C, et al. Eight Americas: investigating mortality disparities across races, counties, and race-counties in the United States. *PLoS Med.* 2006 Sep;3(9):e260.

21. Kochanek KD, Xu J, Murphy SL, et al. Deaths: final data for 2009. *Natl Vital Stat Rep.* 2011;60(3):4. National Center for Health Statistics. Available at: http://www.cdc.gov/nchs/data/nvsr/nvsr60/nvsr60_03.pdf. Accessed January 27, 2013.

22. Hoyert DL, Xu J. Deaths: preliminary data for 2011. *Natl Vital Stat Rep.* 2012;61(6):2. National Center for Health Statistics. Centers for Disease Control and Prevention. Available at: http://www.cdc.gov/nchs/data/nvsr/nvsr61/nvsr61_06.pdf. Accessed January 25, 2013.

23. Hoyert DL, Xu J. Deaths: preliminary data for 2011. *Natl Vital Stat Rep.* 2012;61(6):2. National Center for Health Statistics. Centers for Disease Control and Prevention. Available at: http://www.cdc.gov/nchs/data/nvsr/nvsr61/nvsr61_06.pdf. Accessed January 25, 2013.

24. Heron M. Deaths: leading causes for 2009. *Natl Vital Stat Rep.* 2012;61(7):10. National Center for Health Statistics. Centers for Disease Control and Prevention. Available at: http://www.cdc.gov/nchs/data/nvsr/nvsr61/nvsr61_07.pdf. Accessed January 25, 2013.

25. Howarter AD, Bennett KK. Perceived discrimination and health-related quality of life: testing the Reserve Capacity Model in Hispanic Americans. *J Soc Psychol.* 2013 Jan–Feb;153(1):62–79.

26. What do we mean by "sex" and "gender?" World Health Organization. Available at: http://www.who.int/gender/whatisgender/en. Accessed February 6, 2013.

27. Hoyert DL, Xu J. Deaths: preliminary data for 2011. *Natl Vital Stat Rep.* 2012;61(6):2. National Center for Health Statistics. Centers for Disease Control and Prevention. Available at: http://www.cdc.gov/nchs/data/nvsr/nvsr61/nvsr61_06.pdf. Accessed January 25, 2013.

28. McGinnis JM, Williams-Russo P, Knickman JR. The case for more active policy attention to health promotion. *Health Aff (Millwood).* 2002 Mar–Apr;21(2):78–93. Available at: http://content.healthaffairs.org/content/21/2/78.long. Accessed January 30, 2013.

29. Institute of Medicine. To err is human: building a safer health system. November 1999. Available at: http://iom.edu/~/media/Files/Report%20Files/1999/To-Err-is-Human/To%20Err%20is%20Human%201999%20%20report%20brief.pdf. Accessed January 30, 2013.

30. Classen DC, Resar R, Griffin F, et al. "Global trigger tool" shows that adverse events in hospitals may be ten times greater than previously measured. *Health Aff (Millwood).* 2011 Apr;30(4):581–589. doi:10.1377/hlthaff.2011.0190.

31. McGinnis JM, Foege WH. Actual causes of death in the United States. *JAMA.* 1993;270(18):2207–2212.

32. Khaw K-T, Wareham N, Bingham S, et al. Combined impact of health behaviours and mortality in men and women: the EPIC-Norfolk Prospective Population Study. *PLoS Med.* 2008;5(1):e12. doi:10.1371/journal.pmed.0050012.

33. Horton R. GBD 2010: understanding disease, injury, and risk. *Lancet.* 2012;380:2053–2054.

34. Global burden of mental disorders and the need for a comprehensive, coordinated response from health and social sectors at the country level. World Health Organization. Executive Board, 130th session. EB130/9. December 1, 2011. Available at: http://apps.who.int/gb/ebwha/pdf_files/EB130/B130_9-en.pdf. Accessed February 24, 2013.

35. Rosenbaum L, Lamas D. Facing a "slow-motion disaster"—the UN meeting on noncommunicable diseases. *N Engl J Med.* 2011;365(25):2345–2348.

36. Murray CJL, Vos T, Lozano R, et al. Disability-adjusted life years (DALYs) for 291 diseases and injuries in 21 regions, 1990–2010: a systematic analysis for the Global Burden of Disease Study 2010. *Lancet.* 2012 Dec 13;380:2197–2223. Summary available at: http://www.healthmetricsandevaluation.org/gbd/publications/disability-adjusted-life-years-dalys-291-diseases-and-injuries-21-regions-199. Accessed February 25, 2013.

37. Butler RN, Miller RA, Perry D, et al. New model of health promotion and disease prevention for the 21st century. *BMJ.* 2008;337. doi:http://0-dx.doi.org.skyline.ucdenver.edu/10.1136/bmj.a399.

38. Table 22. Life expectancy at birth, at 65 years of age, and at 75 years of age, by sex, race, and Hispanic origin: United States, selected years 1900–2009. National Center for Health Statistics. Centers for Disease Control and Prevention. Available at: http://www.cdc.gov/nchs/data/hus/2011/022.pdf. Accessed February 24, 2013.

39. Leading causes of death, 1900–1998. Centers for Disease Control and Prevention. National Center for Health Statistics. Available at: http://www.cdc.gov/nchs/data/dvs/lead1900_98.pdf. Accessed February 24, 2013.

40. Ten leading causes of death, United States: 1999–2000, all races, both sexes. National Center for Injury Prevention and Control. Centers for Disease Control and Prevention. Available at: http://webappa.cdc.gov/cgi-bin/broker.exe. Accessed February 25, 2013.

41. Population. AgingStats.gov. Available at: http://www.agingstats.gov/Main_Site/Data/2012_Documents/Population.aspx. Accessed February 24, 2013.

42. Centers for Disease Control and Prevention, the Merck Company Foundation. *The State of Aging and Health in America 2007.* Whitehouse Station, NJ: The Merck Company Foundation; 2007. Available at: http://www.cdc.gov/Aging/pdf/saha_2007.pdf. Accessed August 4, 2011.

43. Centers for Disease Control and Prevention, the Merck Company Foundation. *The State of Aging and Health in America 2007.* Whitehouse Station, NJ: The Merck Company Foundation; 2007. Available at: http://www.cdc.gov/Aging/pdf/saha_2007.pdf. Accessed August 4, 2011.

44. HHS announces the nation's new health promotion and disease prevention agenda. HHS News. US Department of Health and Human Services. December 2, 2010. Available at: http://www.healthypeople.gov/2020/about/DefaultPressRelease.pdf. Accessed January 30, 2013.

45. Anderson G. *Chronic Care: Making the Case for Ongoing Care.* Princeton, NJ: Robert Wood Johnson Foundation; 2010. Available at: http://www.rwjf.org/content/rwjf/en/research-publications/find-rwjf-research/2010/01/chronic-care.html. Accessed February 24, 2013.

46. Overweight and obesity. Centers for Disease Control and Prevention. Available at: http://www.cdc.gov/nchs/fastats/overwt.htm. Accessed February 24, 2013.

47. Overweight in children. American Heart Association. Updated January 16, 2013. Available at: http://www.heart.org/HEARTORG/GettingHealthy/Overweight-in-Children_UCM_304054_Article.jsp. Accessed February 25, 2013.

48. Obesity rates among all children in the United States. Centers for Disease Control and Prevention. Available at: http://www.cdc.gov/obesity/data/childhood.html. Accessed February 24, 2013.

49. Ogden CL, Carroll MD, Kit BK, Flegal KM. Prevalence of obesity and trends in body mass index among US children and adolescents, 1999–2010. *JAMA.* 2012;307(5):483–490.

50. Warner J. Baby boomers may outlive their kids. WebMD. April 9, 2010. Available at: http://children.webmd.com/news/20100409/baby-boomers-may-outlive-their-kids. Accessed February 24, 2013.

51. Lightwood J, Bibbins-Domingo K, Coxson P, et al. Forecasting the future economic burden of current adolescent overweight: an estimate of the coronary heart disease policy model. Am J Public Health. 2009 Dec;99(12):2230–2237.

52. Woolf SH, Aaron L, eds. U.S. Health in International Perspective: Shorter Lives, Poorer Health. Washington, DC: National Academies Press; 2013. Available at: https://download.nap.edu/catalog.php?record_id=13497. Accessed January 11, 2013.

53. Ho JY. Mortality under age 50 accounts for much of the fact that US life expectancy lags that of other high-income countries. Health Aff (Millwood). 2013 Mar;32(3):459–467. doi:10.1377/hlthaff.2012.0574.

54. Hoyert DL, Xu J. Deaths: preliminary data for 2011. Natl Vital Stat Rep. 2012;61(6):2. National Center for Health Statistics. Centers for Disease Control and Prevention. Available at: http://www.cdc.gov/nchs/data/nvsr/nvsr61/nvsr61_06.pdf. Accessed January 25, 2013.

55. Japan. World Health Organization. Available at: http://www.who.int/countries/jpn/en. Accessed February 25, 2013.

56. Woolf SH, Aaron L, eds. U.S. Health in International Perspective: Shorter Lives, Poorer Health. Washington, DC: National Academies Press; 2013. Available at: https://download.nap.edu/catalog.php?record_id=13497. Accessed January 11, 2013.

57. Woolf SH, Aaron L, eds. U.S. Health in International Perspective: Shorter Lives, Poorer Health. Washington, DC: National Academies Press; 2013. Available at: https://download.nap.edu/catalog.php?record_id=13497. Accessed January 11, 2013.

58. Woolf SH, Aaron L, eds. U.S. Health in International Perspective: Shorter Lives, Poorer Health. Washington, DC: National Academies Press; 2013. Available at: https://download.nap.edu/catalog.php?record_id=13497. Accessed January 11, 2013.

59. Woolf SH, Aaron L, eds. U.S. Health in International Perspective: Shorter Lives, Poorer Health. Washington, DC: National Academies Press; 2013. Available at: https://download.nap.edu/catalog.php?record_id=13497. Accessed January 11, 2013.

60. Tapia Granados JA. Health at advanced age: social inequality and other factors potentially impacting longevity in nine high-income countries. Maturitas. 2013 Feb;74(2):137–147. doi:10.1016/j.maturitas.2012.11.013.

61. Stress in America findings. American Psychological Association. November 9, 2010. Available at: http://www.apa.org/news/press/releases/stress/national-report.pdf. Accessed February 24, 2013.

62. Stress in America findings. American Psychological Association. November 9, 2010. Available at: http://www.apa.org/news/press/releases/stress/national-report.pdf. Accessed February 24, 2013.

63. King DE, Mainous AG III, Carnemolla M, Everett CJ. Adherence to healthy lifestyle habits in US adults, 1988–2006. Am J Med. 2009 Jun;122(6):528–534. doi:10.1016/j.amjmed.2008.11.013.

64. American College Health Association. American College Health Association National College Health Assessment II: Reference Group Executive Summary Spring 2011. Hanover, MD: American College Health Association; 2011. Available at: http://www.achancha.org/docs/ACHA-NCHA-II_ReferenceGroup_ExecutiveSummary_Spring2011.pdf. Accessed February 26, 2013.

65. National health expenditure projections 2011–2021. Centers for Medicare and Medicaid Services. Available at: https://www.cms.gov/Research-Statistics-Data-and-Systems/Statistics-Trends-and-Reports/NationalHealthExpendData/Downloads/Proj2011PDF.pdf. Accessed July 30, 2012.

66. Ayanian JZ, Van der Wees PJ. Tackling rising health care costs in Massachusetts. N Engl J Med. 2012;367(9):790–793.

67. Baker SL. U.S. national health spending, 2006. Arnold School of Public Health. University of South Carolina. Available at: http://hspm.sph.sc.edu/Courses/Econ/Classes/nhe06. Accessed January 30, 2013.

68. Centers for Medicare and Medicaid services national health expenditure data. Table 1. National Health Expenditure Tables. Available at: http://www.cms.gov/Research-Statistics-Data-and-Systems/Statistics-Trends-and-Reports/NationalHealthExpendData/downloads/tables.pdf. Accessed January 30, 2013.

69. Health expenditure per capita (current US$). The World Bank. Available at: http://data.worldbank.org/indicator/SH.XPD.PCAP. Accessed January 30, 2013.

70. The power of prevention: chronic disease…the public health challenge of the 21st century. Centers for Disease Control and Prevention. 2009. Available at: http://www.cdc.gov/chronicdisease/pdf/2009-power-of-prevention.pdf. Accessed February 2, 2013.

71. The healthcare imperative: lowering costs and improving outcomes—workshop series summary. Institute of Medicine. February 24, 2011. Available at: http://iom.edu/Reports/2011/The-Healthcare-Imperative-Lowering-Costs-and-Improving-Outcomes.aspx. Accessed July 30, 2012.

72. Alonso-Zaldivar, R. Doctors look for cure to wasteful spending. Associated Press Report. April 4, 2012.

73. Prevalence of heart disease: United States, 2005. MMWR. 2007;56(6):113–118. Centers for Disease Control and Prevention. Available at: http://www.cdc.gov/mmwr/preview/mmwrhtml/mm5606a2.htm. Accessed February 26, 2013.

74. US Department of Transportation, National Highway Traffic Safety Administration (NHTSA). Traffic Safety Facts 2010: Alcohol-Impaired Driving. Washington, DC: NHTSA; 2012. Available at: http://www-nrd.nhtsa.dot.gov/Pubs/811606.PDF. Accessed February 26, 2013.

75. Danaei G, Ding EL, Mozaffarian D, Taylor B, Rehm J, Murray CJ, Ezzati M. The preventable causes of death in the United States: comparative risk assessment of dietary, lifestyle, and metabolic risk factors. PLoS Med. 2009 Apr 28;6(4):e1000058. Available at: http://www.ncbi.nlm.nih.gov/pmc/articles/PMC2667673/?tool=pubmed. Accessed February 26, 2013.

76. Jha P, Ramasundarahettige C, Landsman V, et al. 21st-century hazards of smoking and benefits of cessation in the United States. N Engl J Med. 2013 Jan 24;368(4):341–350. doi:10.1056/NEJMsa1211128.

77. Healthy people 2020 objective topic areas. HealthyPeople.gov. Available at: http://www.healthypeople.gov/2020/topicsobjectives2020/default.aspx. Accessed January 30, 2013.

78. Disparitites. Healthy People. Available at: http://www.healthypeople.gov/2020/about/DisparitiesAbout.aspx. Accessed January 30, 2013.

79. Christakis NA, Fowler JH. Social contagion theory: examining dynamic social networks and human behavior. Stat Med. 2013 Feb 20;32(4):556–577. doi:10.1002/sim.5408.

80. Nakaya ST, Ohmori K, Shimazu T, et al. Sense of life worth living (ikigai) and mortality in Japan: Ohsaki study. Psychosom Med. 2008;70(6):709–715.

81. Rimer BK. Models of individual health behavior. In: Glanz K, Rimer BK, Viswanath K, eds. Health Behavior and Health Education: Theory, Research, and Practice. 4th ed. San Francisco, CA: Jossey-Bass; 2008:42. Available at: http://www.ihepsa.ir/files/h1.pdf. Accessed February 9, 2013.

82. Champion VL, Skinner CS. The Health Belief Model. In: Glanz K, Rimer BK, Viswanath K, eds. Health Behavior and Health Education: Theory, Research, and Practice. 4th ed. San Francisco, CA: Jossey-Bass; 2008:45. Available at: http://www.ihepsa.ir/files/h1.pdf. Accessed February 9, 2013.

83. Prochaska J, DiClemente C, Norcross J. In search of how people change: applications to addictive behaviors. Am Psychol. 1992;47:1102–1114.

CHAPTER 2
Conventional, Complementary, and Integrative Medicine

The practice of medicine is an evolving art and science. Over the millennia, humans have attributed illness to moral weakness, angry gods, witches, imbalances in various bodily fluids, and poor hygiene. The last is a risk factor that has endured. Healers have treated illnesses with prayer, diet, medicinal plants, leeches, maggots, honey, massage, pharmaceutical medications, and surgery.

If you found yourself scoffing at some of those treatments, it might surprise you to know that scientific studies show each have some place in treatment. For instance, maggot therapy has made a comeback for cleaning chronic wounds.[1] Leeches are being used to maintain blood flow and prevent clotting in some types of surgery, such as reattaching a severed finger.[2]

Granted, some treatments used in the past have been discarded. For instance, antibiotics replaced toxins such as arsenic and mercury in the treatment of syphilis. Laudanum, a mixture of opium, water, and alcohol, is no longer used as a cure-all. The media are full of advertisements for remedies. Some have benefits, some do nothing, and some have serious side effects. The trick is keeping an open mind and a healthy skepticism.

Scientific advances have helped us understand the biological causes of many diseases. That knowledge led to strategies for prevention and treatment, thereby saving many lives. What got left out of the equation was the importance of mental, emotional, social, and spiritual factors on health. Take an infectious illness such as strep throat, caused by the bacterium *Streptococcus pyogenes*. Maybe you and a close friend are both exposed, but only one of you becomes ill. Why?

This chapter will explore different approaches to maintaining health and treating diseases: conventional, holistic, alternative, complementary, and integrative. It concludes with tips on helping you to navigate your health care options, research health claims, and make well-informed decisions.

Practice two things in your dealings with disease: either help or do not harm the patient.

- Hippocrates

1. CONVENTIONAL MEDICINE

LEARNING OBJECTIVES

1. Define conventional medicine.
2. Categorize health practitioners based on the type of care delivered.
3. Analyze the objectives of health care delivery systems from sick care to health promotion.

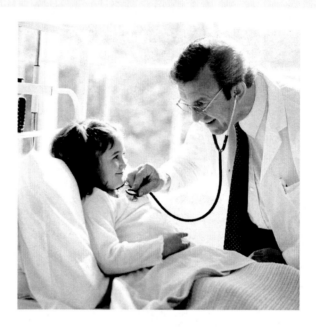

© *Thinkstock*

conventional medicine

A system of medicine in which health care practitioners such as doctors and nurses treat illnesses with medications and surgery.

Because it's the dominant medical system in the United States, most Americans are familiar with the structure of **conventional medicine**. It's also called biomedical medicine, Western medicine, and allopathic medicine. *Biomedical medicine* reflects the premise that identifiable biological agents—genetic defects, microorganisms, chemical toxins—cause physical illness. Consequently, the treatments are mainly biologically based: pharmaceutical medications, radiation therapy, and surgery. *Western medicine* suggests this type of medicine only occurs in the Western hemisphere, which is no longer the case. *Allopathic medicine* means the treatments oppose the processes caused by the disease. For instance, antibiotics kill disease-causing bacteria.

Conventional medicine has strengths and weaknesses. Strengths include high-tech diagnostic tests and treatments, emergency management of physical trauma, critical care for conditions such as heart attacks, and the prevention of illnesses through vaccinations. Weaknesses include emphasis on biological disease factors over social and psychological contributors, insufficient attention to health promotion and disease prevention, and inadequacies in managing chronic disease conditions.

The maxim "If it ain't broke, don't fix it" sums up a societal approach to health. Under that paradigm, a person without significant disease symptoms is considered healthy and the main reason to visit a doctor is the development of worrisome symptoms. That approach makes some sense when you're talking about setting a broken bone, suturing a wound, or combating an infection. Unfortunately, for common diseases such as heart and arterial disease, diabetes, and cancer, obvious symptoms don't occur until the disease is fairly advanced and difficult to reverse. Furthermore, the most common causes of death in America are largely preventable.

Some experts point out that the US health care system needs to move from being reactive to being proactive. Rather than treat symptoms of these diseases once they develop (and try to prevent undesirable risks of these diseases), we should teach people to eat healthy diets, exercise, stress less, and get enough sleep. In other words, we should remove the roots of disease rather than simply prune errant branches.

1.1 Providers of Conventional Medicine

Conventional medicine is a complex system that utilizes a range of professionals. Collectively, these form the *allied health professionals*, credentialed practitioners who undergo formal education and clinical training. Excluding doctors and nurses, there are over 85 occupations in allied health.[3] What follows are the types of providers you're most likely to encounter.

Physicians sit at the top of the hierarchy. They include medical doctors (MDs) and osteopathic doctors (DOs). Their education is similar: typically four years of graduate school, followed by years of postgraduate, in-hospital training. One difference is that osteopathic education includes training in physical manipulation and puts greater emphasis on family medicine and treating the whole person. Physicians are categorized based on emphasis and specialty.

Primary care practitioners provide comprehensive health care. These are the professionals you turn to first for health maintenance and for diagnosis and treatment of common acute and chronic illnesses. In the ideal, primary care also includes patient education and health promotion. Usually a physician performs primary care in collaboration with nurses, physician assistants, and other professionals. Most of the services are rendered in outpatient clinics. However, physicians also see patients in hospitals, long-term care, and home care.

Branches of medical practice that fall under primary care include family medicine, internal medicine (diagnosis and nonsurgical treatment of adult diseases), pediatrics (children's health), and geriatrics (management of the health of elders). Because of the importance of annual exams, many women rely on doctors trained in obstetrics and gynecology (a branch of medicine dealing with conditions related to the female reproductive system). For that reason, these professionals are also often included in the primary care category.

If a condition requires more in-depth evaluation and treatment, primary care physicians refer their patients to a relevant **specialist**. Specialists have training in a limited branch of medicine. Examples of specialties include orthopedics (bone and muscle disorders), rheumatology (joint disorders), dermatology (skin), ophthalmology (eyes), otolaryngology (ears, nose, and throat), gastroenterology (intestinal tract), neurology (nervous system), psychiatric (mental and emotional disorders), cardiology (heart), pulmonology (lungs), infectious disease, and immunology and allergy (immune system disorders). *Surgeons*, doctors who treat ailments with surgical procedures (including lasers), usually also specialize by the bodily system they operate upon.

Nurses include registered nurses (RNs) and nurse practitioners (also called advanced practice nurses). Nurse practitioners undergo graduate-level education and specialized training in an area of medicine (e.g., pediatrics). They function more autonomously than RNs, taking patient histories, ordering some tests, prescribing medications, and performing some procedures.

Physician assistants (PAs) undergo a two-year postbaccalaureate training program and work under the direction of physicians. Their duties and scope of practice is similar to nurse practitioners. However, nurse practitioners can work alone in practice and a PA is supposed to work under a doctor's supervision.

Dentists complete doctoral-level training to become a doctor of dental surgery (DDS) or a doctor of medical dentistry (DMD). Oral surgeons receive further training. Dental hygienists, who receive an associate's degree in dental hygiene, assist dentists by examining patients' oral health, cleaning teeth, and providing preventive care.

Optometrists hold a doctor of optometry degree, which licenses them to examine the eyes to detect vision problems and diseases. They prescribe corrective lenses. **Ophthalmologists**, on the other hand, are medical doctors who specialize in the eye and treat eye diseases medically and surgically.

Podiatrists receive doctoral-level training and specialize in treating foot conditions. They can prescribe medications and perform foot surgeries.

Physical therapists treat physical limitations and pain. They complete either a master's degree or a doctoral degree. **Occupational therapists** receive a master's degree and help people recover the ability to perform everyday activities.

Clinical social workers earn a master's degree. They counsel people to help them overcome mental health and substance abuse problems. **Clinical psychologists** receive doctoral education in mental processes and human behavior, earning either a PhD or a PsyD. **Psychiatrists** are MDs who specialize in mental health. Psychologists do more counseling and psychotherapy; psychiatrists are licensed to prescribe medications and less often engage in therapy.

Public health professionals, who have master's or doctoral degrees, examine population trends; identify disease outbreaks; and work to reduce health hazards, protect health, and improve health care access for entire populations (rather than individuals).

primary care practitioners
Health care providers who deliver comprehensive, continuous medicinal care.

specialist
A medical practitioner with advanced training in a relatively narrow field.

1.2 Trends in Medical Practice: Sick Care versus Health Care

Inequities abound in the current health care system. Many people simply don't have ready access to medical care, mainly because they can't afford it. In 2010, more than 18 percent of Americans under age 65 lacked health insurance.[4] People 65 and up qualify for Medicare. Medicaid, a federal and state program, covers the poor and the disabled. And many people receive insurance that's at least partially subsidized by their employers. The rest pay out of pocket with private insurance or go without. The price tag is enormous. Between 1999 and 2009, salaries rose 38 percent, while health care premiums rose 131 percent.[5] Not surprising, many people fall through the cracks.

Recent statistics show some hopeful signs. The number of people without health insurance fell from 49.9 million (16.3 percent of the population) in 2010 to 48.6 million (15.7 percent of the population) in 2011.[6] That's because passage of President Obama's Patient Protection and Affordable Care Act (ACA) in 2010 led to some immediate changes, such as allowing young adults to remain on their parents' health insurance plans until they turned 26. The number of Americans on Medicaid rose. While Medicaid protects many children, 9.4 percent of kids continued to lack health insurance. One of the ACA's overarching goals is health insurance for all Americans (see the sidebar "Health Care Reform").

Until that mission is fulfilled, the current high number of uninsured Americans presents problems. Polls show that one-third to one-half of Americans put off health care visits to doctors and dentists because of costs, relying instead on over-the-counter drugs and home remedies to manage symptoms.[7] ,[8] Among the uninsured, the proportion swelled to over half. People who do have insurance delay care because of high deductibles (the amount the insured person must pay before the insurer foots the bill).

The next problem lies with the organization of the health care system, which has become increasingly fragmented. That means there are too many decision makers and too little coordination of care. Many of these decision makers are specialists. One patient with a complicated medical history (diabetes, asthma, heart disease) can wind up seeing multiple practitioners—none of whom know the person's whole medical story. Too often, the burden of coordinating a complex system falls to the patient, who may be in no position to take on the task. Diagnostic tests are repeated unnecessarily. And the patient may end up on multiple medications, some of which may interact in undesirable ways.

In addition, our health care system focuses much more on treating illnesses than preventing them. It's reactive rather than proactive. We overemphasize technology (expensive diagnostic tests and treatments) and specialty practices and underemphasize primary care and public health services.

That approach has nearly bankrupted the nation's economy and the collective health of Americans. As discussed in Chapter 1, health care expenditures in the United States have soared, reaching 2.7 trillion dollars in 2011.[9] Seventy-five percent is directed toward the management of chronic diseases. And much of that money goes toward hospital care, physician services, and prescription drugs.

In contrast, public health (population-wide approaches to improve health and prevent illness) spending represents only about 5 percent of total expenditures. Policy experts point out that disease prevention is critical to solving the current crisis in health care.[10]

A closer examination of the three main tiers of medical care will further illuminate the problem and possible solutions. Each level of care has value; the issue is one of balance.

Sick Care and Crisis Care

Under this model, patients enter the health care system because they're ill or wounded. Crisis care refers to the treatment of serious disease and injury. Conventional medicine excels at dealing with medical emergencies involved in unintentional injuries (car crashes, drug and alcohol overdoses, poisonings, falls, burns, drowning), homicides, suicide attempts, natural disasters, terrorist attacks, and other community and national tragedies. Heart attacks, strokes, overwhelming infection, and other life-threatening illnesses require emergency treatment. Crisis care involves professional medical treatment, counseling, the provision of shelter and food (as when a natural disaster strikes), and rehabilitation.

Although health care reform promises to remedy this situation, many people lacking health insurance have relied upon emergency departments for more mundane medical care. Without health insurance, people don't receive routine care and treatment for mild illnesses. By default, the point of access to the health care system becomes the emergency room.

Preventive Care

As the name suggests, preventive medicine's goal is to reduce the likelihood of disease and injury. In theory, people never develop preventable illnesses, don't develop them until much later in life (in the case of chronic diseases), or are diagnosed and treated early to avoid severe illness. There are three types of prevention:

1. **Primary prevention** relies on methods that prevent diseases from occurring in the first place. Examples include vaccinations against infectious diseases and education about following healthy lifestyle habits (whole-foods diet, regular exercise, no smoking) to reduce the risk of heart disease and cancer, wearing a condom to protect against sexually transmitted infections, wearing seat belts and cycling helmets to reduce injuries, and protecting the skin from excessive exposure to ultraviolet radiation.

2. **Secondary prevention** identifies illnesses at their early stages. Early detection and prompt treatment of many conditions can cure the patient, slow the progression of the condition, or otherwise reduce its severity. Screening tests are important because many conditions don't cause signs and symptoms until they're relatively advanced. Examples include cancer screening tests (Papanicolaou ["Pap"] test for cervical cancer, mammogram for breast cancer, and prostate and testicular exams); tests for sexually transmitted infections; blood pressure measurements; urine tests; and blood tests for anemia, cholesterol, and glucose (sugar). Questionnaires and conversations with health practitioners can also screen for depression, substance use disorders, sleep disorders, and stress overload.

3. **Tertiary prevention** targets people who already have the illness in hope of minimizing the harmful effects of disease, controlling symptoms, or preventing recurrence or progression. For instance, people with diabetes can learn to use diet, exercise, and medications to regulate their blood sugar and thereby reduce their risk of diabetes-induced damage to arteries, kidneys, and eyes.

Of the three, primary prevention is the clear winner in terms of longevity, quality of life, and economics. An emphasis on healthy lifestyles and environments thwarts a host of illnesses. These also help achieve what's called *compression of morbidity*, the delay of age-associated illnesses until the end of life.

For decades, however, the emphasis has too often been on secondary and tertiary prevention. The fact that primary preventive care in the United States has lagged behind other developed countries is one explanation for the relatively poorer health of its citizens. Since the late 1980s, the US Preventive Services Task Force has been issuing guidelines for preventive services.[11]

In a positive sign, recent health care reform promises to increase insurance coverage for preventive services. Improved primary prevention of chronic conditions such as obesity, diabetes, and cardiovascular disease will reduce human suffering and health care expenditures.

Health Promotion

The World Health Organization (WHO) defines **health promotion** as "the process of enabling people to increase control over, and to improve their health."[12] The goal is to increase physical, mental, and social well-being. To achieve those goals, people need jobs or other means of securing adequate income, quality working conditions, safe housing and neighborhoods, food security, clean air and water, quality education (including education about personal health), freedom from discrimination, the leisure time to exercise, and access to preventive health services.

This field draws upon diverse disciplines (including medicine, public health, and public policy) to identify factors that determine health and create strategies to optimize health and prevent disease. Governments need to protect the natural environment and ensure social justice, equity, and peace. For instance, government entities can regulate vehicular safety; establish highway speed limits; enforce seat belt laws; ban cell phone use while driving; prohibit smoking in public places; relieve hunger; improve school lunches; improve gun safety laws; mandate universal health insurance; fund services that promote health; and ban discrimination based on race, gender, or sexual orientation. Public health initiatives can create environments that support health.

Health practitioners can educate their patients about lifestyles that promote health and wellness. Some conventional doctors have begun to add elements to their practices such as nutrition counseling and stress management. Some employers, recognizing that healthy employees are happier and more productive, have established workplace wellness programs.

A number of factors have started to push the US system toward prevention and health promotion: the cost of health care (which we all share), the evidence that positive lifestyle changes improve health, and a growing societal interest in wellness. More consumers are willing to take personal responsibility for their health and well-being. They're more informed and more involved in making health care decisions. They're interested in receiving education from their health practitioners.

A recently proposed remedy to the current fragmented system is the **patient-centered medical home**. Under this model, a physician, nurse practitioner, or physician's assistant provides continuous and comprehensive care to each patient.[13] Some aspects of this model harken back to the old-style family doctor who took care of patients from cradle to grave. What's different about the medical home is that the primary care provider also guides and coordinates care when the patient requires treatment from other practitioners. It's more of a team approach, with the primary practitioner acting as the

---

primary prevention

A prevention strategy that uses methods to avoid the development of diseases.

secondary prevention

This second level of prevention catches illnesses in their early stages and attempts to cure or prevent progression.

tertiary prevention

This third level of prevention targets individuals with disease symptoms and attempts to slow progression and prevent further damage.

health promotion

Providing people with tools to improve their health such as information about risk factors and healthy lifestyles and provision of safe working and living environments.

coach. Rather than simply manage disease, medical homes are supposed to help patients meet health care goals.

Another element is that treatments must have evidence of effectiveness. Health information technologies include patient-education tools and electronic health records. These records help practitioners track information about any given patient, which reduces the likelihood of repeating tests unnecessarily, prescribing too many medications, and so on. Medical homes promise to deliver high-quality, cost-effective care.

A number of barriers hamper swift progress. One is the shrinking population of primary care practitioners, who play a critical role in medical homes.[14] Shortages are most pronounced in rural areas.[15] Experts predict that the decline in primary care physicians will create a health care crisis as our population continues to age. Unless many more young doctors enter primary care, the shortage may exceed 52,000 by 2025.[16]

While half of first-year medical students begin their education committed to primary care, the majority switch to specialty training by the time they graduate. Similar trends have occurred in nurses and physician assistants.[17] Several forces drive health practitioners toward specialty care. Primary care is fraught with administrative hassles, high patient loads, and declining income.[18]

Furthermore, practitioners don't have enough time with their patients. Doctors spend, on average, 13 to 16 minutes with each patient.[19] Multiple pressures (high patient loads, administrators and insurance companies, declining revenue) shorten physician visits. Many doctors chafe at the lack of time.[20] Writing a prescription takes seconds; counseling patients takes much longer. Older people may have more than one chronic condition, requiring complex management. The number of diagnostic and treatment options adds to the challenge. Patients likewise may feel rushed and short-changed.

In addition, the current economic system favors reimbursement for sick care (medications and surgical procedure) versus counseling patients in health behavior modifications.[21] Drugs and diagnostic and treatment devices are patentable and therefore profitable.

Lastly, promoting health and preventing chronic noncommunicable diseases requires the participation of individuals, families, communities, the food industry, and government. Medical education will need to change in order to train practitioners with the necessary skills. Patient expectations will have to adapt. At present, many patients expect and prefer a "magic bullet" to reduce symptoms. Swallowing a pill is easy. Undergoing a comprehensive lifestyle overhaul requires a commitment of time and energy and yields gradual, albeit more vital, improvements. In comparison, it's far easier to prevent infectious diseases through vaccinations, personal hygiene, clean water, and food safety.

None of these barriers are insurmountable. Other countries have successfully advanced health promotion. An example is the Victorian Health Promotion Foundation—VicHealth, for short—in Victoria, Australia, which was funded by a tax on tobacco. This entity works with a number of organizations, communities, and individuals to promote health and prevent disease. You can learn more about VicHealth's programs and projects at http://www.vichealth.vic.gov.au/Programs-and-Projects.aspx. Furthermore, in recent years, the United States has taken some significant steps in the right direction.

Health Care Reform

In 2010, President Barack Obama signed into law the Patient Protection and Affordable Care Act (ACA), also dubbed "Obamacare." The goals are to provide health insurance for all Americans, to curb health care spending, and to implement measures designed to prevent illness and promote health. The timeline for putting changes into effect extends from 2010 to 2022. For a timeline summary, go to http://obamacarefacts.com/obamacare-facts.php.

Key provisions of the ACA include the following:

Expanded Access to Health Insurance

- According to the individual mandate, all US citizens need to have health insurance or pay a tax penalty. This provision goes into effect in 2014. Exemptions will be granted to certain low-income individuals. Subsidies would provide assistance to qualifying individuals.

- Medicaid coverage will expand to cover those at 133 percent of the federal poverty level. Medicaid is a state and federal program that provides coverage to people with low incomes, people with disabilities, and some families and children. The 2013 federal poverty level for an individual is $11,490.[22] At 133 percent, the individual threshold is $15,282.

- According to the employer mandate, employers with 50 or more full-time employees need to offer health insurance coverage or pay a fine. Tax credits are also available for small business owners.

- Employers and individuals can purchase insurance policies through state-based American Health Benefit Exchanges and Small Business Health Options Program Exchanges. These exchanges will create a competitive marketplace and more transparency about insurance policies.

- Young adults are now covered under their parents' insurance policies until age 26.

Insurance Reform

- Insurance companies cannot deny coverage to people with preexisting medical conditions. Previously, half of Americans had a health condition that insurance companies could use as a basis for denying coverage.
- Insurance companies can no longer drop from their policies people who become sick.
- Insurance companies can no longer charge copayments (the amount a person pays at the time of service) for preventive services nor apply them to the deductible (the portion a person has to pay before the insurer covers medical expenses).

Disease Prevention, Public Health, and Management of Chronic Diseases

- The Prevention and Public Health Fund will provide greater investment in prevention and public health programs.[23]
- The ACA provides for free preventive care and annual checkups (no copayments or other cost-sharing measures). Examples of preventive services include routine vaccinations; many cancer screening tests; pregnancy counseling and screening tests; blood pressure, cholesterol, and diabetes tests; and counseling about losing weight, quitting tobacco, reducing alcohol, and treating depression.
- The bill adds many preventive services for women and waives copayments for preventive services for seniors. Preventive services for women include well-women checkups, screening for diabetes during pregnancy, screening for domestic violence, contraceptive methods and relevant education and counseling, screening and counseling for sexually transmitted infections, and mammograms.
- Tools are available (including grants for small businesses) to help employers establish workplace wellness programs.
- Prescription drug coverage for Medicare recipients will improve.

Assistance to People Entering Health Care Professions

- The ACA has measures to fund scholarships and loan repayments for people studying to become health professionals.
- Funding will increase the number of primary care practitioners.
- Grants are available to increase training of young doctors in preventive medicine.

Resources: HealthCare.gov, http://www.healthcare.gov; Obamacare Facts, http://obamacarefacts.com/affordablecareact-summary.php; and "Summary of the New Health Reform Law," Kaiser Family Foundation, http://www.kff.org/healthreform/upload/8061.pdf.

 Video Clip 2.1

Health Reform Explained
The Kaiser Family Foundation (KFF) created "Health Reform Hits Main Street," an animated video that explains the basics of the Affordable Care Act. The KFF has more easy-to-understand information at http://healthreform.kff.org/the-basics.aspx.

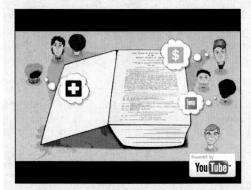

View the video online at: http://www.youtube.com/v/3-llc5xK2_E
Source: Kaiser Family Foundation.

2. COMPLEMENTARY AND ALTERNATIVE MEDICINE

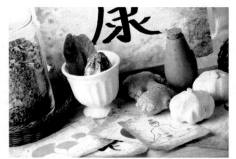

© Thinkstock

complementary and alternative medicine

Treatments that are not considered part of conventional medicine.

complementary therapies

Health practices that are used with conventional medicine.

alternative therapies

Health practices that are used instead of conventional medicine.

Complementary and alternative medicine (CAM) encompasses a diverse group of therapies considered outside of the realm of conventional medicine. **Complementary therapy** refers to practices that are used alongside conventional medicine. For instance, you might add therapeutic massage to treatment recommended by your doctor and physical therapist for a shoulder injury. As the name suggests, the term **alternative therapies** refers to those employed instead of conventional medicine. In this case, you try meditation rather than medication to manage insomnia.

People use CAM for a variety of reasons. Some hope to improve their health, prevent illness, and take a more active role in their health care. Many seek relief from acute and chronic illness. CAM practitioners often provide a holistic approach to health. People lacking health insurance may use CAM because many of these therapies are relatively inexpensive.

In 1992, an increase in the public's use of CAM led to the establishment of the Office of Alternative Medicine (OAM) within the National Institutes of Health (NIH), the government's medical research agency. The OAM's mission was "to investigate and evaluate promising unconventional medical practices."[24] In 1998, Congress established the National Center for Complementary and Alternative Medicine (NCCAM), which replaced the OAM and elevated its status. The mission was similar: facilitate research on CAM, evaluate the effectiveness and safety of CAM, and disseminate accurate, authoritative information to the public.

While one of NCCAM's missions is to fund CAM research, those available funds are relatively small. About 0.4 percent of the NIH budget is appropriated to NCCAM.[25] Pharmaceutical and other private industries are not likely to fund CAM research because, unlike pharmaceuticals, CAM therapies such as herbal medicines, acupuncture, and yoga can't be patented.[26]

Nevertheless, nearly 4 out of 10 American adults regularly use CAM, according to a 2007 National Health Interview Survey. More precisely, 38 percent of adults and 12 percent of children had used CAM within the previous year.[27] They spent nearly $34 billion out of pocket on CAM products, classes, and practitioners' fees.[28] Most people used these therapies as a complement rather than an alternative to conventional care. The conditions most often treated were musculoskeletal problems such as neck and back pain. Unfortunately, two-thirds of them didn't tell their conventional doctors about using CAM.

The popularity of CAM treatments seemed to plateau in about 2008, around the time of the economic recession. While insurance plans cover some CAM services, many people must pay for products and services out of pocket.[29]

FIGURE 2.1   Ten Most Common CAM Therapies among Adults—2007

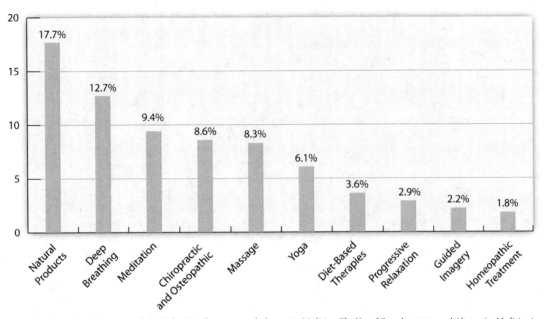

Source: Adapted from CDC/National Center for Complementary and Alternative Medicine. The Use of Complementary and Alternative Medicine in the United States. 2008. Available at: http://nccam.nih.gov/sites/nccam.nih.gov/files/camuse.pdf.

NCCAM divides CAM therapies into several broad categories: mind-body medicine, manipulative and body-based practices, natural products, and whole medicine systems. Excluding prayer, the most commonly used CAM therapies are nonvitamin/nonmineral natural products, deep-breathing exercises, and chiropractic or osteopathic manipulation.

2.1   Mind-Body Medicine

This type of medicine fits the holistic paradigm: mental, emotional, and physical states all interact. Mind-body techniques provide a means to relax all three to restore a sense of well-being. This category includes meditation, breathing exercises, yoga, t'ai chi, chi gong, acupuncture, progressive muscle relaxation, and guided imagery.

Meditation

This ancient practice is a common part of healing techniques around the world. Meditative techniques put you in a state of focused relaxation. There are many types of meditation. Their goal is to quiet the "monkey mind" (the Buddhist term for an unsettled, restless, worried mental state), relax the entire body, and achieve a focused and calm but alert mental state (making it different from a nap).

Physical postures or repetitive movements can produce a meditative state. Some people find that slipping into the flow of jogging, walking, swimming, or cycling creates a focused, relaxed state. Many meditation techniques employ concentrated attention. The focus of concentration could be visual (staring at a candle flame, lava lamp, ocean waves) or auditory (listening to a rhythmic sound like rain, drums, a heartbeat). Many people use chanting, praying, or silently repeating a mantra (word or sound). You can simply repeat "All is well" aloud or silently.

Some meditation practices involve thinking compassionate thoughts and feeling a sense of gratitude or love. Many techniques focus attention on the breath. Some types of meditation have been researched.

Transcendental Meditation (TM) is a type of mantra meditation. A certified TM instructor assigns an individual a mantra, a sound derived from the Vedas (ancient Indian texts) that, while meaningless, is thought capable of creating spiritual transformation. The goal is to empty the mind and transcend ordinary thinking. To practice TM, the person sits in a comfortable position with eyes closed and silently repeats the mantra for about 15 minutes twice a day.

Mindfulness meditation involves paying purposeful attention to the present moment. This ancient Buddhist practice sounds deceptively simple. Small children can do it. By adulthood, most of us have lost the knack. We brood about the past and anxiously speculate about the future. We perform habitual actions automatically. We drive, walk, eat, shower, or sit through a lecture while our minds are preoccupied with other things.

Much credit goes to Jon Kabat-Zinn, PhD, for introducing Americans to the benefits of mindfulness. Kabat-Zinn is an author, researcher, and founding director of the Stress Reduction Clinic and the Center for Mindfulness in Medicine, Health Care, and Society at the University of Massachusetts Medical School. He defined mindfulness as "the awareness that emerges through paying attention on purpose, in the present moment, and non-judgmentally to the unfolding of experience moment by moment."[30] He created a protocol for Mindfulness-Based Stress Reduction (MBSR). Training sessions, which can be conducted online, last eight weeks and involve meditation, stretching, yoga poses, body scans, and discussions.[31]

In mindfulness meditation, you focus on what's going on in real time. In a detached, objective manner, you notice your emotions, thoughts (always bringing them back in a nonjudgmental way to the moment at hand), and physical sensations. The goal isn't a blank mind but a mind that's focused on the present. Once you've centered yourself, you expand your focus to the world around you. With all senses alert, you see, smell, hear, taste, and feel. You deny nothing—your pain, your stress, your anxiety. Your goal is to simply become aware and thoroughly engaged in the reality of the present.

You start with short (15- to 20-minute) practices. For instance, you could mindfully examine, peel, and eat an orange, all the while appreciating the sensory input. With practice, you become aware of thought patterns, which allows you to question and rephrase them. You start to accept rather than run away from uncomfortable thoughts and bodily sensations.

Gradually, you become mindful of everything you're doing—cooking, cleaning, playing music, exercising—which increases your enjoyment and performance. Because energized focus and complete immersion in an activity can make it seem effortless, professionals sometimes refer to this mental state as "flow." Many athletes, musicians, and artists talk about performing their best when in a state of flow.

All types of meditation affect the functioning of several bodily systems. People become more adept at switching from an alert state (as indicated by alpha waves on electroencephalograms) to a relaxed state (as indicated by theta waves). Heart rate, blood pressure, and respiratory rate decrease. Endorphins, natural pain-relieving compounds, are released.[32] Benefits at the cellular level show that regular meditation has the potential to promote healthy longevity.[33]

A regular meditation practice can also reduce high blood pressure[34] and low back pain.[35] Studies in college students show improved attention.[36],[37] Meditation helps relieve emotional distress and improve quality of life in people with chronic illnesses such as diabetes, heart failure, rheumatoid arthritis, and fibromyalgia.[38] Studies show that MBSR and TM relieve stress and mild anxiety.[39] MBSR can act as a useful complement to conventional treatment for anxiety disorders, depression, substance abuse, and eating disorders.[40],[41],[42],[43]

Breathing Exercises

Many healing traditions employ breathing techniques. Most of our breathing occurs without conscious thought. When we're tense or nervous, breathing can become shallow and rapid. On the other hand, conscious awareness and control of breath provide great tools for managing stress, anxiety, pain, and insomnia. If you deliberately slow and deepen your breath, you calm other bodily functions that might be otherwise overstimulated. More specifically, your heart rate slows, blood pressure is reduced,[44] your thoughts become more calm and focused, and you become more aware of sensations coming from within and without.

There are a number of breathing exercises. A simple one is to sit or lie on your back in a comfortable position. Rest one hand on your chest and the other on your abdomen. Inhale deeply and fully, feeling your chest and abdomen rise. Notice how your sides become longer and your back feels fuller with inhalation. Pause briefly. Exhale completely, feeling your chest and abdomen fall. Notice your shoulder blades slide apart and together with deep breathing. Repeat for a full minute. Counting can help regulate the length of your breaths. For example, you can breathe in for a slow count of four, hold four seconds, and exhale to a count of six. Counting acts like a mantra to extinguish distracting thoughts.

Benefits of breathing exercises include the reduction of hot flashes associated with menopause,[45] feelings of nervous tension and fatigue,[46] pain perception,[47] and test anxiety.[48]

Yoga

This ancient practice originated in India some 5,000 years ago.[49] Ancient texts describe eight limbs or aspects of yoga. Hatha yoga, the form most often practiced in the Western world, emphasizes only three of those limbs: *asanas* (physical postures), *pranayama* (breath control), and *dhyana* (meditation). Often, the meditation involves awareness of breathing and concentration on physical postures. Chanting may also be included.

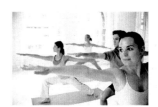

© *Thinkstock*

Hatha yoga comes in various styles. Examples include vinyasa (flowing postures linked to rhythmic breathing), ashtanga (a relatively fast-paced series of postures), and Iyengar (a slower, deeper exploration of postures with or without the use of props).

Yoga didn't become popular in the United States until the middle of the 20th century. Now over 20 million Americans have taken up yoga.[50] A regular practice enhances strength and flexibility—mentally and physically. Studies show it enhances overall well-being, reduces feelings of stress and anxiety,[51] ,[52] improves sleep,[53] eases low back pain,[54] lifts mild depression,[55] augments depression relief when added to antidepressant medications,[56] lessens discomfort during pregnancy,[57] reduces blood pressure,[58] improves quality of life in the face of chronic conditions such as asthma,[59] and more.

A qualified yoga teacher can help students learn to do the postures correctly and without exceeding any one individual's limits. While the rate of injuries is low, they can occur.[60]

 Video Link 2.1

Yoga for Health and Well-Being

The National Center for Complementary and Alternative Medicine created this video on yoga. It includes research-documented information on how people move their muscles and joints in yoga and some of the benefits of yoga.

http://nccam.nih.gov/video/yoga-practice

T'ai Chi Ch'uan and Qigong

Both of these ancient Chinese practices are moving meditations designed to improve the flow of *qi* (pronounced "chee"), the life energy that is thought to move through our bodies. In traditional Chinese medicine (TCM), blockages or imbalances of qi are thought to cause disease. Both practices help regulate movements, thoughts, and breath.

T'ai chi ch'uan (tai chi for short) is derived from the martial arts, though the practice is nonviolent. Qigong involves slow, rhythmic movements timed with breathing. The exercises are designed to open the meridians (energy channels) through which qi travels. People young and old can learn the basic movements, which require low to moderate amounts of exertion.

Tai chi and qigong both tame stress.[61] Studies in older adults indicate that tai chi and qigong may improve balance and strength, reduce falls, lower blood pressure, improve sleep, ease depression, relieve arthritis pain, and enhance immune response.[62] ,[63] ,[64] ,[65] ,[66] ,[67] In addition, tai chi has been shown to improve exercise capacity in people with chronic obstructive lung disease.[68] Qigong has been shown to improve sleep and reduce symptoms associated with menopause.[69] In people with fibromyalgia (a condition characterized by fatigue, pain, and multiple tender areas), qigong can reduce pain and improve sleep, physical function, and mental function.[70]

 Video Link 2.2

Tai Chi and Qigong for Health and Well-Being

This five-part video from NCCAM introduces you to tai chi and qigong and allows you to experience some of the forms.

http://nccam.nih.gov/video/taichidvd-full

Acupuncture

Acupuncture is a primary form of treatment in TCM. Ancient texts describing acupuncture date back to 100 BCE.[71] Acupuncturists insert fine, sterile needles into points along the meridians to restore the normal flow of qi and thereby facilitate healing. Western scientists have trouble explaining how acupuncture works. One theory is that the needles release natural pain relievers called endorphins or otherwise act to relieve pain.

Regardless of how it works, acupuncture has been shown to reduce back pain, labor pains, arthritis pain, headache, menstrual cramps, tennis elbow, carpal tunnel syndrome, and other painful conditions.[72] ,[73] ,[74] Preliminary evidence suggests it may help with other conditions. According to NCCAM, acupuncture is safe if performed correctly.[75]

 Video Clip 2.2

Introduction to Acupuncture
This video briefly explains the Chinese medicine theory behind acupuncture and demonstrates a typical acupuncture session.

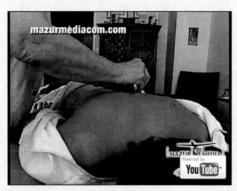

View the video online at: http://www.youtube.com/v/wXgVz4ZqAxo
Source: MazureMedia.

Relaxation Techniques

In addition to deep breathing and mediation, a number of other mind-body practices improve relaxation. They include progressive relaxation, guided imagery, biofeedback, and self-hypnosis. All can release muscle and mental tension, slow breathing and heart rate, lower blood pressure, and enhance well-being. All provide a means to evoke what Herbert Benson, MD, termed the "relaxation response."

Progressive relaxation, also called progressive muscle relaxation, involves sequentially tightening and relaxing each muscle group. It's easiest done lying flat. If you're having trouble falling asleep, start with your feet, pointing your toes as hard as you can and then releasing. Clench and release muscles from toes to face. Each time you let go, appreciate the heaviness and warmth of the muscles. Notice how the floor or mattress supports you.

Guided imagery utilizes your imagination for relaxation. If you find yourself feeling stressed, find a quiet place to sit or recline. Close your eyes. Replace the negative images with something positive. Picture a particular place you find peaceful. Imagine it in all its details. If it's the beach, picture the sky and the expanse of water, feel the sand warm beneath you, smell the seaweed, hear the lapping of waves, the calling of seagulls, the clack of palm fronds moving in the breeze. If you find yourself expecting a bleak outcome, try to visualize the event turning out more positively.

In some ways, guided imagery seems opposite to mindfulness meditation. Rather than focusing on the now, imagine something better. However, what you're changing isn't your circumstances but your negative views about them. The human brain is able to imagine things that haven't happened. It's how we make ourselves miserable and tense and also how we manufacture happiness and contentment. Mental rehearsal helps us improve future performances. Guided imagery allows us a way to change the film we're running in our heads.

Self-hypnosis relies on phrases or nonverbal cues to trigger relaxation. For instance, you might say to yourself, "With each breath, I feel myself become more deeply relaxed. I feel my arms and legs growing heavy." Or you might close your eyes and imagine that you are walking down a flight of steps. With each step, you grow more relaxed. When you're ready, you climb back to the top, feeling refreshed.

Biofeedback requires electronic devices to teach you how to gain conscious control over the relaxation response. For instance, the device might monitor the temperature of your fingertips, heart rate, breathing rate, muscle tension, and/or brain wave patterns. A display shows you how these variables change while using relaxation techniques such as deep breathing or guided imagery. With practice, you can learn to control those processes without the electronic gadgetry. In addition to managing stress, biofeedback can help people reduce high blood pressure and migraine headaches.[76] ,[77] Biofeedback is often used in conventional hospitals and clinics.

 Video Clip 2.3

Biofeedback and Other Strategies for Managing Stress
This narrated slideshow explains biofeedback and other stress-coping strategies.

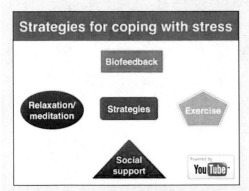

View the video online at: http://www.youtube.com/v/E3GcnGctw2o

Manipulative and Body-Based Practices

Manipulative practices are hands-on practices that address the proper alignment and function for bones, joints, muscles, and other soft tissues. NCCAM divides body-based practices into spinal manipulation, massage therapy, and movement therapies.

In **spinal manipulation**, the practitioner uses hands or other devices to apply gentle force to the spine to improve alignment and physical function and to relieve pain. In addition, practitioners often adjust joints all over the body.

Professionals who employ manipulation techniques include chiropractors, osteopathic physicians, naturopathic physicians, some medical doctors, and physical therapists. Doctoral-level training is required for all these professions. Many of these professions have become so mainstream they're scarcely considered CAM.

The bulk of chiropractic practice is devoted to physical manipulation. Most of the research on manipulation examines chiropractic manipulation. A number of studies show that such treatment can reduce low back pain on par with conventional medical treatment.[78] Manipulative therapy may also reduce crying in infantile colic.[79] It may also relieve chronic headache.[80] Properly performed, spinal manipulation is safe.

Throughout the world, **massage** stands as an ancient form of healing. Gentle touch comforts us. When someone is hurt, we instinctively, literally reach out to that person.

A number of therapeutic massage techniques exist. Most use fingers, hands, and sometimes forearms and elbows to rub the soft tissues. Asian techniques, in theory, stimulate the energy meridians. Application of pressure at acupuncture points is called *acupressure*. In the United States, massage therapists must complete a training program and pass an exam before receiving a license to practice.

Therapeutic massage relaxes tight muscles and improves the local circulation of blood and lymph (tissue fluid and white blood cells that circulate in the lymphatic system). Tight muscles are tender, impair blood flow, and pull on bones and joints to affect postural alignment. Massage has been shown to relieve pain and tension, relax body and mind, and heighten well-being.[81] Massage positively influences people of any age. Giving massage to infants born prematurely enhances immune function, improves weight gain, and shortens hospital stays.[82] ,[83] In adults who have undergone heart surgery, massage can reduce pain, anxiety, and muscular tension.[84]

Some body-based practices involve the active participation of the client. These **movement-based therapies** include the Feldenkrais method, Alexander technique, and Trager psychophysical integration. The therapist may use a combination of gentle manipulation, massage, and education about proper movements to avoid misalignment and unnecessary tension in performing everyday activities. Pilates instructors use machines and mat exercises to train people in motions that improve alignment, balance, and strength.

Natural Products

Echinacea is a popular remedy for the common cold. Research shows that high-quality products taken as recommended modestly shorten cold symptom severity and duration.

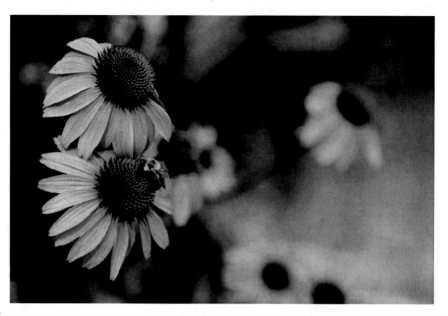

© *Thinkstock*

Natural products are usually sold over the counter as dietary supplements. They include vitamins, minerals, medical herbs, plant and fish oils, amino acids, enzymes, organ tissues, and even some hormones. Some are so often recommended by conventional practitioners that they're not considered CAM. For instance, doctors might recommend multivitamin and mineral formulas, calcium supplements, and fish oil.

The Food and Drug Administration (FDA) regulates dietary supplements under the Dietary Supplement Health and Education Act (DSHEA), passed by the US Congress in 1994. This act defined dietary supplements as products taken by mouth that contain a "dietary ingredient." These ingredients include vitamins, minerals, enzymes, amino acids, certain hormones, organ tissues, and botanicals (medicinal plants, algae, and fungi).[85] The regulatory process is not as rigorous as it is for pharmaceutical medications.

Chapter 8 further discusses vitamins, minerals, and oils from plants and fish. Because references to medicinal plants are scattered throughout the book, more explanation is provided here.

Herbal Medicines

herbal medicines

Preparations derived from medicinal plants.

Humans have probably always relied upon **herbal medicines**, the use of medicinal plants for health and healing. Prehistoric evidence has emerged. The Iceman, a 5,300-year-old mummified body discovered in the Italian Alps in 1991, carried a fungi with antimicrobial properties, which he may have used against the intestinal parasite he was carrying.[86] In 2012, researchers discovered medical plants such as yarrow and chamomile in the tooth scrapings of Neanderthals.[87]

A variety of plants have medicinal properties. The word "herb" is often used, though the botanical definition is a nonwoody plant. Peppermint, oregano, basil, and chamomile are examples of herbs. However, herbalists also make use of shrubs and trees (bark, berries, leaves, nuts, seeds)—plants that aren't, technically speaking, "herbs." They also use fungi (usually mushrooms) and algae (usually seaweeds), which don't belong to the plant kingdom. For purposes of simplicity, the word "herb" will refer to all the living organisms discussed here.

For centuries, herbal medicines represented a primary form of treatment. The Native Americans used over 2,500 medicinal plant species.[88] European settlers, many of whom sailed to the New World carrying seeds of their favorite herbs, learned the native plants from Native Americans. In 1820, the first edition of the *United States Pharmacopeia* (the official authoritative listing of drugs) listed 425 botanical substances, which constituted 67 percent of the entries.[89]

After 1930, pharmaceutical drugs began to replace herbal medicines. However, scientists derived most of these drugs from plants. Examples include morphine and codeine (opium poppy), aspirin (willow bark and meadowsweet), quinine (cinchona), digitalis (foxglove), and menthol (peppermint). Even now, about 40 percent of drugs on the market are either natural products or derived from plants. Adding in synthetic drugs inspired by active plant chemicals, the percentage rises to over 60.[90]

The World Health Organization (WHO) notes, "In some Asian and African countries, 80% of the population depend on traditional medicine for primary health care."[91] Medicinal plants play a huge role in these traditional healing practices. The WHO notes that herbs such as Chinese wormwood (*Artemisia annua*) are traditional remedies against malaria and also the source for the antimalarial drug artemisinin.

Medicinal plants may be sold fresh or dried (fresh ginger and garlic, dried herbs and spices in grocery stores, natural food stores, herb stores) and as teas, tinctures (extractions in water and alcohol), syrups, tablets, and capsules. Capsules can contain ground herb or highly concentrated plant extracts. Topically applied herbal products include creams, oils, salves, and liniments.

There are several advantages of herbal medicines. Our genome evolved with some familiarity of plant chemicals. Herbs contain a complex blend of chemicals, some of which act to together to achieve the desired effect, others of which buffer potential toxic effects. Herbal medicines are also generally inexpensive and accessible. Disadvantages include a generally slower onset and less dramatic effect. Only some herbal products have been standardized to ensure similar potency from batch to batch.

Not all herbs are safe. Some plants are poisonous. Most of these are ingested accidentally (e.g., poisonous mushrooms). Some herbs used medicinally can be toxic in larger amounts or aren't safe in pregnant women and children. Some can't be taken by people with chronic diseases (especially those involving the liver and kidneys). James Duke, PhD, a former botanist for the US Department of Agriculture (USDA), provides a listing of plants considered safe at http://www.ars-grin.gov/duke/syllabus/gras.htm.

With the exception of some weight-loss and sports-endurance products, most herbal products made and sold in the United States are safe when taken within recommended dosage guidelines by otherwise healthy adults. Unfortunately, because dietary supplements form a lucrative market, not all are safe. Other countries may have different standards for contamination with pesticides, microbes, and heavy metals. According to the WHO, "Counterfeit, poor quality, or adulterated herbal products in international markets are serious patient safety threats."[92]

In addition, some otherwise safe herbs—as well as vitamins, minerals, and foods—can interact with prescription and over-the-counter medications. Interactions can be beneficial (enhancing the effectiveness of the drug) or undesirable (lowering blood levels of the drug, increasing the risk of side effects). Dietary supplements that inhibit blood clotting (fish oil and herbs such as ginger, garlic, and ginkgo) should not be taken within two weeks of surgery. Let your health practitioners know about your use of dietary supplements. Section 4 contains recommendations for books and organizations.

After the passage of DSHEA, herb research in the United States boomed. Before then, much of the research occurred in Europe, as well as Asia and the former Soviet Union. Table 2.1 summarizes 10 commonly used herbs.

TABLE 2.1 Commonly Used Herbal Medicines

Common name (Latin name)	Main uses and effectiveness	Safety	Notes

Chamomile, German (*Matricaria recutita*)	Relieves intestinal spasms. Chamomile and other intestinal herbs used in combination have been shown to relieve colic and dyspepsia (indigestion). Chamomile extracts reduce anxiety and depression.[93] ,[94]	Generally recognized as safe.
		    Belongs to the same plant family as ragweed and may cause allergies.
			Commonly consumed as a tea.
			    Research studies use standardized extracts.

Coffee (*Coffea Arabica, C. robusta*, and other species)	Enhances mental alertness. May reduce the risk of colon cancer, type 2 diabetes, gallbladder disease, and Parkinson's disease.	Higher doses cause headache, intestinal distress, anxiety, agitation, nervousness, tremors, and insomnia. Most symptoms are due to caffeine excess.
		    Unfiltered coffee increases cholesterol and triglyceride levels. Coffee may worsen high blood pressure, anxiety disorders, and irritable bowel syndrome.
		    Can increase side effects when combined with stimulant drugs and the asthma drug theophylline.
		    Caffeine is an addictive substance.
			Coffee contains a complex blend of chemicals, many of which have health benefits. If you need caffeine, coffee and tea are healthier choices than sodas and "energy drinks."
			    Research studies suggest moderate doses are two to four cups a day.

Cranberry (*Vaccinium macrocarpon*)	Most research supports use for preventing recurrent urinary tract infections in women.	Safe when used within recommended dosages. High intake (three to four liters a day) of juice can cause upset stomach and diarrhea.	Taken as juice or encapsulated solid extracts.
Chaste tree berry (*Vitex agnus-castus*)	Research supports use for preventing premenstrual syndrome, premenstrual dysphoric disorder (depression around the time of menstruation), and possibly menstrual cycle irregularity.	Safe and well tolerated when taken within recommended dosages. Not recommended for pregnant or nursing women.	Requires daily use (a tincture or standardized extract) for three or more consecutive cycles.
Echinacea (*Echinacea angustiolia, E. purpurea*)	Most studies using high-quality product and adequate dosing show modest reduction in cold symptom duration and severity.	Safe and well tolerated at recommended dosages. Some people are allergic to echinacea, which is in the same plant family as ragweed.	Two preparations consistently show benefit: the preserved juice of the above-ground parts and root extracts. Needs to be started at the first signs of the common cold and continued for one week. The daily dose is divided into three to four doses.
Garlic (*Allium satvum*)	May help prevent and slow progression of atherosclerosis. Modestly reduces blood pressure. Enhances immune function. Has anticancer and antimicrobial activity against numerous bacteria, viruses, fungi, and intestinal parasites.	Safe when used in moderate doses. Gastrointestinal upset possible with higher doses. Causes characteristic "garlic breath." Due to effects on blood clotting, medicinal doses should be discontinued two weeks before surgery.	Cooking deactivates some of the active ingredients. Active forms are raw (minced) garlic, enteric-coated (acid-resistant) garlic tablets, and aged garlic extracts.
Ginkgo (*Ginkgo biloba*)	Research-backed uses include age-related memory impairment, dementia, and peripheral arterial disease. May transiently improve mental function in healthy adults. Does not appear to prevent dementia.	Leaf extracts are well tolerated at recommended dosages. Should not be combined with "blood-thinning" medications. Not recommended during pregnancy. Discontinue two weeks before surgery.	Concentrated, standardized leaf extracts are used in research studies.

Common name (Latin name)	Main uses and effectiveness	Safety	Notes
Peppermint (*Mentha x piperita*)	Studies show success in indigestion and irritable bowel syndrome. Diluted peppermint essential oil is also used topically for headache and muscle ache.	Generally recognized as safe.	Commonly taken as a tea. Research studies typically use encapsulated peppermint oil.
St. John's wort (*Hypericum perforatum*)	Multiple studies in people with mild depression show St. John's wort extracts more effective than placebo and possibly as effective as commonly prescribed antidepressants.	Safe when taken within recommended dosages. Not recommended in people with bipolar disorder or in pregnant and nursing women. Should not be combined with pharmaceutical antidepressants. St. John's wort hastens enzymes that clear many medications (including oral contraceptives, thereby lowering blood levels).	Concentrated, standardized flower and leaf extracts are used in studies. Depressed people should work with a mental health specialist. People taking prescription medications should check with their health practitioners before using St. John's wort.
Tea (*Camellia sinensis*)	Research shows that regular consumption of tea enhances mental alertness and is associated with a lower risk of some cancers and heart disease. Special topical preparations clear genital warts.	Safe when taken in moderate amounts as a beverage. Contains caffeine. Higher doses result in agitation, tremors, insomnia, and upset stomach.	Commonly consumed as a beverage. Green and black tea come from the same species but differ in how they're processed. The latter is higher in caffeine. More research is done on green tea, which is higher in compounds called catechins.

Source: Natural Medicines Comprehensive Database (http://naturaldatabase.therapeuticresearch.com), National Library of Medicine databases, and American Botanical Council databases (http://abc.herbalgram.org).

Plant Essential Oils

Essential oils are usually pure, concentrated extracts of aromatic plants. These small, lipid-soluble molecules pass through skin and across the lung's alveoli, moving quickly into the bloodstream. Because they're volatile, they rise into the air to stimulate olfactory (smell) centers in the brain.

Primitive humans probably burned plant gums and resins as incense and infused anointing oils, such as olive and sesame oil, with fragrant plants. People in ancient Egypt, Greece, Rome, China, India, and the Middle East used fragrant herbs for healing, pleasure, beauty, and ceremony. One of the goals of new trade routes out of Europe was to obtain fragrant, culinary, and medicinal plants.

Smell is the most direct of all the senses. Nerve transmission from other senses is first relayed to the thalamus and then to the cerebrum (higher brain areas). Olfactory receptors are located at the top of the nasal cavities and are the endings of the olfactory nerve, which go straight to the brain's olfactory bulb. From there, nerve connections act to modulate mood and alertness.

Aromatherapy refers to the use of volatile plant essential oils to modulate mood, alertness, relaxation, and general well-being. While the sense of smell plays a big role in how essential oils work, they also exert other effects.

Gently warming essential oils releases their scent. Plant essential oils can also be applied to the skin (usually after first diluting them in carrier oil) to reduce local infection and inflammation. Mixed into massage oil, essential oils can be used to relieve sore muscles and nervous tension. They can be added to hot water to be used in steam inhalation and added to footbaths and full-body baths. The FDA primarily regulates plant essential oils as cosmetics.

Emerging research shows that some plant essential oils reduce objective and subjective measurements of stress and anxiety. Examples include German and Roman chamomile, lavender, rose, and jasmine.[95],[96],[97] Some essential oils (rosemary, lemon, peppermint) may increase cognitive (thinking) skills such as attention and memory.[98],[99],[100] Topical application of diluted peppermint oil reduces headache symptoms.[101] Smelling peppermint or ginger essential oil reduces nausea.[102] Lab studies show that many essential oils are antioxidant, anticancer, anti-inflammatory, antibacterial, antiviral, and antifungal. Tea tree oil is but one example.[103]

Dilution is critical, as these volatile chemicals are highly concentrated. Undiluted topical applications can inflame the skin. Essential oils from citrus trees (lemon, orange, bergamot, lime) increase sensitivity to the sun. Do not take essential oils by mouth or apply them near the nose, eyes, or other sensitive mucous membranes. Bottles containing plant essential oils should be kept out of the reach of children. People may be allergic to some of these plants. If applying to skin, do a test patch first and wait a day to observe skin inflammation.

Energy Medicine

These CAM practices manipulate the body's energy fields to affect health. Some are easier to explain because they use forms of energy scientists are familiar with: electromagnetic fields and visible light. **Magnet therapy** affects the electromagnetic fields. Strong static and dynamic (moving or pulsing) magnets have been used to ease various types of pain in people (neck pain, carpal tunnel syndrome, stroke, and diabetes).[104] ,[105] ,[106] Small, static magnets, such as those embedded in bracelets, do not seem to produce significant relief in people with arthritis.[107] People with pacemakers or insulin pumps should not use commercially available magnets without consulting their physicians.

Light therapy involves exposure to natural light or bright lights. Most of the research involves bright light (light boxes, special lighted visors), which mimics outdoor light. Bright light therapy has been used to help people reset their biological clocks and to combat several types of depression (seasonal affective disorders ["winter blues"]), premenstrual depression, depression during pregnancy, depression in bipolar disorder, and possibly eating disorders.[108] ,[109] Exposure to bright lights at critical times of the day helps regulate circadian (daily) rhythms and restores rhythms and disturbed by night shift or jet travel. Bright light therapy can also help improve sleep in people with certain neurologic diseases.[110] ,[111] ,[112]

Sound energy therapy involves the use of sound waves. Tuning forks, wind chimes, gongs, Tibetan singing bowls, and music are all examples of means of releasing sound energy for therapeutic effects. Music therapy has been studied the longest. Soothing music can reduce blood pressure, pain, and anxiety.[113] ,[114] ,[115]

Some energy therapies are based in a belief that practitioners can affect subtle energy fields in the human body. In **therapeutic touch** (also called healing touch) and **Reiki** (pronounced "ray-kee"), practitioners are said to manipulate these energy fields with their hands, which are placed near or on the person. Qigong and acupuncture are also presumed to affect energy. Intercessory prayer (praying for someone else's health) is another example of a therapy that might work by altering subtle energy.[116] Therapies believed to affect subtle energy (including homeopathy) are controversial because scientists haven't yet measured these energy fields.

Nevertheless, Reiki has been shown in studies to improve relaxation and sleep and reduce anxiety, pain, fatigue, and loneliness in people undergoing cancer chemotherapy.[117] ,[118] ,[119] Reiki therapy and therapeutic touch may also improve memory and reduce behavior problems in people with mild Alzheimer's disease.[120] ,[121] Therapeutic touch reduced stress in college students.[122]

Homeopathy is concerned with energy medicine, even though it involves ingestion or topical use of products. German physician Samuel Hahnemann started homeopathy over 200 years ago. After he graduated from medical school in 1779, Hahnemann began his quest for less toxic treatments than the purging, blood-letting, and heavy metals used at the time. Homeopathy was popular in the United States during the 19th century, after which conventional medicine replaced it. It remains popular in the United Kingdom and Europe.

A central tenet of homeopathy is that "like cures like." In other words, a tiny dose of a substance, that in larger doses causes similar symptoms, jumpstarts healing. This principle became known as the law of similars. While healers as far back as Hippocrates had recognized this principle, Hahnemann was the first to generate an entire system of medicine devoted to it. He named this healing practice "homeopathy," from the Greek words for similar ("homoios") and suffering ("pathos").

Here are some examples. A possible remedy for a rash similar to that caused by poison ivy (*Rhus toxicodendron*) might be homeopathic (very diluted) *Rhus toxicodendron*. Restlessness and insomnia might respond to homeopathic coffee (*Coffea cruda*).

Another homeopathic principle is that the more diluted the remedy, the more potent it is. To create these miniscule doses, the substance in question is diluted, succussed (vigorously shaken), diluted, succussed, diluted, and so on until not one molecule of the original substance remains. Critics are quick to point out that, without a single molecule of the active substance, no biological effect is possible.

Theoretically, what remains is an energetic fingerprint of that substance in the water, the so-called memory of water effect. Experiments have shown that homeopathic solutions can alter the structure of the water in which they're dissolved.[123] Perhaps it's not the content of the water but its structure that produces therapeutic effects.[124]

homeopathy

A system of medicine that treats illnesses with highly diluted substances that, in larger doses, would cause similar symptoms.

Another principle is that a single remedy should clear most of a person's symptoms. In addition, homeopaths view each person as unique. Treatment is highly individualized. That means five people with the common cold may each receive a different remedy. That treatment philosophy makes it tough to design the usual randomized, placebo-controlled clinical trial, wherein people are randomly assigned to receive a placebo (dummy pill) or active treatment. Some studies show benefits and some don't. Critics suggest that positive responses are largely due to the person's belief that the substance will work. On the other hand, benefits have been shown in animals and children, both of whom tend to be less invested in the success of treatment.[125],[126]

While many people confuse homeopathy with herbal medicine, the two are entirely different. Herbal medicines come from plants, as well as algae and fungi. Homeopathy makes use of animal, plant, and mineral substances. Some of them are toxic unless highly diluted. Furthermore, herbal medicines usually concentrate the active ingredients rather than creating infinitesimal dilutions, as happens in homeopathy.

Energy therapies such as therapeutic touch, Reiki, and highly diluted homeopathic remedies are generally considered safe. Homeopaths note that symptoms may initially worsen before improving. The other possible ill effect—one that holds true for any alternative treatment—lies in delaying timely medical treatment.

2.2   Whole Medical Systems

NCCAM defines whole medical systems as "complete systems of theory and practice that have evolved over time in different cultures and apart from conventional or Western medicine."[127] Most of these are traditional forms of medicine. As noted earlier, in Asia and Africa, much of the population relies on traditional forms of healing. The WHO has taken steps "to support and integrate traditional medicine into national health systems," as well as "to ensure safety and quality."[128]

Traditional Chinese Medicine

Traditional Chinese medicine (TCM) dates back more than 2,000 years.[129] Some say it's at least 5,000 years old. The theories behind it are complex. A central tenet is that each person has a limited amount of qi. Qi circulates along 12 meridians, or energy channels, each of which links with internal organs. If qi becomes depleted, stagnant, or blocked, ill health ensues. Another key concept is the importance of balancing of the opposing forces of *yin* and *yang*. Too much or too little yin or yang also rocks the boat of well-being.

To restore yin-yang balance and the healthy flow of qi, TCM practitioners use a variety of treatment modalities. They may recommend dietary changes. They may stimulate meridians with acupuncture needles, moxibustion (the burning of cones or sticks made from herbs near the skin), suction cups, and *tui na* (massage). They may prescribe herbal formulas, meditation, and exercise. Mind-body exercises such as tai chi and qigong focus the mind; manipulate qi; and improve strength, balance, and agility.

In the United States, practitioners complete training programs for either a master of science in oriental medicine (MSOM) or a master of acupuncture (MSAc). The MSOM program usually takes three to four years to complete. During that time, students learn acupuncture, moxibustion, cupping, tui na, Chinese herbal medicine, Chinese nutrition, meditation, movements (qigong, tai chi), and more. Students graduating from accredited acupuncture programs, which take two to three years to complete, can become licensed acupuncturists but do not get significant training in Chinese herbal medicine.

Ayurvedic Medicine

Ayurvedic medicine, or **Ayurveda**, originated in India more than 5,000 years ago, as described in ancient texts called the Vedas. The word "Ayurveda" comes from the Sanskrit *ayuh*, meaning life, and *veda*, meaning knowledge. As with TCM, treatments include dietary modifications, medical herbs and spices, bodywork, movement (yoga), breathing exercises, and meditation, as well as treatments designed to remove toxins.

Ayurvedic practitioners believe health and healing can be found through daily living practices and, when needed, the application of gentle healing modalities. Furthermore, each person has a unique combination of the five primary elements—ether, air, fire, water, and earth. These elements combine in pairs to form *doshas*. A person will have a predominance of one or two of these doshas. Imbalances in these energetic forces can lead to disease.

Although certification programs are available, Ayurveda is not a licensed health care practice in the United States.

The yin and yang symbol represents intertwined duality in nature. In each person, these opposing energies blend: light and darkness, dry and moist, hot and cold, outgoing and reflective. Within the symbol for yang (white) is a circle of black, showing there's a little darkness within the light. The same is true for the black symptom for yin.

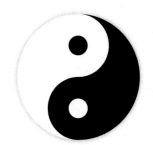

Source: Klem. Yin and yang. 2007.

Available at:

http://commons.wikimedia.org/wiki/ File:Yin_and_Yang.svg.

traditional Chinese medicine

A system of medicine originating in ancient Chinese that employs acupuncture, medicinal plants, massage, meditation, diet, and movement.

Ayurveda

A traditional healing system that originated in India.

Curanderismo and Native American Healing

Curanderismo is a form of Latin American folk healing. Native American healing refers to the techniques used by the first people on this continent. Both are diverse systems, used by a diverse people. For instance, traditional remedies used by the Hopis will differ from those used by Cherokees.

Curanderismo derives from the Spanish word *curar*, to heal. Curanderos (male healers) and curanderas (female healers) may specialize as herbalists, midwives, body workers, or counselors.

Both Native American healing and curanderismo employ techniques for spiritual healing. Spiritual rituals for native traditions can include prayers, cleansing baths, singing, drumming, dancing, and sweat lodge ceremonies. Nature is revered. Every person, animal, plant, and rock, and the earth itself, is imbued with spirit.

Naturopathy

naturopathy

A system of medicine that relies on natural treatments to correct imbalances and allow the body to heal.

Naturopathy, or naturopathic medicine, officially began in the early 1900s when German physician Benedict Lust immigrated to America. He brought with him a European system called the "Nature Cure," which relied upon good diet, exercise (especially outdoors), hot baths, and other nontoxic means to restore health. Later, Lust began calling his system of medicine "Naturopathy."

As with homeopathic colleges, naturopathic colleges proliferated until the 1930s. The decline stemmed from the development of potent pharmaceutical drugs, changes in requirements at medical schools, and pressure from the American Medical Association and government agencies. Today seven naturopathic colleges are accredited in the United States and Canada. Similar to the training of a medical doctor, naturopathic doctors (NDs) undergo four years of graduate training. (Note: Some unaccredited online training programs provide certificates in naturopathy. Such programs do not legitimately prepare anyone to practice medicine.)

Naturopathic physicians work with patients to address imbalances within the domains of wellness. The goal of treatment is to address the root of the illness rather than suppress symptoms. Practitioners employ a unique combination of modern medical science and natural medicines. Treatment is custom tailored to meet the needs of the individual.

To maintain health and manage disease, naturopathic physicians employ a variety of nontoxic, noninvasive therapies such as a healthy diet, exercise, water therapy, physical manipulation, acupuncture, herbs and other nutritional supplements, and homeopathy. NDs may specialize in both the type of therapies they typically recommend (e.g., herbal medicine, acupuncture, homeopathy) and the types of health conditions they treat (e.g., men's health, women's health, pediatrics). In some states, NDs are licensed to prescribe some classes of pharmaceuticals.

Currently, 16 states license naturopathic doctors: Alaska, Arizona, California, Connecticut, Hawaii, Idaho, Kansas, Maine, Minnesota, Montana, New Hampshire, North Dakota, Oregon, Utah, Vermont, and Washington. The District of Columbia also licenses NDs, as do the US territories of Puerto Rico and the US Virgin Islands. In Canada, British Columbia, Manitoba, Nova Scotia, Ontario, and Saskatchewan license NDs. The following states and provinces have legislation pending to license NDs: Colorado, Illinois, Iowa, Massachusetts, New York, North Carolina, Nova Scotia, Pennsylvania, and Wisconsin.[130]

KEY TAKEAWAYS

- Complementary and alternative medicines (CAM) are a diverse group of therapies that fall outside the realm of conventional medical practices. Complementary therapies are used alongside conventional treatments; alternative treatments are used instead of conventional treatments.

- Nearly 40 percent of American adults use CAM. The most commonly used CAM therapies are nonvitamin/nonmineral natural products, deep-breathing exercises, and chiropractic or osteopathic manipulation.

- NCCAM divides CAM therapies into three broad categories: mind-body medicine, manipulative and body-based practices, and natural products.

3. HOLISTIC MEDICINE AND INTEGRATIVE MEDICINE

LEARNING OBJECTIVES

1. Define holistic and integrative medicine.
2. Describe the premises and objectives of both.

3.1 Holistic Medicine

As ancient Greek philosopher Aristotle said, "The whole is greater than the sum of its parts." **Holistic medicine** addresses the health of the whole person—body, mind, and spirit. This view is quite different from a mechanistic, reductionist view that has dominated medical science over the last couple of centuries.

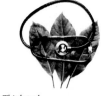

© Thinkstock

holistic medicine

A form of healing that takes into account the whole person—body, mind, emotions, and spirit.

In a mechanistic view (people as machines), the doctor's role is to repair and replace broken parts. The scope of interest is narrowed to the disease part: "The diabetic in room three." Treating bone fractures, heart disease, and infectious diseases isn't quite the same as caring for the people who happen to have these conditions. High-tech diagnostic tests began to replace time-honored clinical diagnosis—listening to and examining the patient. Doctors adopted a paternalistic view, telling their patients what to do.

Furthermore, the scientific method lends itself to a reductionist strategy, controlling as many variables as possible. Rather than study the effect of a food or dietary pattern in populations of humans, it's easier to narrow to the effect of a single vitamin or mineral. The same is true of studying the chemicals medicinal plants contain rather than the entire plant. Doing so provides interesting information but misses out on the interactions of multiple chemicals within foods and herbs. We can't see the forest for the trees.

Granted, this explanation is simplistic and does not intend to malign conventional medicine. In the midst of a heart attack, most of us would want to be rushed to a cardiac care unit. After a car crash, it makes perfect sense to focus on the physical: stop the bleeding, stabilize vital signs, set fractures—worry about the patient's social and spiritual well-being during the rehabilitation period.

For many other conditions, a holistic approach makes sense. Furthermore, it's what many patients and doctors crave. Holistic medicine follows several principles.

1. Humans have an innate ability to heal.

2. In order for a person to feel truly healthy, all the dimensions of wellness—physical, environmental, mental, emotional, social, spiritual, financial—must function optimally. Bringing those domains into balance allows a person to heal and restores well-being.

3. Patients are people, not diseases. Holistic practitioners view each individual as unique and deserving of individualized, compassionate care.

4. The goal of treatment is to correct the underlying cause of illness rather than merely to relieve symptoms. For instance, if a patient has chronic headaches, the practitioner would treat the pain and also investigate the origins of the headaches: allergies, poor posture while working, emotional distress, sinus infection, environmental toxin, and so on.

5. Patients and practitioners are partners. Practitioners act as the guides. Patients participate in the healing process—changing habits related to diet, beliefs, and behaviors. Great value is given to the quality of the practitioner-patient relationship.

Any type of practitioner can practice holistically. Many conventional doctors, nurses, and physician assistants take the whole person into account. Most practitioners of complementary and alternative medicine do as well. Traditional healers have always taken a holistic viewpoint.

In fact, holistic health is nothing new. Ancient Greek and Roman physicians practiced holistic medicine. Traditional healing practices around the world used a holistic approach. Nineteenth-century French physiologist Claude Bernard established the concept that the body seeks to maintain an internal steady. In his book *The Wisdom of the Body*, 20th-century American physiologist Walter Cannon applied the term **homeostasis** to this internal status quo. Advanced age, illness, and stressful events challenge homeostasis. In essence, holistic medicine seeks to restore homeostasis.

Stress researchers such as Hans Selye proved that psychologically and physically stressful events affect multiple bodily systems, including the nervous, immune, hormonal, and cardiovascular systems. In the mid-1970s, Robert Ader and Nicholas Cohen at the University of Rochester coined the term **psychoneuroimmunology** (PNI), the study of how nervous, hormone, and immune systems interact.[131] Thoughts and emotions influence levels of brain chemicals and hormones. Nerve signals and hormones then affect the immune system, as well as other organ systems. Likewise, physical events lead to a pattern of molecular events that affect thoughts and emotions.

When PNI was first introduced, the concept seemed novel and almost radical. Microbes caused infections. Pollen caused hay fever. High cholesterol and high blood pressure caused heart disease. What in the world did thoughts and emotions have to do it? As it turns out, a great deal.

Hundreds of studies have shown that mental and emotional health affect physical health and vice versa. Grieving widowers have suppressed immune function.[132] Perceived lack of social support and more stress accelerate progression in people who have AIDS (acquired immunodeficiency syndrome).[133] Laughter, on the other hand, enhances immune function.[134] Adults who feel their lives have meaning and purpose (elements of spiritual health) have greater longevity.[135] People with major depression are more likely to have heart disease, diabetes, asthma, and strokes.[136] Likewise, having these serious conditions can undermine mental and emotional health.[137]

PNI research also sheds light on how placebos work. A **placebo** is something you wouldn't expect to have a significant effect on the body's functioning. The gold standard of clinical trials (research involving human volunteers) is the placebo-controlled trial. People in one group get the active treatment; people in the other get a placebo. If a drug is the treatment, the placebo group gets a pill without active ingredients (a "sugar pill").

Clinical trials are frequently subject to a **placebo effect**. People who enroll in these studies often have an illness. They know they have a 50-50 chance of getting the new drug or therapy. Researchers ask them how they are, how they're feeling. If the researchers behave in a kind and compassionate manner, that alone can help. So the people in the placebo group often get a bit better. People with depression, anxiety, pain, and insomnia are particularly likely to improve on placebo treatment.[138] PNI research has demonstrated that placebos can produce boosts in immune responsiveness, allergic reactions, changes in blood pressure, and other biological effects—as long as study participants believed they received the "real" treatment. Traumatic injuries and serious ailments are obvious exceptions. (All the positive thinking in the world won't reattach a severed finger.) Medical practitioners of all stripes use the power of placebos in healing. Make a trip to the doctor expecting to get better and you likely will.

homeostasis

The internal state maintained by bodily processes.

psychoneuroimmunology

The study of the interaction of mental and emotional states, nervous system activity, and immune function.

placebo

Anything that is not expected to affect medical treatment.

placebo effect

Any effect that appears to arise from administering a placebo.

Video Clip 2.4

What Is Integrative Medicine?
Andrew Weil, MD, is a Harvard University–trained physician, author, and director of the Center for Integrative Medicine of the College of Medicine, University of Arizona. Here he briefly explains integrative medicine.

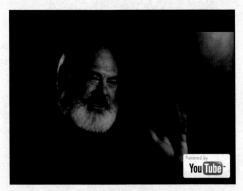

View the video online at: http://www.youtube.com/v/4pXsm3qaFlk

3.2 Integrative Medicine

Over the last few decades, many health care professionals have increasingly returned to the concept of medicine as both science and art. They have recognized that high-tech medicine, despite its merits, can't fully address the rising tide of chronic diseases.[139] What has emerged is a novel model for health care.

Integrative medicine represents the blending of complementary and alternative medicine (CAM) with conventional medicine. Key to this definition is that all therapies have scientific evidence of effectiveness and safety. The goal is to utilize therapies that effectively improve health and well-being while minimizing side effects. It's an inclusive type of holistic medicine that remains sensitive to traditional medical systems.

integrative medicine

A system of medicine that combines evidence-based conventional and CAM treatments.

The principles are similar to those under the holistic model and include additional features:

- Patients and health practitioners work in partnership to affect healing and share in the decision-making process.
- Practitioners consider all the dimensions of wellness when evaluating patients.
- Both conventional and CAM treatments are used, with a goal toward finding the most natural and least invasive treatment.
- In addition to treating disease, practitioners also work to promote healthy lifestyles and prevent illness.
- While science is important, the conventional randomized placebo-controlled trial may not be applicable to some CAM therapies.[140] More pragmatic research models will need to be designed in therapies that lack a suitable placebo control (e.g., acupuncture).

An integrative approach increases the therapeutic options to prevent and manage illness. The choices can seem overwhelming: primary care doctors, medical specialists, and a range of CAM treatments. The trick for consumers and practitioners alike is learning how to make the most of this marriage, how to reap the best of both worlds.

In an integrative model, physicians use a holistic assessment and help their patients design an individualized treatment plan from an array of options. Sometimes a team of experts—dietitians, physical therapists, massage therapist, chiropractors, acupuncturists, conventional doctors—work together to prevent and treat illness. Whenever possible, practitioners recommend the least invasive and least toxic therapies first.

For instance, if you have persistent ankle pain, you might see an orthopedist, rheumatologist, physical therapist, chiropractor, massage therapist, or acupuncturist. Ideally, a primary care practitioner provides the initial evaluation, guides decisions about treatment, and coordinates care.

Integrative medicine offers some advantages for aging populations with increasingly complex conditions. An integrative approach can be used to prevent illness, improve disease symptoms and quality of life, and reduce reliance on medication. For someone with heart disease, integrative treatment might entail meeting with a dietitian, working with an exercise trainer or yoga instructor, learning relaxation techniques, and taking medications to lower cholesterol. Many of the treatments are relatively inexpensive and hold the promise of keeping people healthier longer, which could ultimately reduce health care expenditures. Future studies will need to evaluate the outcomes of integrative treatment approaches.

Most university-based medical centers (including Harvard, Yale, Duke, and Stanford) and freestanding hospitals now have integrative medical centers. Fifty-four academic medical centers and affiliated institutions now belong to the Consortium of Academic Health Centers for Integrative Medicine.[141] Leading cancer centers such as Sloan-Kettering Cancer Center and M. D. Anderson Cancer Center offer integrative medicine services.

The Institute of Medicine of the National Academies (IOM) has convened summits to explore the science and practice of integrative medicine.[142] In 2012, the American College of Preventive Medicine received a government grant to create the National Coordinating Center for Integrative Medicine in Preventive Medicine. So far, 12 preventive medicine residency programs have received funding to incorporate integrative medicine into the training of physicians.[143]

Integrative Medicine Time Capsule

In the 1980s, before the term "integrative medicine" was coined, a young doctor named Dean Ornish embarked with colleagues on a series of groundbreaking experiments. At that point, atherosclerosis (a condition in which fatty material becomes deposited in the arteries) was considered irreversible. The best medicine could do was manage the disease with medications and, if needed, surgery to bypass clogged arteries in the heart. Ornish's experiments proved that intensive lifestyle modifications alone—a vegetarian, low-fat diet; aerobic exercise; smoking cessation; stress-management social support groups; and yoga—lowered cholesterol levels, reduced symptoms such as angina (chest discomfort with exertion), shrank atherosclerotic plaques, and reduced heart attack risk.[144]

Research from the mid-1980s also demonstrated the beneficial effects of social support groups on quality of life and survival in women with breast cancer.[145] Other modalities have since been added to improve the experience of patients undergoing conventional cancer treatment. In China, acupuncture and certain herbs have been shown to offset side effects of anticancer drugs and possibly augment their efficacy.[146],[147],[148],[149] Yoga and meditation can be integrated successfully into cancer treatment, as well as a number of chronic illnesses.[150],[151],[152]

Research at Beth Israel Medical Center in New York has shown that improving the physical environment in treatment areas, using holistic nursing practices (relaxation therapies, visualization techniques, aromatherapy), providing a "patient navigator" to facilitate treatment, and incorporating yoga therapy, heightened cancer patients' quality of life. They had less anxiety, depression, pain, and fatigue.[153] Furthermore, this approach resulted in shorter hospital stays; less use of medications to manage nausea, anxiety, and insomnia; and significant cost savings.[154] The Society for Integrative Oncology has been established to study and facilitate cancer treatment using an integrated approach.[155]

 ### Video Clip 2.5

The Value of Integrative Medicine
Cardiologist Mimi Guarneri, MD, medical director of Scripps Center for Integrative Medicine in La Jolla, California, and one of her patients discuss the value of integrative medicine in helping people with heart disease.

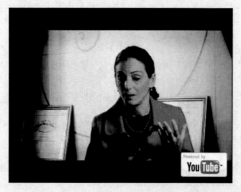

View the video online at: http://www.youtube.com/v/yYEaPZOyiVQ

Source: Scripps Health.

Becoming a Savvy Health Care Consumer

Navigating the health care system has become more complicated. In the old days, people turned to their elders and family physicians for advice. Now bookstore shelves groan with self-help books. The media barrage us with stories and advertisements about the latest cures. Some have credence; others do nothing or produce dangerous side effects. What sources can you trust? How do you separate the wheat from the chaff?

In order to make thoughtful choices, you need to educate yourself. To do that, you need to identify reputable, credible resources for up-to-date information on the treatment's potential benefits and harmful effects. Here are some guidelines to help you make the call.

1. Check the author's credentials. Is this person a credible expert in the health field?

2. Does the author provide evidence for the treatment's efficacy? Look for endnotes (reference citations at the end of the document). Learn how to look up cited sources so you can read the original source. Reference librarians can point you in the right direction.

3. Does the publication, TV show, or website advertise the product or services? If yes, your resource has a conflict of interest and is likely biased toward the treatment. Note that most medical journals contain ads for pharmaceutical drugs. Clearly, that doesn't eliminate them as a source of information.

4. Who operates the website? Does the website's address end in .gov, .edu, or .org? Such sites are generally more objective and accurate than dot-coms, which usually have a commercial interest. Section 4 contains a list of reputable sources for health information.

5. What is the website's purpose? Is it to educate or to sell you something? This litmus test will help you decide whether to trust a dot-com. For instance, webmd.com, emedicinehealth.com, Medscape.com, and medpagetoday.com primarily serve as information sources. Medical experts either write or review the articles.

6. What sources are used to write the information? Sciencedaily.com and ScienceNews.org report on studies published in peer-reviewed journals. (Peer review means professionals evaluate the paper before it's published.) The author should refer to the source in the body of the text and/or include citations to original sources.

7. Does the information sound too good to be true? It likely is.

Self-Care versus Professional Care

Many illnesses are mild, acute, and self-limited, which means they don't last long and go away on their own. You need to observe your signs and symptoms and decide whether you can handle the situation yourself. Then you need to decide what course of action to take. Often the best remedy is rest and extra sleep.

Trust your judgment. You know your body and mind better than anyone. If you sense that something is wrong with your health, get professional help. A medical diagnosis—including the reassurance that you can manage your symptoms at home—can be very helpful.

Whenever you have doubts about your health, contact your primary care practitioner. He or she can help you judge whether self-care (managing symptoms of illness at home) is wise, whether treatments you're interested in trying are safe and effective, and whether your symptoms merit an office visit for evaluation and treatment. Keep in mind that, even if a remedy you read is nontoxic, delaying needed medical treatment can harm your health.

A number of warning signs and symptoms indicate you need professional help. Key among them is the intensity and duration of those symptoms. Specifically, severe, prolonged, or recurrent symptoms deserve an evaluation. Take headaches. If the headache is unlike anything you've ever had, extremely painful, continues for more than a day, or recurs frequently, you should seek medical attention. The same goes for psychological symptoms. If they interfere with function, persist, or recur, see a mental health expert.

You should also call your doctor if you have an adverse reaction to any kind of treatment, conventional or CAM. He or she can file a report and decide whether your symptoms merit treatment.

Emergency warning signs and symptoms include the following:

- high fever (103°F and up), especially if accompanied by a stiff neck or a rash
- shortness of breath at rest
- chest pain (not caused by soreness from physical exertion)

- traumatic injury with suspected bone fractures; ligamentous damage; or possible injury to the spinal cord, brain, or internal organs
- laceration with ragged edges that won't stop bleeding after 10 minutes of steady pressure and gapes open
- venomous snake bite
- animal or human bite that breaks the skin
- severe burn or second-degree burn (the kind that raises blisters) on the hands, feet, face, genitals, or involving a surface area larger than your hand elsewhere on the body
- suspected overdose of alcohol or drugs
- severe allergic reaction that causes swelling of the lips, mouth, and throat
- coughing or vomiting blood
- seizure (convulsions)
- loss of consciousness

KEY TAKEAWAYS

- Holistic medicine addresses the needs of the whole person. The main principles are that the body has an innate ability to heal itself, that removal of underlying causes of illness is necessary for complete healing, that patients and practitioners are partners, and that treatment should be individualized.
- Integrative medicine represents the blending of conventional medicines and CAM (complementary and alternative medicines) with the most evidence for effectiveness and safety. The approach is holistic and inclusive.
- Consumers have a range of diverse health care options and means of acquiring health-related information. In order to make wise decisions, consumers need to maintain a healthy skepticism and learn to evaluate health claims.

DISCUSSION QUESTIONS

1. Explain the differences between conventional, alternative, complementary, and integrative medicine. Give an example of each.
2. Do an Internet search on a health topic that interests you. Examples include treatments for depression, magnets for cancer (or arthritis), supplements for athletic endurance, weight-loss supplements, and causes of chronic fatigue syndrome. Using the criteria listed in the sidebar "Becoming a Savvy Health Care Consumer", critically analyze the credibility of the information you find on three different websites.

4. RECOMMENDED RESOURCES

4.1 Books

Brinker F. *Herbal Contraindications and Drug Interaction*. 4th ed. Sandy, OR: Eclectic Medical Publications; 2010.

Mills S, Bone K. *The Essential Guide to Herb Safety*. Philadelphia, PA: Elsevier; 2005.

Ullman D. *Essential Homeopathy*. Novato, CA: New World Library; 2002.

Wisneski LA, Anderson A. *The Scientific Basis of Integrative Medicine*. 2nd ed. Boca Raton, FL: CRC Press; 2009.

4.2 Websites: Information about Various Health Professions

American Academy of Physician Assistants. http://www.aapa.org.

American Association of Acupuncture and Oriental Medicine. http://www.aaaomonline.org.

American Association of Naturopathic Physicians. http://www.naturopathic.org.

American Chinese Medicine Association. http://www.americanchinesemedicineassociation.org.

American Chiropractic Association. http://www.acatoday.org.

American College for the Advancement of Medicine. http://www.acamnet.org.

American Herbalists Guild. http://www.americanherbalistsguild.com.

American Holistic Medical Association. http://www.holisticmedicine.org.

American Holistic Nursing Association. http://www.ahna.org.

American Medical Association. http://www.ama-assn.org.

American Nurses Association. http://www.nursingworld.org.

American Osteopathic Association. http://www.osteopathic.org.

American Physical Therapy Association. http://www.apta.org.

American Public Health Association. http://www.apha.org.

Ayurvedic Institute. http://www.ayurveda.com.

Consortium of Academic Health Centers for Integrative Medicine. http://www.imconsortium.org/members/home.html.

North American Society of Homeopaths. http://www.homeopathy.org.

4.3   Websites: Credible Sources for Health Information

Agency for Health Care Research and Quality. http://www.ahrq.gov.

American Botanical Council. http://www.herbalgram.org.

Centers for Disease Control and Prevention. http://www.cdc.gov.

Cleveland Clinic. http://my.clevelandclinic.org.

ConsumerLab.com. http://www.consumerlab.com.

Food and Drug Administration: Dietary Supplements. http://www.fda.gov/Food/DietarySupplements/default.htm.

Healthfinder.gov. http://www.healthfinder.gov.

Mayo Clinic. http://www.mayoclinic.com.

MedicineNet.com. http://www.medicinenet.com.

MedlinePlus. http://www.medlineplus.gov.

National Center for Complementary and Alternative Medicine (NCCAM). http://nccam.nih.gov.

National Institutes of Health. http://www.nih.gov.

University of Maryland Medical Center, Complementary Medicine. http://www.umm.edu/altmed.

Victorian Health Promotion Foundation (VicHealth). http://www.vichealth.vic.gov.au.

WebMD. http://www.webmd.com.

World Health Organization. http://www.who.int.

ENDNOTES

1. Gilead L, Mumcuoglu KY, Ingber A. The use of maggot debridement therapy in the treatment of chronic wounds in hospitalised and ambulatory patients. *J Wound Care*. 2012 Feb;21(2):78, 80, 82–85.

2. Whitaker IS, Oboumarzouk O, Rozen WM, et al. The efficacy of medicinal leeches in plastic and reconstructive surgery: a systematic review of 277 reported clinical cases. *Microsurgery*. 2012 Mar;32(3):240–250. doi:10.1002/micr.20971.

3. Allied health. Health Professions Network. Available at: http://www.healthpronet.org/docs/allied_health_fact_sheet.pdf. Accessed February 21, 2013.

4. Ayanian JZ. The Massachusetts journey to expand health insurance coverage. *J Gen Intern Med*. 2012;27:139–141.

5. The healthcare imperative: lowering costs and improving outcomes—workshop series summary. Institute of Medicine. February 24, 2011. Available at: http://iom.edu/Reports/2011/The-Healthcare-Imperative-Lowering-Costs-and-Improving-Outcomes.aspx. Accessed July 30, 2012.

6. Aizenman NC. Number of uninsured Americans drops by 1.3 million, census report shows. *Washington Post*. September 12, 2012. Available at: http://www.washingtonpost.com/national/health-science/number-of-uninsured-americans-drops-by-1-3-million-census-report-shows/2012/09/12/0036c876-fcdc-11e1-a31e-804fccb658f9_story.html. Accessed September 18, 2012.

7. Putting off care because of cost: health tracking poll, August 2011. Figure 14 in Health Care Costs: A Primer. Kaiser Family Foundation. Available at: http://www.kff.org/insurance/upload/7670-03.pdf. Accessed December 8, 2012.

8. Lowes R. One third of Americans postpone care because of cost. Medscape. December 17, 2012. Available at: http://www.medscape.com/viewarticle/776304?src=wnl_edit_medn_fmed&spon=34. Accessed December 22, 2012.

9. National health expenditures by type of service and source of funds, CY 1960–2011. National Health Expenditure Data. Centers for Medicare and Medicaid Services. Available at: https://www.cms.gov/Research-Statistics-Data-and-Systems/Statistics-Trends-and-Reports/NationalHealthExpendData/NationalHealthAccountsHistorical.html. Accessed January 30, 2013.

10. Marvasti FF, Stafford RS. From sick care to health care: reengineering prevention into the U.S. system. *N Engl J Med*. 2012;367:889–891. doi:10.1056/NEJMp1206230.

11. Clarke JL. Preventive medicine: a ready solution for a health care system in crisis. *Popul Health Manag*. 2010;13 Suppl 2:S3–11. doi:10.1089/pop.2010.1382. Available at: http://www.uspreventivemedicine.com/Files/PDFs/In-Line/Supplemental-Article-Population-Health-Management-.aspx. Accessed February 2, 2013.

12. First international conference on health promotion, Ottawa, 17–21 November 1986. The Ottawa Charter for Health Promotion. World Health Organization. Available at: http://www.who.int/healthpromotion/Milestones_Health_Promotion_05022010.pdf. Accessed January 28, 2013.

13. American College of Physicians. *The Advanced Medical Home: A Patient-Centered, Physician-Guided Model of Health Care*. Philadelphia, PA: American College of Physicians; 2005. Position Paper. Available at: http://www.acponline.org/advocacy/where_we_stand/policy/adv_med.pdf. Accessed February 13, 2013.

14. American College of Physicians. The impending collapse of primary care medicine and its implications for the state of the nation's health care: a report from the American College of Physicians. Executive Summary. American College of Physicians. January 30, 2006. ehrCentral @ The Provider's Edge. Available at: http://www.providersedge.com/ehdocs/ehr_articles/The_Impending_Collapse_of_Primary_Care_Medicine_and_Its_Implications_for_the_State_of_the_Nation-s_Healthcare.pdf. Accessed February 2, 2013.

15. Bowman RC. Measuring primary care: the standard primary care year. *Rural Remote Health*. 2008 Jul–Sep;8(3):1009.

16. Petterson SM, Liaw WR, Phillips RL, Rabin DL, Meyers DS, Bazemore AW. Projecting US primary care physician work force needs 2010–2025. *Ann Fam Med*. 2012;10(6):503–509. doi:10.1370/afm.1431. Available at: http://annfammed.org/content/10/6/503.full. Accessed June 4, 2013.

17. Coplan B, Cawley J, Stoehr J. Physician assistants in primary care: trends and characteristics. *Ann Fam Med*. 2013 Jan;11(1):75–79. doi:10.1370/afm.1432.

18. American College of Physicians. The impending collapse of primary care medicine and its implications for the state of the nation's health care: a report from the American College of Physicians. Executive Summary. American College of Physicians. January 30, 2006. ehrCentral @ The Provider's Edge. Available at: http://www.providersedge.com/ehdocs/ehr_articles/The_Impending_Collapse_of_Primary_Care_Medicine_and_Its_Implications_for_the_State_of_the_Nation-s_Healthcare.pdf. Accessed February 2, 2013.

19. Reese SM. Women MDs spend more time with patients: does it matter? Medscape, WebMD. Available at: http://www.medscape.com/viewarticle/744653_print. Accessed June 29, 2011.

20. Cassil A. Physicians: so much to do, so little time: despite more time spent on patient care, more doctors bemoan lack of time with patients. News Release. Center for Studying Health System Change. May 7, 2003. Available at: http://www.hschange.com/CONTENT/558. February 2, 2013.

21. Marvasti FF, Stafford RS. From sick care to health care: reengineering prevention into the U.S. system. *N Engl J Med*. 2012;367:889–891. doi:10.1056/NEJMp1206230.

22. 2012 annual federal poverty guidelines. Families USA. Available at: http://www.familiesusa.org/resources/tools-for-advocates/guides/federal-poverty-guidelines.html. Accessed February 1, 2013.

23. Clarke JL. Preventive medicine: a ready solution for a health care system in crisis. *Popul Health Manag*. 2010;13 Suppl 2:S3–11. doi:10.1089/pop.2010.1382. Available at: http://www.uspreventivemedicine.com/Files/PDFs/In-Line/Supplemental-Article-Population-Health-Management-.aspx. Accessed February 2, 2013.

24. Important events in NCCAM history. National Center for Complementary and Alternative Medicine. Available at: http://www.nih.gov/about/almanac/organization/NCCAM.htm. Accessed February 14, 2013.

25. FY 2009 enacted appropriations. National Institutes of Health. Available at: http://officeofbudget.od.nih.gov/pdfs/FY09/FY%202009%20Enacted%20Appropriations%20%28Final%29.pdf. Accessed February 20, 2013.

26. Frequently asked questions. AlterMed Research Foundation. Available at: http://www.altermedresearch.org/FAQ.html. Accessed February 20, 2013.

27. Barnes PM, Bloom B, Nahin RL. Complementary and alternative medicine use among adults and children: United States, 2007. National Health Interview Survey, no. 12. Hyattsville, MD: National Center for Health Statistics; 2008. Available at: http://www.cdc.gov/nchs/data/nhsr/nhsr012.pdf. Accessed February 14, 2013.

28. Nahin RL, Barnes PM, Stussman BJ, Bloom B. Costs of complementary and alternative medicine (CAM) and frequency of visits to CAM practitioners: United States, 2007. National Health Statistics Reports, no. 18. Hyattsville, MD: National Center for Health Statistics; 2008.

29. Davis MA, Martin BI, Coulter ID, Weeks WB. US spending on complementary and alternative medicine during 2002–08 plateaued, suggesting role in reformed health system. *Health Aff (Millwood)*. 2013 Jan;32(1):45–52. doi:10.1377/hlthaff.2011.0321.

30. Kabat-Zinn J. Mindfulness-based interventions in context: past, present, and future. *Clin Psychol Sci Pract*. 2003;10:144–156.

31. Woods-Giscombé CL, Black AR. Mind-body interventions to reduce risk for health disparities related to stress and strength among African American women: the potential of mindfulness-based stress reduction, loving-kindness, and the NTU therapeutic framework. *Complement Health Pract Rev*. 2010 Dec 14;15(3):115–131. Available at: http://www.ncbi.nlm.nih.gov/pmc/articles/PMC3071547/?tool=pubmed. Accessed June 1, 2012.

32. Meditation. Natural Medicines Comprehensive Database. Available at: http://naturaldatabase.therapeuticresearch.com/home.aspx?cs=&s=ND&AspxAutoDetectCookieSupport=1. Accessed February 14, 2013.

33. Eppel E, Daubenmier J, Moskowitz JT, Folkman S, Blackburn E. Can meditation slow rate of cellular aging? Cognitive stress, mindfulness, and telomeres. *Ann N Y Acad Sci*. 2009 Aug;1172:34–53. doi:10.1111/j.1749-6632.2009.04414.x.

34. Manikonda JP, Stork S, Togel S, et al. Contemplative meditation reduces ambulatory blood pressure and stress-induced hypertension: a randomized pilot trial. *J Hum Hypertens*. 2008;22:138–140.

35. Morone NE, Greco CM, Weiner DK. Mindfulness meditation for the treatment of chronic low back pain in older adults: a randomized controlled pilot study. *Pain*. 2008;134:310–319.

36. Chan D, Woolacott M. Effects of level of meditation experience on attentional focus: is the efficiency of executive or orientation networks improved? *J Altern Complement Med*. 2007;13:651–657.

37. Tang YY, Ma Y, Wang J, et al. Short-term meditation training improves attention and self-regulation. *Proc Natl Acad Sci U S A*. 2007;104:17152–17156.

38. Natural Medicines Comprehensive Database. Meditation. Available at: http://naturaldatabase.therapeuticresearch.com/home.aspx?cs=&s=ND&AspxAutoDetectCookieSupport=1. Accessed February 14, 2013.

39. Chen Y, Yang X, Wang L, Zhang X. A randomized controlled trial of the effects of brief mindfulness meditation on anxiety symptoms and systolic blood pressure in Chinese nursing students. *Nurse Educ Today*. 2012 Dec 19. doi:pii: S0260-6917(12)00387-5.10.1016/j.nedt.2012.11.01.

40. Lee SH, Ahn SC, Lee YJ, et al. Effectiveness of a meditation-based stress management program as an adjunct to pharmacotherapy in patients with anxiety disorder. *J Psychosom Res*. 2007;62:189–195.

41. Pinniger R, Brown RF, Thorsteinsson EB, McKinley P. Argentine tango dance compared to mindfulness meditation and a waiting-list control: a randomised trial for treating depression. *Complement Ther Med*. 2012 Dec;20(6):377–384. doi:10.1016/j.ctim.2012.07.003.

42. Marchand WR. Mindfulness-based stress reduction, mindfulness-based cognitive therapy, and Zen meditation for depression, anxiety, pain, and psychological distress. *J Psychiatr Pract*. 2012 Jul;18(4):233–352. doi:10.1097/01.pra.0000416014.53215.86.

43. Alberts HJ, Thewissen R, Raes L. Dealing with problematic eating behaviour: the effects of a mindfulness-based intervention on eating behaviour, food cravings, dichotomous thinking and body image concern. *Appetite*. 2012 Jun;58(3):847–851. doi:10.1016/j.appet.2012.01.009.

44. Tharion E, Samuel P, Rajalakshmi R, Gnanasenthil G, Subramanian RK. Influence of deep breathing exercise on spontaneous respiratory rate and heart rate variability: a randomised controlled trial in healthy subjects. *Indian J Physiol Pharmacol*. 2012 Jan–Mar;56(1):80–87.

45. Sood R, Sood A, Wolf SL, et al. Paced breathing compared with usual breathing for hot flashes. *Menopause*. 2013 Feb;20(2):179–184. doi:10.1097/gme.0b013e31826934b6.

46. Hayama Y, Inoue T. The effects of deep breathing on "tension-anxiety" and fatigue in cancer patients undergoing adjuvant chemotherapy. *Complement Ther Clin Pract*. 2012 May;18(2):94–98. doi:10.1016/j.ctcp.2011.10.001.

47. Busch V, Magerl W, Kern U, Haas J, Hajak G, Eichhammer P. The effect of deep and slow breathing on pain perception, autonomic activity, and mood processing—an experimental study. *Pain Med.* 2012 Feb;13(2):215–228. doi:10.1111/j.1526-4637.2011.01243.x.

48. Paul G, Elam B, Verhulst SJ. A longitudinal study of students' perceptions of using deep breathing meditation to reduce testing stresses. *Teach Learn Med.* 2007 summer;19(3):287–292.

49. Sengupta P. Health impacts of yoga and pranayam: a state-of-the-art review. *Int J Prev Med.* 2012 July;3(7):444–458. Available at: http://www.ncbi.nlm.nih.gov/pmc/articles/PMC3415184. Accessed February 13, 2013.

50. Levere JL. A moment of Zen, on the go. *New York Times.* January 14, 2013. Available at: http://www.nytimes.com/2013/01/15/business/some-hotel-companies-and-airports-start-to-offer-yoga.html. Accessed February 13, 2013.

51. Alexander GK, Innes KE, Selfe TK, Brown CJ. "More than I expected": perceived benefits of yoga practice among older adults at risk for cardiovascular disease. *Complement Ther Med.* 2013 Feb;21(1):14–28. doi:10.1016/j.ctim.2011.11.001.

52. Smith C, Hancock H, Blake-Mortimer J, Eckert K. A randomised comparative trial of yoga and relaxation to reduce stress and anxiety. *Complement Ther Med.* 2007;15:77–83.

53. Manjunath NK, Telles S. Influence of Yoga and Ayurveda on self-rated sleep in a geriatric population. *Indian J Med Res.* 2005;121:683–690.

54. Sherman KJ, Cherkin DC, Erro J, et al. Comparing yoga, exercise, and a self-care book for chronic low back pain: a randomized, controlled trial. *Ann Intern Med.* 2005;143:849–856.

55. Balasubramaniam M, Telles S, Doraiswamy PM. Yoga on our minds: a systematic review of yoga for neuropsychiatric disorders. *Front Psychiatry.* 2012;3:117. doi:10.3389/fpsyt.2012.00117. Available at: http://www.ncbi.nlm.nih.gov/pmc/articles/PMC3555015. Accessed February 13, 2013.

56. Sharma VK, Das S, Mondal S, et al. Effect of Sahaj Yoga on neuro-cognitive functions in patients suffering from major depression. *Indian J Physiol Pharmacol.* 2006;50:375–383.

57. Chuntharapat S, Petpichetchian W, Hatthakit U. Yoga during pregnancy: effects on maternal comfort, labor pain and birth outcomes. *Complement Ther Clin Pract.* 2008;14:105–115.

58. Damodaran A, Malathi A, Patil N, et al. Therapeutic potential of yoga practices in modifying cardiovascular risk profile in middle aged men and women. *J Assoc Physicians India.* 2002;50:633–640.

59. Bidwell AJ, Yazel B, Davin D, Fairchild TJ, Kanaley JA. Yoga training improves quality of life in women with asthma. *J Altern Complement Med.* 2012 Aug;18(8):749–755. doi:10.1089/acm.2011.0079.

60. Penman S, Cohen M, Stevens P, Jackson S. Yoga in Australia: Results of a national survey. *Int J Yoga.* 2012 Jul;5(2):92–101. doi:10.4103/0973-6131.98217.

61. Skoglund L, Jansson E. Qigong reduces stress in computer operators. *Complement Ther Clin Pract.* 2007;13:78–84.

62. Taylor D, Hale L, Schluter P, et al. Effectiveness of tai chi as a community-based falls prevention intervention: a randomized controlled trial. *J Am Geriatr Soc.* 2012 May;60(5):841–848. doi:10.1111/j.1532-5415.2012.03928.x.

63. Rogers CE, Larkey LK, Keller C. A review of clinical trials of tai chi and qigong in older adults. *West J Nurs Res.* 2009 Mar;31(2):245–279. doi:10.1177/0193945908327529.

64. Irwin MR, Olmstead R, Motivala SJ. Improving sleep quality in older adults with moderate sleep complaints: a randomized controlled trial of Tai Chi Chih. *Sleep.* 2008;31:1001–1008.

65. Tsang HW, Fung KM, Chan AS, et al. Effect of a qigong exercise programme on elderly with depression. *Int J Geriatr Psychiatry.* 2006;21:890–897.

66. Chen K, He B, Rihacek G, Sigal LH. A pilot trial of external Qigong therapy for arthritis. *J Clin Rheumatol.* 2003;9:332–335.

67. Yang Y, Verkuilen J, Rosengren KS, et al. Effects of a Taiji and Qigong intervention on the antibody response to influenza vaccine in older adults. *Am J Chin Med.* 2007;35:597–607.

68. Leung R, McKeough ZJ, Peters MJ, Alison JA. Short-form sun-style an exercise training modality in people with COPD. *Eur Respir J.* 2012. doi:10.1183/09031936.00036912.

69. Yeh SC, Chang MY. The effect of Qigong on menopausal symptoms and quality of sleep for perimenopausal women: a preliminary observational study. *J Altern Complement Med.* 2012 Jun;18(6):567–575. doi:10.1089/acm.2011.0133.

70. Lynch M, Sawynok J, Hiew C, Marcon D. A randomized controlled trial of Qigong for fibromyalgia. *Arthritis Res Ther.* 2012;14:R178. doi:10.1186/ar3931.

71. White A, Ernst E. A brief history of acupuncture. *Rheumatology.* 2004;43(5):662–663.

72. Manheimer E, White A, Berman B, Forys K, Ernst E. Meta-analysis: acupuncture for low back pain. *Ann Intern Med.* 2005;142:651–663.

73. Smith CA, Collins CT, Cyna AM, Crowther CA. Complementary and alternative therapies for pain management in labour. *Cochrane Database Syst Rev.* 2006;18(4):CD003521.

74. Kwon YD, Pittler MH, Ernst E. Acupuncture for peripheral joint osteoarthritis: a systematic review and meta-analysis. *Rheumatology (Oxford).* 2006;45:1331–1337.

75. Acupuncture for pain. National Center for Complementary and Alternative Medicine. Available at: http://nccam.nih.gov/health/acupuncture/acupuncture-for-pain.htm. Accessed February 15, 2013.

76. Tsai PS, Chang NC, Chang WY, et al. Blood pressure biofeedback exerts intermediate-term effects on blood pressure and pressure reactivity in individuals with mild hypertension: a randomized controlled study. *J Altern Complement Med.* 2007;13:547–554.

77. Ciancarelli I, Tozzi-Ciancarelli MG, Spacca G, et al. Relationship between biofeedback and oxidative stress in patients with chronic migraine. *Cephalalgia.* 2007;27:1136–1141.

78. Goertz CM, Pohlman KA, Vining RD, Brantingham JW, Long CR. Patient-centered outcomes of high-velocity, low-amplitude spinal manipulation for low back pain: a systematic review. *J Electromyogr Kinesiol.* 2012 Oct;22(5):670–691. doi:10.1016/j.jelekin.2012.03.006.

79. Dobson D, Lucassen PL, Miller JJ, Vlieger AM, Prescott P, Lewith G. Manipulative therapies for infantile colic. *Cochrane Database Syst Rev.* 2012 Dec 12;12:CD004796. doi:10.1002/14651858.CD004796.pub2.

80. Bronfort G, Assendelft WJ, Evans R, Haas M, Bouter L. Efficacy of spinal manipulation for chronic headache: a systematic review. *J Manipulative Physiol Ther.* 2001 Sep;24(7):457–466.

81. Massage. University of Maryland Medical Center. Available at: http://www.umm.edu/altmed/articles/massage-000354.htm. Accessed February 16, 2013.

82. Ang JY, Lua JL, Mathur A, et al. A randomized placebo-controlled trial of massage therapy on the immune system of preterm infants. *Pediatrics.* 2012 Dec;130(6):e1549–e1558. doi:10.1542/peds.2012-0196.

83. Gonzalez AP, Vasquez-Mendoza G, García-Vela A, et al. Weight gain in preterm infants following parent-administered Vimala massage: a randomized controlled trial. *Am J Perinatol.* 2009 Apr;26(4):247–252. doi:10.1055/s-0028-1103151.

84. Braun LA, Stanguts C, Casanelia L, et al. Massage therapy for cardiac surgery patients—a randomized trial. *J Thorac Cardiovasc Surg.* 2012 Dec;144(6):1453–1459, 1459.e1. doi:10.1016/j.jtcvs.2012.04.027.

85. What is a dietary supplement? Food and Drug Administration. Available at: http://www.fda.gov/Food/DietarySupplements/default.htm#what_is. Accessed November 25, 2012.

86. Wilford JN. Lessons in iceman's prehistoric medicine kit. *New York Times.* December 8, 1998. Available at: http://www.nytimes.com/1998/12/08/science/lessons-in-iceman-s-prehistoric-medicine-kit.html. Accessed February 18, 2013.

87. Hardy K, Buckley S, Collins MJ, et al. Neanderthal medics? Evidence for food, cooking, and medicinal plants entrapped in dental calculus. *Naturwissenschaften.* 2012;99(8):617–626.

88. Moerman DE. *Native American Ethnobotany.* Portland, OR: Timber Press; 1998:12.

89. Blumenthal M. *The ABC Clinical Guide to Herbs.* Austin, TX: American Botanical Council; 2003:xvii.

90. Haffner SM. The insulin resistance syndrome revisited. *Diabetes Care.* 1996;19:275–277. Reported in: Schmidt B, Ribnicky DM, Poulev A, Logendra S, Cefalu WT, Raskin I. *Metabolism.* 2008;57 Suppl 1:S3–S9. doi:10.1016/j.metabol.2008.03.001.

91. Traditional medicine. Fact sheet no. 134. World Health Organization. December 2008. Available at: http://www.who.int/mediacentre/factsheets/fs134/en. Accessed February 18, 2013.

92. Traditional medicine. Fact sheet no. 134. World Health Organization. December 2008. Available at: http://www.who.int/mediacentre/factsheets/fs134/en. Accessed February 18, 2013.

93. Amsterdam JD, Li Y, Soeller I, Rockwell K, Mao JJ, Shults J. A randomized, double-blind, placebo-controlled trial of oral Matricaria recutita (chamomile) extract therapy for generalized anxiety disorder. *Clin Psychopharmacol.* 2009 Aug;29(4):378–382. doi:10.1097/JCP.0b013e3181ac935c.

94. Amsterdam JD, Shults J, Soeller I, Mao JJ, Rockwell K, Newberg AB. Chamomile (Matricaria recutita) may provide antidepressant activity in anxious, depressed humans: an exploratory study. *Altern Ther Health Med.* 2012 Sep–Oct;18(5):44–49.

95. Perry R, Terry R, Watson LK, Ernst E. Is lavender an anxiolytic drug? A systematic review of randomised clinical trials. *Phytomedicine.* 2012 Jun 15;19(8–9):825–835. doi:10.1016/j.phymed.2012.02.013.

96. Lee YL, Wu Y, Tsang HW, Leung AY, Cheung WM. A systematic review on the anxiolytic effects of aromatherapy in people with anxiety symptoms. *J Altern Complement Med.* 2011 Feb;17(2):101–108. doi:10.1089/acm.2009.0277.

97. Setzer WN. Essential oils and anxiolytic aromatherapy. *Nat Prod Commun.* 2009 Sep;4(9):1305–1316.

98. Moss M, Cook J, Wesnes K, Duckett P. Aromas of rosemary and lavender essential oils differentially affect cognition and mood in healthy adults. *Int J Neurosci.* 2003 Jan;113(1):15–38.

99. Moss M, Hewitt S, Moss L, Wesnes K. Modulation of cognitive performance and mood by aromas of peppermint and ylang-ylang. *Int J Neurosci.* 2008 Jan;118(1):59–77.

100. Jimbo D, Kimura Y, Taniguchi M, Inoue M, Urakami K. Effect of aromatherapy on patients with Alzheimer's disease. *Psychogeriatrics.* 2009 Dec;9(4):173–179. doi:10.1111/j.1479-8301.2009.00299.x.

101. Kligler B, Chaudhary S. Peppermint oil. *Am Fam Physician.* 2007 Apr 1;75(7):1027–1030.

102. Lua PL, Zakaria NS. A brief review of current scientific evidence involving aromatherapy use for nausea and vomiting. *J Altern Complement Med.* 2012 Jun;18(6):534–540. doi:10.1089/acm.2010.0862.

103. Pazyar N, Yaghoobi R, Bagherani N, Kazerouni A. A review of applications of tea tree oil in dermatology. *Int J Dermatol.* 2012 Sep 24. doi:10.1111/j.1365-4632.2012.05654.x.

104. Kroeling P, Gross A, Goldsmith CH, Burnie SJ, Haines T, Graham N, Brant A. Electrotherapy for neck pain. *Cochrane Database Syst Rev.* 2009 Oct 7;(4):CD004251. doi:10.1002/14651858.CD004251.pub4.

105. Weintraub MI, Cole SP. A randomized controlled trial of the effects of a combination of static and dynamic magnetic fields on carpal tunnel syndrome. *Pain Med.* 2008 Jul–Aug;9(5):493–504.

106. Weintraub MI, Cole SP. Pulsed magnetic field therapy in refractory neuropathic pain secondary to peripheral neuropathy: electrodiagnostic parameters—pilot study. *Neurorehabil Neural Repair.* 2004 Mar;18(1):42–46.

107. Richmond SJ, Brown SR, Campion PD, et al. Therapeutic effects of magnetic and copper bracelets in osteoarthritis: a randomised placebo-controlled crossover trial. *Complement Ther Med.* 2009 Oct–Dec;17(5–6):249–256. doi:10.1016/j.ctim.2009.07.002.

108. Krysta K, Krzystanek M, Janas-Kozik M, Krupka-Matuszczyk I. Bright light therapy in the treatment of childhood and adolescence depression, antepartum depression, and eating disorders. *J Neural Transm.* 2012 Oct;119(10):1167–1172.

109. Pail G, Huf W, Pjrek E, Winkler D, Willeit M, Praschak-Rieder N, Kasper S. Bright-light therapy in the treatment of mood disorders. *Neuropsychobiology.* 2011;64(3):152–162. doi:10.1159/000328950.

110. Bjorvatn B, Stangenes K, Oyane N, Forberg K, Lowden A, Holsten F, Akerstedt T. Randomized placebo-controlled field study of the effects of bright light and melatonin in adaptation to night work. *Scand J Work Environ Health.* 2007 Jun;33(3):204–214.

111. Burgess HJ, Crowley SJ, Gazda CJ, Fogg LF, Eastman CI. Preflight adjustment to eastward travel: 3 days of advancing sleep with and without morning bright light. *J Biol Rhythms.* 2003 Aug;18(4):318–328.

112. Rutten S, Vriend C, van den Heuvel OA, Smit JH, Berendse HW, van der Werf YD. Bright light therapy in Parkinson's disease: an overview of the background and evidence. *Parkinsons Dis.* 2012;2012:767105. doi:10.1155/2012/767610.

113. Korhan EA, Uyar M, Eyigör C, Hakverdioğlu Yönt G, Celik S, Khorshıd L. The effects of music therapy on pain in patients with neuropathic pain. *Pain Manag Nurs.* 2013 Jan 31. pii: S1524-9042(12)00174-9. doi:10.1016/j.pmn.2012.10.006.

114. Cole LC, Lobiondo-Wood G. Music as an adjuvant therapy in control of pain and symptoms in hospitalized adults: a systematic review. *Pain Manag Nurs.* 2012 Oct 26. doi:pii: S1524-9042(12)00144-0. 10.1016/j.pmn.2012.08.010.

115. Lee EJ, Bhattacharya J, Sohn C, Verres R. Monochord sounds and progressive muscle relaxation reduce anxiety and improve relaxation during chemotherapy: a pilot EEG study. *Complement Ther Med.* 2012 Dec;20(6):409–416. doi:10.1016/j.ctim.2012.07.002.

116. Energy medicine: an overview. National Center for Complementary and Alternative Medicine. Available at: http://www.healthy.net/Health/Article/Energy_Medicine_An_Overview/2407/1. Accessed February 19, 2013.

117. Marcus DA, Blazek-O'Neill B, Kopar JL. Symptomatic improvement reported after receiving reiki at a cancer infusion center. *Am J Hosp Palliat Care.* 2013 Mar;30(2):216–217. doi:10.1177/1049909112469275.

118. Birocco N, Guillame C, Storto S, et al. The effects of Reiki therapy on pain and anxiety in patients attending a day oncology and infusion services unit. *Am J Hosp Palliat Care.* 2012 Jun;29(4):290–294. doi:10.1177/1049909111420859.

119. Tsang KL, Carlson LE, Olson K. Pilot crossover trial of Reiki versus rest for treating cancer-related fatigue. *Integr Cancer Ther.* 2007;6:25–35.

120. Crawford SE, Leaver VW, Mahoney SD. Using Reiki to decrease memory and behavior problems in mild cognitive impairment and mild Alzheimer's disease. *J Altern Complement Med.* 2006;12:911–913.

121. Woods DL, Dimond M. The effect of therapeutic touch on agitated behavior and cortisol in persons with Alzheimer's disease. *Biol Res Nurs* 2002;4:104–114.

122. Dowd T, Kolcaba K, Steiner R, Fashinpaur D. Comparison of healing touch, coaching, and a combined intervention on comfort and stress in younger college students. *Holist Nurs Pract.* 2007;21:194–202.

123. Roy R, Tiller WA, Bell I, Hoover MR. The structure of liquid water; novel insights from materials research; potential relevance to homeopathy. *Mater Res Innov.* 2005;9:577–608. Available at: http://site.fixherpes.com/roy_structure_water.pdf. Accessed February 17, 2013.

124. Milgrom LR. Homeopathy, fundamentalism, and the memory of water. *Curr Oncol.* 2007;14(6):221–222.

125. Mohammadi R, Amini K, Charehsaz S. Homeopathic treatment for peripheral nerve regeneration: an experimental study in a rat sciatic nerve transection model. *Homeopathy.* 2012 Jul;101(3):141–146. doi:10.1016/j.homp.2012.05.002.

126. Bellavite P, Marzotto M, Chirumbolo S, Conforti A. Advances in homeopathy and immunology: a review of clinical research. *Front Biosci (Schol Ed).* 2011 Jun 1;3:1363–1389.

127. What is complementary and alternative medicine? National Center for Complementary and Alternative Medicine. Available at: http://nccam.nih.gov/health/whatiscam. Accessed February 16, 2013.

128. Traditional medicine. Fact sheet no. 134. World Health Organization. December 2008. Available at: http://www.who.int/mediacentre/factsheets/fs134/en. Accessed February 18, 2013.

129. Traditional Chinese medicine. University of Maryland Medical Center. Available at: http://www.umm.edu/altmed/articles/traditional-chinese-000363.htm. Accessed February 16, 2013.

130. Association of Accredited Naturopathic Medical Colleges. New licensure legislation. Naturopathic doctor licensure. Available at: http://www.aanmc.org/careers/naturopathic-doctor-licensure.php. Accessed June 4, 2013.

131. Ader R, Cohen N. Conditioning and immunity. In: Ader R, Felten DL, Cohen H, eds. *Psychoneuroimmunology.* 3rd ed., vol. 2. San Diego: Academic Press; 2001:3–39.

132. Schleifer SJ, Keller SE, Camerino M, Thornton JC, Stein M. Suppression of lymphocyte stimulation following bereavement. *JAMA.* 1983 Jul 15;250(3):374–377.

133. Leserman J, Jackson ED, Petitto JM, et al. Progression to AIDS: the effects of stress, depressive symptoms, and social support. *Psychosom Med.* 1999 May–Jun;61(3):397–406.

134. Bennett MP, Lengacher C. Humor and laughter may influence health IV: humor and immune function. *Evid Based Complement Alternat Med.* 2009 Jun;6(2):159–164. doi:10.1093/ecam/nem149.

135. Tanno K, Sakata K, Ohsawa M, Onoda T, Itai K, Yaegashi Y, Tamakoshi A; JACC Study Group. Associations of ikigai as a positive psychological factor with all-cause mortality and cause-specific mortality among middle-aged and elderly Japanese people: findings from the Japan Collaborative Cohort Study. *J Psychosom Res.* 2009 Jul;67(1):67–75. doi:10.1016/j.jpsychores.2008.10.018.

136. Physical health conditions among adults with mental illnesses. The NSDUH Report. Substance Abuse and Mental Health Services Administration, Center for Behavioral Health Statistics and Quality. April 5, 2012. Available at: http://www.samhsa.gov/data/2k12/NSDUH103/SR103AdultsAMI2012.pdf. Accessed February 16, 2013.

137. Lindén T, Blomstrand C, Skoog I. Depressive disorders after 20 months in elderly stroke patients: a case-control study. *Stroke.* 2007 Jun;38(6):1860–1863.

138. What is the placebo effect? WebMD. Available at: http://www.webmd.com/pain-management/what-is-the-placebo-effect. Accessed February 16, 2013.

139. Maizes V, Rakel D, Niemiec C. Integrative medicine and patient-centered care. Commission for the IOM Summit on Integrative Medicine and the Health of the Public. February 2009. Available at: http://www.iom.edu/~/media/Files/Activity%20Files/Quality/IntegrativeMed/Integrative%20Medicine%20and%20Patient%20Centered%20Care.pdf. Accessed March 6, 2013.

140. Maizes V, Rakel D, Niemiec. Integrative medicine and patient-centered care. Commission for the IOM Summit on Integrative Medicine and the Health of the Public. February 2009. Available at: http://www.iom.edu/~/media/Files/Activity%20Files/Quality/IntegrativeMed/Integrative%20Medicine%20and%20Patient%20Centered%20Care.pdf. Accessed March 6, 2013.

141. Consortium of Academic Health Centers for Integrative Medicine. Available at: http://www.imconsortium.org. Accessed February 16, 2013.

142. Summit on Integrative Medicine and the Health of the Public. Institute of Medicine of the National Academies. November 15, 2012. Available at: http://www.iom.edu/Activities/Quality/IntegrativeMed.aspx. Accessed March 6, 2013.

143. HRSA announces integrative medicine program grants to 12 PMR programs. ACPM Headlines 10/15/12. American College of Preventive Medicine. Available at: http://www.acpm.org/?page=Headlines101512&hhSearchTerms=integrative+and+medicine#1. Accessed March 6, 2013.

144. Ornish D, Scherwitz LW, Billings JH, et al. Intensive lifestyle changes for reversal of coronary heart disease. *JAMA.* 1998;280(23):2001–2007. Available at: http://engine2diet.com/usrfiles/files/publishedstudies/heartdisease/intensive-lifestyle-changes-for-reversal-of-coronary-heart-disease.pdf. Accessed February 13, 2013.

145. Morgenstern H, Gellert GA, Walter SD, Ostfeld AM, Siegel BS. The impact of a psychosocial support program on survival with breast cancer: the importance of selection bias in program evaluation. *J Chronic Dis.* 1984;37(4):273–282.

146. Garcia MK, McQuade J, Haddad R, et al. Systematic review of acupuncture in cancer care: a synthesis of the evidence. *J Clin Oncol.* 2013 [Epub ahead of print]. doi:10.1200/JCO.2012.43.5818.

147. Chen HW, Lin IH, Chen YJ, et al. A novel infusible botanically-derived drug, PG2, for cancer-related fatigue: a phase II double-blind, randomized placebo-controlled study. *Clin Invest Med.* 2012 Feb 1;35(1):E1–E11.

148. Lee JJ, Lee JJ. A phase II study of an herbal decoction that includes Astragali radix for cancer-associated anorexia in patients with advanced cancer. *Integr Cancer Ther.* 2010 Mar;9(1):24–31. doi:10.1177/1534735409935918.

149. McCulloch M, See C, Shu XJ, et al. Astragalus-based Chinese herbs and platinum-based chemotherapy for advanced non-small-cell lung cancer: meta-analysis of randomized trials. *J Clin Oncol.* 2006 Jan 20;24(3):419–430.

150. van Uden-Kraan CF, Chinapaw MJ, Drossaert CH, Verdonck-de Leeuw IM, Buffart LM. Cancer patients' experiences with and perceived outcomes of yoga: results from focus groups. *Support Care Cancer.* 2013 Feb 12 [Epub ahead of print].

151. Cabral P, Meyer HB, Ames D. Effectiveness of yoga therapy as a complementary treatment for major psychiatric disorders: a meta-analysis. *Prim Care Companion CNS Disord.* 2011;13(4). pii: PCC.10r01068. doi:10.4088/PCC.10r01068.

152. Balaji PA, Varne SR, Ali SS. Physiological effects of yogic practices and Transcendental Meditation in health and disease. *N Am J Med Sci.* 2012 Oct;4(10):442–448. doi:10.4103/1947-2714.101980.

153. Kligler B, Homel P, Harrison LB, et al. Impact of the Urban Zen Initiative on patients' experience of admission to an inpatient oncology floor: a mixed-methods analysis. *J Altern Complement Med.* 2011 Aug;17(8):729–734. doi:10.1089/acm.2010.0533.

154. Kligler B, Homel P, Harrison LB, Levenson HD, Kenney JB, Merrell W. Cost savings in inpatient oncology through an integrative medicine approach. *Am J Manag Care.* 2011 Dec;17(12):779–784.

155. Cohen L. Integrative medicine versus alternative medicine: why it's important to know the difference. CancerWise. MD Anderson Cancer Center. September 14, 2010. Available at: http://www2.mdanderson.org/cancerwise/2010/09/integrative-medicine-versus-alternative-medicine-why-its-important-to-know-the-difference.html. Accessed February 19, 2013.

CHAPTER 3
Stress: Staying Sane in a Hectic World

STRESS: THE GOOD, THE BAD, AND THE UGLY

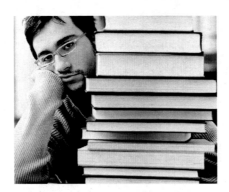

© *Thinkstock*

Stress is unavoidable. A little bit of stress adds spice to life and allows you to learn your potential. As Winston Churchill said, "Kites rise highest against the wind, not with it." Plus, a complete absence of challenge would be boring, and prolonged boredom is stressful. In fact, one study found that bored workers were more likely to die young than their more engaged colleagues.[1]

The ability to react to emergencies is essential to survival. Nerves fire, hormones surge, and—presto—your heart, lungs, and muscles boost their performance. As a result, you might out-ski an avalanche, snatch a toddler out of the way of an oncoming vehicle, carry a wounded friend to safety, or survive a famine. That's great if you're faced with a physical threat. If, on the other hand, you're in the midst of psychological challenges—mired in a traffic jam, stammering through an oral presentation, or receiving a tongue lashing from an employer—stressing out only makes things worse.

Over time, stress overload undermines health and well-being, accelerates aging, and contributes to a long list of illnesses. Many of these diseases rank among the most common conditions afflicting Americans.

By the time you finish this chapter, you should have a basic understanding of the stress response, the short-term survival benefits, and the potential risks of chronic stress. You will also learn simple strategies for taming stress.

There is more to life than increasing its speed.[2]

- *Mohandas "Mahatma" Gandhi*

1. OVERVIEW OF THE STRESS RESPONSE

L E A R N I N G   O B J E C T I V E S

1. Understand the prevalence of stress overload among Americans.
2. Define basic terms: stress, stressor, homeostasis, allostasis, and allostatic load.
3. Discuss the purpose of the stress response.
4. Explain bodily systems that control the stress response.

1.1 Stress in America

Annual Stress in America surveys by the American Psychological Association have uncovered a number of sobering facts.[3] ,[4] In the 2011 survey, the authors write, "Participants' responses have revealed high stress levels, reliance on unhealthy behaviors to manage stress, and alarming physical health consequences of stress—a combination that suggests the nation is on the verge of a stress-induced public health crisis."[5]

- The economic recession has weighed heavily on adults and children.
- Major sources of stress are finances and work—both job stability and excessive demands from employers and finances. Others include family responsibilities, intimate relationships, health concerns, and personal safety.
- Forty-four percent of Americans surveyed said their stress levels had increased over the past five years. Most felt that their stress levels exceeded what was healthy.
- About one-third of people said they felt "routinely overwhelmed by stress." For people with depression or obesity, the number rises to 61 and 55 percent, respectively.
- People living on the East Coast experienced more stress than those living in other regions. West Coasters had the fewest physical manifestations of out-of-control stress.
- Greater than half of people noted that stress had adversely affected their health.
- African Americans experienced more stress than whites, and younger adults experienced more stress than people over age 65.
- Compared to men, women more often reported that they're under excessive stress (28 versus 20 percent) and that their stress level had climbed over the past five years (49 versus 39 percent). Men were more reluctant to admit that stress overload adversely affected personal health and less likely to fend off stress overload with greater attention to diet, social relationships, and adequate sleep. Men more often played sports to manage stress.
- Stress affected children and teens much more than parents realize.
- Almost one-third of children had physical symptoms of stress such as headache, upset stomach, and insomnia.
- Nearly half of teens reported feeling more worried than ever, with 14 percent rating their stress level as extreme. Concerns about physical appearance and future plans, including finding a job and getting into a good college, were frequent preoccupations.
- About a quarter of people felt competent at preventing stress overload; less than a third could reduce feelings of stress when they occurred.
- Adults and teens alike typically turned to sedentary activities such as watching television, playing video games, and listening to music to relieve stress. They also resorted to unhealthy eating patterns: overeating, skipping meals, or eating junk foods. Sadly, compared to older adults, young adults were more likely to smoke and drink alcohol. The good news is they were also more likely to try meditation and yoga.
- About 43 percent of college students experienced more than average stress, and 10 percent experienced "tremendous stress."[6]

1.2 A Historical Overview of Stress Research

While many researchers have advanced the study of stress, two people deserve credit for putting the concept on the scientific map: Walter Cannon and Hans Selye.

In the early 1900s, Cannon originated the term **homeostasis**, from the Greek *homeo* (same) and *stasis* (stable). The century before, French physiologist Claude Bernard called that internal steady state *milieu interior*. The core concept is that your body works to maintain the status quo. Your blood's pH (acidity level) stays about 7.4, your body temperature hovers around 98.6°F, and your arterial blood is at least 94 percent saturated with oxygen. If, for instance, you exercise in a warm environment, you'll flush, sweat, shed clothes, and drink fluids to avoid elevating your body temperature by more than a couple of degrees.

The **stress response** is your body's nonspecific response to any challenge to homeostasis. A **stressor** is the thing that perturbs or threatens to upset that balance. Around 1915, Cannon used the phrase "fight or flight" to describe the body's response to a threat. His research focused on the body's most immediate reaction to a stressor, which prepares it to fight or outrun an opponent. As we'll discuss in more detail, the sympathetic nervous system governs this heart-pounding experience and ensures that the brain, heart, and muscles have enough oxygen and fuel to outsmart, outrun, or outmatch a threat.

While Cannon described stress as a positive adaptation, Selye unveiled the dark underbelly of excessive stress. In the 1930s, he began researching the effects of injecting glandular extracts into rats. Strangely, Selye's experiments yielded the same results: His rats developed stomach ulcers, enlarged **adrenal glands**, and shriveled immune tissues—even those receiving injections of salt water. Fortunately, Selye finally figured out the answer. Because he wasn't adept at handling the animals, he was stressing them out. Stress, not glandular extracts, had caused the disease.

Later, he learned that, no matter the nature of the stressor—heat, cold, pain, or famine—the body's reaction is fairly consistent. He named this nonspecific response the *general adaptation syndrome* and divided it into three stages: the alarm stage, wherein the organism encounters the stressor; the resistance stage, wherein the organism copes with the stressor; and the exhaustion stage, the point at which unremitting stress leads to illness and death. His work eventually led to an understanding of the potentially damaging effects of chronic stress, particularly from high levels of the adrenal hormone cortisol.

Both Cannon and Selye applied the engineering term "stress," which refers to a force that strains or deforms a substance, to the demands on a living organism. Selye further divided stress into *eustress* and *distress*. The prefix "eu-" comes from the Greek for "good." Hence, eustress is a favorable challenge—for example, you enroll in college, fall in love, land a new job, win the lottery, or move to Paris for the year. Such changes are generally exciting and stimulating.

Distress, whose prefix derives from "dys," which is Greek for "bad," entails suffering—for example, an exam doesn't go well, your beloved breaks up with you via text message, your car breaks down, your boss demands that you work weekends. The words "stress" and "stressed out" usually refer to distress.

Both eustress and distress disturb the status quo. The difference is your attitude. Therein lies the secret to managing stress: manipulating your perception of change.

Other researchers recognized that few internal states are truly constant because coping with stressors requires adjustments. In 1988, Peter Sterling and Joseph Eyer coined the term **allostasis**, which takes into account that your body has different set points for different situations. The Greek "allo" means variable. Bruce McEwen, a world-renowned stress researcher and author of *The End of Stress as We Know It*, defines *allostasis* as "the ability to achieve stability, or homeostasis, through change."[7]

In other words, your health and survival depend on your body's ability to adapt. If you hop out of bed and climb two flights of stairs (a mild stressor), your body literally needs to rise to the occasion. Heart rate, blood pressure, and respiratory rate increase to maintain circulation to critical body parts such as your brain. That's why you don't faint at the first landing. You maintain the new steady state until the challenge is over, at which point your body, if healthy, quickly returns to baseline functioning.

Expanding the concept of allostasis, McEwen coined the term **allostatic load**, which he defined as "the price the body pays over long periods of time for adapting to challenges." At this point, the burdens of cumulative stress tax the body, mind, and emotions. At this point, we no longer can respond to the stressor efficiently through allostasis and quickly return to homeostasis. Instead we become like Sisyphus of Greek myth, eternally pushing the boulder uphill. Stress moves from being adaptive to becoming toxic, and health suffers.

homeostasis

The body's internal balance.

stress response

What your body does to cope with change and return to homeostasis.

stressor

Anything that, by perturbing or threatening to perturb homeostasis, activates the stress response.

adrenal glands

Located just above the two kidneys, this gland makes epinephrine, cortisol, and other hormones.

allostasis

The ability to achieve stability through change.

allostatic load

The price the body pays for excessive stress.

How the Stress Response Works

FIGURE 3.1 The Limbic System

This figure indicates the location of the limbic system, which arcs around the center of the brain. It contains key structures in the stress response such as the hippocampus, which is important for memory formation, and the amygdala, which processes strong emotions such as fear, anger, and pleasure. The limbic system communicates with the hypothalamus to regulate hormonal and autonomic nervous system responses.

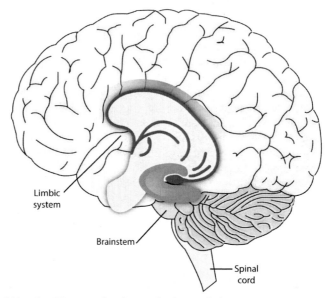

Source: NIDA for Teens. Available at: http://commons.wikimedia.org/wiki/File:Brain_limbicsystem.jpg.

When confronted with a potential threat, your brain initiates a body-wide response. Let's say you're out for a walk and spy a snake in the path. A relatively primitive part of your brain called the **limbic system** reacts swiftly. Two areas of the limbic system are particularly important: the **hippocampus**, an elongated curving structure that interprets and remembers the contextual details (where, when, what) of the situation, and the **amygdala**, an almond-sized structure involved in highly charged emotions such as fear. In the presence of an apparent threat, the amygdala activates the nearby **hypothalamus**, which initiates both a wide-ranging nervous system response and a hormonal cascade.

The nervous system response involves the **autonomic nervous system**, which regulates the activity of visceral organs (e.g., heart, lungs, and intestinal tract), skeletal muscles, and more. Two diametrically opposed nervous systems compose the autonomic nervous system: the **parasympathetic nervous system** (PNS) and **sympathetic nervous system** (SNS). The PNS, also referred to as the rest-and-restoration (or rest-and-digest) system, slows the heart and respiratory rate, increases activity in the intestinal tract, constricts the pupils, and controls other peaceful activities. The SNS, also called the fight-or-flight system, has opposite effects. The SNS also quickly stimulates a surge of epinephrine (also called adrenaline) from the adrenal glands, which sit atop the kidneys. Because of the tight association between the SNS and the adrenal glands, this system is often referred to as the sympathoadrenal system (SAS).

autonomic nervous system

A division of the peripheral nervous system (outside the brain and spinal cord) that controls activities that are mainly unconscious such as digestion, heart rate, and respiratory rate.

parasympathetic nervous system

The branch of the autonomic nervous system that governs restorative processes in the body.

sympathetic nervous system

The branch of the autonomic nervous system that governs the fight-or-flight response.

FIGURE 3.2 The Autonomic Nervous System

The two branches of the autonomic nervous system are the sympathetic nervous system (fight or flight) and the parasympathetic nervous system (rest and restoration). Nerves from each branch go to many of the same areas in the body, though their effects are opposite.

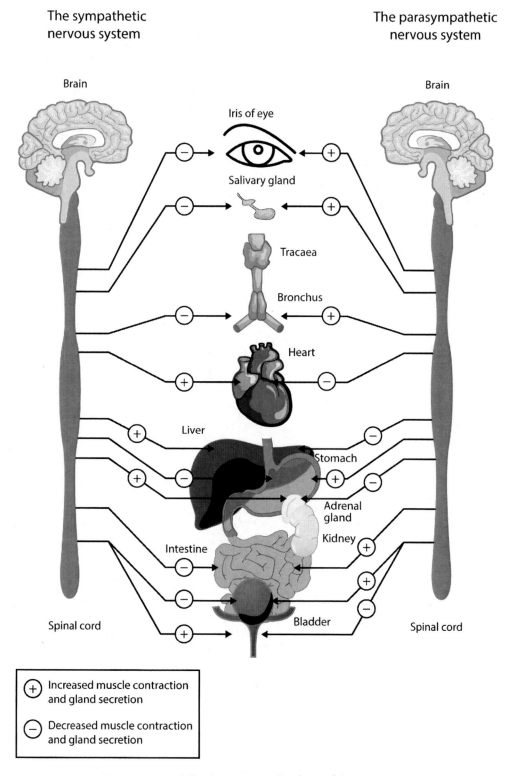

Source: Ruth Lawson Otago Polytechnic. 2007. Available at: http://commons.wikimedia.org/wiki/

File:Anatomy_and_physiology_of_animals_Function_of_the_sympathetic_%26_parasympathetic_nervous_systems.jpg.

With one exception (REM sleep, a sleep stage wherein vivid dreams occur), one system predominates over the other. Otherwise, it would be like simultaneously stomping on the car's brakes and accelerator. It doesn't take a PhD in physiology to imagine what happens in response to a real or imagined threat.

While PNS activity declines, the SNS becomes more active, elevating heart rate, the strength of the heart's contraction, and blood pressure. Blood vessels widen to increase circulation to the heart, brain, and working skeletal muscles, ensuring delivery of nutrients and oxygen to those critical organs. In contrast, blood flow is restricted to other organs and skin. The digestive and reproductive systems become relatively inactive. The eyes' pupils dilate, allowing more light in. The net result is that your thoughts and vision sharpen. You can run faster, fight harder, lift the boulder off a trapped friend, and otherwise survive the challenge.

Meanwhile, the brain's hypothalamus secretes a hormone called cortiotrophin-releasing hormone (CRH), which causes the nearby **pituitary gland** to secrete adrenocorticotrophin-releasing hormone (ACTH) into the bloodstream. Upon reaching the **adrenal glands, ACTH stimulates** them to release glucocorticoids into the blood, which affect cells all over the body. The system is known as the **hypothalamic-pituitary-adrenal axis** (HPA). Glucocorticoids are a group of steroid compounds, the most important of which is **cortisol** (also called hydrocortisone). Cortisol is a potent anti-inflammatory agent. Its derivatives are used in medicine. You may have used topical hydrocortisone cream on a patch of inflamed skin.

hypothalamic-pituitary-adrenal axis

The interactive system that ultimately regulates the release of glucocorticoids such as cortisol from the adrenal gland.

cortisol

The most important glucocorticoid released by the adrenal gland in response to stress; also called hydrocortisone.

FIGURE 3.3 Adrenal Glands

These two glands make several hormones. The most important to the stress response are epinephrine (also called adrenaline), which goes up due to stimulation from the sympathetic nervous system, and cortisol, which is regulated hormones from the hypothalamus and pituitary.

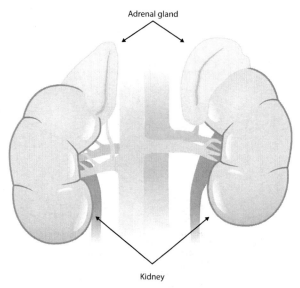

Adrenal gland

Kidney

Source: Adapted from National Cancer Institute. Adrenal gland. SEER Training Modules. Available at: http://commons.wikimedia.org/wiki/File:Illu_adrenal_gland.jpg.

epinephrine

A stress hormone released from the adrenal gland.

Because nerves communicate faster than hormones (which float in the bloodstream until they reach their target), the adrenal gland secretes **epinephrine** almost immediately and cortisol after a lag. A primary action of both hormones is to increase blood levels of glucose (sugar), mainly by breaking down storage molecules of carbohydrate, protein, and fat. The increase in lung and heart function and changes in blood flow ensure the delivery of blood rich with oxygen and glucose to the brain, heart, and muscles—the organs critical to fighting and fleeing.

FIGURE 3.4 The Hypothalamic-Pituitary-Adrenal Axis

During the stress response, the hypothalamus releases the hormone CRH, which stimulates the pituitary gland to release ACTH, which stimulates the two adrenal glands to release glucocorticoids. Once the hypothalamus and pituitary sense blood levels of glucocorticoids are high enough, they reduce secretion of CRH and ACTH, respectively. This type of hormone regulation is called "negative feedback."

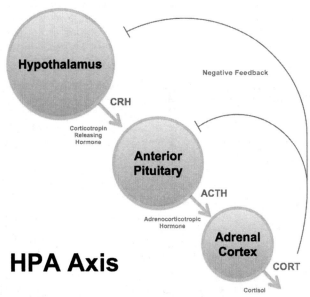

Source: Sweis BM. 2012. Available at: http://upload.wikimedia.org/wikipedia/commons/5/55/ HPA_Axis_Diagram_%28Brian_M_Sweis_2012%29.png.

Clearly, the stress response helps you survive physical challenges. Without it, you wouldn't be able to complete a marathon, escape a rabid dog, or remain alert and active after missing a meal. Unfortunately, more or less the same cascade of events occurs when the stressor is psychological or social in nature. If someone insults you at a dinner party, etiquette restrains you from head-butting your antagonist. If your instructor asks you to explain a scientific principle you scarcely understand, you probably won't bolt from the lecture hall. Ideally, you figure out a way to stay calm in the face of psychological challenges.

That brings us back to the brain, the organ that both starts and has the ability to extinguish the stress response. Let's say that in the snake example, a moment passes and you perceive that the "snake" is actually a stick. A higher brain area called the **prefrontal cortex** (which occupies the space above your eyes) signals to the limbic system to cancel the stress response. In other words, higher brain areas moderate your more primitive reflexes. You can reassess a situation and decide it's not life-threatening and not worth expending needless energy over.

Granted, more extreme stressors will activate the stress response no matter what. Examples include extreme cold or heat, prolonged fasting, protracted exercise, mother-infant separation, severe injury, or illness. In these instances, more positive coping styles soften the blow but don't completely shield you.

However, most of us rarely face life-threatening challenges. More often than not, modern human stress is *psychological. In this case,* our thoughts can provoke the stress response. A key element is the belief that we lack the ability to meet the demands facing us. We worry about whether people like us, whether we ought to bleach our teeth, whether that sunburn will lead to melanoma, whether we'll be able to pay the rent, or whether we'll have a job after graduation.

Of all the animals, we humans excel at thinking our way into a stressed-out frenzy. Our big brains are capable of both *rumination* (turning a thought over and over in our heads) and *anticipation* (forecasting about what may happen). A certain amount of both is useful. Reviewing a past event can provide ideas about how to handle a similar situation better in the future. Likewise, planning a response to something likely to occur soon helps us prepare. (If you have an exam in a week, you'll perform better if you study in advance.)

Nevertheless, worrying won't change the past or the future. Dwelling on unfortunate episodes and forecasting doom make things worse. If you visualize yourself trembling, tongue-tied, and dumbstruck while presenting before an audience, you may fulfill that prophecy. And often the things we worry will happen never do. As author Mark Twain said, "My life has been filled with calamities, some of which actually happened."[8]

No other animal species behaves in this way. That's why renowned Stanford University researcher Robert Sapolsky named his book on stress *Why Zebras Don't Get Ulcers*. A zebra doesn't fret over possible events in the distant future. An immediate potential threat—a lion crouching in the bushes—catches its attention. A menacing twitch from the lion and the zebra springs into action. Once it has successfully outrun the lion, the zebra returns to grazing. It doesn't stay up all night, thinking, "Whew, that was a close one. I really should have started running sooner. Maybe I need to work out more. Why did I dash into the water? Did I forget that lions can swim? What an idiot."

The good news is that, with practice, we can turn our brain power to our advantage. We can learn to let go of minor annoyances, to view challenges as opportunities, to become more confident in our abilities and knowledgeable of our resources, to relax whenever possible, and to avoid potential stressors that aren't worth the physical and emotional cost. It's called wisdom.

Factors That Add to Allostatic Load

- **Sleep deprivation.** A vicious cycle, sleep deprivation activates stress hormones, which interfere with good nighttime sleep. Also worried thoughts triggered by psychological stress can cause insomnia.
- **Overweight and obesity.**[9] In another vicious cycle, perceived social stigma and associated poor physical health add to the stress load. Conversely, the frequent or chronic activation of the stress response promotes central (abdominal) obesity.
- **Alcohol and sedative drugs.** Substances that depress your central nervous system can certainly make you feel more relaxed. However, they don't address your underlying issues. Plus, in excess, they stress the body even more. Excessive amounts of alcohol interrupt sleep. Impairment to physical and mental function can lead to accidents and injuries, legal problems, violence, and sexual indiscretions (including sex without protection against sexually transmitted infections and pregnancy). Chronic use can lead to abuse and addiction.
- **Tobacco.** Cigarette smoke pollutes your body, which causes stress at a cellular level. Nicotine also activates the HPA and SAS axes. Furthermore, smoking interferes with deep sleep. Quitting takes time, patience, and perseverance. Find out about support services on your campus.
- **Caffeine.** Excessive amounts can make you feel tense and nervous and interfere with sleep.
- **Junk food.** Ironically, stress hormones such as cortisol drive you to eat sugary, fatty foods. Unfortunately, junk food actually increases stress hormones.[10]

Common Stressors

What Stresses Americans

The American Psychological Association's Stress in America surveys show that top stressors for Americans mainly have to do with financial concerns.

- money problems covering the cost of housing, food, clothing, college tuition, and medical expenses
- work, particularly overwork and employers who make it difficult to balance work with social relationships
- job instability
- the economy
- relationships with friends, family, and intimate partners
- health problems affecting close family members
- personal physical and mental health problems
- personal safety

Stressors Faced by College Students

The American College Health Association's 2011 National College Health Assessment uncovers a different, though not unsurprising ranking.[11] Here's a list of things that college students find difficult to handle, from most troublesome to least.

1. Academics
2. Finances
3. Intimate relationships
4. Family problems
5. Sleep difficulties

6. Career-related issues

7. Miscellaneous social relationships

8. Personal appearance

9. Health problem of family member or partner

10. Personal health issue

11. Death of a family member

Only a quarter of students reported none of these problems within the past year. Nearly 14 percent had at least one stressor and almost 48 percent (52.4 percent of women and 38.8 percent of men) experienced three or more significant stressors. Students of color experienced social stress due to racism and social isolation. LGBTQIA (lesbian, gay, bisexual, transgender, queer/questioning, intersex, and asexual) students also experienced stress due to perceived discrimination. Working students felt more family pressure, worried more about finances, and had greater difficulty managing their time.[12]

Universal Mammalian Stressors

- extremes of cold or heat
- injury or illness
- unremitting pain
- violence and predation—for humans, sexual and physical assault weigh heavily
- famine and dehydration
- childbirth
- separation of an infant from its mother
- social isolation at any age (in social animals, including humans)
- bereavement

Less Frequently Recognized Stressors Unique to Modern Humans

- pollution of air, water, and soil
- excessive noise and artificial lighting
- lack of access to open space
- calorically adequate but nutritionally deficient diets
- sedentary lifestyles
- sleep deprivation
- information overload and technostress (see "Avoiding Technostress")

Avoiding Technostress

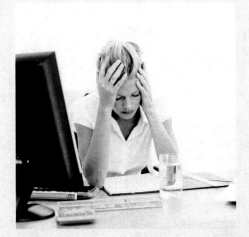

© Thinkstock

The electronic boom has created both conveniences and challenges. Computers have made it easier to do many kinds of research and work efficiently. Mobile devices mean friends, family, employers, professors, and telemarketers can contact you almost any time.

But sometimes the constant flood of information and pinging, eye-popping distractions becomes overwhelming. People often expect instant replies to phone messages, texts, social media posts, and e-mails. Boundaries between work and home blur. As soon as you delete an e-mail, it seems that 10 more take its place.

When it comes to mental activities, your brain can't multitask—it simply toggles attention from one thing to another. Jumping from web page to e-mail to text interferes with the ability to concentrate, complete longer tasks, and sustain a meaningful conversation. Each interruption costs about a minute to refocus.

Is the electronic barrage stressful? It depends on the person and the situation. A 2010 *New York Times*/CBS News poll found that although most Americans think computers, cell phones and smartphones, and personal computers have made it easier to work, nearly 30 percent of adults under the age of 45 reported that these electronic devices had become intrusive, fractured their focus, and increased their feelings of stress.[13] Young people who use their mobile phones a lot and feel pressured to be accessible 24-7 suffer from more sleep problems and depression.[14] Some become addicted to computer activities, texting, e-mailing, chatting, game playing, gambling, and surfing for information.

A study of college students found that high use of mobile phones and computers raised the odds of feeling mentally overloaded, stressed, and socially isolated.[15] They also neglected other activities (including academics) and personal health (missing meals and sleep) and had more symptoms of ill health (muscular pain, headaches, tiredness, depression). Furthermore, "destructive communications" led to misunderstandings, frustration, guilt, anxiety, sadness, and feelings of inadequacy.

Prolonged use of computers, smartphones, and tablets also strains the eyes, particularly when the screen is close to the face. The medical diagnosis is computer vision syndrome.[16] Symptoms include temporary headaches, eye discomfort, dry eyes, and double and blurred vision. Some eye doctors recommend giving your eyes a break for 20 seconds every 20 minutes. Typing causes repetitive-use injuries in hands and wrists. Bending over electronic devices also strains the spine. Take periodic breaks to stretch.

Another issue is that backlit screens emit enough light to suppress the hormone melatonin, which normally rises in the evening and orchestrates a number of daily rhythms, including sleep.[17] That means, when you finally power down your laptop or tablet, you might have trouble dropping off to sleep.

You can take back control. Try a device-free evening. Many people find they're more productive at work if they only read and respond to e-mail once or twice a day. (Turn off alerts for incoming e-mail and texts if they distract you.) When researchers barred office workers from checking e-mails for five days, the employees sustained their focus for longer intervals, switched computer windows less often, interacted with people more on the phone or face-to-face, felt more relaxed, and had less stress, as measured by heart monitors.[18]

Childhood Adversity: Programming the Stress Response

Critical periods in development—during the mother's pregnancy and in early childhood—program the HPA axis.[19],[20] The developing fetus receives clues from its mother about the outside world. The clues come in the form of chemicals such as cortisol that cross easily into the fetal circulation. If a mother is severely stressed, her elevated cortisol programs the fetus for life in a challenging environment. The set-point for the HPA axis shifts, and the newborn enters the world with a hair trigger on the stress response.

If the world is indeed stressful—marked by food scarcity, war, and other physical dangers—the fetus is primed for survival. If instead she grows up with abundant food and mainly psychological aggravations, her higher levels of cortisol raise the risk of high blood pressure, heart disease, diabetes, psychological disorders, substance abuse, and learning and behavioral difficulties. Note that most of the research on prenatal stress has examined children of women undergoing severe stress—famine, war, or abuse, not the daily hassles most pregnant women face.

Childhood trauma (abuse, neglect, maternal depression, parental substance abuse) also produces scars and raises the risk of chronic disorders.[21] Having a protective, responsive, supportive adult buffers the impact of childhood stress. Imagine you're a child and a tornado is spinning your way. If you're alone, that's terrifying. If you're in the basement with an anxious parent, you're only partially reassured. If you're down there with a parent who calmly pulls a deck of cards from a pocket and engages you in a game, you might actually enjoy the adventure. Loving care also takes the sting out of routine childhood challenges.

Pediatric experts advocate early intervention to interrupt the cycle of adverse childhood events perpetuating poverty, low academic achievement, substance abuse, chronic disease, crime, and inadequate parenting. For example, studies show benefits when nurses visit at-risk pregnant women and new mothers to provide education and support.[22]

Assess Yourself: How Vulnerable Are You to Stress?

Check the appropriate spaces below.

I.

- I sleep eight hours a night.
  ____Usually ____Rarely or never
- I feel supported by friends and family.
  ____Usually ____Rarely or never
- When upset, I can express my feelings in a nondestructive way.
  ____Usually ____Rarely or never
- I eat healthfully and avoid junk food.
  ____Usually ____Rarely or never
- I organize my time well.
  ____Usually ____Rarely or never
- I can manage my finances.
  ____Usually ____Rarely or never
- I am physically active for at least 30 minutes a day.
  ____Usually ____Rarely or never
- I take time to relax.
  ____Usually ____Rarely or never
- I do something fun at least once a week.
  ____Usually ____Rarely or never
- I am within five pounds of my ideal weight.
  ____Usually ____Rarely or never
- I restrict my alcohol intake to below the point of intoxication.
  ____Usually ____Rarely or never
- I avoid tobacco smoke.
  ____Usually ____Rarely or never
- I avoid recreational drugs.
  ____Usually ____Rarely or never
- I restrict my intake of caffeinated beverages to three eight-ounce servings a day or less.
  ____Usually ____Rarely or never
- I believe that I can handle most challenges that come my way.
  ____Usually ____Rarely or never
- My spiritual beliefs give me comfort and a sense of purpose.
  ____Usually ____Rarely or never

II.

- I feel impatient with other people.
  _____ Rarely or never ___ Often
- I frequently feel angry or hostile and tend to lash out at others.
  _____ Rarely or never ___ Often
- I check my watch often.
  _____ Rarely or never ___ Often
- I feel time pressured.
  _____ Rarely or never ___ Often
- It seems I work all the time but never accomplish enough.
  _____ Rarely or never ___ Often

III.

- I have suffered trauma (e.g., sexual or physical assault).
  ___ No ___ Yes
- I have been diagnosed with a psychological disorder.
  ___ No ___ Yes

The more check marks you have in the left-hand column of choices the better equipped you are to cope with stress.

The first category gauges whether your behaviors protect or put you at risk for allostatic load. For any item checked in the right-hand column, make a contract with yourself to change at least one of them this semester.

The second category lists traits associated with a type A personality that can ultimately lead to stress-associated ill health. With awareness, an intention to change, and practice, you can replace these undesirable traits with patience, compassion, and a sense of peace.

Checking yes to one or both items in the third category indicates a particular vulnerability to stress. You may need professional help to become more resilient.

Assess Yourself: How Stressful Is Your Life?

The following events are recognized in commonly used rating scales as significant stressors, with the most traumatic life events listed at the top. For any given potential stressor, the impact on you will depend on a variety of factors: your personality, your attitude toward the event, the presence or absence of social support, and so on. Furthermore, you might not perceive some items on the list as stressors. For instance, public speaking may give you a sense of accomplishment or even outright pleasure.

This list doesn't include *daily hassles*—minor irritations and annoyances such as traffic, noise, bad haircuts, skin blemishes, and rude people. Nevertheless, these relatively trivial events can lead to health problems if you allow them to repeatedly and persistently activate your stress response.

With those disclaimers, read over this list and place a check beside events that either have occurred to you in the past 12 months or are looming on the horizon. Underneath, add the things that stress you out, no matter how petty you think they may sound. The fact is they bother you.

The more spaces you check, the greater the potential risk to your health. Your response may be to look for ways to make life easier for yourself, learn to counteract stress symptoms, and possibly seek professional counseling.

- ____ Death of a close family member
- ____ Death of a close friend
- ____ Sexual assault (e.g., rape)
- ____ Physical assault
- ____ Divorce of your parents
- ____ Diagnosis of HIV
- ____ Diagnosis of another sexually transmitted infection
- ____ Unplanned pregnancy (yours or caused by you)
- ____ Major legal violation (jail sentence)
- ____ First or last year of college
- ____ Financial difficulties
- ____ Parenting issues: child care, single parent, special needs child
- ____ Getting married
- ____ Serious personal injury or illness
- ____ Serious illness of close family member
- ____ Feeling unsafe on campus
- ____ Victim of discrimination
- ____ Disagreements with parents
- ____ Failed an important class
- ____ Problems with instructor or boss
- ____ Dropped a class
- ____ Enjoy but feel overwhelmed by a class
- ____ Feel pressured to excel academically
- ____ Disappointed in academic performance
- ____ Problems getting along with roommates
- ____ Feeling friendless and lonely
- ____ Problems with intimate partner or romantic breakup
- ____ New intimate partner
- ____ Difficulty sleeping or insufficient sleep with daytime tiredness

- ▪ _____ Lost a job
- ▪ _____ Have a job you dislike or that interferes with academics
- ▪ _____ Concerned about postcollege job market
- ▪ _____ Rushing a sorority or fraternity
- ▪ _____ Engaged in time-consuming extracurricular activities (e.g., athletics, theater, music)
- ▪ _____ Minor violations of the law (e.g., speeding ticket)
- ▪ _____ Change in living conditions
- ▪ _____ Midterm or final exam week
- ▪ _____ Making an in-class oral presentation

Your daily hassles

- ▪ _____
- ▪ _____
- ▪ _____
- ▪ _____

_Sources: Holmes and Rahe's Social Readjustment Rating Scale. Available at: http://en.wikipedia.org/wiki/Holmes_and_Rahe_stress_scale; Renner and Mackin's College Undergraduate Stress Scale (1998). Available at: http://cwx.prenhall.com/bookbind/pubbooks/morris5/medialib/images/t12_01.pdf; questionnaire comes from a 1992 article: Crandall CS, Preisler JJ, Aussprung J. Measuring life event stress in the lives of college students: the Undergraduate Stress Questionnaire (USQ). Journal of Behavioral Medicine. 1992 Dec;15(6):627–662. Available at: http://concordia.csp.edu/Counseling/_Documents/Student_Stress_Scale.pdf; Feldt RC. Development of a brief measure of college stress: the College Student Stress Scale. Psychological Reports. 2008;102:855–860._

K E Y   T A K E A W A Y S

- ▪ The stress response is designed to help you cope with physical stressors.
- ▪ Modern stressors are more often psychological than physical in nature.
  - ▪ Many Americans, particularly young adults, feel stressed and recognize that their stress levels are not healthy. Few of them effectively cope with stress.
  - ▪ The economic downturn has amplified many Americans' perceptions of stress.
  - ▪ Walter Cannon's research focused on the "fight-or-flight response," which is governed by the sympathetic nervous system.
- ▪ Hans Selye's research revealed that the stress response is fairly nonspecific, meaning that a variety of stressors trigger a similar cascade of bodily changes and that chronic activation can damage health. He expanded our understanding of the hypothalamic-adrenal-pituitary axis.
- ▪ Genetics and experiences with adversity, particularly early in life, can predispose an individual toward excessive responses to stressors and stress-induced illnesses.
- ▪ Maladaptive responses to stress can add to allostatic load.

1. What experimental results led Dr. Selye to call the stress response "the general adaptation syndrome?"

2. Imagine this scenario: You've just driven to the campus on roads congested with cars. You have seven minutes to park and walk to class. You troll the packed parking lot for a space. Finally, you spot red taillights as someone backs out of a spot. You position yourself and wait. An approaching car rolls up and, better positioned to nab the spot, zips into the space before you.

   Write down likely emotions, thoughts, and physical sensations. Next, list your options for responding. Beside each describe the pros and cons (both short and long term). Which option would serve *you* best in the long run?

3. Give an example of a time you've needlessly worried about a future event. What did you imagine? Did an endless loop of anxious thoughts interfere with your sleep? Did fretting affect the outcome? Do you feel anticipatory stress? How might you change this habit?

4. Many people respond to stress by letting lifestyle habits deteriorate. In what ways does your reaction to stress only add to your allostatic load? Which unhealthy responses do you think you could change this semester? How will you do that?

5. Have you become a slave to technology? Do you reflexively respond to every single text, phone call, and e-mail? Do your devices and social networking sites distract you from your work? Do they interrupt your real-time social interactions? Do you want to take back control? Write down at least three ideas for how you will do that.

2. THE DOWNSIDES OF STRESS

LEARNING OBJECTIVES

1. **Investigate the ill effects of overwhelming acute stress and chronic stress on human health.**
2. **Identify common symptoms of stress overload.**

FIGURE 3.5 Stress and the Inverted J Curve

The inverted J curve illustrates the difference between acute and chronic stress on the function of many bodily systems. The vertical axis represents function. You can plug in the nervous, immune, and cardiovascular systems. The horizontal axis measures time. As you see, acute stress causes an improvement above baseline. You think more quickly, mobilize immune cells, and pump blood more efficiently. With time, those processes begin to reverse and eventually descend below baseline into the realm of ill health.

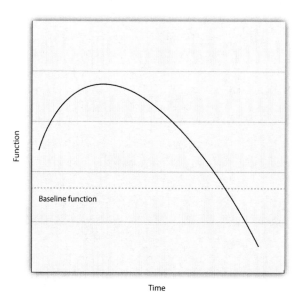

While the stress response protects you in the face of short-term challenges, strong, frequent, or prolonged activation of the stress response becomes toxic. Too much stress can age you, shorten your life, sap your energy, impair most bodily systems, and contribute to a number of diseases. We don't typically die in the jaws of a tiger or at the business end of a rival's spear. Most of us limp around for years with chronic conditions such as heart disease, diabetes, depression, and dementia. Stress contributes to them all.

The main culprits are overactivation of both the **sympathoadrenal system** and the hypothalamic-pituitary-adrenal axis. Cortisol levels become abnormal. One of three patterns can emerge: chronically high cortisol, a flattening of the normal daily rhythm of high morning levels and low evening levels, or, less often, low cortisol.

In surveys, Americans who rate their health as poor are more likely to report higher levels of stress.[23] Stress-induced health problems are costly to individuals and society. People fall ill, miss work, and visit doctors.[24] To add insult to injury, being sick is stressful.

The ways in which stress sickens us vary. Genetics and life experiences dictate our individual vulnerabilities. Stress finds that Achilles' heel—anxiety, depression, eczema, high blood pressure, diabetes, intestinal distress—and exposes it. The **stress-diathesis model** posits that genetics and events occurring during early development (diatheses) predispose us toward a particular condition and that stressful events can manifest the condition. The greater the inherent vulnerability, the smaller the stress necessary to trigger symptoms.

Some problems surface sooner than later. The American College Health Association's 2011 National College Health Assessment found nearly 28 percent of college students reported that stress interfered with **academic performance**.[25] Stress and fatigue also disrupt **social life**.

Stress quickly impairs **sleep**. One, worried thoughts make it hard to relax. Two, sleep requires a predominance of parasympathetic nervous system over sympathetic nervous system. When you're stressed, the reverse is true. Three, stress hormones are alerting. Four, neurotransmitter imbalances and other chemical alterations add to the insomnia. The irony is that sleep deprivation acts as a stressor, activating your sympathetic nervous system and elevating your stress hormones, which can interfere with the next night's sleep.

Mood suffers. Nervousness and irritability rise. If you're vulnerable to a psychological disorder—anxiety, depression, bipolar disorder—excessive stress can activate or worsen the condition.[26] ,[27] ,[28] For some people, significant setbacks (failing a class, a romantic breakup, death) will trigger not just temporary sadness or grief but persistent, serious depression. In vulnerable people, stressful life events both increase the risk of depression and interfere with successful treatment.[29] Just working long hours can increase symptoms of depression and anxiety, particularly in women, as well as decrease productivity.[30] Clearly, attitude toward work and the ability to maintain healthy lifestyle habits matter.

One theory is that recurrences of psychological diseases have to do with "kindling" or "sensitization." The initial triggering event is sufficiently distressing to spark the first episode of the disease. Even without adequate treatment, the fire (illness) eventually dies back to smoldering embers. Afterward, it takes less stress to reignite symptoms. Eventually, symptoms arise even in the absence of life challenges. One reason it's important to receive proper treatment for such conditions is to interrupt this cycle. Chapter 5 explains this concept in more detail.

Bodily systems suffer too. For instance, **immune function** eventually weakens. Acute stress actually enhances immune function, which makes good sense if you're injured while fighting for your life. You don't want those wounds to become infected. However, long-term stress impairs immune function. The immune system's job is to guard against infectious microorganisms and foreign or cancerous cells—without attacking normal cells or benign molecules such as pollen.

A common repercussion is greater susceptibility to upper respiratory infections such as the common cold.[31] Pay attention to the number of students who begin to sniffle and sneeze during final exams or soon after the semester ends. Stressful life events can also hasten the progression of serious infections such as HIV (human immunodeficiency virus).[32] Because of impairment of the immune system and other biological functions, wounds heal slower.[33]

The impact of chronic stress on vulnerability to cancer is harder to prove. So far, research findings are conflicting.[34] Cancer takes many years to develop and the causes are multiple. Also, if you ask a person with newly diagnosed cancer (which is a stressful experience) to reflect upon stressful life events, he or she may be more likely to recall them than someone without cancer. Furthermore, many people cope with stress by smoking or excessive drinking, which can both lead to cancer. Lastly, chronic stress promotes inflammation, obesity, diabetes, and other conditions associated with an elevated cancer risk.[35] Nevertheless, studies do indicate that stress adversely affects defenses against cancer, such as DNA repair and immune system response, and possibly accelerates progression.[36] ,[37]

Chronic stress may also contribute to autoimmunity,[38] wherein the immune system attacks normal cells, as well as immune system hyperactivity and inflammation—hay fever, atopic dermatitis (eczema), and asthma.[39] Chapter 13 discusses the immune system and its disorders in more detail.

sympathoadrenal system

Includes the sympathetic nervous system and the part of the adrenal gland that secretes epinephrine.

stress-diathesis model

A theory that a combination of genetics and early life events predispose an individual toward disease conditions in the face of sufficient stress.

Stress also alters sensitivity to **pain.** Chronic stress heightens pain perception.[40] Anxiety amplifies the problem and also rises as a result of pain.[41] Acute stress, particularly if it's physical in nature, decreases pain perception. That's thanks to the release of natural pain-killing substances such as endorphins. Because of these chemicals, soldiers injured in battle may initially think the blood belonged to someone else.

Attitude also affects pain. If a nurse points a hypodermic needle at your arm, you might think, "This injection will only hurt for a second—less if I relax—and protect me from tetanus." A person who thinks, "I hate needles. This is really going to hurt!" may indeed feel more pain.

Long-term stress can lead to **fatigue.** In addition to interfering with sleep, elevated levels of epinephrine and cortisol break down energy stores (protein, carbohydrate, and fat). After each stressful episode resolves, the body must rebuild those complex molecules. The process entails digesting carbohydrates, proteins, and fats into small, absorbable molecules and then reconfiguring them into storage forms of carbohydrates, protein, and fat. The process requires energy.

Long-term exposure to cortisol is particularly destructive, depleting skeletal muscle and bone. People who are extremely stressed, have cortisol-producing tumors, or take cortisone-based medications may develop chronic fatigue, thin arms and legs (due to the loss of protein stores in skeletal muscles), weakened bones (increasing the risk for a condition called *osteoporosis*), and extra abdominal fat.

Workplace stress—as defined by high demand (too much work), low control (little decision power), inadequate social support, and physical demands—increase both mental and physical fatigue.[42] Rewards and social support cushion workers from psychosocial stress. Chronic overwork can lead to a condition called *occupational burnout,* which is marked by physical and emotional exhaustion, cynicism, apathy, loss of motivation, declining performance, and disengagement from colleagues and friends.

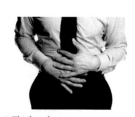

© Thinkstock

A disease whose primary symptom is a debilitating fatigue is *chronic fatigue syndrome.* Cumulative stress over a lifetime and isolated traumatic events, particularly during childhood, raise the risk for this complex, poorly understood condition.[43] In this case, the blunting of the daily rhythm of cortisol secretion (a lower morning peak) results in low levels over a 24-hour period.[44]

Fibromyalgia is a chronic condition characterized by widespread pain and tenderness, as well as fatigue, sleep disruption, worsened mental function, and often depression. The exact cause isn't understood. However, chronic stress and the resultant increased pain perception seem to play a role in fibromyalgia's genesis. This painful, debilitating condition also generates stress. Like chronic fatigue syndrome, the normal patterns of cortisol secretion tend to be suppressed. Many experts now view stress management as important to both prevention and treatment of fibromyalgia.[45]

Reproduction is the ultimate antistress activity. Stress isn't good for that system. Overactivity of the HPA axis disrupts what's called the hypothalamic-pituitary-gonadal axis, which regulates production of sperm and testosterone in men's testes and estrogen and progesterone in women's ovaries.[46] The potential consequence of chronic stress is reduced testosterone and sperm counts in men and absent or irregular menstrual cycles in women. Both sexes often experienced reduced sex drive.

Furthermore, erectile function depends on a delicate balance between the parasympathetic nervous system activity (which orchestrates erection) and sympathetic nervous system (which triggers ejaculation). For all these reasons, fertility can decline. Stressful life events can reduce success for assisted fertility technologies such as in vitro fertilization.[47]

Intimacy (which needn't involve sex), however, buffers against stress, in part by releasing oxytocin, a bonding hormone that is also involved in childbirth and breast-feeding. An acutely distressed man can experience temporary problems developing and maintaining an erection and also with premature ejaculation.

The **gastrointestinal system** is exquisitely sensitive to stress. A key reason is that the stress response diverts blood away from the gut and toward the heart, brain, and skeletal muscles. Furthermore, gastrointestinal function is a rest and restoration activity, meaning the PNS governs it. Because stress decreases PNS activity and increases SNS activity, blood flow to the gut sharply decreases; gastrointestinal motility is impaired; secretions decline. Stress also enhances the perception of pain in the gut.

For many people, stress causes gastrointestinal upset, producing nausea, vomiting, diarrhea, or constipation. It raises the risk of *irritable bowel syndrome,*[48] a condition characterized by cramping, gas, bloating, diarrhea, and constipation. Heartburn (*gastroesophageal reflux*) can also surface. These problems arise from functional rather than structural abnormalities. However, stress can also reveal vulnerabilities for organic (structural) gut problems such as *ulcers* and inflammatory bowel disease.[49]

Stress affects **appetite.** Few of us would pause to eat in an emergency. After the crisis (real or perceived), the hormone cortisol lingers and stimulates appetite,[50] particularly for high-calorie, sugary, fatty foods.[51] That effect serves you well if you've actually expended calories fighting of fleeing. The crisis over, it's time to eat and replenish stores. But if the stressor is an argument with a classmate, eating a bag of chips won't help. If you repeatedly activate the stress response (a traffic jam, a pop quiz, an alarming credit card statement), cortisol can stay elevated.

Note that stress-induced overeating is mainly a problem for "emotional eaters" (people who eat to relieve unpleasant emotions) and "restrained eaters"[52] (people who restrict calories in an effort to lose or maintain weight). While some stressed people skip meals and undereat, they're in the minority.[53] Not surprisingly, chronic stress often leads to being overweight and obesity. Furthermore, cortisol favors the deposition of excess calories as **abdominal fat**, which raises the risk of heart disease, diabetes, and other chronic conditions.[54]

For multiple reasons, stress powerfully contributes to common chronic conditions. Take, for example, the number one killer in America: **heart disease**. Stress elevates blood pressure, unhealthy cholesterol levels, and inflammatory chemicals. The risk of hypertension (abnormally high blood pressure) and atherosclerosis (deposition of fat and other materials harden and narrow the arteries) goes up. The heart has to work harder to pump blood through diseased arteries. All these changes increase the risk of heart attack and stroke (blockage of blood flow to the brain). Serious stress during early development predisposes people to heart disease. So can social stress (divorce, isolation, bereavement) and workplace stress, specifically situations wherein employees face high demands, little control, and relatively low wages.[55],[56]

Like heart disease, **diabetes** has also become epidemic in this country. Again stress plays a role. Epinephrine, cortisol, and other hormones released with stress oppose insulin, the hormone that moves glucose from the blood into cells after a meal. Stress hormones raise blood sugar; insulin lowers it. Stress also favors abdominal obesity, which is a risk factor for diabetes. Childhood trauma can raise the risk of type 1 diabetes, an autoimmune disorder that impairs insulin production.[57] Psychological distress also increases the risk for type 2 diabetes, caused by cellular resistance to insulin. Once diabetes occurs, stress makes it harder to manage blood glucose levels, and stress management can improve blood glucose control.[58]

Acute stress can temporarily disrupt **learning and memory**. Severe stress during intrauterine (within the womb) life and early childhood can change the brain and impair cognitive function and the ability to process thoughts, speech, memory, reason, and focus.[59] Whether or not severe stress contributes to memory-robbing dementia such as Alzheimer's disease is controversial.[60]

Most of these conditions result from chronic wear and tear. However, trauma, even if it is soon over, can create lasting scars. Examples include childhood abuse, rape, witnessing or experiencing violence, or natural disasters—any uncontrollable, overwhelming, terrifying event that threatens the life and well-being of you or a loved one. The result can be **posttraumatic stress disorder (PTSD)**. Symptoms include sleep disturbances, nightmares, flashbacks, avoidance of anything reminiscent of the event, emotional numbing, and social withdrawal. The HPA axis doesn't work normally. The hippocampus, the area of the limbic system critical to memory formation and retrieval, can shrink. Chapter 5 discusses PTSD in more detail.

Lastly, stress accelerates **aging**—right down to the cellular level. A number of things stress cells: heat, cold, toxic chemicals, free radicals—even psychosocial distress. One of the theories of aging has to do with *telomeres*, specialized structures capping the ends of chromosomes. They're akin to the plastic tips that prevent shoelaces from fraying. Every time a cell divides, the chromosomes (which carry the genetic code) also divide and a bit of the telomere is lost. Eventually, the telomeres become too short to permit further cell division and the old cell dies.

Stress hastens telomere shortening. In one study, the telomeres of women with self-perceived high stress suffered a decade's loss relative to low-stress women.[61]

The glass-half-full view is that many people don't suffer ill effects when faced with recurrent or persistent stressors, even traumatic ones. Genetic and environmental factors and psychological skills can work in our favor.

Common Signs and Symptoms of Stress Overload

- irritability and anger
- fatigue
- insomnia—difficulty falling and/or staying sleep
- headache
- upset stomach
- tight, painful muscles, particularly in the neck, shoulders, jaw, and temples
- grinding or clenching teeth (awake or asleep)
- trembling hands
- racing heart
- chest tightness
- anxious or nervous thoughts

- feeling like crying
- change in sex drive, usually decreased
- change in eating habits, usually overeating
- poor concentration
- worrying

Conditions Associated with Chronic Stress

- central obesity (excess fat in the abdomen and the trunk)
- loss of skeletal muscle and bone mass (with persistently high levels of cortisol)[62]
- decreased immune function
- poor wound healing
- sleep disorders
- chronic fatigue
- occupational burnout
- migraine and tension headaches
- cardiovascular disease: hypertension (high blood pressure), atherosclerosis, heart attack, stroke
- ulcers (primarily caused by the bacterium *Helicobacter pylori* but aggravated by stress)
- irritable bowel syndrome
- decreased reproductive function
- diabetes
- depression and anxiety
- accelerated aging

Audio Link 3.1

Stress

This hour-long Radiolab podcast exposes the hazards of chronic psychological stress and offers a few coping strategies. Experts interviewed include author and Stanford University researcher Robert Sapolsky, PhD, and president of the American Institute of Stress Paul J. Rosch, MD.

http://www.radiolab.org/2007/apr/09/
?utm_source=local&utm_media=treatment&utm_campaign=daMost&utm_content=damostcommented

KEY TAKEAWAYS

- Acute stress improves function, particularly in biological systems that allow us to survive physical stress. Thoughts quicken and attention and memory sharpen. The heart beats more strongly. Respiration deepens. Muscles work faster.
- Chronic stress impairs bodily systems, resulting in fatigue, poor wound healing, impaired immunity, suboptimal cognitive function, sleep problems, moodiness, increased pain perception, headaches, reduced fertility, and accelerated aging. Increased appetite and overeating can lead to obesity. Persistently high cortisol levels thin bones and break down muscles. Vulnerability rises for structural and functional gastrointestinal disorders, heart disease, diabetes, and psychological disorders such as anxiety and depression.
- A single episode of overwhelming, terrifying trauma can result in posttraumatic stress disorder.
- The diathesis-stress model posits that stress can unmask vulnerabilities caused by genetic and environmental factors.

DISCUSSION QUESTIONS

1. Apply the diathesis-stress model to your life.
    a. List your suspected diatheses: family history of certain diseases and environmental factors, including stressful life events. You might also mention habits you acquired during childhood that might increase your stress reactivity or add to allostatic load.
    b. List current lifestyle habits that further increase your odds of developing that condition. For example, if you have a family history of heart disease, smoking will elevate that risk.
    c. Note any symptoms or signs you've already developed for conditions you may be at risk for.
    d. Are you motivated to act now to decrease the risk? What's stopping you from doing so?
2. Consider the following scenarios:
    a. A soldier is wounded in battle.
    b. A soldier, wounded last week, learns that he will be sent home.
    c. A soccer player twists his knee scoring the winning goal.
    d. In the middle of the season, a professional soccer player learns that he or she has torn a knee ligament. The repair will require surgery and at least two months of rehabilitation.

For each, discuss how the situation will affect pain perception. Discuss both biological changes associated with stress and the potential effect of mental filters (how these fictitious people might think about the situation).

---

3.   HOW TO BECOME LESS STRESSED

LEARNING OBJECTIVES

1. **Identify your unique stress patterns.**
2. **Learn thinking habits that diminish perceptions of challenges.**
3. **Learn behaviors that help dissipate feelings of frustration and tension.**

Some amount of stress is unavoidable and even desirable. It makes life interesting and promotes personal growth. Coping skills are clearly needed. To learn those skills, you need to meet three main goals:

1. Identify those stressors that should, in fact, be avoided or eliminated.
2. Build psychological **resilience**, the ability to adapt to and recover from stressful events.
3. Learn ways to view challenges as positive events, or at least to minimize the toll they take on you.

Before we expand upon those objectives, let's first examine how Americans attempt to manage stress. Most people recognize that doing so is important. Yet, according to the latest Stress in America survey from the American Psychological Association, less than 30 percent of Americans effectively cope. What gets in their way? Most people blame time constraints. Overwork and stress-induced fatigue interfere with healthy responses such as exercising. Plopping on the couch and pointing the remote at the television is easier. The problem is that sedentary responses can add to allostatic load.

The following strategies can help you become more resilient and feel less stressed.

■ **Recognize how you respond to stress.** Consult the sidebars titled, "Common Signs and Symptoms of Stress Overload" and "Assess Yourself: How Vulnerable Are You to Stress?" These will give you a good idea of the symptoms and behaviors that commonly accompany stress overload. If you become more aware of them, you'll get better at nipping potentially unhealthy situations in the bud. You'll also become more aware of whether your responses to stress (e.g., drinking, smoking, yelling, exercising, problem solving) augment or diminish your allostatic load.

■ **Identify key stressors in your life.** Review the self-assessment sidebar, "Assess Yourself: How Stressful Is Your Life?"

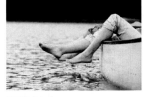
© Thinkstock

resilience

The ability to adapt to and recover from stressful events.

- **Reduce or eliminate.** Are there any stressors, including daily hassles, you could avoid? For example, if traffic aggravates you, could you instead take public transportation, carpool, ride a bike, or walk? If relationships upset you, decide whether you would be better off letting them go or learning skills to improve them. Sometimes hard decisions need to be made about academic schedules, extracurricular activities, and work.

- **Learn cognitive skills.** The goal is not to change the stressor but to adjust your thoughts about the stressor.

  1. **Pause.** Resist reacting immediately. Before you open your mouth, fire off a text or e-mail, or otherwise act, take a moment to breathe slowly and think. If you're initially too upset to reason clearly, the old trick of counting slowly to 10 can work. Unless you're in the midst of a true emergency, you have time to reflect and choose a well-reasoned course of action that serves you best in the short and long run.

  2. **Appraise.** Does the situation pose a significant threat to your well-being? An overflowing e-mail inbox, a boring lecture, a broken mobile phone, an annoying classmate—none of these things will hurt you, unless you mount a full-on stress response. Life needn't be lived as a series of crises.

  3. **Rethink.** This process is also called reappraisal or reframing. Ideally, thoughtful analysis will produce calmness and perhaps optimism, which will lead to an effective response.

     Adopt the objectivity and detachment of a scientist or doctor. You're seeking a second opinion, after all. Ask yourself if you could view the situation in a different way. Could you see it as a challenge or opportunity, something that inspires eagerness, confidence, and hope? For example, you can say, "This class is going to require a lot of work. But I'm excited about how much I'll learn. If I work hard, I believe I'll do well."

     If the stressor is a person, try to understand his or her motivation. Rarely is a person's sole objective to make your life miserable. He or she probably feels threatened (jealous, exhausted, defensive, worried, insecure). A grasp of motivation can lead to a constructive perspective. Even if the person's behavior is unfathomable, you can at least decline to participate in the drama.

  4. **Do a reality check.** Sometimes your best tool is to accept what has happened. As the Zen Buddhist saying goes, "It is what it is." The acceptance is calm, without assigning blame, personalizing, catastrophizing, polarizing, or overgeneralizing. (See sidebar titled "How Thoughts Can Stress Us Out.") Here's an example: You've arrived at the airport only to learn that your plane has been canceled. That's bad news. But you have no control over mechanical failure, inclement weather, or whatever interfered with your travel plans. Yelling at the airline personnel won't do anything but make you and anyone in earshot feel worse.

     The second part of the reality check is taking stock of your internal and external resources. Regardless of whether you can change the situation, you can always cope. Acceptance and faith counter stress.

  5. **Be specific in your assessment.** Let's say a particular subject seems to take you more time to master. This doesn't mean you're unintelligent or that every college class is going to be arduous. The fact that a differential equation makes your head spin shouldn't turn you off from the entire field of mathematics.

  6. **Take responsibility.** Let's say that you're sweating bullets because snarled traffic stands between you and an important appointment. Is traffic really shockingly congested, considering the time of day and the population density? Perhaps, like me, you often underestimate the time it might take to drive to a destination and find a parking space. Or, like me, you think that time will halt as you do one last thing before jumping in the car (check e-mail, answer the phone). In this case, the problem is you (and me), not the density of cars on the road.

  7. **Regain control.** Your honest appraisal, combined with faith in your ability to cope, tells you whether or not you have any control over the situation. A sense of control counters helplessness, anxiety, and stress. Sometimes you have to look for ways, even small ones, that you do have some leverage. Let's say you have a daunting amount of course work. You'll feel more cheerful about tackling it if college was your choice (rather than your parents'), something you view as a privilege and opportunity. You can decide when and where to study, when to take a break, when to turn off the light and sleep, whether to take advantage of tutoring, and possibly whether to drop a class.

  8. **Put predictability on your side.** Academic institutions follow predictable rhythms. Instructors provide syllabi outlining expectations. Dining halls serve during certain hours, classes begin and end at set times, most exams are scheduled, assignments have

due dates, and semesters (or quarters) end. Think how much more stressed you might be if your professor said, "I'm giving you a big exam, but you'll have no way of knowing when." Or, "I will grade these papers by throwing them down the stairs. Those that land on the top steps will receive an A." Take advantage of the known variables and plan accordingly.

9. **Remind yourself of your strengths and resources.** Everyone has strengths. Take stock of yours: ability to problem solve, empathize, communicate, reach out to friends and family, remain optimistic and hopeful, use humor, and so on.

10. **Strategize solutions.** Let's say you're invited to a good friend's wedding in another state but also have an exam and paper due on the same day. You decide you want to go to the wedding. How will you work out the conflicts? Contact your professors? Arrange to take the exam early? Get an extension on the paper?

11. **Create reasonable goals.** A big paper is due in two months. An unreasonable goal would be to attempt to write it the night before it's due. If the project seems overwhelming, break it into bite-sized bits. Set target dates for identifying a topic, creating a rough outline, finding your supportive documents, flushing out your outline, writing a first draft, and polishing a final draft. Recognize your limits. In the optimism of a new semester, it's easy to overcommit, to sign up for too many courses and extracurricular activities.

12. **Learn from your mistakes.** Here's your opportunity for personal growth. You're late for class (and the surprise quiz that took place before your arrival), miss the deadline for turning in an appointment, neglect your sleep, or lose your temper when your roommate asks you to pick up your stuff. Everyone makes mistakes. Personal growth happens when we learn—sometimes after repeated failures—how to do it better next time.

13. **Track your progress.** An appreciation that things are improving deflates stress and builds confidence, a sense of control, and optimism. Maybe you have to have knee surgery. There's the initial pain and restriction on activities. But now the problem's corrected and each day you feel stronger.

14. **Reward your progress.** Overcoming challenges is inherently rewarding. Look what you've accomplished already in college. However, you can also give yourself healthy, inexpensive treats. For instance, you may not look forward to spending a couple of hours studying in the library. But at the end of that time, you've mastered some material and crossed a big item off the to-do list. The carrot at the end of the stick may be a bike ride with a friend, a dance class, sharing dinner with a friend, or watching a funny video.

How Thoughts Can Stress Us Out

Inaccurate, faulty thinking can amplify negative feelings about situations. These so-called *cognitive distortions* amplify rather than relieve stress. Such thought habits can even cause us to perceive threats when none exist. Here are examples of cognitive distortions:

1. **Negative filtering.** Rather than view the world through rose-tinted glasses, people with negative filters mainly see and remember the bad things. A classic college example is to look at a graded term paper and only notice criticisms and overlook praise. Humans tend to do that. Try instead both to learn from errors, perhaps even feeling grateful for those constructive remarks, and to look for the positives. At the end of the day, review the good things from your day. People who thrive despite chronic adversity often experience a cognitive shift that flips the filter from negative to positive. Sometimes hard times make us realize how much we had taken for granted and stimulate a sense of appreciation.

2. **Catastrophizing**, otherwise known as making mountains out of molehills. If something disappoints you, don't make it more than it is. If you do so, you forecast disaster. Here's an example of catastrophic thinking. You get a low mark on a quiz. "I'm going to fail this class. I'll never finish college, much less get into business school, which means I won't get a job and I'm going to end up on a street corner holding out my hand for spare change."

3. **Overgeneralizing.** Take the example of a low mark on a quiz. An overgeneralization is to think, "I'm stupid." If someone turns down a social invitation, an overgeneralization is to think, "Nobody likes me."

4. **Jumping to conclusions.** Sometimes, based on limited information, we make up our minds about an individual's thoughts and motivations. Or we predict a negative outcome without justification. If someone frowns, you may decide the person disapproves or feels angry about something you did. But unless this person verbalized the thoughts and feelings behind the facial expression, you can't know them without asking. For all you know, the person has a brow-furrowing headache.

5. **Personalizing.** This pitfall leads to self-blame, guilt, and low self-esteem. It really isn't all about you. Let's say a friend calls to cancel dinner, saying he feels sick. Personalizing would be to assume the reason is he doesn't want to see you. Consider that he may truly be ill. Even if he feigned illness to avoid you, that's his problem, not yours.

6. **Polarizing.** This type of thinking lumps everything into black and white, good and bad, perfect and flawed, my way or the highway. The world and its inhabitants are full of nuanced hues and contradictions. For a college student, such a viewpoint can lead to feeling that anything less than an A is "bad" or that people with particular political views are evil.

■ **Budget your time and schedule sanely.** First you have to identify the ways in which you get in your own way. Do you procrastinate? Jump from project to project before completing any one of them? Spend too much time on Internet gaming or social networking? Go out too often or too late with friends? Miss enough sleep that you're too tired to concentrate? Work so much that you become inefficient, apathetic, and exhausted? Are you using substances that interfere with your studies? Write down your particular weakness.

The next step is to make a plan for overcoming your foibles.

Now make a to-do list. Prioritize that list from most to least important.

Lastly, create a realistic schedule. Take advantage of biological rhythms. If you're a morning person, tackle your most challenging work first thing and save answering e-mails, exercising, and doing errands for energy lulls. Refrain from overscheduling. Allow for a 10-minute break every hour and a period of relaxation before bed. In addition to the academic tasks and routine chores, be sure to save time for three healthy meals, exercise, adequate sleep, and a social life (but not so much as to interfere with work).

■ **Learn to say no.** This skill is hard if you're an overachiever, feel overly responsible for the welfare of humanity, believe no one else can do the job as well as you, or are vulnerable to guilt. Opportunities are wonderful, but you can share them with other people. If your health suffers because you took on too much, you won't be much good to anyone. You don't need to make excuses. "Sorry. I understand you need help painting your room, getting to the airport, organizing your presidential campaign…but I can't help at this time."

■ **Build stress-busting behaviors.** If you're under stress, you need to take care of yourself, find healthy ways to dissipate tension, and reach out for support.

■ **Eat healthfully.** Stress depletes vitamins and minerals. Make sure you're getting at least five servings of fruits and vegetables a day. Eat modest amounts of nuts, fish, and lean meats. Avoid processed foods (especially those that are greasy or sweet) and excessive amounts of alcohol and caffeine—all of which only serve to increase allostatic load.

■ **Exercise.** Though it doesn't eliminate stressors, physical activity provides an outlet for frustration and tension and counteracts many of the ill effects of stress overload on physical and mental health. You're doing what the stress response was designed to help you do: move. Vigorous activity opens blood vessels to your skin and to muscles, which helps maintain a normal blood pressure. The type of activity is not as important as your enjoyment of it. If you feel moved to turn up the tunes and dance around while cleaning your room, go for it.

■ **Seek social support.** Multiple studies show that positive social ties buffer many types of stress: caregiving, bereavement, workplace pressures, or disease. A University of California study suggested that, while men may be programmed for fight or flight, women are more likely to follow a "tend-and-befriend" pattern when stressed.[63] Theoretically, adaptive responses, at least in the old days, were for men to physically defend the home while women gathered up the children and sheltered them from harm. The bonding hormone, oxytocin, and possibly female reproductive hormones foster such behavior.

Oxytocin has calming, antistress effects. In both men and women, oxytocin promotes social affiliation—cementing bonds between sexual partners and parents and children.[64] Sexual intimacy releases oxytocin, also called the "cuddle hormone." But so does pleasant touch and massage therapy.[65] Women may be more likely to call up a friend to process thoughts and feelings about stress. But men can also use social affiliation to their benefit. That may mean joining an intramural team, for both the physical release and the camaraderie.

■ **Make sure you're getting enough sleep.** Problems often diminish after a good night's sleep. And being rested makes it far easier to cope calmly with challenges. Skimping on sleep simply adds to your allostatic load.

■ **Express yourself.** It's generally better to air your feelings in a socially acceptable manner than to bottle them up. Find a means of expression that works for you: draw, paint, sculpt, dance, make music, or write. Keeping a journal can give you the means to document, analyze, and problem solve stressors.

Locus of Control: Who's Running Your Life?

Locus of control refers to your beliefs about who or what is responsible for future life events. People with an *external locus of control* believe that forces outside of them manipulate their lives. That's dangerous for a couple of reasons. One, it can lead to blaming others for all our disappointments. "I got a D in the class because the professor was inept, unfair, and downright mean." Blame leads to anger and resentment. Two, firmly believing your efforts make little difference in the outcome of events spawns feelings of helplessness and hopelessness, which can lead to depression. Three, placing control elsewhere creates barriers to optimizing your personal health; engaging in local community activities and the political process; and otherwise improving your social, economic, or educational status. Basically, it seems that none of your efforts—to build muscles, lose (or gain) weight, get better grades, make new friends—pay off.

On the other hand, people with an *internal locus of control* believe they have a reasonable amount of control over their destinies. They have an appropriate sense of responsibility for what happens to them and believe their efforts have an impact. A student with an internal locus of control would believe, "The more I study, the better my grades." If she receives a D in class, she might think, "Well, I really didn't put enough work into the class. I registered for too many classes and went out with friends too often. I'm going to meet with an academic advisor about my class schedule for next semester."

Obviously, many events are truly out of your control—natural disasters, war, random acts of violence, the economy. Even so, your response will vary, depending on your personal sense of control. Take, for instance, the plight of the polar bears, whose habitat is literally melting. Someone with an external locus of control might feel despair, anger, or apathy and say, "My parents' generation did this. There's nothing I can do." Someone with an internal locus of control might feel galvanized to join an environmental group or take a class on energy sustainability or find ways to reduce his or her personal consumption of fossil fuel.

 Video Link 3.1

Aimee Mullins: The Opportunity of Adversity

Aimee Mullins, who broke records at the 1966 Paralympic Games, discusses about the concept that adversity isn't something to be avoided or overcome. Adversity does change us. Instead, she recommends that people embrace the opportunities to adapt, test ourselves, and flourish. "Adversity is just change that we haven't adapted ourselves to yet."

http://www.ted.com/talks/aimee_mullins_the_opportunity_of_adversity.html

Source: TEDMED 2009, Filmed October 2009, Posted 2010.

Productivity and Stress: Breaking the Link

Our culture literally labors under the myth that, in order to be productive at school, work, and athletics, we have to rush around with jaws clenched, shoulders hunched, and heart pounding. Americans are notorious for overwork. We take fewer vacations than people in most other wealthy countries, gobble lunch at our desks, or consume caffeine in lieu of a nap. Little if anything is gained from such behavior. Quality of life may well be lost.

Ask yourself these questions: Does mental and physical tension help you accomplish your goals? Might tension instead interfere with productivity? What if you instead learned to relax and work at the same time? Is it possible that the work would go better?

While deadlines are a common source of stress, consider their upsides. They motivate and focus us, right? Plus, you know that after that date, you can celebrate your achievement. Break large projects into manageable portions. When you're completing any one of them, stay present in that task. Avoid thinking about all the other things you have to do tomorrow, next week, or next month. Enter those items on a to-do list or calendar.

No matter the job, see if you can do it peacefully. As you do the necessary work, check in occasionally with your body. Note your posture. If you're slumping, sit up straight and let your shoulders drop away from your ears. How's your breathing? Make it slow, deep, and regular. Does tightening your mouth and jaw contribute anything to the job at hand? Let those muscles relax. You look better now and are less likely to get a headache. Are you having trouble concentrating? Perhaps you need a short break. If you're composed, your projects will likely go more smoothly.

Mini Stress Busters

Unrelenting work can bring anyone down. Procrastination ultimately generates stress. Find a middle ground. Try working for 45 minutes, then taking a break for 10. The following activities take very little time but can nonetheless lighten your load.

- Reset your brain. Some experts say your brain may need brief rests more frequently, perhaps every 20 minutes. I learned the following tricks from a colleague who teaches brain-based learning. Get up and tap the wall at either end of the room. This one you can do seated: holding your arm straight ahead, close your fist but leave your thumb sticking up. Trace the infinity sign (a sideways figure eight) several times with your thumb and let your eyes track it without moving your head. Switch hands. Get back to work.
- Invoke your inner child. Skip, twirl, blow bubbles, play hopscotch, juggle, or hula hoop. Doing something frivolous and goofy can remind you of carefree childhood moments.
- Sing. If you're shy about your voice, turn the music up and sing along. Sing in the shower, the car, or outside in the dead of night. Try "Row, Row, Row Your Boat" in rounds.
- Laugh, even if there's nothing funny. Feelings of foolishness may trigger a genuine giggle. As Woody Allen said, "I am thankful for laughter, except when milk comes out of my nose."[66]
- Watch a funny video.
- Wander. In a safe environment, walk or cycle leisurely without a particular destination. Pay attention to the sights, sounds, smells, textures, and tastes.
- Slowly peel and eat an orange. Engage all your senses. Feel and see the texture of the skin, the squirt of juice as your thumb divides the sections. Smell the citrus aroma. Taste the pulp and the juice. You've just done a mindfulness exercise.
- Hug a friend. If that's not possible, get up and introduce yourself to someone.
- Hug a friendly dog. Stroke a cat. Groom a horse. Research shows that pet therapy reduces stress, including in people with posttraumatic stress disorder (PTSD).[67]
- Spend time outdoors. Natural environments reduce stress and enhance overall well-being.[68] Access to green spaces can buffer the negative health effects of stressful life events.[69]
    - If the weather permits, sit on the ground and mentally catalog everything you see in a square foot.
    - Lie under a tree and watch the leaves and branches and the patches of light between them.
    - Gaze at the stars.
    - Watch the snow fall. Try doing that under a street lamp.
    - Make a snow angel.
    - Hug a tree. Examine the bark, feel the texture, and inhale deeply.

3.1 Mind-Body Therapies

The human stress response illustrates the fact that our perceptions—our thoughts and emotions—have physical consequences. If you're watching a horror film and feel genuinely scared, your stress response is activated. If you've paid good money to ride a roller coaster, you may view the experience as thrilling, especially because it ends after a few minutes.

Many complementary and alternative therapies work, in part, by modulating the autonomic nervous system and hypothalamic-pituitary-adrenal axis. Mind-body therapies are particularly good at that. The sympathetic nervous system quiets and the parasympathetic nervous system has a chance to rebound. Cortisol levels decline. Thoughts slow and shift to a more positive pole. Muscles relax. Herbert Benson, MD, a pioneer in mind-body medicine, called this counterpoint to the stress response the *relaxation response*.

Breath Work

The name autonomic nervous system indicates it runs automatically. In truth, you have some conscious control. Slow deep breathing is the easiest, cheapest method for bringing up the parasympathetic nervous system and dialing down the sympathetic nervous system.

Try the following exercise. Find a quiet place. Sit comfortably or lie on your back. Put one hand on your chest (on the left side so you can feel your heart beat) and the other on your abdomen. Exhale slowly and feel your belly drop. Inhale slowly and feel your belly rise. Start out counting to four slowly for each exhalation and inhalation. If it feels comfortable, lengthen the time for exhalation to a slow count of six or eight. Listen to your breath. If you constrict the back of your throat a little, you start to

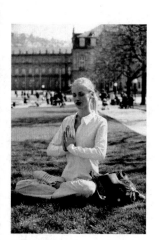

© Thinkstock

sound like an ocean. Try sighing with your exhalations. Can your upper hand feel your heart beat? Has it slowed?

 Video Clip 3.1

The Dalai Lama on Breathing to Decrease Emotional Distress
The Dalai Lama describes how measured, meditative breathing can lead to calm and well-being.

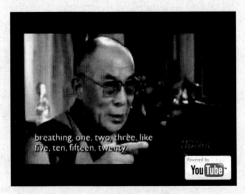

View the video online at: http://www.youtube.com/v/yTCRdM71j2E

Progressive Muscle Relaxation

Find a quiet place and lie on your back. If you can't lie down, sit comfortably. The idea is to start at your head or at your feet, sequentially tightening and relaxing the muscles. I like to start with my feet. Hold the contraction of each muscle group for 10 seconds. Appreciate the feeling of relaxation for another 10 seconds before you move on.

1. Point your toes as hard as you can, as though you were trying to hold a soda can with your arch. If you haven't already, tighten your calves. Relax.
2. Tighten your thighs. Relax.
3. Tighten your buttocks. Relax.
4. Tighten your abdominal muscles. Relax.
5. Clench your fists. Relax.
6. Bending at the elbow, contract the muscles in your arms and shoulders.
7. Tighten your neck. Try angling your head forward, then press the back of your head into the surface you're lying on. Relax.
8. Tighten your jaw. Relax.
9. Purse your lips, then open your mouth and, with your eyes wide open, stick your tongue out as far as it goes. Relax.
10. Scrunch up your forehead. Relax.
11. Tell yourself, "I am completely relaxed." Pay attention to what relaxed feels like. Appreciate the warm, loose muscles.

You can work elements of progressive muscle relaxation into daily life. The postworkout period is an excellent time to take a moment to lie down and feel your whole body go limp. With practice, you'll become more aware of relaxation and tension. Periodically scan for tense muscles—when you're sitting in class, taking an exam, working at your desk, driving, or exercising. Focus on relaxing the muscles not essential to the task at hand. Notice how often the face and neck want to participate when they aren't needed. Even when you're speaking, let go of the facial muscles you don't need to express yourself clearly. Soon, you'll be able to relax within seconds.

Meditation

Meditation couldn't be further from fight-or-flight mode. Chapter 2 described the different types of meditation. Choose a method that works for you. Find 10 to 20 minutes when you won't likely be disturbed. Sit quietly and comfortably. Close your eyes (unless you've chosen to stare at something hypnotic). Become aware of your breathing. Make it slow and even. Scan your body for any tension you can release. Listen to the sounds around you. When your thoughts stray, don't berate yourself, simply come back to your original intention (i.e., repeating a mantra, emptying your mind, focusing on your breath).

Research supports meditation as an antidote to stress. For instance, studies show that Transcendental Meditation, a specific technique for silent repetition of a mantra, enhances parasympathetic control of the heart (more normal heart rate patters and blood pressure) and reduces cortisol spikes in response to an acute stressor.[70] Other types of meditation also improve perceived stress, mood, sleep, and blood pressure in stressed individuals.[71]

Mindfulness-based stress reduction (MBSR), which was pioneered by Jon Kabat-Zinn, has a particularly strong record for building resilience and reducing stress. As described in Chapter 2, mindfulness meditation is about being fully, deliberately aware of the present moment. It's the antithesis of multitasking, ruminating, and fretting. If we're really paying attention, we often recognize that the present moment is tolerable and possibly downright pleasurable.

Research shows MBSR reduces stress and anxiety.[72] ,[73] Regular practitioners become more skilled at accepting reality and appraising stressors positively (a sense of challenge marked by confidence, eagerness, and hope) rather than negatively (with fear and anxiety). The prefrontal cortex (higher reasoning) better governs the primal limbic system.[74] Cortisol levels fall and sleep improves.[75] Emerging research indicates that mindfulness may actually retard the rate of stress-induced cellular aging.[76]

You can practice the mediation as you sit or move about. If you had a handful of raisins, you could start by examining one—see and feel the wrinkles, sniff it, savor the taste. If you're walking, take slow steps and notice each one. If you're folding laundry, do it deliberately, focusing on all the sensory details (rather than absentmindedly working on a math equation). Start with a 15- to 20-minute practice. Gradually extend the time. When you feel rattled during the day, pull yourself back to the here and now.

 Video Clip 3.2

What Is Mindfulness?
Jon Kabat-Zinn, PhD, explains meditation and mindfulness at the University of California, Berkeley's Greater Good Science.

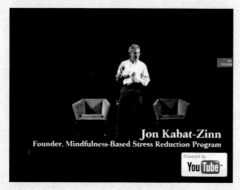

View the video online at: http://www.youtube.com/v/xoLQ3qkh0w0

Using Mindfulness and Compassion to Combat Stress

On a cold and snowy day last winter, Patrick stepped out of the door at 5:30 a.m. As he approached his car, he realized the driver's window was broken. Inside, the glove box hung forlornly open. Personal belongings and shattered glass were scattered. He hadn't left anything of much value in the car.

First he felt disbelief. No way. Really? He passed his hand through where the window used to be. Next was mild annoyance. How would he get to work? He didn't have time to clean up the glass. And it was too cold to drive with no window. Then he felt anger rise. Now he'd have to take the car to an insurance adjuster and a body shop. He'd have to pay the deductible.

He thought about the person who committed this act. It must have been pitch black and even colder. What was he or she thinking? Patrick tried to put himself in the place of someone who felt the need to break into someone's car. He had never felt so out of options as to commit burglary. Suddenly he felt lucky and also sorry for the vandal.

Patrick borrowed a friend's car and made it to work on time. For hours afterward, he marveled how these detached observations had shifted his perspective about this challenge from anger to compassion and gratitude.

Yoga

Hatha yoga, the form popular in the United States, combines three stress-reducing components: physical postures (which provide exercise), controlled breathing, and meditation. A recent review found that, of 35 trials examining the impact of yoga on anxiety and stress, 25 of them resulted in a significant decrease in subjective symptoms.[77] More than half the studies investigated the effects on biological markers of stress and many found improvements. A variety of anxious, stressed-out people have been studied: pregnant women, survivors of natural disasters, musicians, medical students, and fire fighters.

T'ai Chi Ch'uan and Qigong

Chapter 2 describes these two meditative movements. A study of college students found that taking t'ai chi lessons twice a week increased mindfulness, decreased perceived stress, and improved sleep.[78] Numerous other studies have found similar results.[79] Though less studied, qigong has also been shown to improve quality of life, reduce stress, and relieve neck and shoulder pain associated with computer use.[80],[81]

Cognitive Behavioral Stress Management

Cognitive behavioral therapy is a commonly used psychotherapy whose goal is to replace negative thinking patterns and self-defeating behaviors with more positive ones. Cognitive behavioral stress management focuses specifically on reducing stress reactivity. A therapist may incorporate many of the modalities mentioned (breath work, progressive muscle relaxation, meditation) along with skills to restructure thinking patterns, manage anger, become more assertive, and work more efficiently. Studies show that this type of therapy can reduce negative appraisals, lower cortisol levels, and enhance feelings of competent coping.[82],[83]

Harnessing the Senses

Create a sense of beauty and peace in your living space. Play soothing music to unwind stress.[84] Gather or buy flowers to put in a vase. Choose a tranquil image for your screensaver. Post pictures of places and people who make you feel relaxed and happy.

You can also infuse your living space with the calming scents of plant essential oils. Research shows that essential oil of lavender reduces heart rate and blood pressure and induces calm, alert brain activity. [85],[86] Other relaxing essential oils include clary sage, jasmine, bergamot, neroli, and rose. You can add 3 to 5 drops to a diffuser or a bowl of hot water, 5 to 10 drops to bath water, or 10 to 12 drops blended into an ounce of vegetable oil or lotion to massage into your skin. You can also add the drops to a cotton ball, seal in a small jar, and inhale as needed. Do not ingest essential oils. Note that bergamot can make your skin more sensitive to the sun.

Because the sense of smell is closely associated with memory, you can first try inhaling your chosen scent when you are feeling calm. Alternatively, you can pick scents that you associate with serenity in your past—rose, jasmine, or ylang ylang reminiscent of a beach vacation; vanilla because it reminds you of home cooking; and so on. Either way, they'll evoke memories of calmness, security, and perhaps even joy.

For most people, a good massage is a sensory delight. You can try a self-massage. To combine the effects of calming essential oils, blend two to three drops of your favorite oil into a tablespoon of body oil or lotion. Methodically rub into any tight muscles you can reach. Try sitting on the floor or your bed. Bend your knees and pull your feet toward you. Massage them and see if that doesn't help get you out of your head.

You can also swap massages with a friend. If you have the budget for it, have a professional work on you. Students at massage schools usually will work on people at bargain rates. Studies show that massages can reduce stress and increase well-being.[87],[88] Adding pleasing music or aromatherapy to the massage further reduces stress.[89] A possible drawback with massage is that the effects aren't enduring.

Acupuncture

Preliminary research suggests that acupuncture also can improve autonomic nervous system balance, normal-ize cortisol levels, and reduce stress.[90] ,[91] In one study, auriculotherapy—which involves temporarily placing tiny needles in key points on the ears or taping on tiny seeds that a person presses periodically to stimulate the points—reduced stress in nurses.[92]

Adaptogens: Herbs That Modulate Stress

Many healing traditions employ herbs as a defense against stress overload. The term *adaptogen* refers to non-toxic substances that augment resistance to stress. Recent research shows that herbal adaptogens work at the molecular and cellular level to combat stress.[93] In lab studies, they block stress-induced suppression of brain-protective growth factors, normalize cortisol levels, and protect against ailments associated with chronic stress. [94] ,[95] ,[96] ,[97]

Many of the commonly used adaptogens come from the East. Traditional Chinese medicine practitioners have long valued ginseng, astragalus, schisandra, and eleuthero (also called Siberian ginseng).[98] ,[99] Not only do these herbs buffer the stress response; they also enhance immune function. Extracts of ginseng, eleuthero, and astragalus can protect against respiratory infections and possibly cancer. Ginseng also helps fight the fa-tigue associated with cancer.[100] Ginseng and eleuthero reduce blood sugar, which may oppose elevations in-duced by stress hormones.

Two prime adaptogenic herbs used in Ayurvedic (traditional Indian) medicine are bacopa (also called bramhi) and ashwagandha. Both are also calming and are antidepressants.[101] ,[102] Furthermore, recent research sug-gests bacopa improves memory in older adults.[103] That's comforting news, considering the detrimental effect chronic stress has on memory.

Another herb that has caught on in America is the Arctic plant rhodiola (also called roseroot). Preliminary stud-ies indicate that extracts improve cognitive function, reduce fatigue, and have antidepressant and antianxiety effects.[104] In a study of people with stress-related fatigue, a concentrated root extract significantly improved attention and concentration and reduced symptoms of stress burnout and morning cortisol levels.[105]

Stress is best managed by revamping thoughts, emotions, and behaviors. However, these herbs are generally safe when consumed as directed. Don't take if you might be pregnant. If you're being treated for diabetes, consult your doctor before using eleuthero, Asian ginseng, or American ginseng, all of which can lower blood sugar levels. Because many adaptogens also enhance immune system function, they should not be combined with immunosuppressant drugs. Even though the immune suppression caused by chemotherapy (anticancer drugs) is an undesirable side effect, herbs shouldn't be added without working with a doctor.

Taming Performance Anxiety

College is full of performances, even if you're not an athlete, musician, dancer, or thespian. There are quizzes, exams, papers, and presentations. Your performance is graded. Often, instructors point out flaws and how you might improve. It's your job to notice what you did right.

Performance anxiety is normal. Some people feel it more intensely than others. Stress researchers often use public speaking as a stressor, which tells you a lot. Research also shows that people habituate, which means anxiety diminishes with repetition. Research also suggests that you do better if you accept rather than attempt to suppress your feelings.

The first thing to do is let go of any bad feelings about past performances and focus instead on your suc-cesses. Consider the benefits of these college experiences, which give you the opportunity to polish important life skills. Future employers will also judge the way you write, speak, and acquire new information.

Next, strategize how you're going to perform better in the future. Adequate preparation reduces anticipatory anxiety. Create a study schedule for exams. When your mind fatigues or starts to wander, rest or do something physical for a few minutes. If you're having difficulty understanding the material, you have at least three op-tions: (1) meet with a tutor, (2) speak with the instructor, or (3) join a study group.

If you're writing a paper and/or presenting information before the class, you create a timeline for phases of the project. Try "chunking," breaking the project into small, manageable bites. Take it step by step; focus on the task at hand rather than worrying about what else you have to do later. Regardless of whether writing is your strong suit, recruit another pair of eyes to read your paper. Give yourself time to polish the final draft.

Practice oral presentations. Recruit a mock audience. Make sure your talk fits within any time restrictions. Watch videos of people you admire giving talks. (You can find great examples on TED Talks at http://www.ted.com. Keep in mind these speakers had lots of practice before they took the stage.)

The night before an exam or presentation, allow 30 to 60 minutes of relaxation before you get in bed and a good eight hours of sleep. Tell yourself you've done all you could reasonably do. Avoid studying in bed or studying right until the moment you turn off the lights. If you can't fall asleep initially, remain calm. See Chapter 4 for tips on sleeping better.

Just before an exam or presentation do something physical. Walk. Stretch. Flap your lips (which helps relax your face and lighten your spirit). Take some slow, controlled breaths. Remember that performance jitters are normal and that small amounts of stress hormones actually sharpen your thinking.

As you step before your audience, focus on your eagerness to share the information you've learned. Inhale, and as you exhale, let go of muscular and mental tensions. Remind yourself that your instructor and your peers hope you do well. Find a couple of friendly faces to focus on as you speak.

If you're in an exam setting and start to tense up, do a quick body scan. Relax the muscles you don't need to stay upright and push a pencil. Come back to your breathing. Slow it down. Tell yourself you're OK and get back to work.

After an exam or presentation, resist comparing yourself to others. Focus on what went right. For my students who have a really hard time with oral presentations, the fact that they did it seems nothing short of heroic. Any kind of performance becomes easier with repetition. If you didn't prepare sufficiently, don't make it more than it is. You're not a bad person, simply an unprepared person. Sometimes life events get in the way.

If problems persist, seek help. Depending on the problem, you may need an evaluation and support for a learning disability or anxiety disorder. If you do, campus services will help you set up reasonable accommodations with your faculty.

Accessing Your College's Resources

If you routinely feel overwhelmed by stress, get professional help. Most colleges offer a variety of services to help you cope with stress. The student affairs office can help you get started. First, identify your key problem. Otherwise, investigate the following options.

General stress symptoms. See if your health center or counseling center offers individual and/or group classes. You may be able to also sign up for a class for college credit. And you can check with the physical education department to find out about classes in yoga, t'ai chi, or qi gong.

Anxiety and depression. Contact your college health center to find out about meeting with a psychiatrist and/or psychotherapist.

Academic problems. If you're having trouble succeeding in a class, find out about tutoring services. You will probably also want to speak with your instructor.

Troubled relationships. The college counseling center may offer individual and group classes.

Feeling marginalized as a minority. Find out about relevant support services for racial or sexual minorities. Colleges often have support groups for minority groups. If you're concerned about discrimination or other injustices, contact a student judicial affairs officer.

Physical or sexual problems, including infections and pregnancy. Contact the student health clinic. If you opted out of the college's health insurance program, you may need to locate professionals who accept your private health insurance.

Pain in the jaw, clenching or grinding teeth. A dentist can fit you with a night guard. Relaxation classes can also help.

Financial concerns. Contact the financial aid office.

Substance overuse or abuse. Contact the campus psychiatric services and/or counseling center.

Concerns about eating. You can probably start by meeting with a nutritionist or registered dietitian at the student health center. If you're concerned about eating behaviors, make an appointment with a doctor.

Housing problems. If you have a resident advisor, speak to him or her. You may also need to contact the campus housing department.

Sexual harassment. Find out if your college has a sexual harassment officer. When in doubt, call campus security.

Disability. Contact the student disability center to find out about accommodations due to you.

Violence. Dial 911. You need medical and psychological treatment. If you're concerned about future violence, the campus may have a violence prevention program.

KEY TAKEAWAYS

- Your perception of situations has a big impact on whether or not you activate the stress response.
- Cognitive skills, positive emotions, and healthy behaviors build resilience, the ability to adapt to and recover from stressful events.
- A number of cognitive skills can help you view changes as interesting and possibly rewarding challenges rather than as threats. They also help you develop rational, effective responses.
- A sense of reasonable control and predictability reduces stress. So does focusing on positive events, recognizing progress, and believing that actions have meaning and purpose.
- Healthy lifestyle behaviors also protect against stress overload: good diet, regular physical activity, adequate sleep, and supportive friends.
- A number of mind-body exercises promote relaxation and restore balance to the autonomic nervous system and hypothalamic-pituitary-adrenal axis.

DISCUSSION QUESTIONS

1. Imagine that you've recently changed your living situation. Someone in your new dormitory (apartment, condo, house) likes to play music late at night. Last night, you had trouble sleeping and feel tired in class.

    a. Write down the thoughts and emotions you might have the next day.

    b. Do you blame anyone? Where have you placed control over the situation, internally or externally? Is that assessment reasonable? Is there a way to readjust your thinking so that you feel less aggravated?

    c. How would you approach this problem using positive cognitive and behavioral skills? (Assume that changing living situations immediately is not an option.)

2. This experiment works better if you have an assistant. Fill a large cup or small bowl with ice cubes and water. Give your assistant a timer (on a watch, stopwatch, or phone). Ask him or her to time your ability to keep your hand in ice water (or simply hold an ice cube) in the following situations. Stop as soon as the discomfort becomes noticeable. Rest for a full minute or two between each. Feel free to alternate hands.

    a. Get a baseline measurement of your ability to tolerate cold.

    b. Turn on a scary video or think of an upsetting situation. Once your brain is engaged with either experience, immerse your hand.

    c. Start doing abdominal breathing as described in the breath work section. Visualize yourself someplace warm, perhaps on a beach. Immerse your hand and continue to breathe slowly and picture this warm, sunny place.

    d. Compare your times. Discuss the impact, if any, of these activities on your time.

4. RECOMMENDED RESOURCES

4.1 Books

McEwen B, with Norton Lasley E. *The End of Stress As We Know It*. Washington, DC: Joseph Henry Press; 2002.

Sapolsky R. *Why Zebras Don't Get Ulcers*. 3rd ed. New York, NY: Henry Holt; 2004.

Seaward BL. *Managing Stress: Principles and Strategies for Health and Well-Being*. 7th ed. Burlington, MA: Jones & Bartlett; 2012.

4.2 Organizations and Websites

Benson-Henry Institute for Mind Body Medicine. http://www.massgeneral.org/bhi.

Mayo Clinic provides a number of web articles:

"Constant Stress Puts Your Life at Risk." http://www.mayoclinic.com/print/stress/SR00001/METHOD=print.

"Stress Management." http://www.mayoclinic.com/health/stress-management/MY00435.

Stress: Medline Plus from the United States National Library of Medicine National Institutes of Health. http://www.nlm.nih.gov/medlineplus/stress.html#cat57.

American Institute of Stress. http://www.stress.org.

Center for Mindfulness in Medicine, Health Care, and Society. University of Massachusetts Medical School. http://www.umassmed.edu/content.aspx?id=41252.

4.3 Videos

Jon Kabat-Zinn: Coming to Our Senses. Jon Kabat-Zinn, PhD, lectures on mindfulness-based stress reduction at the University of California, San Diego Medical Center. http://health.ucsd.edu/specialties/mindfulness/Pages/default.aspx. http://www.youtube.com/watch?v=qvXFxi2ZXT0. Sponsored by UCSD Center for Mindfulness and part of the series "Health Sciences Journal."

Stress: Portrait of a Killer. National Geographic Society, 2008. This compelling documentary explains the stress response; its benefits; the potential damage of uncontrolled, chronic stress; and how to cope. It features noted stress researchers such Stanford University professor Robert Sapolsky, PhD. Length: 56 minutes. http://www.youtube.com/watch?v=eYG0ZuTv5rs&feature=related.

Using Positivity to Bounce Back from Inevitable Setbacks. Psychologist Barbara Fredrickson, PhD, is the director of the Positive Emotions and Psychophysiology Laboratory at the University of North Carolina at Chapel Hill and the author of *Positivity: Groundbreaking Research Reveals How to Embrace the Hidden Strength of Positive Emotions, Overcome Negativity, and Thrive*. In this 2010 lecture at Boston University, she explains how to access positive emotions to cope with stress. http://www.youtube.com/watch?v=CEEyjTWogiY&feature=related.

ENDNOTES

1. Britton A, Shipley MJ. Bored to death? *Int J Epidemiol*. 2010 Apr;39(2):370–371.

2. Quotations about stress. The Quote Garden. Available at: http://www.quotegarden.com/stress.html. Accessed November 20, 2011.

3. Stress in America 2009. American Psychological Association. Available at: http://www.apa.org/news/press/releases/stress-exec-summary.pdf. Accessed May 29, 2012.

4. Stress in America findings. American Psychological Association. November 9, 2010. Available at: http://www.apa.org/news/press/releases/stress/national-report.pdf. Accessed May 29, 2012.

5. Stress in America: our health at risk. January 11, 2012. Available at: http://www.apa.org/news/press/releases/stress/2011/final-2011.pdf. Accessed May 30, 2012.

6. American College Health Association. *National College Health Assessment II: Reference Group Executive Summary Spring 2011*. Hanover, MD: American College Health Association; 2011. Available at: http://www.achancha.org/docs/ACHA-NCHA-II_ReferenceGroup_ExecutiveSummary_Spring2011.pdf. Accessed May 31, 2012.

7. McEwen BS. Protective and damaging effects of stress mediators. *N Engl J Med*. 1998;338:171–179.

8. Goewey DJ. Worry—the fiction that rarely happens. July 15, 2011. Available at: http://donjosephgoewey.com/worry-the-fiction-that-rarely-happens. Accessed June 4, 2012.

9. Stress in America findings. American Psychological Association. November 9, 2010. Available at: http://www.apa.org/news/press/releases/stress/national-report.pdf. Accessed May 29, 2012.

10. Mitra A, Crump EM, Alvers KM, Robertson KL, Rowland NE. Effect of high-fat diet on stress responsiveness in borderline hypertensive rats. *Stress*. 2011 Jan;14(1):42–52.

11. American College Health Association. *National College Health Assessment II: Reference Group Executive Summary Spring 2011*. Hanover, MD: American College Health Association; 2011. Available at: http://www.achancha.org/docs/ACHA-NCHA-II_ReferenceGroup_ExecutiveSummary_Spring2011.pdf. Accessed May 31, 2012.

12. Grasgreen A. Student stress: whose is worst? *Inside Higher Ed*. Available at: http://www.insidehighered.com/news/2011/06/17/student_stress_factors_and_effects_presented_at_acha_meeting_of_college_health_educators. Accessed May 31, 2012.

13. Connelly M. More Americans sense a downside to an always plugged-in existence. *New York Times*. June 6, 2010. Available at: http://www.nytimes.com/2010/06/07/technology/07brainpoll.html. Accessed May 30, 2012.

14. Thomée S, Härenstam A, Hagberg M. Mobile phone use and stress, sleep disturbances, and symptoms of depression among young adults—a prospective cohort study. *BMC Public Health*. 2011;11:66.

15. Thomée S, Dellve L, Härenstam A, Hagberg M. Perceived connections between information and communication technology use and mental symptoms among young adults—a qualitative study. *BMC Public Health*. 2010;10:66.

16. Rosenfield M. Computer vision syndrome: a review of ocular causes and potential treatments. *Ophthalmic Physiol Opt*. 2011 Sep;31(5):502–515. doi:10.1111/j.1475-1313.2011.00834.x.

17. Cajochen C, Frey S, Anders D, et al. Evening exposure to a light-emitting diodes (LED)-backlit computer screen affects circadian physiology and cognitive performance. *J Appl Physiol*. 2011;110(5):1432–1438.

18. Mark GJ, Voida S, Cardello, AV. A pace not dictated by electrons: an empirical study of work without email. In: Proceedings of the SIGCHI Conference on Human Factors in Computing Systems (CHI 2012, 555–564); May 5–10, 2012; Austin, TX. ACM Press. Full text available at: https://students.ics.uci.edu/~svoida/uploads…/markvoida-chi12.pdf. Accessed May 30, 2012.

19. Essex MJ, Shirtcliff EA, Burk LR, et al. Influence of early life stress on later hypothalamic-pituitary-adrenal axis functioning and its covariation with mental health symptoms: a study of the allostatic process from childhood into adolescence. *Dev Psychopathol*. 2011 Nov;23(4):1039–1058.

20. Pruessner JC, Dedovic K, Pruessner M, Lord C, Buss C, Collins L, Dagher A, Lupien SJ. Stress regulation in the central nervous system: evidence from structural and functional neuroimaging studies in human populations—2008 Curt Richter Award Winner. *Psychoneuroendocrinology*. 2010 Jan;35(1):179–191.

21. Shonkoff JP, Garner AS; Committee on Psychosocial Aspects of Child and Family Health; Committee on Early Childhood, Adoption, and Dependent Care; Section on Developmental and Behavioral Pediatrics. The lifelong effects of early childhood adversity and toxic stress. *Pediatrics*. 2012 Jan;129(1):e232–e246.

22. Kristof ND. A poverty solution that starts with a hug. *New York Times*. January 7, 2012. Available at: http://www.nytimes.com/2012/01/08/opinion/sunday/kristof-a-poverty-solution-that-starts-with-a-hug.html?_r=3&ref=todayspaper. Accessed June 5, 2012.

23. Stress in America findings. American Psychological Association. November 9, 2010. Available at: http://www.apa.org/news/press/releases/stress/national-report.pdf. Accessed May 29, 2012.

24. Kane PP. Stress causing psychosomatic illness among nurses. *Indian Journal of Occup Environ Med*. 2009;13(1):28–32. doi:10.4103/0019-5278.50721.

25. American College Health Association. *National College Health Assessment II: Reference Group Executive Summary Spring 2011*. Hanover, MD: American College Health Association; 2011. Available at: http://www.achancha.org/docs/ACHA-NCHA-II_ReferenceGroup_ExecutiveSummary_Spring2011.pdf. Accessed May 31, 2012.

26. Faravelli C, Lo Sauro C, Lelli L, et al. The role of life events and HPA axis in anxiety disorders: a review. *Curr Pharm Des*. 2012 May 24 [Epub ahead of print].

27. Alvarez MJ, Roura P, Osés A, Foguet Q, Solà J, Arrufat FX. Prevalence and clinical impact of childhood trauma in patients with severe mental disorders. *J Nerv Ment Dis*. 2011 Mar;199(3):156–161.

28. Bender RE, Alloy LB. Life stress and kindling in bipolar disorder: review of the evidence and integration with emerging biopsychosocial theories. *Clin Psychol Rev*. 2011 Apr;31(3):383–398.

29. Hammen C. Stress and depression. *Annu Rev Clin Psychol*. 2005;1:293–319.

30. Virtanen M, Kivimäki M. Saved by the bell: does working too much increase the likelihood of depression? *Expert Rev Neurother*. 2012 May;12(5):497–499.

31. Pedersen A, Zachariae R, Bovbjerg DH. Influence of psychological stress on upper respiratory infection—a meta-analysis of prospective studies. *Psychosom Med*. 2010 Oct;72(8):823–832.

32. Leserman J, Petitto JM, Gu H, et al. Progression to AIDS, a clinical AIDS condition and mortality: psychosocial and physiological predictors. *Psychol Med*. 2002;32(6):1059–1073.

33. Walburn J, Vedhara K, Hankins M, Rixon L, Weinman J. Psychological stress and wound healing in humans: a systematic review and meta-analysis. *J Psychosom Res*. 2009 Sep;67(3):253–271.

34. Psychological stress and cancer. National Cancer Institute. National Institutes of Health. Available at: http://www.cancer.gov/cancertopics/factsheet/Risk/stress. Accessed June 3, 2012.

35. Cohen DH, Leroith D. Obesity, type 2 diabetes and cancer: the insulin and insulin-like growth factor connection. *Endocr Relat Cancer*. 2012 May 16 [Epub ahead of print].

36. Antoni MH, Lutgendorf SK, Cole SW, et al. The influence of bio-behavioural factors on tumour biology: pathways and mechanisms. *Nat Rev Cancer*. 2006;6(3):240–248.

37. Fagundes CP, Glaser R, Johnson SL, et al. Basal cell carcinoma: stressful life events and the tumor environment. *Arch Gen Psychiatry*. 2012;69:618–626.

38. Kemeny ME, Schedlowski M. Understanding the interaction between psychosocial stress and immune-related diseases: a stepwise progression. *Brain Behav Immun*. 2007 Nov;21(8):1009–1018.

39. Chida Y, Hamer M, Steptoe A. A bidirectional relationship between psychosocial factors and atopic disorders: a systematic review and meta-analysis. *Psychosom Med*. 2008 Jan;70(1):102–116.

40. Bardin L, Malfetes N, Newman-Tancredi A, Depoortère R. Chronic restraint stress induces mechanical and cold allodynia, and enhances inflammatory pain in rat: relevance to human stress-associated painful pathologies. *Behav Brain Res*. 2009 Dec 28;205(2):360–366.

41. Sandkuhler J. Models and mechanisms of hyperalgesia and allodynia. *Physiol Rev*. 2009;89(2):707–758. doi:10.1152/physrev.00025.2008.

42. Sembajwe G, Wahrendorf M, Siegrist J, et al. Effects of job strain on fatigue: cross-sectional and prospective views of the job content questionnaire and effort-reward imbalance in the GAZEL cohort. *Occup Environ Med*. 2012;69(6):377–384.

43. Nater UM, Maloney E, Heim C, Reeves WC. Cumulative life stress in chronic fatigue syndrome. *Psychiatry Res*. 2011 Sep 30;189(2):318–320.

44. Papadopoulos AS, Cleare AJ. Hypothalamic-pituitary-adrenal axis dysfunction in chronic fatigue syndrome. *Nat Rev Endocrinol*. 2011 Sep 27;8(1):22–32. doi:10.1038/nrendo.2011.153.

45. Vierck CJ. A mechanism-based approach to prevention of and therapy for fibromyalgia. *Pain Res Treat*. 2012;2012:951354. Available at: http://www.ncbi.nlm.nih.gov/pmc/articles/PMC3200141/?tool=pubmed. Accessed June 4, 2012.

46. Kyrou I, Tsigos C. Chronic stress, visceral obesity and gonadal dysfunction. *Hormones (Athens)*. 2008 Oct–Dec;7(4):287–293.

47. Ebbesen SM, Zachariae R, Mehlsen MY, et al. Stressful life events are associated with a poor in-vitro fertilization (IVF) outcome: a prospective study. *Hum Reprod*. 2009 Sep;24(9):2173–2182.

48. Naeem SS, Siddiqui EU, Kazi AN, Memon AA, Khan ST, Ahmed B. Prevalence and factors associated with irritable bowel syndrome among medical students of Karachi, Pakistan: a cross-sectional study. *BMC Res Notes*. 2012 May 24;5(1):255.

49. Konturek PC, Brzozowski T, Konturek SJ. Stress and the gut: pathophysiology, clinical consequences, diagnostic approach and treatment options. *J Physiol Pharmacol*. 2011 Dec;62(6):591–599.

50. Epel E, Lapidus R, McEwen B, Brownell K. Stress may add bite to appetite in women: a laboratory study of stress-induced cortisol and eating behavior. *Psychoneuroendocrinology*. 2001 Jan;26(1):37–49.

51. Oliver G, Wardle J, Gibson EL. Stress and food choice: a laboratory study. *Psychosom Med*. 2000 Nov–Dec;62(6):853–865.

52. Habhab S, Sheldon JP, Loeb RC. The relationship between stress, dietary restraint, and food preferences in women. *Appetite*. 2009 Apr;52(2):437–444.

53. Nevanperä NJ, Hopsu L, Kuosma E, Ukkola O, Uitti J, Laitinen JH. Occupational burnout, eating behavior, and weight among working women. *Am J Clin Nutr*. 2012 Apr;95(4):934–943.

54. Donoho CJ, Weigensberg MJ, Emken BA, Hsu JW, Spruijt-Metz D. Stress and abdominal fat: preliminary evidence of moderation by the cortisol awakening response in Hispanic peripubertal girls. *Obesity (Silver Spring)*. 2011 May;19(5):946–952.

55. Cohen S, Janicki-Deverts D, Miller GE. Psychological stress and diseases. *JAMA.* 2007;298(14):1685–1687.

56. Kivimaki M, Virtanen M, Elovainio M, et al. Work stress in the etiology of coronary heart disease—a meta-analysis. *Scand J Work Environ Health.* 2006;32(6):431–442.

57. Zung A, Blumenfeld O, Shehadeh N, et al.; Israel IDDM Registry Study Group—IIRSG. Increase in the incidence of type 1 diabetes in Israeli children following the Second Lebanon War. *Pediatr Diabetes.* 2012 Jun;13(4):319–326. doi:10.1111/j.1399-5448.2011.00838.x.

58. Egede LE, Dismuke CE. Serious psychological distress and diabetes: a review of the literature. *Curr Psychiatry Rep.* 2012 Feb;14(1):15–22.

59. Frodl T, O'Keane V. How does the brain deal with cumulative stress? A review with focus on developmental stress, HPA axis function and hippocampal structure in humans. *Neurobiol Dis.* 2012 Mar 9 [Epub ahead of print].

60. Bao AM, Meynen G, Swaab DF. The stress system in depression and neurodegeneration: focus on the human hypothalamus. *Brain Res Rev.* 2008 Mar;57(2):531–553.

61. Epel ES, Blackburn EH, Lin J, et al. Accelerated telomere shortening in response to life stress. *Proc Natl Acad Sci USA.* 2004 Dec 7;101(49):17312–17315.

62. Hasan KM, Rahman MS, Arif KM, Sobhani ME. Psychological stress and aging: role of glucocorticoids (GCs). *Age (Dordr).* 2011 Oct 5.

63. Taylor SE, Klein LC, Lewis BP, Gruenewald TL, Gurung RA, Updegraff JA. Biobehavioral responses to stress in females: tend-and-befriend, not fight-or-flight. *Psychol Rev.* 2000 Jul;107(3):411–429.

64. Feldman R. Oxytocin and social affiliation in humans. *Horm Behav.* 2012 Mar;61(3):380–391.

65. Rapaport MH, Schettler P, Bresee C. A preliminary study of the effects of a single session of Swedish massage on hypothalamic-pituitary-adrenal and immune function in normal individuals. *J Altern Complement Med.* 2010;16(10):1079–1088. doi:10.1089/acm.2009.0634.

66. 7 inspirational quotes for managing stress: or, "Woody's world." Article Dashboard. Available at: http://www.articledashboard.com/Article/7-Inspirational-Quotes-for-Managing-Stress-Or-Woody-s-World/639438. Accessed June 7, 2012.

67. Fike L, Najera C, Dougherty D. Occupational therapists as dog handlers: the collective experience with animal-assisted therapy in Iraq. *US Army Med Dep J.* 2012 Apr–Jun:51–54.

68. Stigsdotter UK, Ekholm O, Schipperijn J, et al. Health promoting outdoor environments—associations between green space, and health, health-related quality of life and stress based on a Danish national representative survey. *Scand J Public Health.* 2010 Jun;38(4):411–417.

69. van den Berg AE, Maas J, Verheij RA, Groenewegen PP. Green space as a buffer between stressful life events and health. *Soc Sci Med.* 2010 Apr;70(8):1203–1210.

70. Maclean C, Walton K, Wenneberg S, et al. Effects of the Transcendental Meditation program on adaptive mechanisms: changes in hormone levels and responses to stress after 4 months of practice. *Psychoneuroendocrinology.* 1997;22:277–295.

71. Innes KE, Selfe TK, Brown CJ, Rose KM, Thompson-Heisterman A. The effects of meditation on perceived stress and related indices of psychological status and sympathetic activation in persons with Alzheimer's disease and their caregivers: a pilot study. *Evid Based Complement Alternat Med.* 2012;2012:927509.

72. Baer RA, Carmody J, Hunsinger M. Weekly change in mindfulness and perceived stress in a mindfulness-based stress reduction program. *J Clin Psychol.* 2012 May 23. doi:10.1002/jclp.21865 [Epub ahead of print].

73. Krusche A, Cyhlarova E, King S, Williams JM. Mindfulness online: a preliminary evaluation of the feasibility of a web-based mindfulness course and the impact on stress. *BMJ Open.* 2012 May 21;2(3):e000803. doi:10.1136/bmjopen-2011-000803. Available at: http://bmjopen.bmj.com/content/2/3/e000803.long. Accessed June 1, 2012.

74. Creswell JD, Way BM, Eisenberger NI, Lieberman MD. Neural correlates of dispositional mindfulness during affect labeling. *Psychosom Med.* 2007 Jul–Aug;69(6):560–565.

75. Brand S, Holsboer-Trachsler E, Naranjo JR, Schmidt S. Influence of mindfulness practice on cortisol and sleep in long-term and short-term meditators. *Neuropsychobiology.* 2012;65(3):109–118.

76. Eppel E, Daubenmier J, Mskowitz JT, Folkman S, Blackburn E. Can meditation slow rate of cellular aging? Cognitive stress, mindfulness, and telomeres. *Ann NY Acad Sci.* 2009;1172:34–53. doi:10.1111/j.1749-6632.2009.04414.x. Available at: http://www.ncbi.nlm.nih.gov/pmc/articles/PMC3057175/?tool=pubmed. Accessed June 7, 2012.

77. Li AW, Goldsmith CA. The effects of yoga on anxiety and stress. *Altern Med Rev.* 2012 Mar;17(1):21–35. Available at: http://www.altmedrev.com/publications/17/1/21.pdf. Accessed June 1, 2012.

78. Caldwell K, Emery L, Harrison M, Greeson J. Changes in mindfulness, well-being, and sleep quality in college students through taijiquan courses: a cohort control study. *J Altern Complement Med.* 2011 Oct;17(10):931–938.

79. Wang C, Bannuru R, Ramel J, Kupelnick B, Scott T, Schmid CH. Tai Chi on psychological well-being: systematic review and meta-analysis. *BMC Complement Altern Med.* 2010 May 21;10:23.

80. Skoglund L, Josephson M, Wahlstedt K, Lampa E, Norbäck D. Qigong training and effects on stress, neck-shoulder pain and life quality in a computerised office environment. *Complement Ther Clin Pract.* 2011 Feb;17(1):54–57.

81. Griffith JM, Hasley JP, Liu H, Severn DG, Conner LH, Adler LE. Qigong stress reduction in hospital staff. *J Altern Complement Med.* 2008 Oct;14(8):939–945.

82. Gaab J, Blättler N, Menzi T, Pabst B, Stoyer S, Ehlert U. Randomized controlled evaluation of the effects of cognitive-behavioral stress management on cortisol responses to acute stress in healthy subjects. *Psychoneuroendocrinology.* 2003 Aug;28(6):767–779.

83. Gaab J, Sonderegger L, Scherrer S, Ehlert U. Psychoneuroendocrine effects of cognitive-behavioral stress management in a naturalistic setting—a randomized controlled trial. *Psychoneuroendocrinology.* 2006 May;31(4):428–438.

84. Holm L, Fitzmaurice L. Emergency department waiting room stress: can music or aromatherapy improve anxiety scores? *Pediatr Emerg Care.* 2008 Dec;24(12):836–838.

85. Kim S, Kim HJ, Yeo JS, Hong SJ, Lee JM, Jeon Y. The effect of lavender oil on stress, bispectral index values, and needle insertion pain in volunteers. *J Altern Complement Med.* 2011 Sep;17(9):823–826.

86. Sayorwan W, Siripornpanich V, Piriyapunyaporn T, et al. The effects of lavender oil inhalation on emotional states, autonomic nervous system, and brain electrical activity. *J Med Assoc Thai.* 2012 Apr;95(4):598–606.

87. Airosa F, Andersson SK, Falkenberg T, et al. Tactile massage and hypnosis as a health promotion for nurses in emergency care—a qualitative study. *BMC Complement Altern Med.* 2011 Oct 1;11:83.

88. Hanley J, Stirling P, Brown C. Randomised controlled trial of therapeutic massage in the management of stress. *Br J Gen Pract.* 2003;53:20–25.

89. Cooke M, Holzhauser K, Jones M, Davis C, Finucane J. The effect of aromatherapy massage with music on the stress and anxiety levels of emergency nurses: comparison between summer and winter. *J Clin Nurs.* 2007;16(9):1695–1703. doi:10.1111/j.1365-2702.2007.01709.x.

90. Park HJ, Park HJ, Chae Y, Kim JW, Lee H, Chung JH. Effect of acupuncture on hypothalamic-pituitary-adrenal system in maternal separation rats. *Cell Mol Neurobiol.* 2011 Nov;31(8):1123–1127.

91. Hollifield M. Acupuncture for posttraumatic stress disorder: conceptual, clinical, and biological data support further research. *CNS Neurosci Ther.* 2011 Dec;17(6):769–779. doi:10.1111/j.1755-5949.2011.00241.x.

92. Kurebayashi LF, Gnatta JR, Borges TP, et al. The applicability of auriculotherapy with needles or seeds to reduce stress in nursing professionals. *Rev Esc Enferm USP.* 2012 Feb;46(1):89–95.

93. Panossian A, Wikman G, Kaur P, Asea A. Adaptogens stimulate neuropeptide y and hsp72 expression and release in neuroglia cells. *Front Neurosci.* 2012;6:6.

94. Xu Y, Ku B, Tie L, Yao H, Jiang W, Ma X, Li X. Curcumin reverses the effects of chronic stress on behavior, the HPA axis, BDNF expression and phosphorylation of CREB. *Brain Res.* 2006 Nov 29;1122(1):56–64.

95. Liu L, Luo Y, Zhang R, Guo J. Effects of ginsenosides on hypothalamic-pituitary-adrenal function and brain-derived neurotrophic factor in rats exposed to chronic unpredictable mild stress. *Zhongguo Zhong Yao Za Zhi.* 2011 May;36(10):1342–1347.

96. Rai D, Bhatia G, Sen T, Palit G. Anti-stress effects of Ginkgo biloba and Panax ginseng: a comparative study. *J Pharmacol Sci.* 2003 Dec;93(4):458–464.

97. Rai D, Bhatia G, Palit G, Pal R, Singh S, Singh HK. Adaptogenic effect of Bacopa monniera (Brahmi). *Pharmacol Biochem Behav.* 2003 Jul;75(4):823–830.

98. Eleutherococcus senticosus. *Altern Med Rev.* 2006 Jun;11(2):151–155.

99. Astragalus membranaceus. *Altern Med Rev.* 2003 Feb;8(1):72–77.

100. Barton DL, Soori GS, Bauer BA, et al. *Phase III Evaluation of American Ginseng (Panax quinquefolius) to Improve Cancer-Related Fatigue: NCCTG Trial N07C2.* American Society of Clinical Oncology. 2012.

101. Calabrese C, Gregory WL, Leo M, Kraemer D, Bone K, Oken B. Effects of a standardized Bacopa monnieri extract on cognitive performance, anxiety, and depression in the elderly: a randomized, double-blind, placebo-controlled trial. *J Altern Complement Med.* 2008 Jul;14(6):707–713.

102. Withania somnifera. *Altern Med Rev.* 2004 Jun;9(2):211–214. Available at: http://www.altmedrev.com/publications/9/2/211.pdf. Accessed March 22, 2012.

103. Morgan A, Stevens J. Does Bacopa monnieri improve memory performance in older persons? Results of a randomized, placebo-controlled, double-blind trial. *J Altern Complement Med.* 2010 Jul;16(7):753–759.

104. Panossian A, Wikman G, Sarris J. Rosenroot (Rhodiola rosea): traditional use, chemical composition, pharmacology and clinical efficacy. *Phytomedicine.* 2010 Jun;17(7):481–493.

105. Olsson EM, von Schéele B, Panossian AG. A randomised, double-blind, placebo-controlled, parallel-group study of the standardised extract shr-5 of the roots of Rhodiola rosea in the treatment of subjects with stress-related fatigue. *Planta Med.* 2009 Feb;75(2):105–112.

CHAPTER 4
Sleep

ALL ANIMALS SLEEP: HUMANS JUST DON'T SLEEP ENOUGH

Sleep is a readily reversible state of relative unawareness of external stimuli. When you really think about it, sleep is rather inconvenient, although not as much of a nuisance as being in a coma. You can't study, balance your checkbook, play tennis, tend the fire, eat, hunt down prey, or watch out for predators. It's a time of relative inactivity and vulnerability.

Yet even birds that migrate across the ocean and sea mammals like dolphins manage to sleep. Instead of falling to sleep in the usual fashion, the whole brain oblivious to the outside world, these creatures allow half their brain to sleep while the other half continues to direct activities such as flapping or paddling.

While most members of the animal kingdom bed down when they're sleepy, we modern humans chronically mismanage our sleep schedules in a futile attempt to get along with less and less sleep. While most adults need an average of eight hours of sleep a night, surveys show that more than one-third of Americans sleep fewer than seven hours a night.[1],[2] The 2011 Sleep in America poll from the National Sleep Foundation found that 43 percent of Americans aged 13 to 64 rarely or never got a good night's sleep on weekdays.[3] Furthermore, 95 percent of respondents used electronic devices (cell phones, music devices, computers, video games) in the hour before bed. A few nights each week, cell phones beeping with texts and phone calls fractured the sleep of 18 percent of teens and 20 percent of those 19 to 29 years old.

Many of us compensate with caffeine. Sixty percent of teens 13 to 18 are already hooked on the stuff. However, the only remedy for sleepiness is sleep. As you're about to learn, shortchanging your sleep needs can have potentially disastrous consequences.

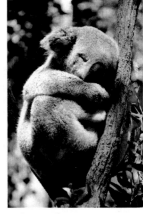

© *Shutterstock*

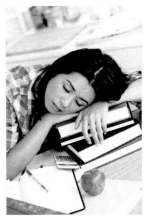

© *Shutterstock*

1. THE FUNCTION OF SLEEP

LEARNING OBJECTIVES

1. Discuss whether scientists have identified the function of sleep.
2. Explore possible theories about the function of sleep.

Given that we spend about a third of our lives slumbering, you would think that scientists would have figured out why we need so much of it. Curiously they haven't. Sleep remains one of nature's great mysteries. Most of what we know about sleep comes from experiments investigating the consequences of not getting enough. Theories abound, though none have been proven. What seems most likely is that sleep fulfills multiple functions.[4]

Some scientists believe that sleep helps animals conserve energy. During sleep, *metabolic* rate (the amount of energy expended over a period of time) falls.[5] As a result, body temperature declines and fewer calories are expended. Predators sleep during the time of day when it's harder to hunt. Prey animals sleep when it's safer to lie low. Either way, the animal has found a way to conserve resources. Of course, humans can eat whenever they want. The evolutionary drive to sleep clearly hasn't caught up to the era of pantries, refrigerated food, and 24-hour grocery stores.

Clearly, food isn't the only thing that nourishes. Sleep is restorative. Without nightly sleep feasts, we feel depleted. Indeed, hormones and cellular processes related to repair and restoration peak at night. For instance, levels of the stress hormone cortisol, which promotes breakdown of energy stores, ebb at night. Growth hormone levels are higher at night.[6]

If you want to watch near-overnight growth, observe an infant. Babies sleep more than half the day. Half their sleep time is spent in an active stage of sleep called rapid eye movement (REM) sleep. In comparison, adults sleep less and spend only 25 percent of the night in REM sleep.

Sleep may be critical for an infant's rapid growth and development, particularly for brain development. Babies are born with about 200 billion brain cells, only about half of which are needed. As they learn about the world, their brains rewire, reinforcing useful nerve connections and pruning back those that aren't used. Perhaps sleep supports these processes.

Evolutionary studies provide further support for the importance of sleep for brain development. More highly evolved animals have more organized sleep patterns. Most mammals have REM sleep. In most species, REM sleep is highest in the first weeks following birth, after which time the duration tapers. Another possible driving force behind longer sleep duration in mammals is immune system hardiness. As it turns out, animal species that sleep for longer periods have higher blood levels of immune cells.[7]

memory consolidation

The stabilization of recently acquired information from short-term to long-term storage.

For humans and other animals of any age, sleep seems to be important for **memory consolidation**, the stabilization of recently acquired information from short-term to long-term storage. Theories conflict about which stages of sleep are most important for learning and which types of learning benefit most from sleep. Nevertheless, studies in humans and other animals show that brain regions involved in learning "replay" nerve activation patterns during sleep.[8],[9] A person's expectation that some new bit of information might be useful in the near future enhances memory consolidation during sleep.[10] While insufficient sleep impairs certain types of learning and memory, recovery sleep eventually restores those deficits.[11]

The adage to "sleep on it" has legs. Several studies show that students recall information better after a period of sleep. In one experiment, high school students were given lists of vocabulary words in English and German. Students recalled the words better if they learned them at 8 p.m. than at 8 a.m.—provided a full night's sleep followed the nighttime study session. Students who stayed up all night watching TV and playing games had lower recall, even though they did get to sleep before the test.[12]

Lastly, sleep provides respite from the day's cares. Whereas stress increases sympathetic (fight or flight) nervous system activity and decreases parasympathetic (rest and restoration) nervous system activity, the opposite is true for sleep (with the exception of the active dreaming stage). Most of the time you're asleep, blood pressure is low, and heart rate and respiratory rate are slow and regular. A good night's sleep fortifies you for the next day's triumphs and challenges. Without it, we trudge ragged and bruised into the next round.

With Macbeth as his mouthpiece, Shakespeare said it better:

Sleep that knits up the ravell'd sleeve of care,

The death of each day's life, sore labour's bath,

Balm of hurt minds, great nature's second course,

Chief nourisher in life's feast… (2.2.34–37)

KEY TAKEAWAY

- Scientists still don't know for certain why we need to sleep. Quite likely the functions are multiple. Dominant theories are that sleep is important for energy conservation, tissue growth and repair, and learning and memory.

1. What is the evidence that sleep is restorative? (Hint: Blood levels of what kind of hormone are lower at night? Blood levels of what kind of hormone are higher at night?)
2. What facts support the theory that sleep is important for brain development?
3. Why do scientists think that sleep improves memory consolidation?

2. REGULATION OF SLEEP AND WAKEFULNESS

LEARNING OBJECTIVES

1. Explain the basics of the brain's regulation of sleep and wakefulness.
2. Discuss the central concepts behind the two opposing processes that determine your overall level of alertness.
3. Explain how circadian processes allow humans to consolidate periods of wakefulness and sleep within a 24-hour period.
4. Name key brain structures and hormones that regulate circadian rhythms.

Your life is divided into two main states: wakefulness and sleep. Because we're diurnal animals, we are active by day and sleep at night. **Zeitgebers** (German for "time givers") help synchronize our biological clock to the earth's 24-hour cycle, or **circadian cycle**. (Circadian comes from the Latin words *circa*, which means "around," and *dia*, or "day.")

The strongest zeitgeber is light. Light enters your eye, stimulating receptors on the back of the eye (the retina). Nerves from the eye convey information about the brightness to a specialized part of your brain called the *hypothalamus*. Within the hypothalamus are two **suprachiasmatic nuclei (SCN)**. Consider the SCN as control central for your circadian rhythms. Even if you spent a month in a pitch-black cave, your circadian clock would still run.

In the presence of light, nerves from the SCN go to the **pineal**, a pea-sized gland in the center of the brain, to suppress that gland's secretion of **melatonin** into the blood. Melatonin levels are normally low during the day and high at night. This hormone regulates a number of rhythmic processes, including sleep, body temperature, and the onset of puberty. It also has antioxidant and anticancer properties.

While all animals follow circadian rhythms, most species don't stay awake for 16 hours and then sleep for 8 solid hours. If you've ever lived with a cat, dog, hamster, or human infant, you may have noticed that such creatures take many naps.

In the quest to understand sleep-wake processes, scientists figured out that the brain keeps track of how long you're awake. Every hour you're awake is another hour of sleep deprivation. As the hours of wakefulness mount, so does the pressure to sleep. This process is called the homeostatic process. Recall from Chapter 3 that homeostasis reflects your body's drive to maintain physiologic equilibrium.

With the homeostatic process under their belts, scientists then smacked up against a paradox. If the pressure to sleep rises during the day, why don't we collapse of exhaustion after lunch? Many of us are indeed sleepier after the midday meal. And in many countries, humans take an afternoon siesta.

zeitgebers

Environmental cues such as light that influence the biological clock.

circadian cycle

A pattern of oscillations in physical, mental, and behavioral processes that roughly follows the earth's 24-hour cycle.

suprachiasmatic nuclei (SCN)

Twin areas in the hypothalamus thought to control circadian rhythms.

pineal

A pea-sized gland in the center of the brain that produces melatonin, a hormone that regulates sleep and other bodily processes.

melatonin

A hormone manufactured by the pineal gland from the amino acid tryptophan. It regulates circadian rhythms, including sleep, and acts as a natural antioxidant, antitumor, and immune-enhancing agent.

FIGURE 4.1 Anatomical Structure of the Brain

Key brain structures involved in regulating circadian rhythms.

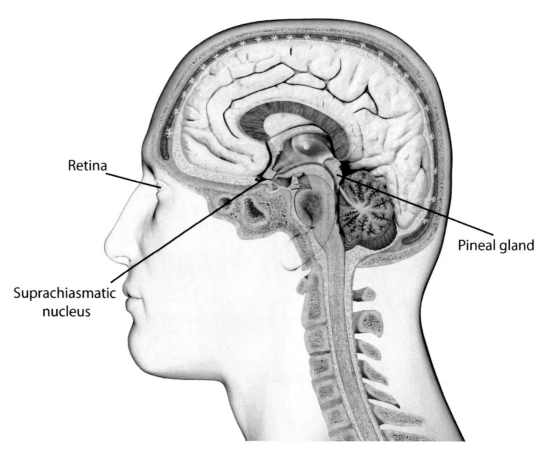

Retina

Pineal gland

Suprachiasmatic
nucleus

© Thinkstock

Yet, even without a nap, most of us start to feel *more alert* in the evening. How can that be when the sleep load has grown ever heavier? How many times have you stayed up too late socializing or studying, staggered bleary-eyed to class, resorted to drinking caffeinated beverages and digging your fingernails into your palms to appear awake in afternoon lecture, or considered cancelling your evening plans, only to get a seemingly heroic "second wind" around dinnertime?

A Swiss scientist came up with an explanation. Two processes influence sleep and wakefulness.[13] Process one is the **homeostatic process**, with sleep pressure building for each hour of wakefulness. Process two is the **circadian process**, which is *independent* of your sleep load and instead dependent on the time of day. During the day, areas of your brain responsible for wakefulness are active, and stimulating hormones such as the stress hormone cortisol run high. At night, other brain areas inhibit the activating centers, cortisol falls, and melatonin rises.

homeostatic process

The pressure to sleep. This process depends on how long you've been awake, rather than the biological clock.

circadian process

Changes in alertness governed by the biological clock rather than the number of hours of wakefulness. It's also called clock-dependent alerting.

FIGURE 4.2 The Circadian Process and the Homeostatic Process

The top graph illustrates the two peaks in your circadian process at about 9 a.m. and 9 p.m. The bottom graph shows how the pressure to sleep mounts for every hour you are awake.

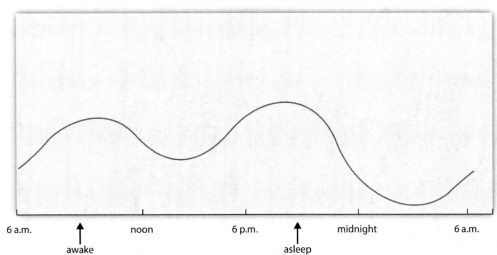

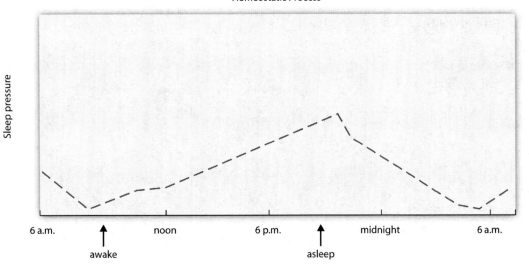

From here the process gets even more elegant. The circadian process rises in the morning, dips a bit in the midafternoon (allowing you to take a nap if you need it), then gets even stronger into the evening. It craters at your regular bedtime. At this point, the homeostatic process has risen above the circadian process and resisting sleep becomes more arduous. The inactivity of the circadian process at night allows you to sleep 8 to 10 hours straight—longer if your sleep debt hasn't been paid back.

KEY TAKEAWAYS

- Your body follows a circadian rhythm.
- Zeitgebers such as light and melatonin levels influence your circadian clock.
- The circadian clock's headquarters is located in the suprachiasmatic nuclei.
- Two opposing processes—the homeostatic process and the circadian process—determine whether you are awake or asleep.
- The homeostatic process is always on, keeping track of your sleep debt.
- The circadian process is active during the day and inactive during the dead of night.
- Some hormones fluctuate over a 24-hour cycle. Melatonin, which regulates sleep, is high at night. The stress hormone cortisol rises in the morning and declines at night.

DISCUSSION QUESTIONS

1. A friend tells you that he's always sleepy after lunch. He attributes his sleepiness to the diversion of blood from his brain to his gut and to the energy required to digest the food. How might you politely respond?

2. At about 2 p.m., a classmate complains of sudden sleepiness and worries she won't be able to study for an exam that evening. What advice might you offer?

3. Another friend admits that she is sleep deprived. The previous night, in an effort to pay back her sleep debt, she went to bed at 9 p.m. But she couldn't fall asleep until 11 p.m. How do you respond to her frustration?

4. Short naps have been shown to increase work productivity. After examining Figure 4.2, explain when the ideal time to take a nap might be.

3. STATES AND STAGES OF SLEEP

LEARNING OBJECTIVES

1. Identify the two states and five stages of sleep and the characteristics that distinguish them.
2. Debunk the myth that the brain is inactive during sleep.
3. Define polysomnography.

States of Being

- Awake
- Asleep
    - NREM Sleep—Occupies 75 percent of the night and contains four stages.
        - Stage 1—Light sleep. Brain waves of calm wakefulness (alpha) give way to the brain waves of early sleep (theta).
        - Stage 2—Sleep spindles and K complexes appear on the EEG.
        - Stage 3—Rolling brain waves called delta waves appear.
        - Stage 4—Delta waves dominate to produce a pattern called slow-wave sleep. Breathing rate, heart rate, and blood pressure are slow and steady. The sleeper is very relaxed, not easily awakened, and quite likely confused if something does awaken him.
    - REM Sleep—Occupies 25 percent of the night. Brain activity increases. Heart rate and respiratory rate may accelerate. The eyes move rapidly. Most other skeletal muscles can't move. Most dreaming occurs in this stage.

Sleep is divided into two states: non-rapid eye movement (non-REM or NREM) and rapid eye movement (REM). REM sleep is also considered one of the five stages of sleep. NREM sleep is divided into four stages.

Researchers learned that sleep is divided into stages by observing sleeping people and their electroencephalograms (EEGs). (In an EEG, electrodes placed on the scalp measure the electrical activity generated by the brain's nerve cells.) They first noticed that the electrical patterns characteristic of alert wakefulness disappeared during sleep and that people's eyes sometimes moved rapidly under their closed eyelids.

During the 1950s, William C. Dement, MD, PhD, discovered and named the five stages of sleep. Dr. Dement devoted his life to sleep research and founded the Stanford University Sleep Disorders Division, which was the world's first sleep disorders clinic.

EEG patterns and physiologic and behavioral changes define these stages. Stage 1 through stage 4 belong to **non-rapid eye movement (NREM) sleep**. The sleeper progresses from light sleep (stage 1) to the deepest sleep (stage 4). The body relaxes, body temperature declines, heart rate and breathing rate slow, blood pressure declines, stress hormones fall, restorative hormones like the growth hormone rise, and the sleeper becomes increasingly difficult to awaken.

non-rapid eye movement (non-REM or NREM) sleep

Encompasses sleep stage 1 through stage 4.

By stage 3 and stage 4, brain waves take on a slow, rolling appearance. It's like all the brain cells are drowsily doing "the wave" together. That's why deep, restorative sleep is also called **slow-wave sleep (SWS)**. After an all-nighter, you have more of this type of sleep.

After stage 4, sleep becomes lighter again before moving into a different type of sleep called **rapid eye movement (REM) sleep**. This stage is characterized by intense brain activity on par with an awake, alert state. At the same time, voluntary muscles (except those needed to move air and the eyes) are paralyzed. Heart rate, breathing rate, and blood pressure may rise. Sexual arousal occurs, with clitoral engorgement in women and penile erection in men. Under the closed eyelids, the eyes sometimes move rapidly. Most of your dreaming happens during REM sleep. Dreams can occur in other stages, but they lack the rich plots and vividness of REM dreams.

After REM, the brain descends back to deeper sleep, rises back to another REM, and so on. In other words, the pattern of stage changes is 1, 2, 3, 4, 3, 2, REM, 2, 3, 4, 3, 2, REM, and so on. The cycle repeats at about 90-minute intervals. NREM sleep occupies 75 percent of the night; REM sleep takes up the other 25 percent. (The split is 50:50 in infants.)

Most of your deep sleep happens at the beginning of the night. REM sleep dominates toward morning. If you're awakened earlier in the night, you may be groggy and confused. If you're awakened toward morning, you may find yourself smack in the midst of an intense dream.

FIGURE 4.3   The Cycle of the Sleep Stages during a Typical Night

Notice that stage 4 sleep occurs in the first part of the night and that REM sleep predominates toward morning.

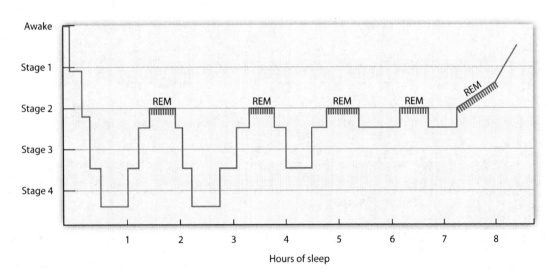

Sleep labs now use **polysomnography**, which tests multiple parameters, including eye and leg movements, muscle tone, airflow, respiratory effort, heart rate, blood pressure, blood oxygen levels, and the sounds the sleeper makes (such as snoring).

A pediatric patient prepared for a polysomnogram by a respiratory therapist, St. Louis Children's Hospital, St. Louis, Missouri, 2006.

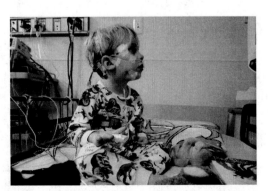

Source: Lawton R. 2006. Available at: http://commons.wikimedia.org/wiki/File:Pediatric_polysomnogram.jpg.

slow-wave sleep (SWS)

The deep sleep characterized by the delta waves that predominate in stage 3 and stage 4.

rapid eye movement (REM) sleep

A stage of sleep during which most skeletal muscles are paralyzed, the eyes move rapidly, the brain is active, and the sleeper dreams.

polysomnography

A sophisticated sleep study in which multiple parameters are monitored.

DISCUSSION QUESTIONS

1. From which stage of sleep are you most easily awakened? From which stage would a friend have the hardest time waking you?
2. During which stage do you do most of your dreaming? Why don't you act out your dreams?
3. During what part of the night do you have more slow-wave sleep (SWS)?
4. How might you feel the next day if frequent nighttime noises prevented you from getting much SWS, even if you managed to snooze a collected eight hours? Explain your answer.
5. During what part of the night do you have more REM sleep? If your alarm goes off during this time, what might be going on in your head just before you rise to consciousness?
6. During what stage of sleep is the brain active, with EEG patterns that resemble wakefulness?

4. HOW SLEEP CHANGES WITH AGE

LEARNING OBJECTIVES

1. Describe changes in sleep needs and sleep stages over the life cycle.
2. Debunk the myth that adolescents and young adults need far less sleep than children.
3. Explain why children tend to be "morning larks" and teens and young adults tend to be "night owls."

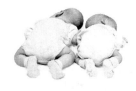

© *Shutterstock*

As we progress from infancy to adulthood, sleep needs and the amount of time spent in the various sleep stages change. As mentioned earlier, newborns don't have consolidated periods of sleep. Once the pressure to sleep builds, they fall asleep, cycling in and out of sleep multiple times over a 24-hour period. They nap like cats but are more demanding than felines while awake. Total sleep time averages 16 to 18 hours. At first, they don't have five defined sleep stages. By three months, they have distinctive NREM and REM sleep stages, spend about 50 percent of their sleep time in REM, sleep 14 to 15 hours a day, and do more of it during the dark of night.

Sleep needs decline steadily until about the age of five. School-aged children still need a good 10 hours of sleep a night. Unfortunately, one survey found that 15 million American children don't get enough sleep.[14] These kids are less likely to live up to their academic potentials and face the same risks of sleep deprivation as adults.

Many people think that sleep needs decrease markedly with adolescence. Not so. Teens and young adults still require between 8.5 and 9.5 hours a night. However, only about 15 percent of teens actually get the minimum of 8.5 hours.[15] The circadian clock is delayed during adolescence. In other words, they're not physiologically ready for sleep until around 11 p.m. Sleep debt mounts Monday through Friday, when early school times clash with biological rhythms. Sleeping late on the weekend pays back some of the debt but makes it even harder to get to sleep early enough Sunday nights. Plus, even when their schedule allows for sleep, teens tend to be sleepier by day than adults.[16] High schools progressive enough to start later in the morning reap the benefits of more alert students, as well as reduced truancy and drop-out rates.[17]

Not surprisingly, teens and young adults are at high risk for extreme daytime sleepiness and the problems associated with sleep deprivation. College students are particularly vulnerable. Psychological and financial stressors, overconsumption of stimulants, and noisy living situations may disturb sleep. Social activities and academic activities may encroach on sleep time. Nighttime use of backlit electronic devices such as laptops can suppress the normal nighttime rise in melatonin and feelings of sleepiness.[18]

FIGURE 4.4

Older adults often have lighter, more easily interrupted sleep. To make up for lost nighttime sleep, they may nod off during the day.

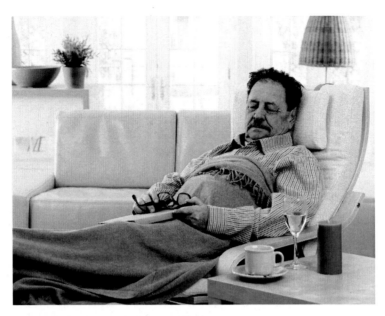

© Shutterstock

Once past this stage, adults typically need between seven to nine hours of sleep a night. Although sleep needs don't change, **sleep architecture** (the structure of the sleep stages) does. SWS and REM sleep decline steadily. Do the math and you'll see that leaves older adults with relatively more of stage 1 and stage 2 sleep—the least restorative, more easily interrupted stages. Medical disorders and the medications to treat them can thwart sleep. As a result, **sleep efficiency** (the amount of time asleep relative to the time in bed) drops. The circadian clock advances. Older adults typically fall asleep relatively early in the night and pop awake at the crack of dawn.[19]

sleep architecture

The structure of the sleep stages.

sleep efficiency

Amount of time asleep relative to time in bed.

KEY TAKEAWAYS

- Sleep needs vary across the life cycle. Infants sleep more than half the day. Children and teens still need a lot of sleep, though they don't get enough.
- Circadian rhythms shift. Circadian phase advances cause children and older adults to be morning larks. Phase delays make many adolescents and young adults into night owls.
- Sleep architecture changes with age too. Slow-wave sleep (SWS) and rapid eye movement (REM) sleep decline slowly and steadily. Older adults sleep less efficiently, with more time in stage 1 and stage 2.

DISCUSSION QUESTIONS

1. A new mother proudly tells you she plans on training her newborn to sleep through the night by the age of one month. Why is her plan likely to fail?
2. Many people believe teenagers need the same amount of sleep as adults. They also think teenagers should adapt to an adult schedule. What's wrong with starting the high-school day at 7:15 a.m.? What benefits might occur if the start time was delayed?
3. Ben is 30, and Harold is 80. Both spend eight hours a night in bed. How might their sleep differ? Who gets more deep sleep? Which one is more likely to go to bed early and wake early? Why?

5. SLEEP DEPRIVATION: RUNNING ON EMPTY

LEARNING OBJECTIVES

1. Define sleep debt.
2. Explain microsleeps and our conscious awareness of these events.
3. Explain the relationship between stress overload and sleep deprivation.
4. Discuss the impact of sleep deprivation on mental and physical function.
5. Describe the relationship between sleep deprivation and common chronic diseases.
6. Explore the impact of sleep deprivation on the risk of accidents.
7. Explain the interaction of sleep deprivation and alcohol.

sleep debt

The difference between the amount of sleep you get and the amount of sleep you need to feel alert during the day. It accumulates over time.

Night after night, millions of Americans don't get enough sleep. Chronic sleep deprivation is particularly common among adolescents and young adults (high school and college students).[20] Too many people regard sleep as a commodity freely exchangeable for daytime activities. Too few people recognize the potentially dire consequences of this trade. You're about to be initiated into this select tribe. This knowledge will give you a chance to change your ways—or at least provide you with a handy topic when dinnertime conversation falters.

Sleep is so important that your brain keeps track of how long you're awake. Normally you need one hour of sleep for every two hours you're awake. **Sleep debt** is the difference between the hours of sleep you get and the amount of sleep you need to feel alert during the day. Like the national deficit, it accumulates over time. Most Americans run a debt during the workweek and partially pay it back on weekends.

If you're not sure how much sleep you need, use eight hours. Every morning subtract the number of hours you sleep from eight. At the end of the week, add the difference. That's your weekly sleep debt.

The main symptom of insufficient sleep is **excessive daytime sleepiness**. The brain keeps track of how much sleep you're missing. The weightier this sleep debt, the more irresistible sleep becomes, especially if it outwrestles the circadian alerting process. Like hunger, sleepiness is a basic drive that cannot be ignored indefinitely. The brain, as though muttering "enough already," simply flips a sleep switch.

In general, sleep deprivation impairs **mental function**. Attention, concentration, vigilance, motivation, and alertness wane.[21] More errors are made. It's harder to make decisions, think quickly, solve problems, and memorize and recall information.

Compared to their rested peers, college students limping along on insufficient sleep and irregular sleep-wake schedules tend to have lower grade point averages.[22] In sleep-deprived, school-aged kids, inattention, poor impulse control, and hyperactivity can lead to a misdiagnosis of attention deficit disorder.[23]

Cognitive problems surface after one night of insufficient sleep. These deficits accumulate. However, people get used to a certain level of sleepiness and can fail to notice that processes like memory and thinking speeds have steadily declined over a single workweek.[24] Furthermore, one big sleep on the weekend may not be enough to recover those deficits.[25]

Physical function declines too. While you can continue to perform automatic, routine actions, they may feel more arduous. Indeed, heart rate and respiratory rates rise, suggesting it takes more work. Reaction times diminish. You can still drive and ride a bike, but your ability to veer out of the way of the squirrel darting across the road may not be as swift. Performance in sports that require closer attention and agility suffer more.[26] You may swim laps just as well after an all-nighter but have trouble playing a game of tennis.

No doubt you've noticed that feeling stressed makes sleep more elusive. But the reverse is true too: Sleep deprivation adds to your **stress** load. When you don't sleep, you miss that nighttime nadir in cortisol and sympathetic nervous system activity (fight or flight). Furthermore, sleep deprivation acts as a stressor. Activation of the stress response elevates the stress hormones, which can disrupt the next night's sleep.[27] Talk about a vicious cycle.

Like stress overload, sleep deprivation contributes to many of the **chronic conditions** that have become so common: obesity,[28] type 2 diabetes,[29] and cardiovascular disease. In one study, daytime sleepiness in older people was associated with a greater risk of death from any cause, particularly from cardiovascular disease.[30]

Chronic sleep deprivation impairs **immune function**, increases inflammatory chemicals,[31] and increases sensitivity to pain.[32] Disruptions in sleep are a common trigger for migraine and tension **headaches**[33] and may aggravate chronic **inflammatory diseases** such as asthma, inflammatory bowel disease, rheumatoid arthritis, and lupus.[34]

In addition, sleep deprivation worsens **mood**. You may be more irritable and short-tempered, more easily stressed, and less able to cope with even minor hassles.

If you're sleep deprived, **social skills** can flag. You don't communicate as well. Speech becomes monotonous and unclear. Judgments tend to be more negative. In other words, you drag your exhausted self to the party only to slump into the couch and make snarky remarks about the food, the music, the other guests…until you find yourself alone.

In vulnerable people, chronic sleep deprivation can do more than make a person cranky. Recent decades have seen a parallel rise in **mental health problems** and chronic sleep deprivation among young adults. A study of young Australian adults found that each hour of missed sleep ramped up the risk of experiencing psychological distress by 14 percent.[35] Chronic sleep deprivation contributes to work burnout and raises the risk of depression and anxiety.[36],[37] Depression and anxiety also interfere with sleep, making it hard to distinguish the chicken from the egg. Scrimping on sleep does not, however, cause psychosis.[38]

Even when sleep deprivation doesn't trigger a disease, it can make you feel lousy. What's sad is that many people don't understand that their chronic **malaise** has a simple cure: sleep. Spread the word.

FIGURE 4.5

Being sleep deprived can make you feel moody, out of sorts, and uncommunicative.

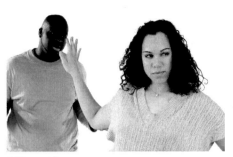

© *Shutterstock*

Asleep at the Wheel

Sleep deprivation causes a lot of accidents. Sleepy nurses, doctors, pilots, and air-traffic controllers make more errors on the job. All of us become dimmer witted, clumsier, and slower to react. Eventually, *drowsiness*, the sense that the eyelids are heavy and need to close, sets in. At this point, we may involuntarily go to sleep. We can experience **microsleeps**: brief episodes of sleep lasting from less than a second to 30 seconds. Often, we don't even realize we nodded off.

Yet a lapse in conscious awareness for even a few seconds can be enough to miss a critical announcement in a lecture, nail-gun a hand instead of the two-by-four, or veer a car across a couple lanes of traffic.

Too many of us are getting behind the wheel under the influence of excessive sleepiness. In one survey, some 38 percent of American adults had unintentionally dozed off during the day at least once in a month's time, and almost 5 percent had fallen asleep at the wheel.[39] A sampling of commercial bus drivers revealed that 20 percent were very sleepy, 8 percent admitted to falling asleep at the wheel once a month, 7 percent had gotten into an accident, and 18 percent had narrowly avoided a collision.[40] Given that teens and young adults are at particular risk for sleep deprivation, it's not surprising that one analysis found that people 25 and under caused 25 percent of sleepiness-related car crashes.[41]

Sleep loss can impair driving on par with alcoholic intoxication. In one experiment, volunteers either missed a night's sleep, slept only five hours a night for seven days, or drank enough alcohol to reach blood alcohol levels close to 0.10 percent.[42] (In all states, it's a crime to drive with a blood alcohol concentration [BAC] at or above 0.08 percent. In some states, it's illegal to drive with a BAC between 0.05 and 0.08, which qualifies as driving while ability impaired [DWAI].[43]) The results? All three groups drove equally badly. The only difference was that the sleep-deprived people were irritable and "fitful," while the drunks were "frivolous and carefree."

Other experiments show that the combination of moderate sleep restriction (four hours of sleep the previous night) plus low-dose alcohol (enough to elevate blood alcohol levels to about 0.03 percent) produced a double-whammy deterioration of alertness and driving performance.[44] Worse still, this impairment can continue in sleep-deprived people, even after blood alcohol content drops to zero.[45] It's almost as though alcohol flips a sleepiness switch in the brain—a switch that only sleep can flip back. One of the more dangerous things you can do is pull an all-nighter to study for an exam, celebrate with a few drinks, and get into your car.

TABLE 4.1 The Dangers of Chronic Sleep Deprivation

Excessive daytime sleepiness
Cognitive impairment: poor concentration, memory, attention
Impaired physical function for tasks requiring quick reaction times
Easily overwhelmed, harder to handle daily hassles
Reduced pain threshold
Negative mood, depression, and anxiety
Cardiovascular disease
Diabetes
Weight gain
Absenteeism from work, school, and social gatherings
Diminished quality of life
Note: Compare this to the sidebar "Conditions Associated with Chronic Stress" in Chapter 3. How much overlap do you notice between disorders associated with sleep deprivation and those linked to stress overload?

Assess Yourself: How's Your Sleep?

Most adults need between 7 and 9 hours of sleep a night, with an average of about 8.25 hours. Genetics influences your sleep need, your tendency to be a morning lark or a night owl, and the impact of sleep deprivation on your daytime function. Americans tend to get 6.5 hours of sleep on weekdays and 7.5 hours on weekends.

If you're getting enough sleep, you wake up feeling refreshed and ready to start your day. You feel alert all day, without resorting to stimulants. You can stay awake during the midafternoon trough in your circadian alerting process, even if that dip coincides with a boring lecture in a dimly lit, warm room. You also don't need to sleep in on the weekends.

To find out how much you really need, you have two main options.

- Go on a vacation. Sleep as much as you want. It may take several days to pay back your sleep debt. After that, notice how long you sleep each night.
- Go to bed 15 minutes earlier or sleep in 15 minutes later for several nights running. If you still don't feel alert by day, add another 15 minutes. Keep it up until you feel wide awake all day.

Can you train yourself to function well on less sleep? No. In experiments where people attempt to do so, volunteers may think they're functioning adequately on less sleep, but tests of mental and physical performance indicate otherwise.[46]

FIGURE 4.6 Measuring Sleepiness

Tests have been designed to determine just how sleepy you are. You can check yourself against one of the Epworth Sleepiness Scales several times over the course of the day. Try rating yourself an hour or two after you wake up, midafternoon, and early evening. See if you can determine the peaks and valleys in your circadian alerting system. Understanding your own biological rhythms will help you schedule classes, study times, and naps. **Multiple Sleep Latency Test (MSLT)** is the best test of sleepiness, though completing it requires spending a day in a sleep lab. No stimulants such as coffee or tea are allowed the day of the test. A person has to lie down in a dim, quiet room for 20 minutes every 2 hours during the day. Brain waves and eye movements are monitored to record sleep. The time to fall asleep (*sleep latency*) is measured. Around 20 minutes indicates the person is alert. Five minutes and under indicates serious sleep deprivation.

Name: ______________________________ Today's date: ______________

Your age (Yrs): ____________ Your sex (Male = M, Female = F): ______

How likely are you to doze off or fall asleep in the following situations, in contrast to feeling just tired?

This refers to your usual way of life in recent times.

Even if you haven't done some of these things recently try to work out how they would have affected you.

Use the following scale to choose the **most appropriate number** for each situation:

0 = would **never** doze
1 = **slight chance** of dozing
2 = **moderate chance** of dozing
3 = **high chance** of dozing

It is important that you answer each question as best you can.

Situation	**Chance of Dozing (0-3)**
Sitting and reading ____________	___
Watching TV ____________	___
Sitting, inactive in a public place (e.g. a theatre or a meeting) ____________	___
As a passenger in a car for an hour without a break ____________	___
Lying down to rest in the afternoon when circumstances permit ____________	___
Sitting and talking to someone ____________	___
Sitting quietly after a lunch without alcohol ____________	___
In a car, while stopped for a few minutes in the traffic ____________	

THANK YOU FOR YOUR COOPERATION

Source: Reprinted with permission © MW Johns, 1990–1997.

What to Do If You're Sleepy

If you can, take a nap. Short (15- to 30-minute) naps enhance subsequent alertness and performance.[47] If you're a caffeine consumer, you can have a cup of tea or coffee just before the nap. It will take about a half hour for your caffeine level to peak. Don't do either of these things—the nap or the caffeine—past midafternoon, or else you'll have a hard time getting to sleep that night.

KEY TAKEAWAYS

- Chronic sleep deprivation has become epidemic in America.
- If you restrict your sleep, you lose mental and physical performance and risk accidents.
- Missing sleep activates the stress response and also makes it harder to cope with daily hassles.
- Over time, the risk of conditions such as obesity, heart disease, diabetes, anxiety, and depression rises.
- Drowsiness is the last step before falling asleep. If you feel drowsy, get off the road. You may fall asleep at any minute, despite your best efforts. Let someone who's alert drive while you take a nap.

DISCUSSION QUESTIONS

1. Is it possible to have a microsleep and not notice? In what way might microsleeps be dangerous?
2. Discuss the two-way relationship between stress overload and sleep deprivation. It may help to refer to Chapter 3 (Signs and Symptoms of Stress Overload, Conditions Associated with Stress) with The Dangers of Chronic Sleep Deprivation (Table 4.1). Note the symptoms and diseases both conditions can cause or aggravate.
3. What impact might your sleep habits have on your college GPA?
4. Is drowsiness the first step or the last step before falling asleep? If you suddenly feel drowsy while driving, what should you do? Can chewing gum, opening a window, and turning up the music guarantee that you'll stay awake?
5. Which is more dangerous, driving drunk or driving drowsy?
6. Why might drinking even a small amount of alcohol be a problem if you're sleepy?
7. Jennifer is a premed college student who wants to become a pediatrician. She's heard that doctors don't get much sleep when they're on night duty. But she also thinks that she can adapt to getting less sleep. Based on the facts you just learned, what would you tell Jennifer?

6. SLEEP DISORDERS

LEARNING OBJECTIVES

1. Discuss the prevalence of disordered sleep in America.
2. Define dyssomnia and parasomnia.
3. Identify the key characteristics of the most common sleep disorders.
4. Discuss insomnia—its prevalence, causes, and potential solutions.

Some 50 to 70 million American adults struggle with chronic sleep disorders.[48] A study at the University of North Carolina found that, based on answers to questionnaires, 27 percent of college students were at risk for sleep disorders.[49] Most of them are either preventable or treatable. Despite the consequences of poor-quality sleep, the public doesn't know how important it is to seek treatment, and the average health care practitioner doesn't screen patients for sleep problems.

Parasomnias, from the Latin meaning "around sleep," are abnormal events that accompany sleep and may interfere with normal sleep. Most of the parasomnias listed here arise during NREM sleep and are aggravated by sleep deprivation.

parasomnias

Abnormal events that accompany sleep, often without awakening the sleeper.

- **Sleepwalking**, also called somnambulism, occurs in 17 percent of children and 4 percent of adults. The behavior begins during NREM stage 3 and stage 4. Sometimes a sleepwalker will simply shuffle around the room, then crawl back into bed. Other times, people engage in more complex and potentially dangerous activities like driving, jumping out of windows, and running barefoot into the snow. Sleepwalkers usually have a glassy-eyed, zombie-like appearance. Afterward, they have no memory of the event. Attempts to wake a sleepwalker can trigger confused and even violent actions. If you encounter such a person, it's better to lead him or her gently back to bed. Safety-proof the bedroom to prevent injuries.

- **Sleep-talking** is common and often accompanies sleepwalking. Usually the talk is meaningless.

- **Sleep terrors** not uncommonly bedevil children 3 to 12 years old. Within an hour or two of falling asleep, the child begins to scream and flail about, eyes wide with terror but unseeing. Attempts to calm or awaken the child are usually fruitless. In the morning, the child remembers nothing of the event. Sleep deprivation, stress, and a change in routine may *trigger* but don't cause sleep terrors. While sleep terrors arise during NREM sleep, **nightmares** occur during REM sleep and often awaken the sleeper, who can relay the complex details of the bad dream.

- **Periodic limb movement disorder** is characterized by recurrent, rhythmic jerking of the limbs (usually the legs). This condition may or may not wake the sleeper.

- **REM sleep behavior disorder** is an unusual condition in which the usual muscle paralysis associated with REM sleep fails to occur, allowing the sleeper to act out violent dreams. The person may run, punch, shout, swear, and throw things. Both the sleeper and bed partner may be injured. Most cases occur in older men, many of whom later develop a brain disease such as Parkinson's disease or dementia.

Dyssomnias are conditions that interfere with sleep. From the Latin for "difficult sleep," these disorders derail the initiation or maintenance of sleep.

Occlusion of the airway during sleep in someone with obstructive sleep apnea. During sleep, the tissues in the upper airway relax and sag inward. If enlarged tonsils and adenoids or excess fat narrow the airway, the blockage can become complete.

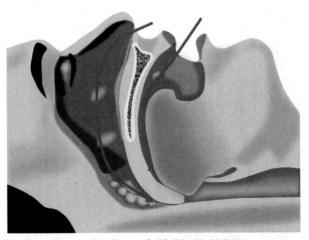

Source: M'henni H. 2011. Available at: http://commons.wikimedia.org/wiki/File:OSA_No_MAS.svg.

sleepwalking

Also called somnambulism, a condition in which the sleeper arises and walks around or does other activities without conscious awareness.

sleep-talking

An extremely common occurrence, wherein people talk, usually in a meaningless ramble, during their sleep. May accompany sleepwalking.

sleep terrors

Sudden, partial arousals from SWS in which the person behaves in a frightened manner. Also called night terrors, these occurrences are different from *nightmares*, which arise from REM sleep.

periodic limb movement disorder

A condition characterized by recurrent, rhythmic jerking of the limbs (usually the legs) during sleep.

REM sleep behavior disorder

Lack of adequate muscle paralysis during REM sleep allows the acting out of violent, aggressive dreams.

dyssomnias

Conditions that interfere with sleep.

- **Sleep apnea** is a serious condition in which a person stops breathing during sleep. There are two types: **central** (a rare condition in which the brain periodically fails to send the signal to breathe) and **obstructive** (an all-too-common condition in which tissues in the upper airway obstruct airflow). Obstructive sleep apnea (OSA) is the most common sleep disorder, affecting about 4 percent of Americans. An estimated 80 percent of Americans with OSA aren't diagnosed.[50]

In OSA, sleep can be interrupted many times in a single hour. In the deeper stages of NREM and also REM sleep, the muscles of the upper airway relax so much that no air can pass into the lungs. A full minute may go by before the person briefly wakes to gasp for breath—often without conscious awareness of the sleep interruption. He or she then falls back to sleep, starts snoring, stops breathing, gasps, or snores. Bed partners don't sleep well either.

The main risk for OSA is being overweight. The excess tissue in the neck narrows the airway, a situation that becomes exaggerated as muscles in the throat relax during sleep. Not surprisingly rates of OSA have gone up in tandem with the obesity epidemic. However, thin people and children can have OSA, particularly if they have recessed chins or enlarged tonsils and adenoids.

OSA undermines quality of life. Overwhelming daytime sleepiness makes it difficult to work and socialize. Sexual function declines.[51] Worse, OSA can be life threatening. People can fall asleep at the wheel and suffer heart attacks, heart arrhythmias,[52] and strokes.[53] If you know anyone who snores loudly, especially if the person sometimes stops breathing during sleep, advise a medical evaluation.

The main treatments are losing weight and wearing a mask at night that delivers continuous positive airway pressure (CPAP) to ensure delivery of fresh air to the lungs. People with OSA should avoid central nervous system depressants such as alcohol and sleeping pills. Some people sew a tennis ball to the back of their pajamas to prevent them from sleeping on their backs—a tactic that may or may not work. Children with OSA may need to have their tonsils and adenoids removed.

- **Narcolepsy** is a condition characterized by daytime sleep attacks, **cataplexy** (sudden loss of muscle tone), hallucinations, and/or muscle paralysis during the transition from sleep to wakefulness, and fragmented sleep at night. Even if nighttime sleep is sufficient, daytime sleepiness remains overwhelming. REM sleep seems to intrude into normal waking life. Strong emotions can trigger cataplexy. The disorder seems to result from a deficiency of an alerting brain chemical called hypocretin (also called orexin).[54]

 Video Clip 4.1

Narcoleptic Dog Video
This video shows a narcoleptic poodle.

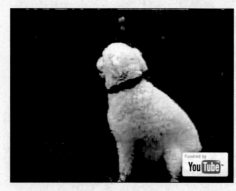

View the video online at: http://www.youtube.com/v/X0h2nleWTwl

- **Restless legs syndrome** (RLS) is a condition in which unpleasant sensations in the limbs (usually the legs) compel a person to move, which temporarily relieves the sensation. Ironically, these annoying feelings are worse with rest. The person may lie still, get the creepy-crawly feeling, move about, lie down, get the feeling, move…sleeping only once exhaustion overwhelms the unpleasant sensations. RLS affects 10 to 15 percent of the population. The condition tends to run in families. Iron deficiency raises the risk. Some but not all RLS sufferers have low brain levels of iron.[55] A number of medications can provide relief.

Video Clip 4.2

Amazing Domino Video for Restless Legs Syndrome
An interesting video with dominoes and restless legs syndrome.

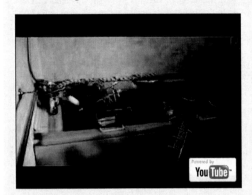

View the video online at: http://www.youtube.com/v/2bBMKtRm898

- **Sleep bruxism** involves clenching or grinding the teeth during sleep. This behavior can damage teeth and cause jaw pain and morning headache. People can also clench during daytime hours. Dentists can fit a person with a guard to protect the teeth. Stress-reduction therapies such as progressive muscle relaxation may help.[56]

- **Circadian rhythm disturbances** have a number of underlying causes. Here are the main types of biological rhythm upheavals:

    Jet-lag disorder results from rapidly crossing time zones. You fly to Paris full of excitement to tour the Eiffel Tower, shop along the Champs-Élysées, stroll along the Seine River, and hang at outdoor cafes. But when you straggle off the plane at 9 a.m. local time, your body insists it's the middle of the night and propels you toward the nearest bed. Resist that urge. Expose yourself to the Parisian sunlight. If you nap, keep it short. Don't sleep until dark. Jet lag tends to be worse when traveling east. It can take a day to recover from each time zone crossed.[57]

    Shift-work disorder occurs when a job requires a person to work when he or she ought to be asleep. Shift work, which has become more common in our 24-hour society, can entail permanent night shifts, rotating schedules, or occasionally having to work overnight. Because we're diurnal mammals, we don't adjust to topsy-turvy schedules. The internal clock continues to run on a diurnal schedule. Alerting chemicals foil daytime sleep and sleep-inducing chemicals make it difficult to resist nighttime sleep. Some people cope better than others.[58] Most feel continually jet lagged, only without the benefit of suddenly finding themselves in the Caribbean. People who work shifts face a huge risk of disorders associated with sleep deprivation.[59]

    Delayed sleep-phase disorder occurs when a person habitually keeps very late bedtimes—2 a.m. or later. Falling asleep earlier is nearly impossible because the circadian clock is still on alert. The problem comes when school, work, or social engagements require the person to be awake and functional before 10 a.m.

    Advanced sleep-phase disorder produces the opposite situation: staying awake past dinnertime is difficult to impossible. People with this disorder fall asleep early in the evening and awaken at dawn or earlier. If they manage to stay awake for a nighttime engagement, they still pop awake at the usual time.

For all the circadian rhythm disturbances, manipulating zeitgebers can help reset the biological clock. Low-dose melatonin can be taken in the morning to delay the clock and in the evening to advance the clock. Exposure to bright light in the morning advances the clock, while evening light delays the clock. Chronotherapy—gradually, systematically shifting the bedtime toward a more acceptable schedule—is sometimes also used.

sleep bruxism

Clenching or grinding the teeth during sleep.

circadian rhythm disturbances

Conditions that arise from a mismatch between a person's biological clock and the dark-light cycle.

jet-lag disorder

A transient circadian rhythm disorder that arises after rapid travel across time zones.

shift-work disorder

A type of circadian rhythm disorder caused when people work during the normal sleep period.

delayed sleep-phase disorder

A condition wherein people fall asleep and wake up at times later than is conventional.

advanced sleep-phase disorder

A condition wherein people feel compelled to go to sleep and wake up much earlier than most of the rest of society.

6.1   Banishing Insomnia

insomnia

Difficulty falling asleep and/or staying asleep.

Insomnia, much like fever, is a symptom, not a disease. Most people have spent at least one night tossing and turning. For some, it's an all too common occurrence; chronic insomnia affects 10 to 15 percent of the population.[60] Insomniacs can have difficulty falling asleep and/or staying asleep. They may experience frequent awakenings or awaken too early. A night of tossing and turning is less than refreshing.

The hyperarousal of our 24-7 lifestyle and stress, particularly psychological stress, are common causes. A number of other factors can also interfere with sleep (see Table 4.2). Furthermore, some people, after a few sleepless nights, can develop anxiety about sleep itself, thus perpetuating the problem.

TABLE 4.2   Things That Disrupt Sleep

Medical disorders: painful conditions (including fibromyalgia,[61] respiratory conditions [asthma, coughs, colds, chronic obstructive lung disease], heart conditions [heart failure], urinary conditions [bladder infections, prostate enlargement], gastrointestinal conditions [gastroesophageal (acid) reflux disease, inflammatory bowel disease, irritable bowel syndrome])
Sleep disorders: all the dyssomnias interfere with sleep
Psychiatric disorders: depression, anxiety, bipolar disorder, schizophrenia
Stress overload, especially when accompanied by worry and anxiety
Medications: some of the drugs to treat pain, asthma, psychiatric disorders, and ADHD
Substances: caffeine, alcohol, tobacco, marijuana, amphetamines, opioids
Incandescent lighting, as well as the light emitted by backlit electronic screens, suppresses nighttime melatonin release.
Overwork, overscheduling
Circadian rhythm disruptions: shift work, jet travel
Environmental factors: noise, light, room too hot or too cold, ascending rapidly to high altitudes
Roommates, bed partners, pets, children

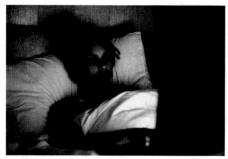

Working on electronic devices at night can delay melatonin and stimulate the brain.

© Shutterstock

Ideally, treatment should address the underlying problem. However, too few chronic insomniacs seek treatment and too few of those who do see a doctor receive adequate treatment. Perhaps it's not surprising that about a third of insomniacs self-medicate with alcohol or over-the-counter medications.[62] Improving sleep habits is a first step for people whose own behaviors are sabotaging sleep. Section 7 discusses sleep hygiene.

A number of **nondrug treatments** have been shown to correct insomnia. They include cognitive behavioral therapy (learning to replace self-defeating thoughts, feelings, and behaviors with healthy ones), biofeedback (using monitors of functions like heart rate and brain activity to learn to control them), progressive muscle relaxation, acupuncture and acupressure (use of blunt pressure on acupuncture points), yoga, and tai chi (a Chinese form of slow, meditative exercises).[63],[64]

Prescription medications such as benzodiazepines (a group of drugs that includes Valium, Restoril, Halcion, Serax, and others) and imidazopyridines (a group of drugs that includes Ambien, Sonata, and Lunesta) are effective and relatively safe. The risk for abuse with these drugs is quite low.

However, discontinuation of the sleep-inducing drugs can trigger a resurgence of insomnia.[65] Both drug categories can produce anterograde amnesia (loss of memory for short periods of time while on the drug).[66] Ambien has also been linked to sleep-related behaviors such as sleepwalking, though the risk seems to be greater with higher doses (more than 10 mg) and not going to bed right after taking the pill.[67] Some experts point out that the hazards associated with chronic insomnia's sleep deprivation outweigh those associated with these drugs.

Over-the-counter medications are of limited value for insomniacs. They contain antihistamines (drugs used for allergies and colds) and can produce side effects such as dry mouth and nose, dizziness, blurred vision, and residual morning sedation.[68]

Before the advent of pharmaceuticals, insomniacs turned to **medicinal plants**. The best-researched hypnotic herb is valerian (*Valeriana officinalis*). More than 20 studies, most of them with positive results, have investigated this herb's ability to promote sleep. Some studies show that extracts of the root decrease sleep latency (the time to fall asleep) and the number of nighttime awakenings, and improve overall sleep quality.[69] Extracts have been successfully used to improve the sleep of chronic insomniacs who stopped taking benzodiazepines.[70]

Valerian has also been shown effective in combination with hops (*Humulus lupulus*)[71] and/or lemon balm (*Melissa officinalis*).[72],[73] That same combination also neutralized the arousing effects of caffeine on the central nervous system.[74] Less well-researched but promising herbs include California poppy (*Eschscholzia californica*) and passion flower (*Passiflora incarnata*).[75]

Because the smell of the valerian root has been likened to old gym socks, most people prefer to take this herb as a concentrated product extracted into water and alcohol (tincture) or as an encapsulated standardized extract. Research supports doses of 400 to 900 mg valerian extract taken about 30 minutes before bedtime. One study found that, while a single dose didn't help chronic insomniacs, a two-week regimen did.[76] Side effects are rare and mild. The herb doesn't cause morning "hangover." It's not recommended for pregnant and nursing women and children under the age of three years. Theoretically, the herb could augment the effects of alcohol and sedative drugs.

Aromatherapy with calming essential oils from plants such as lavender, chamomile, and ylang-ylang may also improve sleep. One study found that smelling lavender essential oil helped seniors maintain sleep as they withdrew from benzodiazepines.[77] These highly concentrated plant essential oils should not be taken internally. Rather, they are inhaled or diluted with a carrier oil and applied topically. (See Chapter 2 for more information on this therapy.)

Melatonin, the pineal gland hormone that rises at night, regulates several physiologic processes, including sleep-wake cycles. In many people, this hormone declines with age. Blood levels have been shown to be lower in elderly insomniacs than in people the same age who didn't have insomnia.[78]

The question is whether taking melatonin as a supplement improves sleep. Studies show that, in elderly people with low levels, supplemental melatonin can improve sleep. Not all studies, however, are positive, and most experts don't consider it an effective remedy for run-of-the-mill insomnia.

As mentioned earlier, melatonin can help reset the biological clock. While the efficacy in people who do shift work isn't impressive, supplements may help people who travel by jet, are blind, or have delayed sleep phase syndrome (habitually going to bed very late).[79] Interestingly, a new category of sleep medication involves using an altered version of melatonin.[80]

The specific dose for melatonin has yet to be clearly defined. Low doses (0.3 to 0.5 mg) are taken to reset the clock. To induce sleep, the usual recommendations are 1 to 5 mg one-half hour to one hour before bed. Side effects are few and mild and may include morning grogginess, dizziness, and headaches. Use is discouraged in children (though research studies exist in children with developmental disabilities) and in women who wish to become or are pregnant.[81]

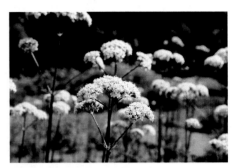

Flowers of valerian (*Valeriana officinalis*). Extracts made from the root of this plant are a traditional remedy against insomnia.

© *Shutterstock*

KEY TAKEAWAY

- Sleep disorders are all too common. Worse, too many people don't receive adequate treatment for these conditions. The consequences are excessive daytime sleepiness, reduced quality of life, and also the other disorders associated with chronic sleep deprivation.

DISCUSSION QUESTIONS

1. Can people who work the night shift adjust completely to working at night and sleeping during the day? Defend your answer.

2. Your aunt jokes about your uncle's loud snoring. It's clear she thinks his noisy sleep is annoying but not serious. What do you think?

3. Whenever Angela is still, her calves begin to ache. As soon as she moves her legs, the feeling subsides, only to return again when she stops moving. The problem interferes with her ability to study and sleep. What condition does Angela have?

4. Five-year-old Nate sometimes awakens screaming in the night. How would his parents know whether he's having a sleep terror or a nightmare? How might the response differ for each of these conditions?

5. Trudy brings Ralph, her 80-year-old husband, to the doctor. She says that the night before, she awoke with Ralph's hands around her neck. When she screamed, he awakened and apologized repeatedly. He said he had dreamed that someone was trying to kill her. Over the past months, Ralph has had other nighttime episodes when he swears, kicks, and breaks things. He has bruises on his forearms and shins. During the day, he's kind and even-tempered. What sleep disorder does he likely have?

6. Rachel feels extremely sleepy all day and frequently falls asleep. She doesn't dare drive. She guards her emotions because laughter, tears, or rage can trigger an embarrassing loss of muscle control. What sleep disorder might she have?

7. Xavier is a high-school senior who's always been a night owl. His tendency to stay up late has gotten so extreme that his parents can't get him to wake up at 6:30 a.m. He snoozes through his first couple of classes. The summer before, he lost a job as a house painter because he kept showing up late. A teacher advises that his parents simply force Xavier to go to bed by 10 p.m. Would that strategy work? If not, why not?

8. Think about a time when you were unable to sleep. Do you remember what might have interfered with your sleep? How many nights did the insomnia last? What did you do? Did your actions (or inactions) help you get to sleep? Now that you've read this chapter, what might you do differently?

7. HOW TO SLEEP BETTER

LEARNING OBJECTIVES

1. List steps involved in improving sleep hygiene.
2. Explain why substances such as caffeine, alcohol, and tobacco can interfere with normal sleep.

Myriad factors can interfere with sleep, including physical and psychological maladies, disturbances in circadian rhythm, and drugs that affect the central nervous system. More commonly, we simply don't schedule enough time to sleep.

The key to sleeping better and feeling better is to rank adequate sleep high on your priority list. Put it up on the pedestal with food, shelter, and intimacy. Identify the things that interfere with a good night's sleep, and see if you can steadily eliminate them.

The next step is to clean up your **sleep hygiene**, those behaviors and environmental factors relevant to good sleep. The term may conjure the image of a nurse marching into your bedroom to snatch away laptops and cell phones, sharply tuck in the sheets, and snap off the light. Nevertheless, adopting healthy sleep habits can work wonders. Try these strategies yourself.

- **Maintain a regular schedule for bedtime and awakening time.** This step is probably the most important of all. Irregular bedtimes put you out of sync with your biological clock and produce less refreshing sleep.

- **Keep naptimes short and limit them to one a day.** Time them to the afternoon dip in your circadian alerting process. Set an alarm so that you don't snooze more than 30 to 45 minutes. Otherwise, you'll have trouble sleeping that night.

- **If you drink alcohol, drink moderately.** Most experts recommend you avoid alcohol four to six hours before bedtime. Most adults ignore that advice, given that they'd be fired if they had a cocktail at work. Alcohol is problematic for a number of reasons. One, in terms of central nervous system impairment, alcohol and sleep deprivation have an additive effect.[82] Two, alcohol in higher amounts *interferes* with sleep. Although it can make people sleepy, that effect fades quickly with habitual use. High doses of alcohol lead to light, restless sleep, particularly in the second half of the night.[83]

- **Chill on the caffeine.** While caffeine helps maintain alertness, the downsides are temporary increases in heart rate and blood pressure, jitteriness, insomnia, and dependency. Much of the morning fuzziness habitual users experience represents withdrawal symptoms. Blood levels of caffeine peak within 30 minutes to an hour of consumption. The average time to eliminate *half* the caffeine consumed is *5 hours*. The clearance time is longer in women on birth control pills[84] or in the latter months of pregnancy.[85] Because caffeinated sodas and "energy" drinks like Red Bull and Monster are sweet and cold, people tend to gulp them rather than sip them, leading to spikes in caffeine rather than a smooth, steady rise. Consider drinking green tea instead, which has much less caffeine.

- **Nix the nicotine.** It stimulates the nervous system. Cigarette smokers tend to sleep less well than nonsmokers. Some of the disruption may stem from cravings as nicotine levels fall.[86]

- **Avoid heavy late-night meals.** Consider a bedtime snack if episodes of low blood sugar interrupt your sleep. According to the National Diabetes Information Clearinghouse, symptoms of hypoglycemia during sleep include crying out and nightmares, waking up in sweaty bedclothes, and feeling irritable or confused.

- **Exercise daily.** This will help you sleep more deeply. Gentle stretching and relaxing yoga poses can be part of your bedtime routine. Avoid strenuous exercise before bed, as it can make it harder to fall asleep.

- **Create a cozy sleep environment.** The temperature should be just right—not too warm and not too cold. Select comfortable bedding. Block out the light with window shades and coverings over electronic devices that emit light. Turn up the quiet—turn off the television and silence your cell phone and your music player. (Even quiet music can disrupt sleep.) If your environment is noisy, invest in good earplugs.

- **Use the bed for sleep and sex only.** Don't work, study, chat, play games, watch videos, argue, balance your checkbook, or do anything mentally stimulating in that sacred space. If you're a worrier, set aside a time earlier in the evening to vent your frustrations, review the day, plan for the next day, and make lists.

- **Create soothing bedtime rituals.** Light a candle (but remember to blow it out before you close your eyes). Take a warm bath with 10 to 15 drops of calming plant essential oils. Alternatively, use a diffuser to scent the bedroom with calming essential oils or blend a few drops into lotion/oil and apply to your hands, neck, forehead, and chest (avoid eyes).

- **Let go.** When you lie down, mentally scan your body for areas of tension. Inhale and deliberately tighten that muscle; with an exhalation, release. Appreciate the support of the bed and pillows; visualize restful sleep and sweet dreams. To calm your mind, focus on your breathing. Inhale through your nose to a slow count of four, exhale to a count of eight. Notice your belly rises with inhalation and falls with exhalation.

Try This at Home: Create a Sleep Diary

To better understand your sleep patterns and behaviors, try keeping a sleep diary for a week or two. It may help you identify the root cause of daytime sleepiness and poor nighttime sleep. Each day, record the following things:

- the time you went to bed the night before
- roughly how long it took to fall asleep
- the number of times you awakened in the night and the duration of each awakening
- the overall quality of your sleep
- the time you got up in the morning
- the number of hours asleep during the night
- timing and duration of naps
- your dreams. For this optional task, keep a bedside notebook, as the details of dreams fade quickly.
- your level of alertness at several times over the day (midmorning, noon, midafternoon, early evening, late evening). You can either use the Epworth Sleepiness Scale or simply describe whether you feel bright-eyed, fuzzy-headed, dog-tired, or semicomatose.
- lifestyle habits or environmental influences that might affect your nighttime sleep (e.g., the times of day you consumed caffeinated beverages or drank alcohol, performed mentally stimulating activities late at night, and so on)

When to Seek Help

Chronic exhaustion can be a sign of an underlying condition that deserves medical attention. Call the clinic if you have any of the following signs or symptoms:

- You feel tired most days, despite taking steps to get sufficient sleep.
- You snore loudly or have been told that you do. If you want confirmation, set a tape recorder while you sleep. Be particularly concerned if you hear a pattern of snoring, no sound, then a gasp—a pattern suggestive of obstructive sleep apnea.
- You have signs or symptoms of restless legs syndrome, narcolepsy, or periodic limb movement disorder as described in this chapter.
- You have more than occasional episodes of sleepwalking, particularly if you have injured yourself or someone else.
- You have chronic insomnia or a condition such as heartburn, nightmares, or discomfort that often fragments your sleep.

KEY TAKEAWAYS

- Stress overload, overscheduling, noise, ambient light, some substances, insomnia, and a number of health challenges can keep you from getting enough good-quality sleep.
- You can, however, control a number of factors that influence sleep. Maintaining regular sleep-wake schedules, avoiding sleep-spoiling substances, and creating a peaceful sleep environment are key.

DISCUSSION QUESTION

1. After you read the following case, write an analysis of this student's sleep behaviors and make suggestions for how she might improve her sleep.

   Alison is a theater major on a partial scholarship. To supplement her finances, she works the morning shift at the college coffee house. A large latté in hand, she runs to her afternoon classes. No matter what, she usually nods off in lecture. In the evenings, she grabs a quick dinner and a diet soda and rushes to play rehearsal. At about 10 p.m., she returns to the dorm to study and relax with friends. At 1 p.m., she gets in bed but usually has trouble getting to sleep. When that happens, she drinks a beer, smokes a cigarette, turns on her MP3 player, jams her headset into her ears, and closes her eyes. Her sleep is fitful and sometimes interrupted by texts and calls from friends. By Friday night, she's exhausted but parties anyway. Saturday and Sunday, she sleeps until about 1 p.m. Sunday night, she has a hard time getting to sleep. Early Monday morning, the week begins again as she trudges grimly off to work.

8. RECOMMENDED RESOURCES

8.1 Books

Dement WC. *The Promise of Sleep*. New York, NY: Dell; 1999.

Epstein L, Mardon S. *The Harvard Medical School Guide to a Good Night's Sleep*. New York, NY: McGraw-Hill; 2006.

Hauri P, Linde S. *No More Sleepless Nights*. New York, NY: Wiley & Sons; 1996.

Moorcroft WH. *Understanding Sleep and Dreaming*. New York, NY: Kluwer Academic/Plenum; 2003.

Schenck C. *Sleep: The Mysteries, the Problems, and the Solutions*. New York, NY: Avery; 2007.

8.2 Organizations and Websites

American Academy of Sleep Medicine. http://www.sleepeducation.com.

Centers for Disease Control and Prevention. Sleep. http://www.cdc.gov/sleep/index.htm.

Howard Hughes Medical Institute has lectures and video demonstrations, such as this video on the biological clock: http://www.hhmi.org/biointeractive/clocks/SCN.html, as well as lectures such as "Clockwork Genes: Discoveries in Biological Time." Available at http://www.hhmi.org/biointeractive/clockwork-genes-discoveries-biological-time.

Information about Sleep. National Institutes of Health. http://science.education.nih.gov/supplements/nih3/sleep/guide/info-sleep.htm.

National Institute of Neurologic Disorders and Stroke. Brain basics: understanding sleep. http://www.ninds.nih.gov/disorders/brain_basics/understanding_sleep.htm.

National Sleep Foundation. http://www.sleepfoundation.org.

Sleep Home Pages. http://www.sleephomepages.org. Within this site is a syllabus with explanations of many aspects of sleep. Available at http://www.sleephomepages.org/sleepsyllabus.

The Sleep Well. There's a wealth of information on the personal site of pioneer sleep researcher Dr. William C. Dement. http://www.stanford.edu/~dement.

University of Maryland Sleep Disorders Center. This site has useful information on sleep. http://www.umm.edu/sleep/index.htm.

8.3 Podcasts

Sleep. WNYC's Radiolab. http://www.radiolab.org/2007/may/24. Or go to iTunes, search for WNYC's Radiolab, and listen for free to the May 24, 2007, episode on sleep. You can also subscribe to Radiolab for free on iTunes.

ENDNOTES

1. Centers for Disease Control and Prevention. Unhealthy sleep-related behaviors—12 states, 2009. *MMWR Morb Mortal Wkly Rep.* 2011 Mar 4;60(08):233–238. Available at: http://www.cdc.gov/mmwr/preview/mmwrhtml/mm6008a2.htm. Accessed April 22, 2011.

2. Centers for Disease Control and Prevention. Effect of short sleep duration on daily activities—United States, 2005–2008. *MMWR Morb Mortal Wkly Rep.* 2011 Mar 4;60(08):239–242.

3. Sleepy Connected Americans. National Sleep Foundation. Available at: http://www.sleepfoundation.org/alert/sleepy-connected-americans. Published March 7, 2011. Accessed April 22, 2011.

4. Vassalli A, Dijk DJ. Sleep function: current questions and new approaches. *Eur J Neurosci.* 2009 May;29(9):1830–1841.

5. Siegel JM. Clues to the functions of mammalian sleep. *Nature.* 2005;437(27):1264–1271. doi:10.1038/nature04385.

6. Steiger A. Sleep and endocrinology. *SRS Basics of Sleep Guide.* Westchester, IL: Sleep Research Society; 2005:100–101.

7. Preston BT, Capellini I, McNamara P, Barton RA, Nunn CL. Parasite resistance and the adaptive significance of sleep. *BMC Evol Biol.* 2009;9:7.

8. Vassalli A, Dijk DJ. Sleep function: current questions and new approaches. *Eur J Neurosci.* 2009 May;29(9):1830–1841.

9. Wamsley EJ, Perry K, Djonlagic I, Reaven LB, Stickgold R. Cognitive replay of visuomotor learning at sleep onset: temporal dynamics and relationship to task performance. *Sleep.* 2010 Jan 1;33(1):59–68.

10. Wilhelm I, Diekelmann S, Molzow I, Ayoub A, Mölle M, Born J. Sleep selectively enhances memory expected to be of future relevance. *J Neurosci.* 2011 Feb 2;31(5):1563–1569. Available at: http://www.jneurosci.org/content/31/5/1563.long. Accessed December 19, 2012.

11. Banks S, Dongen H, Maislin G, Dinges DF. Neurobehavioral dynamics following chronic sleep restriction: dose-response effects of one night of recovery. *Sleep.* 2010;33(8):1013–1026.

12. Gais S, Lucas B, Born J. Sleep after learning aids memory recall. *Learn Mem.* 2006 May–Jun;13(3):259–262.

13. Moorcroft, WH. *Understanding Sleep and Dreaming.* New York, NY: Kluwer Academic/Plenum; 2003:53.

14. Smaldone A, Honig JC, Byrne MW. Sleepless in America: inadequate sleep and relationships to health and well-being of our nation's children. *Pediatr.* 2007 Feb;119(suppl 1):29–37.

15. Wolfson AR, Carskadon MA. Sleep schedules and daytime functioning in adolescents. *Child Dev.* 1998;69(4):875–887.

16. Tarokh L, Raffray T, Van Reen E, Carskadon MA. Physiology of normal sleep in adolescents. *Adolesc Med*: State of the Art Reviews. 2010 Dec;21(3):401–417, vii.

17. Wahlstrom KL. Accommodating the sleep patterns of adolescents within current educational structures: an uncharted path. In: Carskadon MA, ed. *Adolescent Sleep Patterns: Biological, Social, and Psychological Influences.* Cambridge, UK: Cambridge University Press; 2002:172–197.

18. Cajochen C, Frey S, Anders D, et al. Evening exposure to a light emitting diodes (LED)-backlit computer screen affects circadian physiology and cognitive performance. *J Appl Physiol.* doi:10.1152/japplphysiol.00165.2011. Revised March 17, 2011.

19. Ancoli-Israel S. Normal human sleep at different ages: sleep in the older adult. *SRS Basics of Sleep Guide.* 1st ed. Westchester, IL: Sleep Research Society; 2005.

20. Breslau N, Roth T, Rosenthal L, Adreski P. Daytime sleepiness: an epidemiological study of young adults. *Am J Public Health.* 1997;87:1649–1653.

21. Orzeł-Gryglewska J. Consequences of sleep deprivation. *Int J Occup Environ Health.* 2010;23(1):95–114.

22. Peters BR, Joireman J, Ridgway RL. Individual differences in the consideration of future consequences scale correlate with sleep habits, sleep quality, and GPA in university students. *Psychol Rep.* 2005 Jun;96(3 Pt 1):817–824.

23. Chang SJ, Chae KY. Obstructive sleep apnea syndrome in children: epidemiology, pathophysiology, diagnosis and sequelae. *Korean J Pediatr.* 2010 Oct;53(10):863–871.

24. Van Dongen HP, Maislin G, Mullington JM, Dinges DF. The cumulative cost of additional wakefulness: dose-response effects on neurobehavioral functions and sleep physiology from chronic sleep restriction and total sleep deprivation. *Sleep.* 2003;26:117–126.

25. Banks S, Van Dongen HP, Maislin G, Dinges DF. Neurobehavioral dynamics following chronic sleep restriction: dose-response effects of one night for recovery. *Sleep.* 2010 Aug 1;33(8):1013–1026.

26. Moorcroft, WH. *Understanding Sleep and Dreaming.* New York, NY: Kluwer Academic/Plenum; 2003:38.

27. Sapolsky R. Stress and a good night's sleep. *Why Zebras Don't Get Ulcers.* 3rd ed. New York, NY: Owl/Henry Holt; 2004.

28. Garaulet M, Ordovás JM, Madrid JA. The chronobiology, etiology and pathophysiology of obesity. *Int J Obes.* 2010 Dec;34(12):1667–1683.

29. Tsujimura T, Matsuo Y, Keyaki T, Sakurada K, Imanishi J. Correlations of sleep disturbance with the immune system in type 2 diabetes mellitus. *Diabetes Res Clin Pract.* 2009 Sep;85(3):286–292.

30. Newman AB, Spiekerman CF, Enright P, et al.; The Cardiovascular Health Study Research Group. Daytime sleepiness predicts mortality and cardiovascular disease in older adults. *J Am Geriatr Soc.* 2000 Feb;48(2):115–123.

31. Bollinger T, Bollinger A, Oster H, Solbach W. Sleep, immunity, and circadian clocks: a mechanistic model. *Gerontology.* 2010;56(6):574–580.

32. Haack M, Sanchez E, Mullington JM. Elevated inflammatory markers in response to prolonged sleep restriction are associated with increased pain experience in healthy volunteers. *Sleep.* 2007 Sep 1;30(9):1145–1152.

33. Bruni O, Russo PM, Ferri R, Novelli L, Galli F, Guidetti V. Relationships between headache and sleep in a non-clinical population of children and adolescents. *Sleep Med.* 2008 Jul;9(5):542–548.

34. Ranjbaran Z, Keefer L, Stepanski E, Farhadi A, Keshavarzian A. The relevance of sleep abnormalities to chronic inflammatory conditions. *Inflamm Res.* 2007 Feb;56(2):51–57.

35. Glozier N, Martiniuk A, Patton G, et al. Short sleep duration in prevalent and persistent psychological distress in young adults: the DRIVE study. *Sleep.* 2010;33(09):1139–1145.

36. Gangwisch J, Babiss L, Malaspina D, Turner J, Zammit G, Posner K. Earlier parental set bedtimes as a protective factor against depression and suicidal ideation. *Sleep.* 2010;33(01):97–106.

37. Bourdet C, Goldenberg F. Insomnia in anxiety: sleep EEG changes. *J Psychosom Res.* 1994;38(1)(suppl):93–104.

38. Kahn-Greene ET, Killgore DB, Kamimori GH, Balkin TJ, Killgore WD. The effects of sleep deprivation on symptoms of psychopathology in healthy adults. *Sleep Med.* 2007 Apr;8(3):215–221.

39. Centers for Disease Control and Prevention. Unhealthy sleep-related behaviors—12 states, 2009. *MMWR Morb Mortal Wkly Rep.* 2011 Mar 4;60(08):233–238. Available at: http://www.cdc.gov/mmwr/preview/mmwrhtml/mm6008a2.htm. Accessed April 22, 2011.

40. Vennelle M, Engleman HM, Douglas NJ. Sleepiness and sleep-related accidents in commercial bus drivers. *Sleep Breath.* 2010 Feb;14(1):39–42.

41. Pack AI, Pack AM, Rodgman E, Cucchiara A, Dinges DF, Schwab CW. Characteristics of crashes attributed to the driver having fallen asleep. *Accid Anal Prev.* 1995 Dec;27(6):769–775.

42. Powell NB, Schechtman KB, Riley RW, Kasey L, Troell R, Guilleminault C. The road to danger: the comparative risks of driving while sleepy. *Laryngoscope.* 2001;111(5):887–893.

43. Colorado DUI & DWAI Laws: Fines & Penalties. DrivingLaws.org. Available at: http://dui.drivinglaws.org/colorado.php. Accessed May 1, 2011.

44. Vakulin A, Baulk SD, Catcheside PG, et al. Effects of moderate sleep deprivation and low-dose alcohol on driving simulator performance and perception in young men. *Sleep.* 2007 Oct 1;30(10):1327–1333.

45. Roehrs T, Beare D, Zorick F, Roth T. Sleepiness and ethanol effects on simulated driving. *Alcohol Clin Exp Res.* 1994 Feb;18(1):154–158.

46. Moorcroft, WH. *Understanding Sleep and Dreaming.* New York, NY: Kluwer Academic/Plenum; 2003:209.

47. Lumley M, Roehrs T, Zorick F, Lamphere J, Roth T. The alerting effects of naps in sleep-deprived subjects. *Psychophysiology.* 1986 Jul;23(4):403–408.

48. Institute of Medicine. *Sleep Disorders and Sleep Deprivation: an Unmet Public Health Problem.* Washington, DC: The National Academies Press; 2006.

49. Gaultney JF. The prevalence of sleep disorders in college students: impact on academic performance. *J Am Coll Health.* 2010 Sep–Oct;59(2):91–97.

50. Young T, Evans L, Finn L, Palta M. Estimation of the clinically diagnosed proportion of sleep apnea syndrome in middle-aged men and women. *Sleep.* 1997 Sep;20(9):705–706.

51. Subramanian S, Bopparaju S, Desai A, Wiggins T, Rambaud C, Surani S. Sexual dysfunction in women with obstructive sleep apnea. *Sleep Breath.* 2010 Feb;14(1):59–62.

52. Shah NA, Yaggi HK, Concato J, Mohsenin V. Obstructive sleep apnea as a risk factor for coronary events or cardiovascular death. *Sleep Breath.* 2010;14(2):131–136. doi:10.1007/s11325-009-0298-7.

53. Yaggi HK, Concato J, Kernan WN, Lichtman JH, Brass LM, Mohsenin V. Obstructive sleep apnea as a risk factor for stroke and death. *N Engl J Med.* 2005 Nov 10;353(19):2034–2041.

54. Cao M, Guilleminault C. Hypocretin and its emerging role as a target for treatment of sleep disorders. *Current Neurol Neurosci Rep.* 2011 Apr;11(2):227–234.

55. Trotti LM, Rye DB. Restless legs syndrome. *Handb Clin Neurol.* 2011;100:661–673.

56. Ommerborn MA, Schneider C, Giraki M, et al. Effects of an occlusal splint compared with cognitive-behavioral treatment on sleep bruxism activity. *Eur J Oral Sci.* 2007 Feb;115(1):7–14.

57. Moorcroft, WH. *Understanding Sleep and Dreaming.* New York, NY: Kluwer Academic/Plenum; 2003:215.

58. Van Dongen HP, Belenky G. Individual differences in vulnerability to sleep loss in the work environment. *Ind Health.* 2009 Oct;47(5):518–526.

59. Chung SA, Wolf TK, Shapiro CM. Sleep and health consequences of shift work in women. *J Womens Health (Larchmt).* 2009 Jul;18(7):965–977.

60. Drake CL, Roehrs T, Roth T. Insomnia causes, consequences, and therapeutics: an overview. *Depress Anxiety.* 2003;18(4):163–176.

61. Harding SM. Sleep in fibromyalgia patients: subjective and objective findings. *Am J Med Sci.* 1998 Jun;315(6):367–376.

62. Roehrs T, Hollebeek E, Drake C, Roth T. Substance use for insomnia in Metropolitan Detroit. *J Psychosom Res.* 2002 Jul;53(1):571–576.

63. Sarris J, Byrune GJ. A systematic review of insomnia and complementary medicine. *Sleep Med Rev.* 2011;15(2):99–106.

64. Taylor DJ, Roane BM. Treatment of insomnia in adults and children: a practice-friendly review of research. *J Clin Psychol.* 2010 Nov;66(11):1137–1147.

65. Roth T. Sedative hypnotics. *SRS Basics of Sleep Guide.* Westchester, IL: Sleep Research Society; 2005:148.

66. Tsai JH, Yang P, Chen CC, et al. Zolpidem-induced amnesia and somnambulism: rare occurrences? *Eur Neuropsychopharmacol.* 2009 Jan;19(1):74–76.

67. Hwang TJ, Ni HC, Chen HC, Lin YT, Liao SC. Risk predictors for hypnosedative-related complex sleep behaviors: a retrospective, cross-sectional pilot study. *J Clin Psychiatry.* 2010 Oct;71(10):1331–1335.

68. Zhang D, Tashiro M, Shibuya K, et al. Next-day residual sedative effect after nighttime administration of an over-the-counter antihistamine sleep aid, diphenhydramine, measured by positron emission tomography. *J Clin Psychopharmacol.* 2010 Dec;30(6):694–701.

69. Salter S, Brownie S. Treating primary insomnia—the efficacy of valerian and hops. *Aust Fam Physician.* 2010 Jun;39(6):433–437.

70. Poyares DR, Guilleminault C, Ohayon MM, Tufik S. Can valerian improve the sleep of insomniacs after benzodiazepine withdrawal? *Prog Neuropsychopharacol Biol Psychiatry.* 2002;26(3):539–545.

71. Morin CM, Koetter U, Bastien C, Ware JC, Wooten V. Valerian-hops combination and diphenhydramine for treating insomnia: a randomized placebo-controlled clinical trial. *Sleep.* 2005 Nov 1;28(11):1465–1471.

72. Dressing H, Reimann D. Insomnia: are Valeriana/Melissa combinations of equal value to benzodiazepine? [Article in German.] *Therapiewoche.* 1992;42:726–736.

73. Dressing H, Kohler S, Muller W. Improvement in sleep quality with a high dose valerian-melissa prepartion. *Psychopharmacotherapy.* 1996;3:123–130. In: Blumenthal M, ed. *The ABC Clinical Guide to Herbs.* Austin, TX: American Botanical Council; 2003.

74. Schellenberg R, Sauer S, Abourashed EA, Koetter U, Brattström A. The fixed combination of valerian and hops (Ze91019) acts via a central adenosine mechanism. *Planta Med.* 2004;70(7):594–597.

75. Hoffmann, David. *Complete Illustrated Guide to the Holistic Herbal.* London: Element; 1996:208.

76. Donath F, Quispe S, Diefenbach K, Maurer A, Fietze I, Roots I. Critical evaluation of the effect of valerian extract on sleep structure and sleep quality. *Pharmacopsychiatry.* 2000 Mar;33(2):47–53.

77. Hardy M, Kir-Smith MD, Stretch DD. Replacement of drug treatment for insomnia by ambient odour. *Lancet.* 1995;346(8976):701.

78. Leger D, Laudon M, Zisapel N. Nocturnal 6-sulfatoxymelatonin excretion in insomnia and its relation to the response to melatonin replacement therapy. *Am J Med.* 2004;116(2):91–95.

79. Buscemi N, Vandermeer B, Hooton N, et al. The efficacy and safety of exogenous melatonin for primary sleep disorders. A meta-analysis. *J Gen Intern Med.* 2005;20(12):1151–1158. doi:10.1111/j.1525-1497.2005.0243.x.

80. McGechan A, Wellington K. Ramelteon. *CNS Drugs.* 2005;19:1057–1065.

81. Melatonin. Natural Medicines Comprehensive Database. Available at: http://naturaldatabase.therapeuticresearch.com/nd/Search.aspx?cs=&s=nd&pt=100&id=940. Accessed May 9, 2011.

82. Zwyghuizen-Doorenbos A, Roehrs T, Lamphere J, Zorick F, Roth T. Increased daytime sleepiness enhances ethanol's sedative effects. *Neuropsychopharmacology.* 1988 Dec;1(4):279–286.

83. Roehrs T, Roth T. Sleep, sleepiness, and alcohol use. *Alcohol Res Health.* 2001;25(2):101–109.

84. Balogh A, Klinger G, Henschel L, Börner A, Vollanth R, Kuhnz W. Influence of ethinylestradiol-containing combination oral contraceptives with gestodene or levonorgestrel on caffeine elimination. *Eur J Clin Pharmacol.* 1995;48(2):161–166.

85. Knutti R, Rothweiler H, Schlatter C. The effect of pregnancy on the pharmacokinetics of caffeine. *Arch Toxicol.* 1982;5:187–192.

86. Drugs of abuse and sleep. *SRS Basics of Sleep Guide.* Westchester, IL: Sleep Research Society; 2005.

CHAPTER 5
Psychological Health

Take a look at the following *New York Times* headlines:

"SAT and ACT to Tighten Rules after Cheating Scandal"

"Gas Leak on Offshore Platform Forces Evacuation in North Sea"

"911 Tapes Released in Killing of Florida Teenager"

"Japan—Earthquake, Tsunami and Nuclear Crisis"

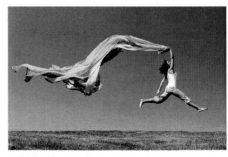
© *Thinkstock*

How frequently does good news appear in the news media? Not often. Does that mean good things don't happen? Of course not. But you'll have to admit that a headline such as "President Plays Tag with Schoolchildren" wouldn't sell many papers. Disaster and drama hook us. Just make sure they don't drag you down.

Pay attention to whether your thoughts tend toward the negative or the positive, whether your friends talk about their triumphs or their disappointments, whether they and other people around you smile or frown, and whether you listen to upbeat or depressing music. Ideas and moods are contagious. Try to catch happiness. If you look carefully, you'll see glimmers of positivity everywhere. Even in the newspaper, you can find glad tidings like this one: "Lunch-Break Dance Spreads in Europe."[1]

You can learn to become a more positive person. As with any skill, it takes practice. The first part of this chapter will discuss the elements of psychological health and provide tips on how to improve yours. Following that, we'll explore the major psychological disorders: what's known about potential causes, risk factors, warning signs and symptoms, and treatment options.

Happiness is not something ready made. It comes from your own actions.

- Dalai Lama

1. A FALSE DICHOTOMY

LEARNING OBJECTIVES

1. Discuss the interrelationship between physical and mental health.
2. Review the basic anatomy and physiology of the nervous system.
3. Define psychology and the assorted mental health specialists.
4. Outline the tenets of positive psychology.
5. Examine the effects of lifestyle and habits of thought and behavior on psychological function.

The words "mental health" suggest a distinction from physical health. But mental and physical health intertwine. The structure and function of your physical body, including your brain, influence your thoughts and emotions. A number of things—habits of thought, diet, stress, sleep patterns, physical activity, social and spiritual connectedness—modify that biology. If you consume too much caffeine, your pulse rises, your fingers tremble, and your brain generates anxious, irritable thoughts. If you're upset or frightened, your heart rate accelerates and your palms sweat. Depression causes physical and psychological symptoms. Physical processes (a heart attack), outside influences (alcohol, certain foods, influenza viruses, a blow to the head), and interior processes (psychological stress, muscle tension) can lower your mood and make your head ache.

In a nutshell, we're back to the holistic model—back to the concept that body, mind, and spirit influence one another.

1.1 Nervous System Tutorial

Before we go further, it helps to understand some brain basics. The brain belongs to the nervous system. You can divide that system into the central nervous system (spinal cord and brain) and peripheral nervous system (the nerves outside the central nervous system). Some nerves (effectors) send impulses from the central nervous system to peripheral tissues. Others (affectors) send impulses about sensory stimuli from periphery to the central nervous system.

Each individual nerve cell is called a **neuron**. Some are short and some are very long and skinny. For instance, the nerve that tells the muscles in your big toe to flex runs the full length of your leg. Neurons transmit information in a two-step process. First, an electrical wave spreads down the neuron. Second, chemicals called **neurotransmitters** are released into the *synapse*, the tiny gap separating one neuron from another. Depending on the type and amount of neurotransmitter released, the next neuron's electrical impulse is stimulated or inhibited.

In the brain, various neurotransmitters are associated with learning, attention, pleasure, mood, sleep, and other functions. Chemicals made by other organs also affect the brain. For instance, the immune system generates inflammatory chemicals that make you feel sleepy. Also nerve growth factors in the central and peripheral nervous system protect and support neurons.

Perhaps you're wondering whether having a bigger brain makes you smarter and more successful? Not necessarily. If that were the case, the average professional basketball player (six foot six inches tall) could outsmart someone like Albert Einstein (five foot nine inches). Large animals such as whales, elephants, walruses, and camels have much heavier brains than humans.[2]

Here's another reason brain size is less critical than you might think: Not all the cells in your brain are neurons. Support cells called *neuroglia* tend to the neurons. Furthermore, you don't use the full potential of your brain. That *reserve capacity* helps offset loss of cells that happens with age. Lastly, more is not necessarily better. For example, studies suggest that small children with autism have too many neurons crowded into the part of the brain responsible for language development and social and emotional communication.[3]

What's most important are the connections among the brain's neurons. At birth, the skull is crammed with about 100 billion neurons. But compared to the adult brain, the connections among these neurons are sparse. The infant's experiences facilitate the formation of groups of connected neurons called *neural networks*. Much-used neurons branch to form synapses with other neurons in that pathway. Unused neurons wither and die. You end up with fewer but better-connected neurons to help you function optimally.

This branching and pruning demonstrates the principle of *neural plasticity*: your brain can change in response to your experiences. Experiences in the womb and in early childhood powerfully influence brain development. Throughout life, your thoughts and actions continually remodel your brain. That means you can't fall back on excuses like "My brain isn't good at math" or "My brain is wired to be pessimistic."

There's more good news. Not long ago, scientists thought that once the brain fully develops, it couldn't make new neurons (a process called *neurogenesis*). In 1998, researchers provided evidence that an area of the brain called the hippocampus can generate neurons throughout life.[4] This brain area has numerous functions, including memory formation and retrieval. You may remember from Chapter 3 that the hippocampus is involved in the stress response and is damaged by chronically high levels of the stress hormone cortisol. How fortunate that, given a reprieve, the hippocampus is capable of recovery.

One last principle is that the brain develops from inner layers to outer layers, from a more primitive to a more sophisticated area. A primitive area called the brain stem is basically an extension of the spinal cord. It controls automatic processes such as heartbeat and breathing. The crowning glory is the cerebrum, the outermost part of the brain. Wrinkled as a walnut to maximize surface area, the outermost layer of the cerebrum is the cortex, also referred to as the gray matter. Compared to other animals, humans have relatively thick cortices. The cerebrum is key in processing all the information coming into the brain, including the five senses: taste, touch, vision, hearing, and smell. From the constant barrage of incoming data, the cerebrum synthesizes our perception of the world. (To some extent, "reality" is all in your head.)

neuron

A nerve cell.

neurotransmitter

A chemical released upon arrival of a nerve impulse at the end of a neuron that transmits the impulse to adjacent neurons.

FIGURE 5.1 The Nervous System

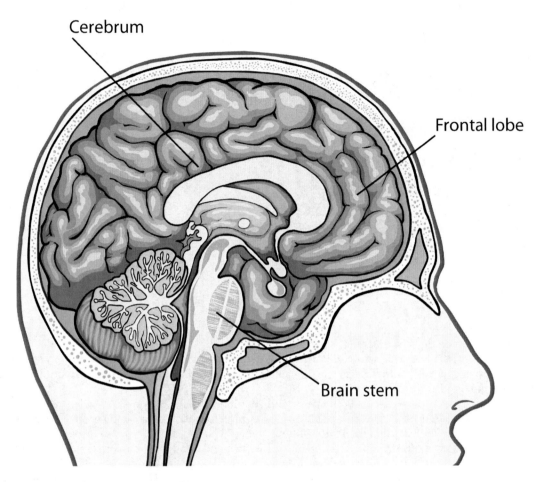

© *Thinkstock*

The cerebrum develops from back to front. The very last area to mature is the prefrontal cortex, an area just above your eyes.[5] This lofty area contributes to personality and the regulation of thoughts, emotions, and behaviors. It allows you to focus your attention, solve problems, analyze, make decisions, judge situations, and predict outcomes based on available data. It suppresses urges arising from lower brain areas. Thanks to your prefrontal cortex, you can refrain from urinating in public, kissing attractive strangers, eating all the cookies in the bag, and smacking the person who cuts in line ahead of you. Some degenerative brain diseases attack this brain area. Alcohol and other sedatives inhibit prefrontal cortex function. The fact that the prefrontal cortex doesn't finish developing until well into adulthood explains why children and adolescents sometimes behave in irrational ways.

  Video Link 5.1

Brain Basics

The National Institute of Mental Health has produced a video that explains the basic structure and function of the brain, the way it grows, the way depression can affect the brain, and techniques involved in studying the brain.

http://www.nimh.nih.gov/brainbasics/index.html

Video Clip 5.1

Neurons and How They Work
This video shows neurons and how they work.

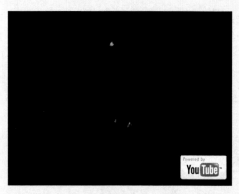

View the video online at: http://www.youtube.com/v/FR4S1BqdFG4

1.2 Psychology

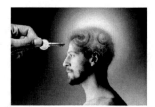

© Thinkstock

psychology

The study of the mind and behavior.

psychologist

A professional with doctoral training in psychology.

psychotherapy

The nondrug treatment for mental disorders under the care of a mental health provider.

psychiatrist

A medical doctor with specialized training in psychiatry.

psychiatry

The science of diagnosing and treating mental, emotional, and behavioral problems.

Interest in human thought processes, emotional responses, and behaviors dates back to ancient Greece. Greek philosopher Aristotle wrote about the *psyche*, the conscious and unconscious human mind. Formal experimental inquiries began in the late 19th century, birthing the field of **psychology**, the study of the mind and behavior.

Psychological health includes both mental and emotional health. *Mental health* refers to our ability to think, process information, reason, judge, problem solve, formulate plans, and perceive life events in realistic ways. *Emotional health* has to do with our feelings and subjective response to events. Thoughts and emotions then motivate our behaviors. Ideally, we respond in rational, measured, peaceful, and appropriate ways.

Within the discipline of psychology lie many specialty areas. People with doctoral training in the field are called **psychologists**. Some do research, some teach, some counsel patients. During counseling sessions, psychologists generally use **psychotherapy**. A variety of therapies exist to help people understand and resolve their issues. However, other types of professionals also provide services to address mental, emotional, and behavioral health.

Psychiatrists are medical doctors (MDs) with specialty training in **psychiatry**, the science of diagnosing, preventing, and treating mental, emotional, and behavioral problems. Although most do little if any psychotherapy, they can diagnose mental health disorders (also called psychiatric disorders) and prescribe medications. Primary care physicians such as family doctors, pediatricians, and internists can also prescribe psychiatric medications, though they lack in-depth training in psychiatric disorders.

Psychiatric nurses have specialized training in psychiatry and some forms of psychotherapy. In some states, they may also be able to prescribe medications.

Clinical social workers have a master's degree in social work (MSW). Additional specialty training leads to the Licensed Counselor of Social Work (LCSW) designation. They can counsel and perform some forms of psychotherapy but cannot prescribe medications.

Marriage and family therapists usually have a master's degree with training in psychology.

1.3 Mental Wellness: Positive Psychology

Just as medicine concentrates on disease, psychologists and psychiatrists have, for many years, focused on mental illness. That study has clarified the risk factors for mental illness so we can attempt to avoid them. Furthermore, a better understanding of the biological changes associated with psychiatric illness has led to new treatments for many conditions.

For a time, scientists and doctors were so wrapped up in understanding mental illnesses, they neglected to study mental health. The World Health Organization (WHO) recognizes that it's more than a lack of mental illness. The Declaration of Independence lists the "pursuit of happiness" as one of our "unalienable rights." Why then does happiness sometimes seem so elusive, so transient? How do we infuse our life with more joy? Why do some people consistently see the glass half full? How do they manage to flourish, despite the obstacles? The million-dollar question is, can anyone learn to be happier?

In 1998, the scientific spotlight shifted toward an investigation into well-being when psychologist Martin Seligman launched the field of **positive psychology**. He urged his colleagues to join him in studying the nature of positive emotions and the conditions that make life more fulfilling. He and like-minded colleagues did just that.

First they established their objectives. A key goal is to have more positive than negative emotions, to enhance an overall sense of well-being. Some positive emotions pertain to the immediate moment: contentment, happiness, joy, ecstasy, and serenity. Emotions such as optimism, confidence, hope, trust, and faith reflect an affirmative attitude about the future. Another goal is to learn to derive pleasure from everyday experiences. Satisfying either goal nourishes the other. Feeling joy renders even the most commonplace experience pleasurable. An appreciation of the beauty and meaning in daily life fuels happiness and contentment.

Perversely, many of us have been raised to believe that joy follows success. We hurry along, telling ourselves we have to check off tasks X, Y, and Z before we can enjoy ourselves. However, it seems we have been putting the proverbial cart before the horse. Psychologists now believe that happiness leads to success.[6] ,[7] Positive people invest in important resources, especially social relationships. Compared to gloomier peers, they tend to get higher grades, have healthier friendships and marriages, enjoy more career success, and make more money. They're more resilient in the face of stress and, at the end of the day, glean more life satisfaction. Rather than simply survive, they thrive.

Furthermore, expectations about what makes us happy are often wrong. It's not the grand events: getting into a good college, landing a lucrative job, acquiring a luxury car, and so on. Such things typically fire up a fleeting, unsustainable glory. Soon, we're back at our baseline, whether that's generally cheerful or glum. Likewise, seemingly devastating events—breaking a leg, losing the crown jewels—may not feel as tragic as we might imagine. Sometimes setbacks are actually liberating. Again, it depends on your ability to spin straw into gold.

As it turns out, the small things bring us joy: a colorful sunset, a baby's smile, a dog's tail wagging, a shared meal. More specifically, choosing to appreciate and feel gratitude for such blessings engenders well-being. This "noticing" necessitates being aware of the present moment, a practice called mindfulness.

Here's the exciting news: You can learn to be happier. Personality, like your brain, is not set in stone. The skills are simple but take practice. Even better, this cultivation of positive emotions not only makes you feel great but also boosts performance in all arenas.

At this point, you may be asking whether prioritizing happiness isn't a bit superficial and self-involved. Most people, if asked whether they would swallow a pill that would make them joyful each and every moment, would say no. One, perpetual ecstasy would be exhausting. Two, life would become monochromatic. It would be like a month of Sundays. It would be like eating your favorite food at every single meal—boring.

Plus, while the ability to feel pleasure is desirable and healthy, out-and-out hedonism is not. A hedonist simply wants to have as much pleasure as possible: food, sex, alcohol, drugs, spa services, new clothes, ski days, and beach vacations. The problem is these activities often lack meaning and therefore ultimately fail to provide a sense of life satisfaction. As Dr. Seligman notes, positive psychology is not "happiology." Ideally, you engage with life in such a way that both positive and negative events have value.

Furthermore, the goal is not to avoid negative emotions. Feelings should be authentic. However, rumination, on the other hand, perpetuates distress. Suppressing strong emotions like anger can create a toxic stew that nourishes depression[8] and eating disorders[9] and lowers pain thresholds.[10]

Clearly, some situations call for negative emotions. The loss of a loved one naturally triggers grief. Anger in response to social injustice can motivate a corrective action. A rattlesnake coiled near your feet strikes a ripple of fear, which activates a life-preserving, hasty retreat. If someone betrays you, your distrust can protect you from further hurt.

Nevertheless, those emotions can be uncomfortable. Talking to a trusted friend, writing about thoughts and feelings, creating expressive art, exercising—such outlets diffuse and provide perspective on inner turmoil.

Occasional struggle and pain stimulate personal growth and provides a contrast against which we appreciate happiness and joy. Better yet, we can learn to appreciate the silver lining in setbacks, to grow stronger rather than give up, to learn from these experiences so we rise even higher from those ashes.

Here's an example: While riding their bicycles to class, two college students collide at a busy intersection. Neither is severely injured. One student screams profanities at the other. She rejects bystanders' attempts to help and limps off to class, grumbling about being late. For days, she complains to everyone who will listen about the other cyclist and repeatedly states that nothing is going well for her this semester.

The other student apologizes to the angry cyclist. She thanks the people who flock around to help her up, wash her wound, or ask if she needs a ride. She vows to be more careful in the future and feels grateful that nothing worse happened. She forgives the other student and continues on with her day.

positive psychology

A branch of psychology devoted to the study of the elements that allow individuals to thrive.

Which student do you imagine generally feels happier? Which do you think is more likely to find success and fulfillment in life?

 Video Link 5.2

The State of Psychology

Martin Seligman, PhD, provides an overview of the history of psychology, defines positive psychology, and explains the elements that contribute to psychological health: positive emotion, signature strengths, flow, and meaning.

http://www.ted.com/talks/martin_seligman_on_the_state_of_psychology.html

1.4 Factors That Promote Psychological Well-Being

Experiences during intrauterine life and early childhood profoundly influence psychological makeup. Protective factors include maternal physical and mental health during the pregnancy and family harmony. It also helps to grow up with parents and other caregivers who are kind, reliable, and upbeat and know how to establish limits, discipline with love and logic, recognize a child's strengths, and gradually transfer control to the child. Raised in this way, a child has a good chance of becoming an independent, self-assured, and appropriately assertive individual.

Adults also teach children to regulate emotions. Ideally, kids learn that, although strong emotions are normal, these feelings need to be articulated in socially acceptable fashions. The goal is to recognize emotions, examine them, articulate them, express them (in writing, nondestructive speech, art, music, movement), and find healthy ways to release them.

Parents also can teach children to recognize their strengths and to apply those skills. They teach children to utilize internal and external resources to cope with setbacks. Challenging situations often form the crucible from which personal health arises.

Kids acquire from their mentors their baseline traits and values. Positive traits include integrity, honesty, trust, creativity, tolerance, empathy (the ability to understand another person's emotions and motives), optimism, compassion, altruism (concern for the welfare of others), and forgiveness.

Parents also shape lifestyle habits that promote psychological health: nutritious diet, adequate sleep, regular exercise, social activity, stress management, and spiritual practices.

In addition to nurturing families, other institutions that promote our psychological well-being include good schools, accessible health care, and safe communities.[11] Social services that support those in need improve our collective welfare. A democratic government also tends to produce happier citizens.

Through all these avenues, you developed a *self-concept*—ideally one that's healthy. This perception of yourself is comprised of several components that also begin with "self."

- **Self-awareness** means you notice what you do and think and recognize the impact on yourself and the world around you.
- **Self-respect** allows you to honor your thoughts and feelings and not put up with others trying to bring you down.
- **Self-confidence** is a feeling of security about yourself.
- **Self-esteem** describes a sense of your value or self-worth. You feel both compassion for yourself and pride for the successes you've earned. It's better if your sense of reward and mastery comes from inside rather than from external accolades.
- **Self-efficacy** is faith in your competence. You possess a can-do attitude and believe that your actions will be successful in attaining a certain goal.
- **Self-acceptance** is self-explanatory. No one's perfect, not even you. Perfectionists set unrealistic standards for themselves. An inability to mute the inner critic can lead to chronic doubt and dissatisfaction.
- **Self-forgiveness** gives you the grace to accept those shortcomings without losing your motivation for improvement.
- **Self-acceptance** can blossom into **self-love**, which gives you the ability to love and forgive others. And healthy social relationships are critical to psychological health.

Can You Choose Your Emotional Response?

Sometimes it may seem as though you have no choice about your emotional response. Indeed, responding to a tragic situation with laughter is inappropriate. But oftentimes, you can make a choice. You can go out for a walk and focus on the tattered trash bags fluttering from power lines, the toxic oil sheen on puddles, or the smell of diesel exhaust. Or you can notice the grass pushing through the sidewalk cracks, the man walking his cat, or the two children giggling and skipping. You can grunt and silently complain through an exercise class or think, "This is great! I'm getting stronger."

See if you can make your sense of happiness and contentment less dependent upon things and events. Rather than thinking, "I'll be so happy once I finish the semester," try, "I'm lucky to have this opportunity to learn about new subjects and new people. I'm going to savor every moment."

1.5 Simple Ways to Feel Happier Now

As mentioned earlier, it's often the small things that give us joy. Practicing positive activities—thoughts, emotions, and behaviors—improves well-being, which enhances your social interactions, work productivity, and mental and physical health. They're all free, cheap, and convenient.

Count Your Blessings and Express Your Gratitude

Repeated studies have shown that expressing gratitude increases positive emotions[12] and decreases symptoms of depression.[13] For instance, researchers divided undergraduates into three groups, all of which made weekly records for 10 weeks.[14] Students in group one wrote down five things that made them feel grateful. Group two noted five hassles. Group three listed any five events of their choosing. At the end, the gratitude group rated their lives more optimistically, enjoyed greater well-being, exercised more, and experienced fewer symptoms of physical illness.

Express your thanks to the people in your life aloud and in writing. Open appreciation strengthens intimate relationships. At school and at work, positive acknowledgments foster collegiality and enhanced performance. Reward even the smallest acts of kindness. If someone holds the door for you, say thank you. Thank the people who cook and serve your food. Notice their response. Notice how you feel.

Smile and Laugh

Humor has been used as medicine for millennia. Watching comedic videos can reduce pain, decrease stress hormones, enhance immune function, buoy mood, and heighten alertness and creativity. Apparently your body doesn't know the difference between spontaneous mirth and simulated laughter. Either way, health benefits occur.[15],[16] Emerging evidence hints that, though it's harder to laugh when depressed, doing so can counteract symptoms. "Laughter therapy" decreases chronic pain and symptoms of depression[17] and improves quality of life and resilience in cancer survivors.[18]

Try laughing for no reason. It may evolve into genuine giggles. Smile at friends and total strangers (unless you're concerned about your safety). Crack jokes. (If you don't know many, search the Internet.)

Relish Present and Past Moments

Look for pleasure and beauty in your life. Enjoy the patter of rain on the roof, the breeze against your skin, the perfume of spring blossoms, the taste of blueberries bursting on your tongue, the friendship in a friend's eyes. Put flowers on your desk. Choose an inspiring screensaver for your computer. Play joyous music. Post pictures of happy moments. When your spirits flag, recall those happy moments.

Discover Your Strengths

Discover your strengths and capitalize on them. Perhaps you have a knack for picking up languages, enjoy learning, find pleasure in helping others, or often come to the defense of others less fortunate than you. Maybe you're creative, responsible, reliable, diligent, punctual, kind, or generous. Emphasize your assets. If you notice a potential flaw, detach from it emotionally and consider how your strengths can mend that defect.

Dwell on the Positive

Happier people tend to interpret their experiences in a brighter light. Let's say you got an A on a paper. Congratulate yourself on a job well done, rather than chalking it up to luck or your professor's generosity. Mentally store those positive events. If something doesn't go as well as you hoped, remember past successes and remain optimistic about the future. Notice ways in which you and your life have improved.

Nurture Your Friendships

People who are generally upbeat and successful have many friends and know how to maintain intimate relationships.[19] Likewise, having caring friends and family support correlates with happiness and success.[20] Both giving and receiving social support enhances well-being, though giving seems to provide even greater personal satisfaction.[21] When we're stressed, anxious, and unhappy, we tend to withdraw from the company of others, which often intensifies negative emotions. Taking a moment for friends can lift you out of those dark moods.

Practice Kindness

Whenever possible, choose to respond with kindness. See a child stumble and fall? Ask if you can help. Find a stray (and obviously friendly) dog? Look on the tags for a phone number to call. Think a fellow student looks stressed or sad? Offer emotional support. Help friends cook, clean, and pack. Slip a quarter into a parking meter that's about to expire. Buy coffee for the person behind you in line.

Keep Hope Alive

A study of college students found those with greater hope were less likely to become depressed after a negative life event.[22] After natural disasters, volunteers show up with clothing, food, and building materials. People plant gardens in the grittiest parts of cities. Trees spring from sidewalk cracks. Psychological and physical injuries heal. Keep on the lookout for hopeful signs in your own life.

Serve Others

Positive people enjoy helping others and are less likely to be self-absorbed. Also, service provides a sense of meaning, creates an awareness of others who are less fortunate, and offers a chance to interact with people from different backgrounds. Kindness and service often overlap. An example is massaging your roommate's shoulders after he or she complains of pain from hours of computer work.

Forgive

When someone does you wrong, it's normal to feel sadness, betrayal, and outrage. Holding grudges perpetuates bad feelings and hinders the healing of psychological wounds. Whether you give the person a second chance depends on the situation. True forgiveness can take time. See if you can at least let go of your anger and hostility. Not only will you feel more at peace, but you will protect your cardiovascular system from the damaging effects of those negative emotions.[23]

Experience Solitude

Rich social networks keep us well. But that doesn't mean you should spend every waking moment with other people. Moments of quiet introspection allow us to recharge, reflect, and process events.

Exercise

self-efficacy

Faith in one's ability to achieve one's goals.

Physical activity improves mental health for several reasons. It relieves frustration, stress, and tension. It provides a sense of accomplishment and **self-efficacy**. An activity that requires concentration and focus takes your mind off your worries. Some types of exercise give you an opportunity to socialize. Strenuous exercise releases endogenous opioids (naturally occurring pain relievers such as endorphins) and increases mood-lifting neurotransmitters. The postexercise glow enhances feelings of relaxation.

Go Outside

Whether you live in the city or the country, spending time in nature enhances well-being and overall health.[24] Also, in response to the ultraviolet rays in sunlight, your skin makes vitamin D, which is important for mental function and mood.[25] Take outdoor study breaks. Run around or be still. Use all your senses to appreciate the experience.

Allow Yourself Childlike Moments

Skip, blow bubbles, make chalk drawings on the sidewalk, dress like a superhero. These things can make you feel downright gleeful.

Sleep Sufficiently

Sleep deprivation corrodes mood. It's important both to sleep enough and to maintain a regular sleep-wake rhythm. College life challenges that balance. Disruptions in these daily rhythms predispose people to anxiety, impulsive behavior, depression, and its polar opposite, mania.[26] In turn, difficulty sleeping is an early sign of mood disorders.

Tend Your Spiritual Life

As discussed in Chapter 2, spiritual pursuits provide a sense of purpose, connection, values, personal strength, and, often, community spirit—all of which contribute to mental health. Greater engagement with religious and spiritual practices protects mental health. Planning activities with friends, playing music, creating art, running in a race, fund-raising for cancer research, raising a puppy—many things give us a reason for being and make us feel connected to the web of life.

Cultivating Optimism: The Glass *Is* Half Full

Optimism turns out to be a particularly valuable and learnable psychological trait. It has to do with how you perceive and interpret what's going on around you. Not only do you notice what's positive in your world, but you also expect a bright future and view negative events as temporary, surmountable setbacks. Pessimists, on the other hand, adhere to Murphy's Law: "If anything can go wrong, it will."

Regardless of your worldview, you'll find evidence to back you up. Why not stack those expectations on the positive side? Part of doing so requires that you have a healthy self-concept, that you view yourself as lovable, capable of achieving those goals, and deserving (but not entitled) of those hard-earned rewards. You can feel motivated to accomplish great things. If your parents didn't bolster your self-esteem during childhood, it's worth the effort to create a more optimistic style now.

Optimism is good for your health. Compared to pessimists, optimists live longer,[27] report better quality of life, and enjoy greater physical and mental function over the long haul,[28] including cardiovascular health.[29] Optimists are more likely to embrace healthy lifestyle habits—to eat well and exercise. They cope better with stress. They're more extroverted, expect to be liked, and have friends.

Of course, it's possible to be overly optimistic. For instance, most people are overly confident in their ability to drive—including when under the influence. Remaining realistic is important.

So how do you become more optimistic? Act it. Get up in the morning and say, "It's going to be a great day." See the sidebar "Thinking Compassionately about Yourself", which is about shifting your thoughts toward the positive. Identify the upbeat people in your life and hang with them. If you're not yet optimistic by nature, you may have to "fake it till you make it." Soon you'll *feel* optimistic and automatically see the glass half full.

Thinking Compassionately about Yourself

Regardless of whether you're aware of the interior patter, you're silently talking to yourself. It's how you process the world. Take random samples of your thoughts, particularly when something unsettles you. We humans have a tendency to hang onto negative things. Have you ever gotten a paper back and only noticed the criticisms? Have you ever had a fun evening—marred only by one rude comment—and spent the night thinking of the stinging reply you wished you'd uttered? While these are normal responses, they don't serve us.

Catch those negative thoughts and put them under a microscope. "I can't write papers." "I'm stupid." "I'm never going to succeed at college or anything else." "So-and-so's a complete jerk." "No one likes me." Are these thoughts realistic? Fair? Kind? Have you made the event bigger than it is? Are you jumping to (unfounded) conclusions? Have you misinterpreted something? Are you overgeneralizing? (What's the evidence that no one in your social sphere likes you?) Are you letting your thoughts cause you unnecessary distress and set you up for failure?

Tell yourself, "Stop!" If you can't derail the negative thoughts, write them down. Now write down something positive about that situation. Shift your attention to the present. Look out the window until you observe at least one beautiful thing. Go outside and walk until you see something that amuses you. Exercise and congratulate yourself. Fix yourself a healthy meal and consider the plants, animals, and laborers who made it possible. Clean your desk and admire the shiny surface, the order. Each day, identify your attainable goals and record your progress in meeting them.

Expect good things and look for confirmation. Tell yourself as you walk into a lecture, "I am going to learn something this next hour." As you leave, try saying to a classmate, "I thought it was interesting that…" Study. When you finish, notice something you feel happy about learning. Before you begin an exam, tell yourself, "I am as prepared as I could be." When you get back an exam or a paper, focus on the things you did right. View errors as opportunities for improvement. Allow yourself self-compassion and self-forgiveness.

Practice changing negative thoughts to positive ones. Make two columns. In the left-hand column, note the negative thought. In the right-hand column, rephrase that statement to the positive. Here are some examples. Try adding three negative thoughts of your own and changing them to a positive, realistic statement.

Negative thought	Positive thought
I'm bad at math.	I can learn what I set my mind to and will find out about getting a math tutor.
I hate my roommate.	My roommate seemed upset last night. Maybe I didn't handle things well. I'll try to talk to him/her and find out what's going on. If that doesn't work, I'll see if the resident advisor has ideas.
Drat. It's raining. I'm going to get wet and cold. I hate rain.	I enjoy the sound of rain on the roof. I'm glad I have a raincoat. The birds seem to be enjoying the rain.
The traffic here is horrible.	I'm going to learn more about the public transportation system here. If I need to drive, I can listen to an audio book.

Smartphone Apps

You can find a number of smartphone apps aimed at increasing well-being, gratitude, and happiness. I recommend Live Happy, which is grounded in research from renowned positive psychologist Sonja Lyubomirsky, PhD, professor at the University of California, Riverside, and author of *The How of Happiness: A New Approach to Getting the Life You Want.* Some free apps include http://www.trackyourhappiness.org and http://itunes.apple.com/us/app/healthy-habits-health-happiness/id416687813?mt=8.

 ## Video Link 5.3

The Happy Secret to Better Work

In this TED talk, Shawn Achor gives an entertaining and informative discussion about positive psychology. The winner of distinguished teaching awards for his positive psychology classes at Harvard University, Achor continues speaking and researching at his consulting firm in Cambridge, Massachusetts.

TEDxBloomington, filmed May 2011; posted February 2012. Available at: http://www.ted.com/talks/shawn_achor_the_happy_secret_to_better_work.html

Brain Food

A general rule is that a whole-foods diet based on vegetables, fruit, whole grains, fish, and limited amounts of high-quality meat promotes overall health and supports brain function. Such diets provide critical vitamins, minerals, amino acids, antioxidants, and healthy fats. Particularly important micronutrients include B and C vitamins, magnesium, zinc, the amino acid L-tryptophan, and omega-3 fatty acids. Whole-foods diets also protect the heart and blood vessels, thereby ensuring good blood circulation to the brain. Healthy eating reduces the risk of depression, anxiety, stroke (bleeding or blood clots in the brain), and dementia (progressive loss of mental function and the ability to perform daily activities).[30] People who follow a Mediterranean diet—which emphasizes vegetables, fruits, nuts, whole grains, fish, and olive oil—enjoy some protection against depression, stroke, and dementia, including Alzheimer's disease.[31],[32],[33]

Antioxidants help protect the brain from free-radical damage. Flavonoids act as potent antioxidants and also decrease inflammation. While all plants contain them, particularly rich sources include berries, red grapes, and green tea. Regular consumption helps preserve brain function through the years.[34],[35] In countries such as India, where people regularly eat curried foods, dementia is less common. Turmeric, the key ingredient in curry spice, contains a flavonoid called curcumin, which lab studies show has an anti-Alzheimer's effect.[36]

Healthy fats are also critical. The brain is 60 percent fat (dry weight). Monounsaturated fats (found in olive oil, avocado, and nuts) and polyunsaturated fats (found in leafy greens, nuts, seeds, and fish) promote brain circulation, reduce inflammation, and build nerve cell membranes and their insulating myelin sheaths. Adequate consumption protects against depression and stroke.

Oily fish such as salmon, herring, and mackerel are rich in a type of polyunsaturated fat called omega-3 fatty acids. In susceptible people, low levels seem to increase the risk of attention deficit hyperactivity disorder (ADHD), depression, suicide, and psychosis.[37] ,[38] ,[39] Deficits also correlate with accelerated brain aging and cognitive (which relates to intellectual ability like thinking, reasoning, remembering, and learning) decline.[40] Supplementation with omega-3 fatty acids modestly improves ADHD and may augment conventional drug treatment.[41]

Coffee and tea do more than kick-start your day. Moderate consumption of coffee (two to three cups a day) is associated with a lower risk of depression and stroke.[42] ,[43] Keep your intake in check. Although caffeine increases alertness, it also can heighten feelings of anxiety and drive up heart rate and blood pressure. Green tea contains a lesser amount of caffeine, as well as an amino acid called L-theanine, which has antianxiety effects.[44] Regular consumption of green tea (three or four cups a day) is associated with a reduced risk of depression,[45] psychological distress,[46] age-related cognitive decline,[47] and stroke.[48]

Meditation and Exercise

Meditation provides multiple brain benefits. For one, it is antithetical to the stress response. Stress elevates the hormone cortisol, which, when elevated in the long term, damages the hippocampus (a brain area key to memory). It may also elevate the brain-derived growth factor (BDNF), which stimulates nerve cell growth and protects and repairs nerve cells. There's more good news: Regular meditation may strengthen nerve circuits (useful connections between nerve cells), maintain good brain circulation, enhance mental function, and reduce the gradual loss in gray matter that comes with age.[49] It also makes it easier to cope with stress with an even keel.

Physical activity is important for a well-functioning brain. Like meditation, it stimulates BDNF, promotes nerve cell growth, enhances learning and memory, and elevates mood. Movement provides a release from nervous tension and stress. Regular physical activity protects against cognitive decline and dementia, including Alzheimer's disease.[50] Aerobic exercise stimulates release of pain-relieving chemicals called endorphins as well as mood-enhancing neurotransmitters such as serotonin and norepinephrine. It also aids recovery from depression.[51]

KEY TAKEAWAYS

- The pillars of good health overall also protect the brain, reducing the risk of mental illness, cognitive decline, and stroke.
- An offshoot of psychology called positive psychology explores factors that allow people not simply to escape disease but to thrive.
- A number of simple, inexpensive practices foster robust mental and emotional health.

1. Keep a gratitude journal for one week. Before you go to bed, write down three things that made you feel appreciative that day. Follow each item with a description. Rather than simply writing "water," briefly describe your experience of drinking a glass of it, diving into it, showering, or watching a public fountain. Try to use as many of the five senses as possible (touch, taste, smell, hearing, vision) and to feel genuinely thankful. After you finish your description, record how you feel emotionally. The next morning, note whether you slept any differently with those visions in your head.

2. Write a thank you note to someone. The event you express gratitude about could be in the recent or distant past. Perhaps you never let someone know how much you appreciated something he or she did for you during your childhood. If you can, deliver the letter.

3. Write about a time when you performed at your best. The activity doesn't matter. What counts is that you experienced "flow"—the sense that you were in the present moment and that your thoughts and actions seemed nearly effortless. What personal strengths did you exhibit at the time? How can you continue to capitalize on these strengths?

4. Greet at least five strangers as you make your way to your next class. Say whatever comes naturally—"Hello," "Howdy," "Hiya," "Good day." Mix it up. Have some fun. Salute nonhuman animals, if you feel like it. Smile. Watch people's reactions. Notice your own. How did you feel at the end?

5. Make a list of things that made you happy as a child. Try doing three of them now. Finger-paint. Make snow angels. Fly a kite. Blow bubbles. Skip. Sing. Dance.

6. Go to http://www.authentichappiness.sas.upenn.edu and register for free. Then take the Authentic Happiness survey. How do you compare with other people your age? What do you think you could do to feel better?

2. PSYCHOLOGICAL DISORDERS

LEARNING OBJECTIVES

1. Define mental illness.
2. Gain an appreciation of the magnitude of psychological illness in the world and the United States.
3. Identify risk factors for mental ill health.
4. Describe key points about common psychological disorders: potential causes, symptoms, conventional treatment, and promising complementary therapies.
5. List the warning signs for suicide.

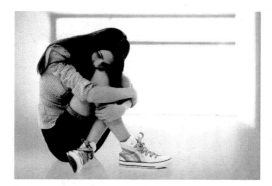

© Thinkstock

Of the many psychological disorders, all have one thing in common: a sustained alteration in thoughts, emotions, or behaviors that causes distress and impairs normal functioning. According to the World Health Organization (WHO), mental illnesses affect some 450 million people and cause more disability in the developed world than any other chronic condition, including heart disease and cancer.[52] Over 46 percent of Americans experience some form of mental illness during their lives.[53] In 2004, some 25 percent of American adults reported a mental illness during the previous year. These conditions cost the United States over $300 billion a year.

A nationwide survey of college students found that about a third had a mental health problem and just over a third of them received any kind of treatment the previous year.[54] When asked what stopped them from getting help, students expressed skepticism that treatment would work or noted that they didn't believe treatment was urgent.

Furthermore, people suffering from mental illnesses too often endure social stigma and discrimination. The perceived stigma, as well as lack of insurance or inadequate insurance coverage for mental health services and insufficient screening of mental health problems, hinders treatment. Only 30 percent of American adults with mood disorders and anxiety receive even minimally adequate treatment. That leaves a lot of people suffering needlessly.[55] Furthermore, *comorbidity*—having more than one concurrent condition—is not uncommon.

Professional help is important. Psychiatric conditions are illnesses, not signs of personal weakness. Most are biologically based. You can't wish or will them away. And you shouldn't blame yourself for having them. Too many people try to hide or ignore symptoms. Too many self-medicate with substances and withdraw from the very social support they need. If you're one of these, ask yourself whether you'd ignore an infected wound, self-treat diabetes, or attempt to hide a broken leg. Would you limp around, thinking, "I should just pull myself together and get over it"? Probably not. Respond to signs of psychiatric illness as you would a serious medical condition: get help.

We've come a long way in the diagnosis and treatment of mental illness. We've discarded demonic possession, imbalance of humors, and malingering as the primary causes. The treatment is no longer exorcism, stoning, and bleeding. But we have a way to go before mental illness is treated on par with physical illness. Too many severely ill people fall through the health care cracks. Those who do risk drug addiction, homelessness, and incarceration. Rather than lock people in state-run mental institutions (many of which have closed), we increasingly put our drug-addicted and mentally ill citizens behind bars.

As noted in a 2011 editorial in the *New England Journal of Medicine*, "The largest facilities housing psychiatric patients in the United States are not hospitals but jails. More than half of inmates have symptoms of a psychiatric disorder…yet only 22 percent of state prisoners and 7 percent of jail inmates receive mental health treatment while incarcerated."[56] Clearly, this problem represents a public health challenge—one that we can and should overcome.

  Video Clip 5.2

Stigma Reduction: Celebrities Speak Out
This public service announcement shows a number of celebrities encouraging people to come out of the closet about mental health disorders.

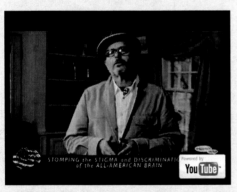

View the video online at: http://www.youtube.com/v/KwLjAsal13l

2.1 Risk Factors

Mental illnesses represent a diverse group of conditions. Even though most of their causes continue to elude scientists, several factors stand out as contributing to poor mental health.

Family History

Many mental illnesses run in families, suggesting a genetic basis. However, we share more than genes with close family members. Our families influence diet, activity levels, substance use, education, the way we mentally and emotionally process our experiences, and other factors that shape mental health. If a close relative (parent or sibling) has a mental illness, you may be more vulnerable. However, history doesn't equate to destiny.

Stress

Stressful life events raise the risk of a number of depression and anxiety disorders. Children born to mothers who are severely stressed (malnourished, very ill, traumatized) during pregnancy face an increased probability of mental health challenges.[57] Early childhood trauma—death of a parent, abandonment, abuse, neglect—also tip the scales toward rockier mental health. Physical and sexual assault at any age pose a risk.[58] Other childhood stressors—divorce, school bullies, gang violence, drug-riddled neighborhoods—take a toll as well.

Stressful events later in life, such as job loss, financial uncertainty, family discord, or loss of a loved one, can wear down mental and emotional reserves. Everyday hassles, overwork, sleep deprivation, lack of social support, poor nutrition, physical inactivity, and substance abuse add to the stress load.

Military service, though it has its rewards, can also fray mental health. One in five soldiers returning from Iraq or Afghanistan has suffered from major depression or posttraumatic stress disorder (PTSD).[59] Worse, many veterans worry about losing their job if they report mental illness, which further increases the risk of depression.

Chronic Illness

Coping with a serious illness is stressful and can generate anxiety and low mood. Conditions such as cardiovascular disease and diabetes raise the risk of depression.[60] Likewise, depressed people are more at risk for cardiovascular disease and cancer. Nevertheless, many people manage chronic illnesses with grace and optimism.

Obesity

Excess body fat is linked to an increased risk of mental illnesses and substance abuse. The cause isn't clear. Inflammatory chemicals associated with excessive weight affect the brain. Also the social stigma obesity carries makes life more difficult.[61] In turn, mental illnesses such as depression and bipolar disorder may lead to weight gain.

Social Isolation

Humans need gentle touch and kindness to flourish. A lack of healthy relationships promotes depression and anxiety.

Substance Abuse

Alcohol in excess, tobacco, and illicit drugs can adversely affect the brain. In turn, untreated mental illness can drive people to use substances in an attempt to self-medicate.[62]

Malnutrition

Just as a whole-foods diet protects mental health, the "Western" diet of processed meat, high-fat dairy products, refined grains, and fried, sugary foods correlates with more depression and anxiety, as well as a higher risk of stroke.[63],[64] Fast-food diets (think hamburgers, French fries, pizza, and soda) increase the risk of depression.[65] Teens who consume a lot of junk food often experience deteriorating mental health over time.[66] High intake of salt, saturated fats, and trans fats impairs mental function and raises the risk of stroke.[67]

Deficiencies of nutrients needed for nervous system functioning are particularly problematic. These include amino acids such as L-tryptophan, omega-3 fatty acids, magnesium, vitamin D, and certain B vitamins.

Assess Yourself: Mental Health

How do you know if your mental and emotional state is normal? All humans feel at least occasional anxiety, sadness, and euphoria. No line demarcates normal from abnormal. Intensity and duration help to determine whether symptoms and signs indicate illness. Ask yourself the following questions:

- Do you have trouble deriving satisfaction and pleasure from your life?
- Have any members of your family struggled with a mental/emotional disorder?
- Do your moods seem extreme? Do you often feel unwarranted anger, sadness, or euphoria?
- Do you feel agitated? Do these feelings interfere with your sleep?
- Do you have so many thoughts you can't speak fast enough to articulate them?

- Do you have uncomfortable, recurrent thoughts? For instance, you might keep thinking you've done something wrong (despite evidence to the contrary), that you have germs on your hands, or that something bad is about to happen to a loved one.

- Have you started drinking heavily or using drugs to mask uncomfortable emotions?

- Do you cling to unusual rituals? Examples include frequent hand washing, avoiding sidewalk cracks, tapping, or ordering things. Do you feel anxious unless you perform them?

- Do you repeatedly act before you think, sometimes with unhappy consequences?

- Has it become more difficult to concentrate, make decisions, and remember things?

- Do you hear voices or see things others don't?

- Do you feel like hurting yourself or someone else?

- Have you ever considered ending your life?

A family history of mental illness indicates vulnerability and serves as a motivating force for taking steps to bolster your mental health. Contact a mental health professional if any of these signs and symptoms persist beyond two weeks or become severe enough to interfere with your ability to function at work, school, and play. Ask your family doctor or the student health clinic for a referral. If you currently have thoughts of ending your life, seek emergency medical assistance.

Is Being Plugged In Bad for Mental Health?

The Internet has changed our lives in many ways. Clearly, much good has come of this technology. However, excessive use can sap mental health. Paradoxically, despite the fact that teens and young adults overuse the Internet primarily to connect to social media sites, they become more disconnected from actual humans. Compulsive use of computers and wireless mobile devices comes at the expense of other pillars of health: sleep, nutrition, exercise, and spiritual activities. As a result, social, spiritual, physical, mental, and emotional health decline. Anxiety disorders, depression, and anger management problems have all been linked to overuse of electronic devices. What's confusing is that moodiness and feelings of emptiness both stimulate us to use the Internet and arise from overusing (or being blocked from using) it.[68]

If you find that you have difficulty unplugging from your devices, contact a mental health specialist. Even if you don't, set boundaries around use of electronic devices, particularly nonacademic uses (Tweeting, texting, e-mailing, browsing social media sites). When you're studying, take a 5- to 10-minute break each hour to do something unrelated to books and computers. Stretch; sing; play music; go outside; take a walk; appreciate nature; interact with a flesh-and-blood human; or pet a friendly, furry creature.

2.2 Anxiety Disorders

Of all the psychiatric conditions, **anxiety disorders** are the most common. According to the American Psychiatric Association, these conditions affect more than 25 million Americans.[69] The lifetime chances of having an anxiety disorder are nearly 29 percent.[70] While everyone has occasional moments of nervousness and fearfulness, people with anxiety disorders experience these uncomfortable thoughts and feelings most of the time. They can, in fact, be so severe as to interfere with normal functioning.

Anxiety produces fearful thoughts that may or may not be grounded in reality. When the worries aren't likely to happen, the person recognizes them as such but still can't relax. Physical symptoms include rapid heart rate, sweaty palms, muscle tension, "butterflies" in the stomach, nausea, and diarrhea. Depression may accompany anxiety.

The cause of anxiety disorders isn't clear, but seems to involve a combination of genetics and environmental factors. They can run in families. Stress can unmask the underlying vulnerability.

There are five main types of anxiety disorders.

anxiety disorder

A group of conditions characterized by severe, persistent anxiety.

generalized anxiety disorder

Unremitting, excessive worries about nonspecific things.

panic disorder

Recurrent panic attacks.

panic attack

A sudden episode of terror or dread with pounding heart, rapid breathing, dizziness, sweating, faintness, chest discomfort, and a sensation that breathing is difficult. In panic disorder, a person has recurring panic attacks.

phobia

A morbid, irrational fear of a particular object or situation: spiders, heights, closed spaces, social situations.

obsessive-compulsive disorder

Persistent, recurrent doubts and worries about a particular issue (germs, order, intruders, violence, sex) that are temporarily relieved by a ritual (hand washing, ordering, locking and relocking doors, praying).

posttraumatic stress disorder (PTSD)

The development of anxiety, irritability, flashbacks, nightmares, difficulty sleeping, emotional numbing, social withdrawal, hypervigilance, and social withdrawal after a traumatic event.

1. **Generalized anxiety disorder** (GAD). People with GAD worry constantly about everything from whether they'll be able to keep on top of schoolwork to whether they can get their laundry done. If a family member didn't respond immediately to a text, they might imagine something horrible may have happened. A headache may trigger concerns about a brain tumor. Molehills become mountains. Life becomes one big emergency. Muscle tension and fretting fray sleep. Concentration fractures. Irritability mounts. The condition can affect people of any age, race, or gender.

2. **Panic disorder**. People with this disorder have recurrent **panic attacks**. Symptoms often start suddenly—sometimes in the middle of the night. They include a pounding heart or chest pain, shortness of breath, sweating, shaking, nausea and vomiting, light-headedness or dizziness, chills or sweating, and feelings of doom or of "going crazy." The first attack can send someone to the emergency room.

3. **Phobias** are intense and excessive fears about a particular thing, activity, or situation. Often the object of the phobia would not cause the person harm. For example, people with *social phobias* (also called *social anxiety disorder*) fear the potential embarrassment of trying to interact with others so much that they avoid parties and other situations. This condition is distinguished from shyness in that social phobia significantly impairs normal function.[71] *Specific phobias* involve more narrow fears. For instance, people with arachnophobia fear spiders so much they may not be able to look at photos or videos of them without undue anxiety. *Agoraphobia* involves a fear of any situation in which the person believes he or she might not be able to escape or may become humiliated by the development of a panic attack. In extreme cases, people become so fearful they confine themselves to their homes.

4. **Obsessive-compulsive disorder** (OCD) involves two main problems: obsessive thinking and compulsive behaviors. The worried thoughts are persistent and intrusive and usually follow a theme. A common concern is "germs." In this case, a person with OCD might walk to the classroom, eye the doorknob, begin worrying about the bacteria swarming on it, and wait until someone else opens the door. Sitting down, she considers the microorganisms crawling over the seat and desk. Her mind jumps to news reports of flesh-eating bacteria. She's so preoccupied and anxious she can't focus on the lecture.

   Other common obsessions may center on perfectionism, religious or superstitious thoughts, and taboo thoughts ("If I think about wanting that necklace in the store window, am I a shoplifter?"). Many of the worries could happen to anyone. Someone with OCD, however, can't push them out of his mind; the thoughts run around and around and are associated with fear of harm to oneself or others.

   Compulsions are the ritualized behaviors that relieve the intense anxiety generated by obsessions. Examples include excessive hand washing; ordering items in a precise way; touching things in a particular pattern; reciting specific prayers; and checking that the stove is off, the door is locked, or the wallet is in the purse. Occasionally engaging in such behaviors is normal. However, in someone with OCD, the behavior only temporarily relieves the worries. Soon doubts about whether his hands are truly clean, the pencils are perfectly aligned, or the door is properly locked drive him to repeat the ritual. The vicious cycle of obsessions and compulsions makes it difficult to concentrate on other matters and complete tasks.

5. **Posttraumatic stress disorder (PTSD)** can occur after experiencing or witnessing terrifying events. The person or someone he or she loves is threatened. The situation usually involves a sense of helplessness—child abuse, rape, armed robbery, war, kidnapping, accidents, natural disasters. Not everyone exposed to a traumatic event will develop PTSD. Symptoms and signs, which develop within three months, include flashbacks (reliving the event), nightmares, trouble sleeping, emotional numbing, social withdrawal, jitteriness, irritability, hypervigilance (always feeling on alert for a threat), and avoidance of anything reminiscent of the event.

Treatment varies for the different anxiety disorders but usually involves psychotherapy plus or minus medications. Not only does treatment relieve symptoms; it can positively change brain structure and function.[72] Psychotherapy can help people learn to manage their anxious thoughts, modify behaviors, and improve lifestyle habits. People can learn to do reality checks to remind themselves that their worries may be ill founded. Reappraising the situation can help someone see potential opportunities and benefits. Instead of dreading an oral presentation, a person might instead remind herself that no actual threat to life and limb exists and try to view it as an opportunity to share useful information. Attempting to suppress worried thoughts and feelings often perpetuates the uncomfortable feelings. Sometimes mindful, nonjudgmental acceptance of one's feelings without any attempt to control them can actually reduce them.[73]

Nevertheless, medication may also be needed. Although sedatives such as benzodiazepines (Ativan, Xanax, Valium) can reduce anxiety, they are not recommended for long-term treatment due to undesirable side effects and the risk of dependence. Instead, Buspar (buspirone), which is not sedating, is used. Antidepressant drugs such as serotonin reuptake inhibitors (Prozac, Zoloft, Celexa, Paxil, Lexapro) also address anxiety.

Exposure and response prevention, a type of therapy used both in OCD and phobias, involves an actual or imagined encounter with the dreaded object. The goal is to steadily build tolerance to the resultant anxiety. Gradually, the person becomes desensitized. For instance, someone worried about germs may start with looking at photos of doorknobs and gradually progress to touching a doorknob—without rushing to wash her hands. She learns that doorknobs are not threatening her life, that nothing bad happens after touching them, and that the anxious thoughts and feelings related to them dissipate with time.

Studies have shown that expressive writing (writing about thoughts and feelings) can reduce feelings of anxiety and depression[74] and can also improve intimate relationships in returning war veterans.[75] These exercises, when done regularly (some studies assign 15-minute writing exercises for three days running), can help someone get in touch with his emotions, organize thoughts, and imbue traumatic events with a sense of meaning. Putting it down on paper may also help stop rumination, the cycle of repeatedly running the same thoughts through one's brain. Research suggests that it's better to let a month or two elapse before writing about a trauma, as doing so immediately afterward may intensify discomfort.[76]

Exercise can also dissipate anxious thoughts and feelings. Regular participation in brisk walking, yoga, and tai chi all can help manage anxiety.[77],[78] Meditation can also reduce symptoms.[79],[80] Relaxation training and breathing exercises can restore a sense of calm and may help manage panic disorders.[81]

 Video Clip 5.3

Anxiety Overview
This segment of "The Answered Patient" from answerstv.com provides an overview of the five main anxiety disorders.

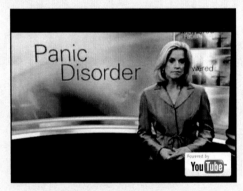

View the video online at: http://www.youtube.com/v/_Cr7lomSy8s

2.3 Mood Disorders

Several psychiatric conditions disturb mood, chiefly: depression, bipolar disorder, and anxiety disorders. In addition to straining emotions, they also cause physical symptoms. Granted, we all occasionally dip into sadness, anxiety, and elation. Mood disorders, however, plunge us so deeply into the undertow we feel we're drowning and can scarcely function well enough to perform everyday activities. Surveys estimate that nearly 21 percent of Americans experience a mood disorder at some point in their lives.[82]

As with most psychiatric conditions, no objective tests—blood tests or brain scans—detect mood disorders. However, an interview with a qualified mental health practitioner unveils important clues. A physical exam and lab tests can identify treatable physical disorders that produce similar symptoms. Unfortunately, mood disorders are substantially underdiagnosed and undertreated.

Depression

depression

A mood disorder with sad mood, loss of interest, inability to feel pleasure, feelings of guilt and shame, low energy, and poor sleep.

If you fail an exam or have a falling out with a friend, sadness is normal. For most people the gray mood lifts in a matter of days. **Depression**, on the other hand, afflicts people with persistent unhappiness and an inability to derive pleasure from activities, even those that once brought joy. It afflicts people regardless of age, race, sex, and socioeconomic status. It's so prevalent that Seligman has labeled depression the common cold of psychological problems.

According to the WHO, the condition affects 121 million people around the globe and places second behind heart disease as a leading cause of disability.[83] Overall, depression affects 10 to 15 percent of the United States population. At any one time, 5.6 percent of teens 13 to 18 have serious depression; 20 percent may become depressed sometime during adolescence.[84] About 16.3 million Americans over the age of 18 experience some type of depression. Major depression strikes 20 percent of women and 13 percent of men.[85]

The first episode usually occurs before age 18 and can last nine months. The college years are a common time to develop depression perhaps because of the stress associated with greater academic challenges, inadequate sleep, being away from home, and adjusting to dorm life.

Depression does more than make people feel sad; it also warps thinking and generates physical symptoms. For children and teens, irritation and verbal outbursts may overshadow sadness. Compared to women, men are more likely to "act out" and express anger. Sleep disturbances create daytime sleepiness and fatigue. Children and elders may complain primarily of stomachaches, headaches, and other pains.

During depression, the brain works differently. Show a depressed person a series of human faces and she'll remember the sad faces more than the happy ones. The same goes if given a series of adjectives, with better recall for negative words (tragic, sad, devastating). It's as though the glass can only be viewed as half empty. Depressed people may fail to recognize personal progress and accomplishments. "Sure, I got an A on the test, but the professor made it too easy." "That award? It was just a fluke."

The following are signs and symptoms of depression:

- Persistent sad mood and, often, excessive crying.

- Irritability, anxiety, and restlessness.

- *Anhedonia*—an inability to feel pleasure, even for things that formerly brought joy and satisfaction. For example, a depressed person may recognize that she should feel delighted her friends planned a surprise birthday party but instead feels nothing or only sadness.

- Sleep disturbances. Sometimes problems sleeping precede mood changes. Insomnia is common, especially with early morning awakenings. However, some depressed people sleep more than usual.

- Fatigue. Depression is exhausting. Regardless of whether the person sleeps less or more than usual, he or she feels tired during the day.

- Increases or decreases in appetite.

- Weight loss or gain.

- Increased pain.

- Difficulty concentrating, remembering, and making decisions.

- Feelings of worthlessness, hopelessness, and guilt. These feelings, in addition to exhaustion, hamper the ability to seek help. A depressed person may feel like a burden and that he or she doesn't deserve help or may assume that nothing will make him or her feel better.

- Suicidal thoughts and actions. A bleak outlook that life is no longer worth living and will never improve can lead people to contemplate, plan, attempt, and actually commit suicide.

Types of Depression

- **Major depressive disorder.** Persistence of five or more symptoms of depression for two weeks or more with resultant distress and impairment of function.

- **Dysthymia.** Low-level depression that does not significantly impair function and lasts for two years or longer.

- **Seasonal affective disorder.** Occurs in the Northern Hemisphere when the days are short in fall and winter.

- **Premenstrual dysphoric disorder.** Depression that appears during the days preceding menstruation.

- **Postpartum depression.** Depression following the birth of a child.

Cause

Just as each person's experience of depression is unique, no single thing causes depression in all people. Rather, a number of aggravating factors can conspire to provoke the classic symptoms. A unifying theme is the link between many of these factors and reduced levels of certain neurotransmitters, notably serotonin, norepinephrine, and dopamine. Brain scans also reveal alterations in patterns of nerve activation in the brain. The neurotransmitters associated with depression are serotonin, norepinephrine, and dopamine. Other hormones, nerve growth factors, inflammatory chemicals, and chemical imbalances also figure in.

Risk Factors for Developing Depression

- **Genetics.** A number of genes regulate mood-related neurotransmitters and other relevant brain functions. That's why depression may "run in the family." Family history suggests predisposition, not predetermination.

- **Female Gender.** Until puberty, the rate of depression is similar in boys and girls. After that time, women are nearly twice as likely as men to become depressed.[86] Hormones and gender roles may contribute. Times of particular vulnerability include puberty, the days before menses, pregnancy, the period just after birth, and the years before menopause—times characterized by hormonal fluctuation, other physical changes, and emotional challenges.

- **Diet.** As noted earlier, processed foods increase the risk and whole-foods diets are protective. Low levels of omega-3 fatty acids and folate increase the risk of depression. Folate supplements may augment response to antidepressants.[87] Insufficient vitamin D levels correlate with an elevated risk of depression, suicide, and anxiety.[88] Although few foods contain vitamin D, exposure to the sun's ultraviolet rays triggers vitamin D production in the skin. Nevertheless, indoor lifestyles and use of sunscreen have made vitamin D insufficiency common. While vitamin D supplements can restore normal blood levels, it's not yet clear whether they relieve depression symptoms.[89]

- **Alcohol.** Alcohol quite literally depresses the central nervous system. Heavy drinking engenders depression.

Risks Associated with Depression

Depression raises the risk for other medical conditions. It unbalances immune function, increasing the risk of infection[90] and poor wound healing and elevating levels of inflammatory chemicals, which, in turn, worsens mood and raises the stakes for a number of chronic diseases.[91]

Heart disease and stroke (a blood clot or hemorrhage in the brain) have a bidirectional relationship with depression. Blood vessel disease raises the risk of depression, either directly or indirectly via associated lifestyle factors (poor diet, smoking, stress overload). In kind, depression, especially when it occurs later in life, increases the risk of heart disease,[92] including fatal heart attacks and strokes.[93]

Depression adversely affects brain areas associated with memory. Long-standing depression is a risk factor for cognitive decline and dementia.[94] The bottom line is that depression degrades overall quality of life, contributes to general ill health, and shortens life expectancy,[95] which is why it's important to get treatment.

- **Diagnosis.** Even though no objective test detects depression, the diagnosis is easily made in an interview with a qualified health care practitioner. A physician can also differentiate between depression and conditions that cause similar symptoms, such as an underactive thyroid. Unfortunately, many people go undiagnosed because they don't recognize the nature of their symptoms, don't think they deserve help, worry about the stigma, or doubt that treatment will help them recover.

Video Clip 5.4

Signs, Symptoms, and Treatment of Depression
Learn about depression in this National Institute of Mental Health video.

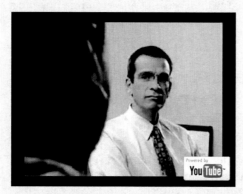

View the video online at: http://www.youtube.com/v/mINCavst2EU

- **Treatment.** Depression usually resolves on its own, though the process can take several miserable months. Treatment can hasten the process and reduce the likelihood of recurrence. The combination of antidepressant drugs and psychotherapy provides relief for 60 to 80 percent of depressed people.[96] However, no one-size-fits-all therapy exists—as befits a complex condition with multiple risk factors and varying symptom patterns. Unfortunately, fewer than a quarter of depressed people receive effective treatment.

  If you are diagnosed with depression, be patient and hopeful. It can take a few weeks to identify the best treatment and for mood to improve. After that, expect slow but steady gains. There is no such thing as snapping out of depression. Accept the support of friends and family. Confide in trusted friends. Each day, find some pleasurable activity. Get a massage. Buy yourself flowers. Download a song that makes you happy.

Treatment Options

- **Psychotherapy.** Therapy alone can lift mild depression and, in combination with antidepressant medications, more serious depression. There are several types of group and individual therapies. A commonly practiced method is *cognitive-behavioral therapy*, which addresses the thoughts and behaviors that contribute to the condition. A therapist can help an individual identify self-defeating, negative thoughts and take gradual steps toward rephrasing them into positive statements. A therapist can also help the client improve behaviors that affect mood. Other types of therapy focus on remedying interpersonal relationships, family dynamics, and life situations contributing to low moods. Therapy gives people tools to mend their depression and to avoid falling back into harmful patterns.

  Mindfulness-based cognitive therapy is a relative newcomer. Rather than attempting to change a depressed person's way of thinking, a therapist would instead encourage her to observe her thoughts in a more detached way, exhibit more self-compassion, and embrace positive ways of being in the world. This therapy shows promise in improving symptoms of depression and preventing relapse.[97]

- **Antidepressant Medications.** Up to 11 percent of Americans 12 years old and up take antidepressants.[98] They're the third most commonly used prescription drug. Used primarily to treat depression, these medications are also prescribed to manage anxiety disorders, chronic pain, and other conditions. However, only a third of severely depressed people take them. And among people who do go on antidepressants, only about a third respond favorably.[99] Some people respond to one drug but not to another.

  Antidepressants are categorized based on which of three key neurotransmitters they increase. The selective serotonin reuptake update inhibitors (SSRIs) increase serotonin; serotonin and norepinephrine reuptake inhibitors (SNRIs) increase norepinephrine; and tricyclic antidepressants (TCAs) increase serotonin, norepinephrine, and dopamine. Bupropion (Wellbutrin) raises dopamine and norepinephrine. Doctors often prescribe the SSRIs first, because they're relatively safe and help many of the people who try them. SSRIs include fluoxetine (Prozac), citalopram (Celexa), escitalopram (Lexapro), fluvoxamine (Luvox), paroxetine (Paxil), and sertraline (Zoloft). SNRIs include venlafaxine (Effexor) and duloxetine (Cymbalta).

How antidepressants work isn't clear. The simple explanation is that they lift depression by increasing levels of the neurotransmitters that are low in depression. However, that augmentation happens quickly, as does a subtle shift from negative to positive emotional processing,[100] yet major symptoms don't significantly improve for several weeks. Presumably, other molecular changes are going on in the meantime. While theories abound, none have been proven.

Antidepressants are generally safe. Possible side effects include upset stomach, nervousness, dizziness, weight change, headache, sleepiness, insomnia, and sexual problems (decreased sex drive, delayed ejaculation, and decreased orgasm). Most of these bothersome symptoms decline after the initial days and weeks. Sexual side effects do not, although some antidepressants are less likely to cause such problems than others. Furthermore, depression dampens sex drive too. If you are prescribed antidepressants and side effects seem intolerable, contact your physician. He or she may have an easy solution.

Also, it's important that a mental health specialist monitor reactions to these medications, especially during the first weeks. Rarely, depressive symptoms can worsen. Worse, people may become agitated and develop suicidal thoughts, symptoms that warrant immediate medical treatment. However, lack of treatment also raises the risk of suicidal thoughts and behaviors. One long-term study found that antidepressant therapy decreased the risk of suicide by 20 percent.[101]

Abruptly stopping many of the antidepressants can trigger what's called a "discontinuation syndrome." Associated symptoms include insomnia, muscle aches, headache, fatigue, nausea, dizziness, anxiety, and weird sensations.[102] Furthermore, recurrence of depression is a risk. Discuss any desires to stop a medication with your psychiatrist, who can help you slowly taper off the medication and monitor your progress.

- **Positive Activity Interventions.** Positive psychology experts now advocate moving beyond simply relieving symptoms of depression to fostering well-being.[103] To that end, they recommend activities described earlier: counting one's blessings; focusing on one's strengths; meditating (with positive thoughts toward oneself and others); and practicing gratitude, optimism, and kindness. The fact that these activities are free, easy to learn, and within a person's control increases self-efficacy and autonomy and shifts the locus of control from external to internal (though they aren't intended to replace professional monitoring). Significant improvements can occur within a week of consistent practice.[104] Well-being therapies also blend well with psychotherapy and antidepressant treatment in people with anxiety and/or depression[105] and also protect against relapse.[106]

- **Bright-Light Therapy.** Light boxes, which simulate outdoor light, were first shown to improve seasonal affective disorder. Subsequent research found that it also helped major depression, depression in bipolar disorder, depression during pregnancy, and premenstrual depression.[107] You can buy light boxes at drugstores and Internet retailers. A doctor's prescription is only necessary for insurance coverage. Columbia University provides useful information about this kind of therapy at http://www.columbia.edu/~mt12/blt.htm.

- **Brain Stimulation Therapies.** These therapies, which are reserved for severe depression unresponsive to medication or therapy, activate the brain with electricity, magnets, or implants.[108] Once called "shock therapy," electroconvulsant shock therapy (ECT) conjured images from the book and movie *One Flew Over the Cuckoo's Nest*. Recently the procedure, which involves passing a strong electrical current through the brain, has improved and provides relief for deep-seated depression. Performed under light anesthesia, the procedure takes only minutes. Short-term side effects include muscle aches, confusion, disorientation, and memory loss from events around the time of treatment. Sometimes mild memory loss persists.

  Newer, experimental stimulation therapies include transcranial magnetic stimulation (TMS). Compared to ECT, the current is magnetic rather than electrical. TMS doesn't require anesthesia and doesn't produce memory loss. It is, however, expensive and may not improve symptoms for several weeks.

- **Physical Activity.** A number of studies confirm that exercise reduces symptoms of depression.[109] In one study, researchers compared the effect of four months of aerobic exercise, the antidepressant sertraline, and a placebo pill in a group of sedentary adults with major depression. Compared to the placebo, both sertraline and exercise were similarly effective in diminishing symptoms. When the researchers checked in on them a year later, the proportion of depression-free people had increased from an average of 46 percent to 66 percent. More time spent exercising led to greater symptom relief—up until three hours a week, at which point benefits plateaued.[110]

Suicide

According to the WHO, nearly one million people commit suicide annually.[111] Compared to men, women attempt suicide two to three times as often men. Men, on the other hand, are four times more likely to commit suicide.

While all untreated mental illnesses increase the risk, depression is the most common cause of suicide. Feeling alone and hopeless further ramp up the risk. Bullying and abuse represent dangers too. According to one survey, nearly half of war veterans who return home and attend college harbor suicidal thoughts. Not surprisingly, many of them had psychiatric symptoms such as anxiety, depression, and PTSD.[112]

Protective factors include effective mental health care, restricted access to lethal weapons (especially firearms), robust connections to friends and family, and religious and cultural beliefs against suicide.[113]

Suicide warning signs include feeling hopeless, trapped, and without purpose; engaging in high-risk activities (with no apparent thought); increasing use of alcohol or drugs; expressions of rage or agitation; withdrawing from friends and family; having thoughts of suicide; looking for ways to commit suicide; and talking or writing about a wish to die.[114]

If you or someone you know exhibits such signs, get help immediately. Call a mental health provider or 911 or proceed immediately to the emergency room of the nearest hospital. Your campus may have a crisis hotline.

Other resources include the following:

- 24-hour National Suicide Prevention Lifeline, 1-800-273-TALK (8255)
- Veterans Crisis Line, 800-273-8255, press 1
- Suicide Prevention Resource Center, http://www.sprc.org, 877-GET-SPRC (438-7722)
- Suicide Hotlines, http://www.suicidehotlines.com, 1-800-SUICIDE (1-800-784-2433)

Audio Link 5.1

Prevent Suicide in Young Adults

This audio recording from the National Institute of Mental Health discusses the risk of mental illness and suicide on college campuses. The narrator notes that among college students, 13 percent have been diagnosed with mental illness and 10 percent have a friend who attempted suicide within the last year.

http://www.nimh.nih.gov/news/media/audio/prevent-suicide-in-young-adults.shtml

Video Link 5.4

Suicide Prevention and Research

This National Institute of Mental Health video discusses risk factors for suicide and efforts to prevent and treat suicide.

http://www.nimh.nih.gov/news/media/video/suicide-prevention-and-research.shtml

Yoga and Acupuncture as Complementary Therapies

The ancient Indian practice of yoga is thought to enhance the connection between mind and body. Awareness of emotions, thoughts, and bodily sensations increases. You learn tools for coping with challenges, both on and off the yoga mat. You learn to quiet the stress response—both nervous system activation and hormones.[115] Yogic breathing exercises, meditation, and poses all help alleviate mental and emotional distress. An analysis of 10 studies investigating yoga as adjunct treatment judged the practice helpful in anxiety, PTSD, and schizophrenia.[116] It may help resolve symptoms that linger despite conventional treatment.

Preliminary studies suggest promise for the use of acupuncture as a complement to the conventional treatment of anxiety,[117] PTSD,[118] schizophrenia,[119] and depression.[120] More rigorous research is needed to confirm the efficacy.

Bipolar Disorder

Bipolar disorder (BPD) was formerly more descriptively called manic-depressive disorder. People with this condition have episodes of depression and its polar opposite: *mania*. A manic episode is marked by an abnormally elevated mood, racing thoughts, rapid speech, grandiose ideas, and increased activity and energy. The initial euphoria and increased energy may, at first, feel exhilarating. But symptoms and behaviors can spiral out of control. Ideas come so quickly that confusion replaces clarity. Irritability, impatience, agitation, and anger uproot tranquility. Manic people may not sleep for days. During that time, they may accomplish brilliant work or they may do weird things like talk to truckers all night on a CB radio. Poor judgment and impulsiveness can lead to risky sexual activities, drinking, substance abuse, fighting, gambling, and ruinous spending sprees. For example, someone without means may buy a Porsche on credit, only to lose it in a bet or total it in an accident. Or he might fill shopping carts with things he doesn't even like and has no use for. Sometimes depression and mania can overlap in what's called a "mixed state." In that case, a person can feel highly energized and agitated and also empty, sad, and hopeless.

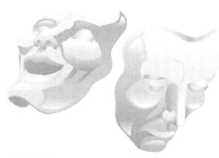

© *Thinkstock*

bipolar disorder (BPD)

Also known as manic-depressive illness, a condition that results in both depression and mania, which is characterized by high energy, decreased sleep, euphoria, restlessness, agitation, rapid thoughts, and impulsive behavior.

FIGURE 5.2 Mood Scale

Everyone has a range of moods. In bipolar disorder, the swings are extreme.

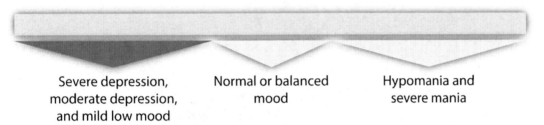

| Severe depression, moderate depression, and mild low mood | Normal or balanced mood | Hypomania and severe mania |

Source: Adapted from National Institute of Mental Health. 2008. Available at: http://www.nimh.nih.gov/images/pubs/r2_bipolar-adults-scale.jpg.

Typically, periods of normal mood—often lasting two to three years—intervene between the two opposing poles of depression and mania. Some people, however, slip from mania into depression or vice versa. Some even rapidly cycle between the two over the course of days or hours. Often people first develop symptoms of depression. Because bipolar disorder is biologically different from unipolar depression (depression without mania), antidepressant medication may trigger mania.

According to the National Institute of Mental Health, 2.6 percent of adults have bipolar disorder.[121] Symptoms usually surface during late adolescence or early adulthood. But children can also have this disorder. The cause isn't known. The condition does run in families, suggesting genetic origins. However, while having a parent or sibling with the disease raises the risk by a factor of four to six, not every child born into such a family will become bipolar.[122]

Treatment is critical. Without it, abnormal moods can last days, weeks, or even months. Also the condition can worsen, with symptoms becoming more intense and more frequent. Relationships fall apart and jobs are lost. People may abuse substances in an attempt to self-treat.

Severe mania or depression necessitates hospital admission. Milder symptoms can be managed on an outpatient basis. Either way, medications and psychotherapy manage symptoms and the behaviors that may trigger those symptoms. They also reduce the risk of relapse. Mood-stabilizing medications include the element lithium and anticonvulsant drugs such as valproic acid, divalproex sodium (Depakote), and lomtrigine (Lamictal). It's important that a mental health specialist monitor for adverse effects, symptom progression, or the development of suicidal thoughts.

Video Clip 5.5

Bipolar Disorder
A student at the University of Texas talks about his experience with bipolar disorder. He refers to SSD, which stands for Services for Students with Disabilities. Most colleges and universities offer such supportive services.

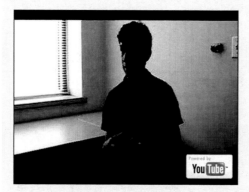

View the video online at: http://www.youtube.com/v/b-qQVG-OnHs

Herbs and Other Dietary Supplements

St. John's Wort

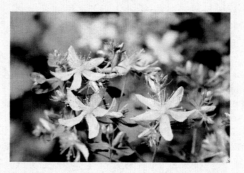

© *Thinkstock*

Mental illness is just as serious as heart disease and diabetes. No matter the condition, self-care is always a good idea. However, while scientific evidence supports the use of some supplements for mental health, it's nonetheless important to work with a mental health expert.

That said, the best-researched supplement for depression is *St. John's wort*. People used it for centuries to lift mood. Studies show that, for mild to moderate depression, standardized extracts work better than placebo (dummy pill) treatment and on par with synthetic antidepressants, though with fewer side effects.[123]

Because it can increase sun sensitivity, fair-skinned people should take precautions to avoid sunburn. Also, this herb speeds up the body's breakdown of many medications, including oral contraceptives and drugs used to treat conditions such as asthma, HIV infection, heart disease, seizures, and cancer. As a result, blood levels of medications can fall below therapeutic levels. Check with your doctor before combining St. John's wort with medications. Do not combine this herb with antidepressant drugs and avoid it if you have bipolar disorder.

Two lesser known herbs, rhodiola and saffron, also show promise in managing mild depression.[124],[125] Rhodiola also has antianxiety action. A number of other herbs reduce anxiety and nervous tension, including valerian,[126] passionflower, skullcap, hops, lemon balm, passionflower,[127],[128] and German chamomile.[129] German chamomile has been shown to provide relief for people with generalized anxiety disorder.[130] A few studies suggest that essential oils such as lavender, bergamot, ylang ylang, and sandalwood can temporarily reduce feelings of anxiety.[131],[132] These concentrated plant extracts can be inhaled or diluted into a carrier oil and massaged into the skin but are not taken internally.

The best-researched herb in anxiety disorders is the South Pacific plant *kava*. Several studies have shown kava superior to placebo.[133] When compared to sedative drugs, kava reduces anxiety but without impairing mental and physical function. Unfortunately, case reports have linked use of kava extracts with liver damage. To date, the cause is not clear. Theories include using the wrong plant parts or varieties of the plant, moldy plant parts, taking kava along with substances that injure the liver (alcohol, Tylenol), or atypical breakdown of plant chemicals in the body.[134] Test-tube studies suggest damage to liver cells is possible. However, research studies lasting up to six months have not reported serious side effects. Many experts recommend that people refrain from taking kava extracts until further research confirms both its effectiveness and safety.

A nonherbal product is *S-adenosyl methionine* (SAMe), which occurs naturally in the body. Studies indicate that supplements can improve depression symptoms.[135] While SAMe has been shown to improve response to conventional treatment,[136] it should not be combined with antidepressant drugs without physician monitoring. Because of the risk of triggering mania, people with bipolar disorder shouldn't take it. Otherwise, its main drawback is expense.

Omega-3 fatty acids are a type of polyunsaturated fat abundant in cold-water fish. Low levels correlate with an increased risk of depression and ADHD. People who regularly eat fish have a lower risk of depression and suicide.[137] Preliminary research suggests that fish oil supplements improve symptoms of depression[138] and ADHD[139],[140] and lengthen the time in remission in bipolar disorder.[141] Preliminary research suggest that supplementation with fish oil (plus or minus evening primrose oil) improves ADHD symptoms in children.

2.4   Psychotic Disorders

A person in the grips of **psychosis** has lost touch with reality. It becomes difficult to distinguish between what is real and what isn't. He or she may have auditory hallucinations (e.g., hear voices), visual hallucinations, and *delusions*, ideas the person believes to be true but are not. For instance, a man may believe he is King Arthur or Superman. The delusions may be paranoid, in which the person suspects he is being persecuted or betrayed. A woman might believe her dentist has implanted tiny transmitters in her teeth that will allow blood-thirsty aliens to track her down. The hallucinations and delusions seem quite real and, depending on their nature, terrifying.

The causes of psychosis divide into three broad categories.

1. **Substances.** Examples include alcohol, cocaine, amphetamines, MDMA (Ecstasy), cannabis (marijuana), psilocybins (from a particular species of mushroom), lysergic acid (LSD), and ketamine. Once the substance wears off, the psychosis resolves.

2. **Medical conditions.** Parkinson's disease, Alzheimer's disease, and Lewy body dementia directly affect the central nervous system. Depending on location and size, brain tumors can lead to psychotic symptoms. Serious infections with fevers such as malaria can produce hallucinations. In the case of brain tumor and infection, treating the underlying cause can clear the psychosis.

3. **Psychiatric conditions.** Severe depression or the mania associated with bipolar disorder can produce symptoms of psychosis. Cases of extreme stress such as PTSD can lead to moments of psychosis. **Schizophrenia** is a chronic, debilitating condition whose primary symptoms are hallucinations and delusions. Thoughts and speech become disorganized. Worldwide, about 4 in 1,000 people have schizophrenia.[142] Symptoms begin during adolescence and early adulthood and can make it difficult to impossible to function in school and work and to maintain social relationships. Brain abnormalities exist, though the cause is not well understood. Antipsychotic medications diminish symptoms and prevent relapses.[143]

psychosis

A severe psychological disorder wherein radical changes in personality and impairment of thoughts and emotions lead to loss of contact with reality.

schizophrenia

A chronic, debilitating condition marked by hallucinations and delusions.

2.5   Attention Deficit Hyperactivity Disorder

Attention deficit hyperactivity disorder (ADHD) is classified as a behavior disorder. Children and adults with ADHD exhibit some degree of inattention and distractibility, restlessness and hyperactivity, and impulsivity (trouble restraining their urges). They may become easily bored or frustrated with tasks. They mentally drift off. Tasks remain unfinished. Homework and other items get lost. Problems sleeping are also common.

ADHD varies in its presentation and exists along a spectrum. Some scientists believe that it's not a single disorder.[144] Some people predominantly express symptoms related to marshaling and sustaining inattention. They daydream, move slowly, have trouble completing directions, forget things, and seem not to listen. Other people exhibit more symptoms of hyperactivity and impulsivity. They can't sit still, talk a blue streak, interrupt, and cut in line. Often kids and adults have a combination of all these symptoms.

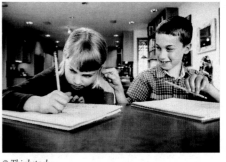

© *Thinkstock*

Behaviors typical of ADHD can interfere with a child's ability to function successfully at home and at school and challenge relationships with family and peers. Likewise, adults may have problems at work and in their personal lives. It's difficult to manage time, stay organized, keep on task, and meet goals. Inadequate treatment results in repeated reprimands and failures in school and work, damaged self-esteem, substance abuse, accidents, and trouble with the law.

According to a large national survey, 9 percent of teens 17 to 18 years old have ADHD.[145] Overall, 4 percent of girls and 13 percent of boys have it. Troublesome behaviors surface before age seven. While symptoms and signs can change with age, they can often persist into adulthood.

Scientists don't know exactly what causes ADHD. Genetics play a role, as do environmental and social factors.[146] Some experts believe that television overstimulates the brain. A recent study found that for every hour of daily television viewing, kids aged one to three faced a 10 percent increased risk of developing problems with attention by age seven.[147] A related theory is that insufficient exercise plays a role in ADHD. Television takes the place of physical activity, compounding reduced physical education in schools.

No objective tests for ADHD exist. Diagnosis hinges upon a child's history and physical exam, reports from parents and teachers, and subjective rating scales. Sometimes children are misdiagnosed with ADHD when they actually have an anxiety disorder, a sleep disorder, unmet emotional needs, a conflict-ridden home life, or other problems that interfere with sustained attention and composure. Occasionally, adults' expectations are unreasonably rigid or the child is lagging in developmental maturity. That's why it's important to meet with a mental health specialist.

This heterogeneity of ADHD means a one-size-fits-all treatment simply doesn't work for all people. Conventional treatment centers on stimulant medications to control symptoms. Examples include methylphenidate (Ritalin) and amphetamine salts (Adderall). These medications can improve grades and behavior at home and at school.[148] Side effects for the first few days include nausea, dizziness, abdominal pain, and headaches. Reduced appetite with resultant weight loss may persist. People with preexisting heart problems are at a slightly higher risk of heart attack and stroke.[149] Nonstimulant drugs such as atomoxetine (Strattera) have also successfully been used. Side effects include upset stomach, decreased appetite, and dizziness.

In addition, education and therapy are important. Kids need to learn life skills to help with focus, attention, and planning. Parents, caregivers, and teachers need to learn effective, humane means to counter unruly behavior and structure activities. The combination of therapy plus drugs is thought to be the ideal treatment—more effective than either treatment alone.[150]

Lifestyle changes may also help. In the 1970s, allergist Dr. Ben Feingold posited that diet could affect behavior. More specifically, he linked color additives and other artificial ingredients in foods and beverages to hyperactivity and believed that a hypoallergenic, additive-free diet could be therapeutic.[151] Many practitioners dismissed his theories, although some practitioners and families reported success. The debate continues today. A 2011 study linked "Western" diets (lots of processed foods, fat, and sugar) with double the risk of ADHD compared to a "healthy" diet, one low in junk foods and rich in fruits, vegetables, legumes, whole grains, and fish.[152] A 2012 review of the literature reiterated the protective effects of healthy diets.[153] Kids with ADHD can have low levels of polyunsaturated fats; supplementation with omega-3 fatty acids (plus or minus omega-6 fats) may improve symptoms. The review study's authors also noted that, in the face of known deficiency of zinc or iron, supplementation may help.

Exercise not only helps dissipate frustration and pent-up energy; it may also improve higher thinking functions in kids with ADHD.[154] Learning to relax and focus the mind takes practice for us all. Preliminary research indicates benefits for modalities such as massage,[155] meditation,[156] yoga,[157] biofeedback,[158] and progressive muscle relaxation[159] can help children and adolescents with ADHD.

Video Clip 5.6

Brain Changes in ADHD
Dr. Gerald Chodak discusses changes in brain structure and function associated with ADHD. From Answers.com TV.

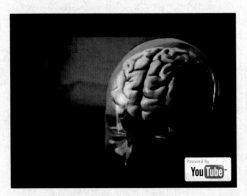

View the video online at: http://www.youtube.com/v/u82nzTzL7To

Accessing Student Support Services

If you're a college student with a mental or behavior health condition, find out what support services are available on campus. If your college is far from home, you will probably need to find a new mental health specialist. The college student health center may have someone on staff or at least be able to refer you. Also, many psychological conditions qualify you for disability accommodations. Find out about your college's center for students with disabilities and book an appointment. Try to do that before the start of the semester. Normally, professors can't make accommodations retroactively.

Another resource is Children and Adults with Attention Deficit Disorders (http://www.chadd.org/), an advocacy group that disseminates information about ADHD, including how to find support for this condition; training and conferences; and relevant books, videos, and audios.

2.6   Autism Spectrum Disorders

Autism spectrum disorders (ASD) are a group of developmental disabilities characterized by problems with social interactions, communication, and peculiar repetitive behaviors. Autism is perhaps the best known of these disorders.

Children with ASD typically avoid eye contact, dislike being touched, don't play well with others, and don't speak or have delayed development of speech. When they can feel emotions and affection, they don't display them. They also display narrow interests. For instance, a child may be interested in dinosaurs and little else. Physical movements tend to be clumsy. Repetitive movements include hand clapping, arm flapping, rocking, and head rolling. Rigid adherence to daily rituals—dressing, food choices, and so on—is common.

Children with autism also often have some degree of mental retardation. *Asperger syndrome* is a mild form of autism. Language typically develops late. Speech is often stilted and formal. Impairments in nonverbal communication skills (gestures, facial expressions, eye contact, body posture, touch) suggest indifference toward others, including family members. Social impairments render the person awkward. Intelligence, however, is normal to above average. The latest version of the American Psychiatric Association's *Diagnostic and Statistical Manual of Mental Disorders* eliminated Asperger's syndrome as a distinct illness within ASD.

As you can see, the degree of impairment in ASD varies widely. Some individuals don't speak and exhibit severe mental retardation. Some are highly intelligent with only mildly impaired social skills. Such people may complete advanced degrees and excel in careers that don't require charisma.

Obvious signs of developmental delays show up before affected children reach their third birthdays. There are no objective diagnostic tests such as blood tests or brain scans for ASD. Instead, health professionals, along with the help of parents and other caregivers, observe that the child isn't developing normally.

autism spectrum disorders

A group of developmental disabilities beginning in early childhood and characterized by difficulty forming relationships and communicating and repetitive activities.

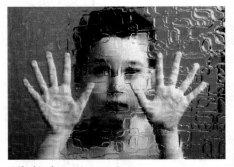

© *Thinkstock*

Alarmingly, autism spectrum disorders are on the rise, though scientists don't know why. Some of the apparent escalation in the incidence of ASD may be due to increased awareness and diagnosis of these conditions. Between 2006 and 2008, the prevalence increased 23 percent. According to a government survey, ASD affects 1 out of every 88 children eight years of age.[160] That's nearly 1 percent of kids. Four times more boys than girls develop ASD. White children are at greater risk than black or Hispanic children. The estimated annual cost is $126 billion.

Researchers have identified subtle differences in the brains of people with autism compared to those without it. These changes may explain why a person with ASD has trouble integrating sensory stimuli. However, the cause of these developmental disorders is unknown. Genetics and environmental factors both seem to contribute.[161],[162] Identical twins share the same genes, yet autism may only affect one of the pair. Environmental risks seem to begin as early as the mother's pregnancy. Scientists have researched heavy metals and pesticides as possible causative agents—to no avail. Studies have linked ASD with older parental age, obesity and diabetes in pregnant women, small size at birth, and premature birth.[163],[164],[165] However, association doesn't prove causation.

Contrary to myth, the measles, mumps, and rubella (MMR) vaccine does not increase the risk of autism.[166] Multiple studies fail to show any association. In fact, the opposite is true. Babies exposed to rubella (German measles) while in the womb, a condition called congenital rubella syndrome, are at risk for ASD and other devastating consequences. Vaccinations against rubella (the R in the MMR vaccine) prevent congenital rubella syndrome and therefore protect against ASD.[167]

While there is no cure for ASD, a number of nondrug treatments can help, particularly if begun early in a child's life. Special education and therapy are essential to improve social and communication skills and manage potentially destructive behaviors. Studies show that early, intensive therapy improves outcomes.[168] Parents, other caregivers, siblings, and teachers all need support. Prescription drugs are sometimes used to manage aggressive, hyperactive, and self-injurious behavior.

 Video Clip 5.7

What Is Autism?

An Overview Provided by Children's Hospital Los Angeles.

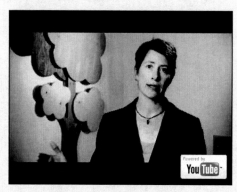

View the video online at: http://www.youtube.com/v/IbUTx-GHMao

KEY TAKEAWAYS

- Psychological disorders are common and can lead to chronic disability.
- Mental illness is underdiagnosed and undertreated.
- Oftentimes, treatment can markedly decrease and even eliminate symptoms.
- Although symptoms of psychological distress can arise in anyone, persistence and impairment of daily function indicate significant disorder.
- Anxiety disorders are the most common type of mental illness and include generalized anxiety disorder, panic disorder, phobias, obsessive-compulsive disorder, and posttraumatic stress disorder.
- Mood disorders include depression and bipolar disorder, a condition wherein mood can swing between depression and mania.
- Some psychological disorders, other medical conditions, and drugs and other substances can lead to psychosis, a disconnection from reality.
- Attention deficit hyperactivity disorder is a behavioral problem with some combination of inattention, excessive physical activity, and impulsive behavior.
- Autism spectrum disorder is an umbrella term for a group of neurodevelopmental disabilities that impair social interactions and interpersonal communication. People with these disorders usually engage in rigid, repetitive behaviors.

DISCUSSION QUESTIONS

1. Discuss the connection between stress and psychological disease.
2. Explain the difference between normal anxiety and generalized anxiety disorder.
3. Ralph seemed sad and withdrawn at the start of the semester. He rejected invitations to go out with his friends and spent hours alone in his room. After a few weeks, he appeared better. However, just before finals, his roommate reported that Ralph wasn't sleeping at night. On the way to class, he danced through campus. He scaled the wall of the student center and, from the roof, tossed dollar bills below. He stopped attending class and talked incessantly about various half-baked projects. What do you think might be Ralph's problem? List the warning signs you notice that led you to that conclusion.
4. Sandrine was raped as a child and has since struggled with PTSD and depression. She did pretty well her first year of college, but then she stopped going to therapy and taking her medications and fell in with a group that partied heavily on weekends. Someone posted pictures of her looking drunk and disheveled on a social media site. Sandrine's grades fell. She didn't think she could possibly turn her grade point average around. Her parents, she was sure, wouldn't forgive her. College—even her whole life—seemed pointless. She started smoking. She drank during the day. She had sex with anyone who asked. When friends commented, she flew into a rage and isolated herself from them even further. She gave away her cat, saying he was better off without her. She stole her roommate's sleeping pills and hid them under her bed. Analyze this case and include a list of all the warning signs that support your opinion. If you were Sandrine's roommate or friend, what would you do?

3. RECOMMENDED RESOURCES

3.1 Books

Achor S. *The Happiness Advantage: The Seven Principles of Positive Psychology That Fuel Success and Performance at Work*. New York, NY: Crown Business; 2010.

Jamison KR. *An Unquiet Mind: A Memoir of Moods and Madness*. New York, NY: Vintage; 1997.

Keim J. *The Joy of Appreciative Living*. New York, NY: Tarcher; 2008.

Lyubomirsky S. *The How of Happiness*. New York, NY: Penguin; 2007.

Schiller L. *The Quiet Room: A Journey Out of the Torment of Madness*. New York, NY: Grand Central Publishing; 1996.

Seligman MEP. *Authentic Happiness: Using the New Positive Psychology to Realize Your Potential for Lasting Fulfillment*. New York, NY: Free Press; 2003. Available at: http://www.authentichappiness.sas.upenn.edu.

Seligman MEP. *Learned Optimism: How to Change Your Mind and Your Life*. Vintage; 2006.

Seligman MEP. *Flourish: A Visionary New Understanding of Happiness and Well-being*. New York, NY: Free Press; 2011.

Stangor, C. *Introduction to Psychology*. Available at: http://catalog.flatworldknowledge.com/bookhub/reader/127.

3.2 Organizations and Websites

American Psychiatric Association. http://www.psych.org.

American Psychological Association. http://www.apa.org.

HOPES Brain Tutorial. Huntington's Outreach Project for Education at Stanford University. https://hopes.stanford.edu/sites/hopes/files/brain.swf.

National Alliance on Mental Illness. http://www.nami.org.

National Institute of Mental Health. http://www.nimh.nih.gov.

Neuroscience for Kids. http://faculty.washington.edu/chudler/functional.html.

3.3 Videos

For those of you who want to understand more about the structure and function of the nervous system, check out The Human Nervous System Part 1, http://www.youtube.com/watch?v=4M82WwFACLg&feature=related, created by Michael Chin for his 12th grade biology class.

Renowned researcher, author, and Stanford University professor Robert Sapolsky, PhD, speaks engagingly about the biological basis of major depression. This video is 52 minutes long. http://www.youtube.com/watch?v=NOAgpIgTxfc&feature=relmfu.

ENDNOTES

1. Kallgren J; Associated Press. Lunch-break dance spreads in Europe. *USA Today*. April 1, 2012. Available at: http://usatoday30.usatoday.com/money/workplace/story/2012-04-01/sweden-lunch-beat/53887376/1. Accessed May 27, 2013.

2. Chudler EH. Brain facts and figures. University of Washington. Available at: http://faculty.washington.edu/chudler/facts.html. Accessed April 7, 2012.

3. Courchesne E, Mouton PR, Calhoun ME, et al. Neuron number and size in prefrontal cortex of children with autism. *JAMA*. 2011 Nov 9;306(18):2001–2010.

4. Eriksson PS, Perfilieva E, Björk-Eriksson T, Alborn AM, Nordborg C, Peterson DA, Gage FH. Neurogenesis in the adult human hippocampus. *Nat Med*. 1998 Nov;4(11):1313–1317.

5. Raznahan A, Shaw P, Lalonde F, et al. How does your cortex grow? *J Neurosci*. 2011 May 11;31(19):7174–7177.

6. Lyubomirsky S, King L, Diener E. The benefits of frequent positive affect: does happiness lead to success? *Psychol Bull*. 2005 Nov;131(6):803–855.

7. Cohn MA, Fredrickson BL, Brown SL, Mikels JA, Conway AM. Happiness unpacked: positive emotions increase life satisfaction by building resilience. *Emotion*. 2009 Jun;9(3):361–368.

8. Cheung RY, Park IJ. Anger suppression, interdependent self-construal, and depression among Asian American and European American college students. *Cultur Divers Ethnic Minor Psychol*. 2010 Oct;16(4):517–525.

9. Norwood SJ, Bowker A, Buchholz A, Henderson KA, Goldfield G, Flament MF. Self-silencing and anger regulation as predictors of disordered eating among adolescent females. *Eat Behav*. 2011 Apr;12(2):112–118.

10. Quartana PJ, Bounds S, Yoon KL, Goodin BR, Burns JW. Anger suppression predicts pain, emotional, and cardiovascular responses to the cold pressor. *Ann Behav Med*. 2010 Jun;39(3):211–221.

11. Olives EV, Forero CG, Maydeu-Olivares A, et al. Environmental risk and protective factors of adolescents' and youths' mental health: differences between parents' appraisal and self-reports. *Qual Life Res*. 2013 Apr;22(3):613–622. doi:10.1007/s11136-012-0167-x.

12. Wood AM, Froh JJ, Geraghty AW. Gratitude and well-being: a review and theoretical integration. *Clin Psychol Rev*. 2010 Nov;30(7):890–905.

13. Lambert NM, Fincham FD, Stillman TF. Gratitude and depressive symptoms: the role of positive reframing and positive emotion. *Cogn Emot*. 2011. doi:10.1080/02699931.2011.595393.

14. Emmons RA, McCullough ME. Counting blessings versus burdens: an experimental investigation of gratitude and subjective well-being in daily life. *J Pers Soc Psychol*. 2003 Feb;84(2):377–389.

15. Mora-Ripoll R. Potential health benefits of simulated laughter: a narrative review of the literature and recommendations for future research. *Complement Ther Med*. 2011 Jun;19(3):170–177.

16. Bennett MP, Lengacher C. Humor and laughter may influence health: III. Laughter and health outcomes. *Evid Based Complement Alternat Med*. 2008 March;5(1):37–40. doi:10.1093/ecam/nem041. Available at: http://www.ncbi.nlm.nih.gov/pmc/articles/PMC2249748/?tool=pubmed. Accessed May 18, 2012.

17. Shahidi M, Mojtahed A, Modabbernia A, Mojtahed M, Shafiabady A, Delavar A, Honari H. Laughter yoga versus group exercise program in elderly depressed women: a randomized controlled trial. *Int J Geriatr Psychiatry*. 2011 Mar;26(3):322–327. doi:10.1002/gps.2545.

18. Cho EA, Oh HE. Effects of laughter therapy on depression, quality of life, resilience and immune responses in breast cancer survivors. *J Korean Acad Nurs*. 2011 Jun;41(3):285–293. doi:10.4040/jkan.2011.41.3.285.

19. Diener E, Seligman ME. Very happy people. *Psychol Sci*. 2002 Jan;13(1):81–84.

20. Demir M, Ozdemir M, Marum KP. Perceived autonomy support, friendship maintenance, and happiness. *J Psychol*. 2011 Nov–Dec;145(6):537–571.

21. Deci EL, La Guardia JG, Moller AC, Scheiner MJ, Ryan RM. On the benefits of giving as well as receiving autonomy support: mutuality in close friendships. *Pers Soc Psychol Bull*. 2006 Mar;32(3):313–327.

22. Visser PL, Loess P, Jeglic EL, Hirsch JK. Hope as a moderator of negative life events and depressive symptoms in a diverse sample. *Stress Health*. 2012 May 2. doi:10.1002/smi.2433 [Epub ahead of print].

23. Lawler-Row KA, Karremans JC, Scott C, Edlis-Matityahou M, Edwards L. Forgiveness, physiological reactivity and health: the role of anger. *Int J Psychophysiol*. 2008 Apr;68(1):51–58.

24. Saulle R, La Torre G. Good quality and available urban green spaces as good quality, health and wellness for human life. *J Public Health (Oxf)*. 2012 Mar;34(1):161–162.

25. Garcion E, Wion-Bardot N, Montero-Menei C, Berger F, Didier W. New clues about vitamin D functions in the nervous system. *Trends Endocrinol Metab*. 2002;13:100.

26. Salgado-Delgado R, Tapia Osorio A, Saderi N, Escobar C. Disruption of circadian rhythms: a crucial factor in the etiology of depression. *Depress Res Treat*. 2011;2011:839743.

27. Brummett BH, Helms MJ, Dahlstrom WG, Siegler IC. Prediction of all-cause mortality by the Minnesota Multiphasic Personality Inventory Optimism-Pessimism Scale scores: study of a college sample during a 40-year follow-up period. *Mayo Clin Proc*. 2006;81(12):1541–1544.

28. Maruta T, Colligan RC, Malinchoc M, Offord KP. Optimism-pessimism assessed in the 1960s and self-reported health status 30 years later. *Mayo Clin Proc*. 2002;77(8):748–753.

29. Boehm JK, Kubzansky LD. The heart's content: the association between positive psychological well-being and cardiovascular health. *Psychol Bull*. 2012 Apr 16 [Epub ahead of print].

30. Parrott MD, Greenwood CE. Dietary influences on cognitive function with aging: from high-fat diets to healthful eating. *Ann NY Acad Sci*. 2007 Oct;1114:389–397.

31. Sánchez-Villegas A, Delgado-Rodríguez M, Alonso A, Schlatter J, Lahortiga F, Serra Majem L, Martínez-González MA. Association of the Mediterranean dietary pattern with the incidence of depression: the Seguimiento Universidad de Navarra/University of Navarra follow-up (SUN) cohort. *Arch Gen Psychiatry*. 2009 Oct;66(10):1090–1098.

32. Fung TT, Rexrode KM, Mantzoros CS, Manson JE, Willett WC, Hu FB. Mediterranean diet and incidence of and mortality from coronary heart disease and stroke in women. *Circulation*. 2009;119:1093–1100.

33. Solfrizzi V, Frisardi V, Seripa D, et al. Mediterranean diet in predementia and dementia syndromes. *Curr Alzheimer Res*. 2011 Aug;8(5):520–542.

34. Andrade JP, Assunção M. Protective effects of chronic green tea consumption on age-related neurodegeneration. *Curr Pharm Des*. 2012;18(1):4–14.

35. Ramassamy C. Emerging role of polyphenolic compounds in the treatment of neurodegenerative diseases: a review of their intracellular targets. *Eur J Pharmacol*. 2006 Sep 1;545(1):51–64.

36. Ahmed T, Enam SA, Gilani AH. Curcuminoids enhance memory in an amyloid-infused rat model of Alzheimer's disease. *Neuroscience*. 2010 Sep 1;169(3):1296–1306.

37. Hedelin M, Löf M, Olsson M, et al. Dietary intake of fish, omega-3, omega-6 polyunsaturated fatty acids and vitamin D and the prevalence of psychotic-like symptoms in a cohort of 33,000 women from the general population. *BMC Psychiatry*. 2010;10:38.

38. Lucas M, Mirzaei F, O'Reilly EJ, et al. Dietary intake of n-3 and n-6 fatty acids and the risk of clinical depression in women: a 10-y prospective follow-up study. *Am J Clin Nutr*. 2011;93:1337–1343.

39. Lewis MD, Hibbeln JR, Johnson JE, Lin YH, Hyun DY, Loewke JD. Suicide deaths of active-duty US military and omega-3 fatty-acid status: a case-control comparison. *J Clin Psychiatry*. 2011;72:1585–1590.

40. Tan ZS, Harris WS, Beiser AS, et al. Red blood cell omega-3 fatty acid levels and markers of accelerated brain aging. *Neurology*. 2012;78:658–664.

41. Bloch MH, Qawasmi A. Omega-3 fatty acid supplementation for the treatment of children with attention-deficit/hyperactivity disorder symptomatology: systematic review and meta-analysis. *J Am Acad Child Adolesc Psychiatry*. 2011 Oct;50(10):991–1000.

42. Lucas M, Mirzaei F, Pan A, et al. Coffee, caffeine, and risk of depression among women. *Arch Intern Med*. 2011;171:1571–1578.

43. Larsson SC, Virtamo J, Wolk A. Coffee consumption and risk of stroke in women. *Stroke*. 2011;42:908–912.

44. Ritsner MS, Miodownik C, Ratner Y, et al. L-theanine relieves positive, activation, and anxiety symptoms in patients with schizophrenia and schizoaffective disorder: an 8-week, randomized, double-blind, placebo-controlled, 2-center study. *J Clin Psychiatry*. 2011 Jan;72(1):34–42.

45. Niu K, Hozawa A, Kuriyama S, et al. Green tea consumption is associated with depressive symptoms in the elderly. *Am J Clin Nutr*. 2009 Dec;90(6):1615–1622.

46. Hozawa A, Kuriyama S, Nakaya N, et al. Green tea consumption is associated with lower psychological distress in a general population: the Ohsaki Cohort 2006 Study. *Am J Clin Nutr*. 2009 Nov;90(5):1390–1396.

47. Kuriyama S, Hozawa A, Ohmori K, et al. Green tea consumption and cognitive function: a cross-sectional study from the Tsurugaya Project 1. *Am J Clin Nutr*. 2006 Feb;83(2):355–361.

48. Arab L, Liu W, Elashoff D. Green and black tea consumption and risk of stroke: a meta-analysis. *Stroke*. 2009 May;40(5):1786–1792.

49. Xiong GL, Doraiswamy PM. Does meditation enhance cognition and brain plasticity? *Ann NY Acad Sci*. 2009 Aug;1172:63–69.

50. Buchman AS, Boyle PA, Yu L, Shah RC, Wilson RS, Bennett DA. Total daily physical activity and the risk of AD and cognitive decline in older adults. *Neurology*. 2012;78:1290–1291,1323–1329.

51. McGovern MK. The effects of exercise on the brain. Serendip Studio. Available at: http://serendip.brynmawr.edu/bb/neuro/neuro05/web2/mmcgovern.html. Accessed May 20, 2012.

52. World Health Organization. *Promoting Mental Health: Concepts, Emerging Evidence, Practice (Summary Report)*. Geneva, Switzerland: World Health Organization; 2004. Available at: http://www.who.int/mental_health/evidence/en/promoting_mhh.pdf. Accessed May 7, 2012.

53. Kessler RC, Berglund P, Demler O, Jin R, Merikangas KR, Walters EE. Lifetime prevalence and age-of-onset distributions of DSM-IV disorders in the National Comorbidity Survey Replication [published erratum appears in *Arch Gen Psychiatry*. 2005;62:768]. *Arch Gen Psychiatry*. 2005;62:593–602.

54. Eisenberg D, Hunt J, Speer N, Zivin K. Mental health service utilization among college students in the United States. *J Nerv Ment Dis*. 2011 May;199(5):301–308.

55. National Institutes of Health, National Institute of Mental Health, Collaborative Psychiatric Epidemiology Surveys, 2001–2003. Online document at: http://www.ahrq.gov/qual/qrdr08.htm. Accessed April 14, 2012.

56. Rich JD, Wakeman SE, Dickman SL. Medicine and the epidemic of incarceration in the United States. *N Engl J Med*. 2011;364(22):2081–2083.

57. de Rooij SR, Veenendaal MV, Räikkönen K, Roseboom TJ. Personality and stress appraisal in adults prenatally exposed to the Dutch famine. *Early Hum Dev*. 2012 May;88(5):321–325.

58. Rees S, Silove D, Chey T, et al. Lifetime prevalence of gender-based violence in women and the relationship with mental disorders and psychosocial function. *JAMA*. 2011;306(5): 513–521.

59. Veterans struggle with war trauma. *Los Angeles Times* website. Available at: http://articles.latimes.com/2008/apr/18/nation/na-stress18. Accessed August 28, 2011.

60. World Health Organization. *Investing in Mental Health*. Geneva, Switzerland: World Health Organization; 2003. Available at: http://www.who.int/mental_health/en/investing_in_mnh_final.pdf. Accessed May 7, 2012.

61. Barry D, Pietrzak RH, Petry NM. Gender differences in associations between body mass index and DSM-IV mood and anxiety disorders: results from the National Epidemiologic Survey on Alcohol and Related Conditions. *Ann Epidemiol*. 2008;18:458–466.

62. Cargiulo T. Understanding the health impact of alcohol dependence. *Am J Health Syst Pharm*. 2007 Mar 1;64(5 Suppl 3):S5–S11.

63. Jacka FN, Pasco JA, Mykletun A, et al. Association of Western and traditional diets with depression and anxiety in women. *Am J Psychiatry*. 2010 Mar;167(3):305–311.

64. Akbaraly TN, Brunner EJ, Ferrie JE, et al. Dietary pattern and depressive symptoms in middle age. *Br J Psychiatry*. 2009 Nov;195(5):408–413.

65. Sánchez-Villegas A, Toledo E, de Irala J, Ruiz-Canela M, Pla-Vidal J, Martínez-González MA. Fast-food and commercial baked goods consumption and the risk of depression. *Public Health Nutr*. 2012;15:424–432.

66. Jacka FN, Kremer P, Berk M, et al. A prospective study of diet quality and mental health in adolescents. *PLoS One*. 2011;6:e24805.

67. Fiocco AJ, Shatenstein B, Ferland G, et al. Sodium intake and physical activity impact cognitive maintenance in older adults: the NuAge Study. *Neurobiol Aging*. 2012 Apr;33(4):829.e21–e28.

68. Flisher C. Getting plugged in: an overview of Internet addiction. *J Paediatr Child Health*. 2010;46(10):557–559. doi:10.1111/j.1440-1754.2010.01879.x.

69. Anxiety disorders: let's talk about facts brochure. American Psychiatric Association. Available at: http://www.healthyminds.org/Document-Library/Brochure-Library/Anxiety.aspx. Accessed April 22, 2012.

70. Kessler RC, Berglund P, Demler O, Jin R, Merikangas KR, Walters EE. Lifetime prevalence and age-of-onset distributions of DSM-IV disorders in the National Comorbidity Survey Replication. *Arch Gen Psychiatry*. 2005;62:593–602.

71. Burstein M, Ameli-Grillon L, Merikangas KR. Shyness versus social phobia in US youth. *Pediatrics*. 2011 Nov;128(5):917–925.

72. Hoexter MQ, de Souza Duran FL, D'Alcante CC, et al. Gray matter volumes in obsessive-compulsive disorder before and after fluoxetine or cognitive-behavior therapy: a randomized clinical trial. *Neuropsychopharmacology*. 2012 Feb;37(3):734–745. doi:10.1038/npp.2011.250.

73. Hoffmann SG, Heering S, Sawyer AT, Asnaani A. How to handle anxiety: the effects of reappraisal, acceptance, and suppression strategies on anxious arousal. *Behav Res Ther*. 2009;47(5):389–394.

74. Gortner EM, Rude SS, Pennebaker JW. Benefits of expressive writing in lowering rumination and depressive symptoms. *Behav Ther*. 2006 Sep;37(3):292–303.

75. Baddeley JL, Pennebaker JW. A postdeployment expressive writing intervention for military couples: a randomized controlled trial. *J Trauma Stress*. 2011 Oct;24(5):581–585. doi:10.1002/jts.20679.

76. Writing about emotions may ease stress and trauma. Harvard Health Publications. Harvard Medical School. October 22, 2011. Available at: http://www.health.harvard.edu/healthbeat/writing-about-emotions-may-ease-stress-and-trauma?utm_source=review&utm_medium=email&utm_campaign=OCTOBER2011&j=27937255&e=lwhite27@mscd.edu&l=16278673_HTML&u=321965855&mid=148797&jb=0. Accessed April 22, 2012.

77. Smith C, Hancock H, Blake-Mortimer J, Eckert K. A randomised comparative trial of yoga and relaxation to reduce stress and anxiety. *Complement Ther Med*. 2007 Jun;15(2):77–83.

78. Jin P. Efficacy of Tai Chi, brisk walking, meditation, and reading in reducing mental and emotional stress. *J Psychosom Res*. 1992 May;36(4):361–370.

79. Carmody J, Baer RA. Relationships between mindfulness practice and levels of mindfulness, medical and psychological symptoms and well-being in a mindfulness-based stress reduction program. *J Behav Med*. 2007 Sep 25 [Epub ahead of print].

80. Srivastava M, Talukdar U, Lahan V. Meditation for the management of adjustment disorder anxiety and depression. *Complement Ther Clin Pract*. 2011 Nov;17(4):241–245. doi:10.1016/j.ctcp.2011.04.007.

81. Sánchez-Meca J, Rosa-Alcázar AI, Marín-Martínez F, Gómez-Conesa A. Psychological treatment of panic disorder with or without agoraphobia: a meta-analysis. *Clin Psychol Rev*. 2010 Feb;30(1):37–50.

82. Kessler RC, Berglund P, Demler O, Jin R, Merikangas KR, Walters EE. Lifetime prevalence and age-of-onset distributions of DSM-IV disorders in the National Comorbidity Survey Replication. *Arch Gen Psychiatry*. 2005;62:593–602.

83. Depression. World Health Organization. Available at: http://www.who.int/mental_health/management/depression/en/. Accessed April 1, 2012.

84. Jane Costello E, Erkanli A, Angold A. Is there an epidemic of child or adolescent depression? *J Child Psychol Psychiatry*. 2006;47:1263–1271.

85. National Comorbidity Survey Replication (NCS-R). Table 1. Lifetime prevalence of DSM-IV/WMH-CIDI disorders by sex and cohort (n=9282). 2007. Available at: http://www.hcp.med.harvard.edu/ncs. Accessed May 7, 2012.

86. Bromet E, Andrade LH, Hwang I, et al. Cross-national epidemiology of DSM-IV major depressive episode. *BMC Med*. 2011 Jul 26;9:90.

87. Morris DW, Trivedi MH, Rush AJ. Folate and unipolar depression. *J Altern Complement Med*. 2008 Apr;14(3):277–285.

88. Tariq MM, Streeten EA, Smith HA, et al. Vitamin D: a potential role in reducing suicide risk? *Int J Adolesc Med Health*. 2011;23(3):157–165.

89. Bertone-Johnson ER. Vitamin D and the occurrence of depression: causal association or circumstantial evidence? *Nutr Rev*. 2009 Aug;67(8):481–492.

90. Irwin M, Costlow C, Williams H, et al. Cellular immunity to varicella-zoster virus in patients with major depression. *J Infect Dis*. 1998 Nov;178 Suppl 1:S104–S108.

91. Kiecolt-Glaser JK, Glaser R. Depression and immune function: central pathways to morbidity and mortality. *J Psychosom Res*. 2002;53(4):873–876.

92. Whang W, Kubzansky LD, Kawachi I, et al. Depression and risk of sudden cardiac death and coronary heart disease in women: results from the Nurses' Health Study. *J Am Coll Cardiol*. 2009;53:950–958. doi:10.1016/j.jacc.2008.10.060. Available at: http://www.ncbi.nlm.nih.gov/pmc/articles/PMC2664253/?tool=pubmed. Accessed August 12, 2011.

93. Pan A, Okereke OI, Sun Q, et al. Depression and incident stroke in women. *Stroke*. 2011. doi:10.1161/strokeaha.111.617043 [Published online ahead of print]. Available at: http://stroke.ahajournals.org/content/early/2011/08/11/STROKEAHA.111.617043.abstract. Accessed August 12, 2011.

94. Jorm AF. Is depression a risk factor for dementia or cognitive decline? A review. *Gerontology*. 2000 Jul–Aug;46(4):219–227.

95. Paulson D, Bowen ME, Lichtenberg PA. Successful aging and longevity in older old women: the role of depression and cognition. *J Aging Res*. 2011;2011:912680.

96. Depression. World Health Organization. Available at: http://www.who.int/mental_health/management/depression/definition/en. Accessed April 1, 2012.

97. Sipe WE, Eisendrath SJ. Mindfulness-based cognitive therapy: theory and practice. *Can J Psychiatry*. 2012 Feb;57(2):63–69.

98. Pratt LA, Brody DJ, Gu Q. Antidepressant use in persons aged 12 and over: United States, 2005–2008. National Health and Nutrition Examination Surveys. Centers for Disease Control and Prevention. Available at: http://www.cdc.gov/nchs/data/databriefs/db76.htm. Accessed April 1, 2012.

99. Rush AJ, Trivedi MH, Wisniewski SR, et al. Acute and longer-term outcomes in depressed outpatients requiring one or several treatment steps: a STAR*D report. *Am J Psychiatry*. 2006;163(11):1905–1917.

100. Harmer CJ, O'Sullivan U, Favaron E, et al. Effect of acute antidepressant administration on negative affective bias in depressed patients. *Am J Psychiatry*. 2009 Oct;166(10):1178–1184.

101. Leon AC, Solomon DA, Li C, Fiedorowicz JG, Coryell WH, Endicott J, Keller MB. Antidepressants and risks of suicide and suicide attempts: a 27-year observational study. *J Clin Psychiatry*. 2011;72(5):580–586.

102. Warner CH, Bobo W, Warner C. Antidepressant discontinuation syndrome. *Am Fam Physician*. 2006;74:449–456, 457.

103. Layous K, Chancellor J, Lyubomirsky S, Wang L, Doraiswamy M. Delivering happiness: translating positive psychology intervention research for treating major and minor depressive disorders. *J Altern Complement Med*. 2011;17(8):675–683. doi:10.1089/acm.2011.0139.

104. Seligman MEP, Steen TA, Park N, Peterson C. Positive psychology progress: empirical validation of interventions. *Am Psychol*. 2005;60:410–421.

105. Fava GA, Ruini C. The sequential approach to relapse prevention in unipolar depression. *World Psychiatry*. 2002 Feb;1(1):10–15.

106. Fava GA, Ruini C. Development and characteristics of a well-being enhancing psychotherapeutic strategy: wellbeing therapy. *J Behav Ther Exp Psychiatry*. 2003;34:45–63.

107. Pail G, Huf W, Pjrek E, Winkler D, Willeit M, Praschak-Rieder N, Kasper S. Bright-light therapy in the treatment of mood disorders. *Neuropsychobiology*. 2011;64(3):152–162.

108. Brain stimulation therapies. National Institute of Mental Health. Available at: http://www.nimh.nih.gov/health/topics/brain-stimulation-therapies/brain-stimulation-therapies.shtml. Accessed May 16, 2012.

109. Dirmaier J, Steinmann M, Krattenmacher T, Watzke B, Barghaan D, Koch U, Schulz H. Non-pharmacological treatment of depressive disorders: a review of evidence-based treatment options. *Rev Recent Clin Trials*. 2012 May;7(2):141–149.

110. Hoffman BM, Babyak MA, Craighead WE, et al. Exercise and pharmacotherapy in patients with major depression: one-year follow-up of the SMILE study. *Psychosom Med*. 2011 Feb–Mar;73(2):127–133.

111. Investing in mental health. World Health Organization. 2003. Available at: http://www.who.int/mental_health/en/investing_in_mnh_final.pdf. Accessed May 7, 2012.

112. Rudd MD, Goulding J, Bryan CJ. Student veterans: a national survey exploring psychological symptoms and suicide risk. *Prof Psychol Res Pr*. 2011 Oct;42(5):354–360. doi:10.1037/a0025164.

113. Risk and protective factors for suicide. Suicide Prevention Resource Center. Available at: http://www.sprc.org/sites/sprc.org/files/library/srisk.pdf. Accessed May 17, 2012.

114. Warning signs of suicide. National Institute of Mental Health. Available at: http://www.nimh.nih.gov/health/topics/suicide-prevention/suicide-prevention-studies/warning-signs-of-suicide.shtml. Accessed May 17, 2012.

115. Riley D. Hatha yoga and the treatment of illness. *Altern Ther Health Med.* 2004 Mar–Apr;10(2):20–21.

116. Cabral P, Meyer HB, Ames D. Effectiveness of yoga therapy as a complementary treatment for major psychiatric disorders: a meta-analysis. *Prim Care Companion CNS Disord.* 2011;13(4). pii:PCC.10r01068. Available at: http://0-http://www.ncbi.nlm.nih.gov.skyline.ucdenver.edu/pmc/articles/PMC3219516/?tool=pubmed. Accessed May 17, 2012.

117. Errington-Evans N. Acupuncture for anxiety. *CNS Neurosci Ther.* 2012 Apr;18(4):277–284. doi:10.1111/j.1755-5949.2011.00254.x.

118. Hollifield M. Acupuncture for posttraumatic stress disorder: conceptual, clinical, and biological data support further research. *CNS Neurosci Ther.* 2011 Dec;17(6):769–779. doi:10.1111/j.1755-5949.2011.00241.x.

119. Ronan P, Robinson N, Harbinson D, Macinnes D. A case study exploration of the value of acupuncture as an adjunct treatment for patients diagnosed with schizophrenia: results and future study design. *Zhong Xi Yi Jie He Xue Bao.* 2011 May;9(5):503–514.

120. Ernst E, Lee MS, Choi TY. Acupuncture for depression? A systematic review of systematic reviews. *Eval Health Prof.* 2011 Dec;34(4):403–412.

121. Bipolar disorder among adults. National Institute of Mental Health. Available at: http://www.nimh.nih.gov/statistics/1BIPOLAR_ADULT.shtml. Accessed May 15, 2012.

122. Nurnberger JI Jr, Foroud T. Genetics of bipolar affective disorder. *Curr Psychiatry Rep.* 2000 Apr;2(2):147–157.

123. Kasper S, Caraci F, Forti B, Drago F, Aguglia E. Efficacy and tolerability of Hypericum extract for the treatment of mild to moderate depression. *Eur Neuropsychopharmacol.* 2010 Nov;20(11):747–765.

124. Panossian A, Wikman G, Sarris J. Rosenroot (Rhodiola rosea): traditional use, chemical composition, pharmacology and clinical efficacy. *Phytomedicine.* 2010 Jun;17(7):481–493.

125. Akhondzadeh Basti A, Moshiri E, Noorbala AA, Jamshidi AH, Abbasi SH, Akhondzadeh S. Comparison of petal of Crocus sativus L. and fluoxetine in the treatment of depressed outpatients: a pilot double-blind randomized trial. *Prog Neuropsychopharmacol Biol Psychiatry.* 2007 Mar 30;31(2):439–442.

126. Andreatini R, Sartori VA, et al. Effect of valepotriates (valerian extract) in generalized anxiety disorder: a randomized placebo-controlled pilot study. *Phytother Res.* 2002;16:650–654.

127. Awad R, Levac D, Cybulska P, Merali Z, Trudeau VL, Arnason JT. Effects of traditionally used anxiolytic botanicals on enzymes of the gamma-aminobutyric acid (GABA) system. *Can J Physiol Pharmacol.* 2007 Sep;85(9):933–942.

128. Kennedy DO, Little W, Haskell CF, Scholey AB. Anxiolytic effects of a combination of Melissa officinalis and Valeriana officinalis during laboratory induced stress. *Phytother Res.* 2006 Feb;20(2):96–102.

129. Sarris J, Panossian A, Schweitzer I, Stough C, Scholey A. Herbal medicine for depression, anxiety and insomnia: a review of psychopharmacology and clinical evidence. *Eur Neuropsychopharmacol.* 2011 Dec;21(12):841–860. doi:10.1016/j.euroneuro.2011.04.002.

130. Amsterdam JD, Li Y, Soeller I, Rockwell K, Mao JJ, Shults J. A randomized, double-blind, placebo-controlled trial of oral Matricaria recutita (chamomile) extract therapy for generalized anxiety disorder. *J Clin Psychopharmacol.* 2009 Aug;29(4):378–382.

131. Kyle G. Evaluating the effectiveness of aromatherapy in reducing levels of anxiety in palliative care patients: results of a pilot study. *Complement Ther Clin Pract.* 2006 May;12(2):148–155.

132. Perry N, Perry E. Aromatherapy in the management of psychiatric disorders: clinical and neuropharmacological perspectives. *CNS Drugs.* 2006;20(4):257–280.

133. Sarris J, LaPorte E, Schweitzer I. Kava: a comprehensive review of efficacy, safety, and psychopharmacology. *Aust N Z J Psychiatry.* 2011 Jan;45(1):27–35.

134. Teschke R, Qiu SX, Xuan TD, Lebot V. Kava and kava hepatotoxicity: requirements for novel experimental, ethnobotanical and clinical studies based on a review of the evidence. *Phytother Res.* 2011 Mar 28. doi:10.1002/ptr.3464 [Epub ahead of print].

135. Papakostas GI. Evidence for S-adenosyl-L-methionine (SAM-e) for the treatment of major depressive disorder. *J Clin Psychiatry.* 2009;70 Suppl 5:18–22.

136. Papakostas GI, Mischoulon D, Shyu I, et al. S-adenosyl methionine (SAMe) augmentation of serotonin reuptake inhibitors for antidepressant nonresponders with major depressive disorder: a double-blind, randomized clinical trial. *Am J Psychiatry.* 2010;167:942–948.

137. Tanskanen A, Hibbeln JR, Hintikka J, et al. Fish consumption, depression, and suicidality in a general population. *Arch Gen Psychiatry.* 2001;58:512–513.

138. Su KP, Huang SY, Chiu CC, Shen WW. Omega-3 fatty acids in major depressive disorder: a preliminary double-blind, placebo-controlled trial. *Eur Neuropsychopharmacol.* 2003;13:267–271.

139. Richardson AJ, Puri BK. A randomized double-blind, placebo-controlled study of the effects of supplementation with highly unsaturated fatty acids on ADHD-related symptoms in children with specific learning difficulties. *Prog Neuropsychopharmacol Biol Psych.* 2002;26:233–239.

140. Sinn N, Bryan J. Effect of supplementation with polyunsaturated fatty acids and micronutrients on learning and behavior problems associated with child ADHD. *J Dev Behav Pediatr.* 2007;28:82–91.

141. Stoll AL, Severus WE, Freeman MP, et al. Omega 3 fatty acids in bipolar disorder: a preliminary double-blind, placebo-controlled trial. *Arch Gen Psychiatry.* 1999;56:407–412.

142. Bhugra D. The global prevalence of schizophrenia. *PLoS Med.* 2005:2(5):e151. doi:10.1371/journal.pmed.0020151.

143. Lieberman JA, Stroup TS. The NIMH-CATIE schizophrenia study: what did we learn? *Am J Psychiatry.* Aug 2011;168(8):770–775.

144. Fair DA, Bathula D, Nikolas MA, Nigg JT. Distinct neuropsychological subgroups in typically developing youth inform heterogeneity in children with ADHD. *Proc Natl Acad Sci USA.* 2012 Apr 24;109(17):6769–6774. doi:10.1073/pnas.1115365109.

145. Merikangas KR, He JP, Burstein M, et al. Lifetime prevalence of mental disorders in U.S. adolescents: results from the National Comorbidity Survey Replication—Adolescent Supplement (NCS-A). *J Am Acad Child Adolesc Psychiatry.* 2010 Oct;49(10):980–989.

146. Lichtenstein P, Carlström E, Råstam M, Gillberg C, Anckarsäter H. The genetics of autism spectrum disorders and related neuropsychiatric disorders in childhood. *Am J Psychiatry.* 2010 Nov;167(11):1357–1363.

147. Christakis DA, Zimmerman FJ, DiGiuseppe DL, McCarty CA. Early television exposure and subsequent attentional problems in children. *Pediatrics.* 2004 Apr;113(4):708–713.

148. Yang P, Chung LC, Chen CS, Chen CC. Rapid improvement in academic grades following methylphenidate treatment in attention-deficit hyperactivity disorder. *Psychiatry Clin Neurosci.* 2004 Feb;58(1):37–41.

149. Medications. Attention Deficit Hyperactivity Disorder. National Institute of Mental Health. Available at: http://www.nimh.nih.gov/health/publications/attention-deficit-hyperactivity-disorder/medications.shtml. Accessed May 18, 2012.

150. MTA Cooperative Group. A 14-month randomized clinical trial of treatment strategies for attention-deficit/hyperactivity disorder. *Arch Gen Psychiatry.* 1999;56:1073–1086.

151. Feingold BF. Hyperkinesis and learning disabilities linked to artificial food flavors and colors. *Am J Nurs.* 1975 May;75(5):797–803.

152. Howard AL, Robinson M, Smith GJ, Ambrosini GL, Piek JP, Oddy WH. ADHD is associated with a "Western" dietary pattern in adolescents. *J Atten Disord.* 2011;15(5):403–411.

153. Millichap J, Yee MM. The diet factor in attention-deficit/hyperactivity disorder. *Pediatrics.* 2012. doi:10.1542/peds.2011–2199.

154. Chang YK, Liu S, Yu HH, Lee YH. Effect of acute exercise on executive function in children with attention deficit hyperactivity disorder. *Arch Clin Neuropsychol.* 2012 Mar;27(2):225–237.

155. Field T, Quintino O, Hernandez-Reif M, Koslovsky G. Adolescents with attention deficit hyperactivity disorder benefit from massage therapy. *Adolescence.* 1998;33(129):103–108.

156. Black DS, Milam J, Sussman S. Sitting-meditation interventions among youth: a review of treatment efficacy. *Pediatrics.* 2009 Sep;124(3):e532–e541.

157. Mehta S, Mehta V, Mehta S, Shah D, Motiwala A, Vardhan J, Mehta N, Mehta D. Multimodal behavior program for ADHD incorporating yoga and implemented by high school volunteers: a pilot study. *ISRN Pediatr.* 2011;2011:780745. doi:10.5402/2011/78074

158. Bakhshayesh AR, Hänsch S, Wyschkon A, Rezai MJ, Esser G. Neurofeedback in ADHD: a single-blind randomized controlled trial. *Eur Child Adolesc Psychiatry.* 2011 Sep;20(9):481–491.

159. Denkowski KM, Denkowski GC. Is group progressive relaxation training as effective with hyperactive children as individual EMG biofeedback treatment? *Biofeedback Self Regul.* 1984 Sep;9(3):353–364.

160. Autism and Developmental Disabilities Monitoring Network Surveillance Year 2006 Principal Investigators; Centers for Disease Control and Prevention. Prevalence of autism spectrum disorders—autism and developmental disabilities monitoring network, United States, 2006. *MMWR Morb Mortal Wkly Rep.* 2009;58:1–24. Available at: http://www.cdc.gov/mmwr/preview/mmwrhtml/ss5810a1.htm. Accessed March 29, 2012.

161. Chamak B. Autism: overestimation of the genetic origins. *Med Sci (Paris).* 2010 Jun–Jul;26(6–7):659–662.

162. McCanlies EC, Fekedulegn D, Mnatsakanova A, et al. Parental occupational exposures and autism spectrum disorder. *J Autism Dev Disord.* 2012 Mar 8 [Epub ahead of print].

163. Croen LA, Najjar DV, Fireman B, et al. Maternal and paternal age and risk of autism spectrum disorders. *Arch Pediatr Adolesc Med.* 2007;161:334–340.

164. Tanne JH. Maternal obesity and diabetes are linked to children's autism and similar disorders. *Br Med J.* 2012 Apr 17;344:e2768. doi:10.1136/bmj.e2768.

165. Krakowiak P, Walker CK, Bremer AA, Baker AS, Ozonoff S, Hansen RL, Hertz-Picciotto I. Maternal metabolic conditions and risk for autism and other neurodevelopmental disorders. *Pediatrics.* 2012 Apr 9 [Epub ahead of print].

166. Miller E. Measles-mumps-rubella vaccine and the development of autism. *Semin Pediatr Infect Dis.* 2003 Jul;14(3):199–206.

167. Berger BE, Navar-Boggan AM, Omer SB. Congenital rubella syndrome and autism spectrum disorder prevented by rubella vaccination—United States, 2001–2010. *BMC Public Health.* 2011 May 19;11:340. Available at: http://www.ncbi.nlm.nih.gov/pmc/articles/PMC3123590/?tool=pubmed. Accessed August 17, 2011.

168. LeBlanc LA, Gillis JM. Behavioral interventions for children with autism spectrum disorders. *Pediatr Clin North Am.* 2012 Feb;59(1):147–164, xi–xii.

CHAPTER 6
Social and Gender Health

What do humans need to survive? Most people will answer water, food, oxygen, and protection from extremes of heat and cold—the usual mammalian necessities. We also require social interaction. Infants perish without gentle touch. Neglected or abused children stop growing for lack of kindness. Socially isolated adults can survive without it, though loneliness takes a toll on health. Solitary confinement represents a severe punishment in prisons; carried out long term, it constitutes torture.

Under the influence of love and tender touch, humans flourish. Our relationships birth our greatest joys and our greatest sorrows. Material possessions and personal accomplishments seem hollow and meaningless without someone with whom to share them. Even when pain, disappointment, and loss threaten to sink us, our friends are there to buoy us up.

This chapter will explore the determinants and benefits of social health, types of relationships, and ways to improve social health and recognize dysfunctional relationships. It will also examine the influence of gender on health behaviors.

The most terrible poverty is loneliness, and the feeling of being unloved.

- Mother Teresa

1. DEFINING SOCIAL HEALTH

LEARNING OBJECTIVES

1. Examine determinants of social health for individuals and groups.
2. Define the types of social relationships.

Our relationships form the core of our life experiences. We are born into a family, play with friends, and spend weekdays with classmates and, later, with coworkers. At some point, we may commit ourselves to an intimate partner and start a family. These relationships mean so much to us that we would defend a loved one with our very lives. Sometimes we even make sacrifices for complete strangers.

Social health applies to individuals and groups, including society at large. A socially healthy person gets along easily with others and has a robust network of supportive friends and family. Social groups can include families, a band of friends, workplaces, other organizations, entire regions, and countries. In the ideal, such groups function under an ethos of kindness, equality, tolerance, and respect.

The health of society profoundly affects its citizens' well-being. A strong social order provides basic services such as education, health care, and assistance for the needy. It also ensures basic civil rights: personal liberty, freedom of expression, legal justice, and democratic governance.

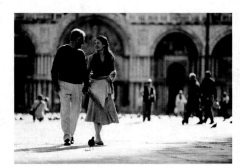

© *Thinkstock*

According to the World Health Organization (WHO), "The social determinants of health are the circumstances in which people are born, grow up, live, work and age, and the systems put in place to deal with illness. These circumstances are in turn shaped by a wider set of forces: economics, social policies, and politics."[1] The term *socioeconomic status* refers to a person's rank within the social hierarchy as determined by variables such as education, occupation, wealth, and living situation.

The following critical factors shape collective social health:

- **Family.** Our families do the lion's share of socializing us. Beginning in infancy, parents and other caregivers provide us with trust and security. We learn that when we cry out, someone will, time after time, assist and comfort us. We understand the meaning of loyalty, the importance of sticking together through thick and thin. Family members reward good behaviors and discourage those that threaten our safety and our ability to attract friends. They teach us empathy, compassion, and tolerance. If they don't, we may emerge from childhood distrustful, hostile, selfish, or overly dependent.

- **Daily living conditions.** Safe, affordable housing and food security free us to be productive members of society. In the ideal, neighbors greet and look out for one another. More dystopian neighborhoods are riddled with graffiti; trash; substance abuse; and hostile, violent people. In such a stressful climate, residents may become reactive rather than proactive and productive.

- **Work conditions.** The work environment affects not just income but also social status, overall happiness, and self-esteem. At the very least, workplaces should be clean, well-lit, and safe. Employers should treat workers fairly and pay them decent wages. In the ideal, workplaces foster a sense of community and purpose and motivate employees to improve their health.

- **Income.** In a perfect world, all adults who want to work are employed, treated fairly, and paid decently. Equal work receives equal pay. Poverty is extremely stressful, increasingly so as the gap widens between the very poor and very rich. Within any given country, those on the bottom rungs of the economic ladder are the least healthy.

- **Education.** Higher education correlates with financial success, better health, and greater longevity. All citizens—rich and poor, male and female, majority and minority—should have access to quality education.

- **Health care.** All people deserve access to health care. Inequities constitute a social injustice and contribute to health disparities. The WHO recommends universal health care, noting that catastrophic health care costs plunge some 100 million people into poverty each year.[2]

- **Freedom from discrimination.** Some people are treated unfairly based on gender, race, ethnicity, income, religious beliefs, sexual orientation, disability, age, or body shape or size. Discrimination lies at the root of many inequities: income, education, health care, legal justice, and political decision making. It's demoralizing, oppressive, and stressful, and it diminishes society as a whole. Tolerance and respect for others are hallmarks of a healthy society.

- **Distribution of power.** Democratic societies tend to be healthier than countries ruled by despots. Granted, political leaders have more power than the average citizen. But when all citizens have representation in the decision-making process, they are more likely to receive social justice. For that reason, it's important to exercise your civic duties and participate in the political process (i.e., vote). Members of any group—family, college communities, businesses, nursing homes—have a better quality of life if they feel they have a voice. If one person in any partnership has all the power, dysfunction develops.

Social Health in the United States

To assess a society's health, researchers measure indicators of poor social health such as homicides, food insecurity, lack of affordable housing, income inequality, and alcohol-related motor vehicle fatalities. They also quantify indicators by stage of life, tracking things like infant mortality, child abuse, child poverty, teen suicide and drug abuse, high school dropout rates, adult unemployment, weekly wages, health insurance coverage, poverty among the elderly, and out-of-pocket health care expenses.

According to the Institute for Innovation in Social Policy at Vassar College, a 2009 analysis revealed that the index of social health had dropped to the lowest point in 13 years, presumably due to the economic recession of 2007.[3] Since the institute began tracking social health data in 1970, indices such as child poverty and abuse, teen suicide, and income inequality have steadily worsened. In terms of global infant mortality rates, 40 other countries boast rates lower than ours, including Canada, Western Europe, New Zealand, Australia, and Japan.[4] On a brighter note, many groups in the United States and around the world are working to improve social health policies.

1.1   Types of Social Relationships

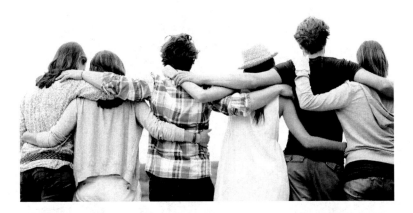

© *Thinkstock*

Just as social policies affect an individual's health, so do our collective interpersonal relationships shape society. That means each of us has the power to steadily transform society for the better. While overall societal health may lag behind other countries, the majority of Americans have meaningful social relationships. In a 2008 survey on social connectedness, 97 percent responded that they have people in their lives whom they trust and whom they can rely on for support.[5] Over half of respondents had at least five such people in their lives.

Social relationships vary in the depth of their **emotional intimacy**, the feeling of connectedness and closeness. Physical intimacy may or may not be present. Men and women differ somewhat in terms of the kind of activities that promote attachments. Women may need to talk more to bond. Men may feel close when doing something with another person.

While the following list runs from acquaintances to significant others, that spectrum doesn't necessarily follow a linear path. We can be close to different people in different ways. Your family members may know you the longest. But you may share certain personal details only with dear friends. Sexual partners may be close physically but guarded emotionally.

Acquaintances are people we know but with whom we haven't developed a close friendship.

Friends are characterized by reciprocal trust, acceptance, loyalty, and affection. They provide companionship and boost self-confidence. While friends share core values and beliefs, they should also tolerate different points of view. They maintain their support through tough times and provide assistance when needed. They give us a sense of belonging to a larger tribe than the nuclear family.

Family members help us develop basic social skills. It's within the home that we learn how to become intimate. To explain how this process proceeds in stages, psychologist Abraham Maslow developed a hierarchy of human needs. The most basic needs have to be met sequentially in order for a person to become self-actualized or develop to his or her full potential. For instance, an infant needs food, water, and shelter to survive. She or he has to feel safe and secure to progress to a sense of belonging and reciprocal love. Love and belonging, in turn, provide the foundation for confidence and self-esteem, which then allows the person to become tolerant, fair, moral, and creative.

People with strong family ties continue to rely on those relationships for lifelong support and satisfaction. However, not everyone is so fortunate. If your family didn't meet your needs, know two things. One, humans are resilient. The tremendous personal growth that occurs during adolescence and young adult life provide another opportunity to establish intimate relationships. Two, you can build a supportive community of friends and significant others. You don't have to be biologically related to people for them to feel like family.

emotional intimacy

A close, connected, bonded relationship with another person or group of people.

FIGURE 6.1 Maslow's Hierarchy of Needs

Maslow's hierarchy of needs is often depicted as a pyramid, with the most basic needs at the bottom and the most highly evolved needs at the top. Lower-level needs must be met before a person can progress upward.

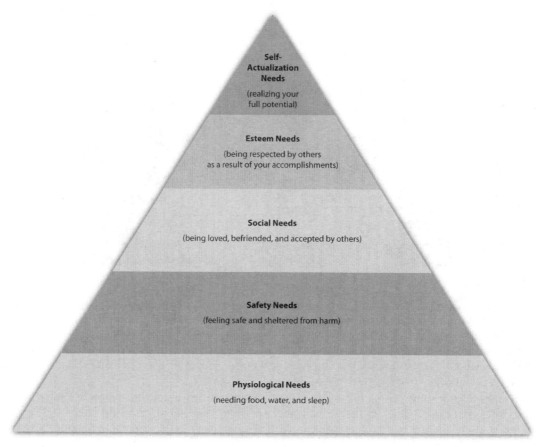

Source: Adapted from Maslow AH. A theory of human motivation. Psychological Review. 1943;50(4):370–396.

Significant others are people with whom we have a long-term romantic or sexual relationship. They can provide a sense of stable support, the safety to be completely vulnerable and to give and express love. Romantic relationships proceed by stages and not all of them endure. That's okay. From these experiences, you learn how to be a good partner and discover the qualities you desire in a partner.

In his **triangular theory of love**, psychologist Robert Sternberg identified three components that exist to varying degrees in close relationships: intimacy, passion, and commitment.

1. **Intimacy** encompasses feelings of closeness, connectedness, and attachment. It has both physical and emotional aspects and requires a sense of mutual trust, safety, and affection. Infants bond with sensitive and responsive primary caregivers and feel outright anxiety upon separation from loved ones. We can also become attached to companion animals, friends, and lovers.

2. **Passion** involves romantic and sexual attraction. Passion generates excitement and energy. When starting a new relationship, you may think involuntarily and frequently about the person. Perhaps against your better judgment, you want to write poetry and sing ballads outside your beloved's window. It turns out that the brain of someone in the throes of passion bears some similarities to that of someone with obsessive compulsive disorder or a drug addiction.[6] In long-term romantic relationships, passion may fade or may wax and wane. When relationships fall apart, passion can spark negative emotions such as anger and jealousy.

3. **Commitment** indicates a dedication to remain connected with the other person. You share stories, experiences, good times, and hard times. You may desire the commitment or feel obligated to stand by the person, even without love. With healthy commitment, two people feel reciprocal love.

The presence or absence of these components characterizes different relationships as follows.

- Good friends and family members enjoy a **companionate** relationship that combines intimacy and commitment.

- **Fatuous love** (also called infatuation) involves an ill-advised combination of passion and commitment. Fatuous means foolish. This type of love is intense, exhausting, and difficult to sustain.

- **Romantic love** contains passion and intimacy but without commitment.

- **Consummate love** refers to the ideal combination of love, passion, and commitment. This blend creates strong, enduring, and satisfying partnerships. Consummate used as an adjective means perfect or complete in every respect. The verb *consummate* means "to bring to completion." If you close a business deal, you consummate it. Consummating a relationship suggests that sexual intercourse occurred.

consummate love

The ultimate form of love, which combines intimacy, passion, and commitment.

FIGURE 6.2 Sternberg's Triangular Theory of Love

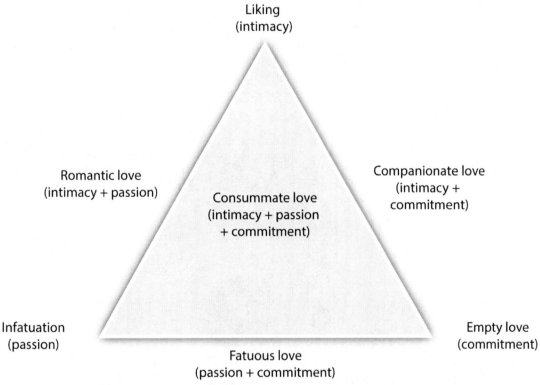

Source: Adapted from Robert JS. Triangulating love. In: Oord TJ, ed. The Altruism Reader. West Conshohocken, PA: Templeton Press; 2007:332.

1.2   The Influence of Social Connectedness on Health

In the United States, family size has decreased, more children spend time alone at home, and more people live alone. Granted, being alone and loneliness are two different things. Likewise, it's possible to feel lonely in a crowd or to be alone and not feel lonely. In fact, many of us seek solitude in small doses. Feeling lonely implies sadness due to a lack of social support.

Socially isolated young adults tend to cope poorly with stress. Everyday hassles are more stressful to them. In response to a stressor, they have greater arterial constriction, thus elevating their risk for high blood pressure. They also sleep less and exhibit slower wound healing.[7] Perceived social isolation makes us more vulnerable to physical and mental illness, substance abuse, eating disorders,[8] and premature death. It's a risk factor for the top killers in America—heart attack, stroke, cancer, and diabetes. Unfortunately, chronic illness can contribute to social marginalization and isolation.

On the other hand, numerous studies show that people with rich social connections live longer, happier, healthier lives. A diverse network of friends and family give us a sense of belonging, security, and purpose. Scholars, recognizing the value of social networks, coined the term *social capital*. As the name implies, monetary wealth factors in. Who you know and how well you work with others does influence career success. But rich social networks also endow people with broader and more profound benefits.

Participation in community organizations, both religious and secular, correlates with better health—in large part because of the inherent social support.[9] A diversity of acquaintances and casual friendships certainly has value. Emotionally intimate relationships allow us to be vulnerable, drop our masks, and be ourselves. They provide an emotional support, an outlet for stress and frustration, and a lifeline in times of crisis. Responding to stress by reaching out to friends—talking, hugging—releases stress-reducing hormones.[10] Satisfying social connections protects against chronic diseases such as heart disease, depression, and dementia.

Social support also enhances immune function and improves outcomes in the face of serious conditions such as HIV infection and cancer. Programs such as Alcoholics Anonymous help people overcome addictions in part because they provide social and emotional support.[11] Furthermore, caring friends and family may encourage us to adopt healthy lifestyles and intervene when risky behaviors appear to be getting out of control.

Ideally, you pick friends who influence you in positive ways. Studies suggest that thoughts, moods, and behaviors spread through social networks in a manner akin to an infectious disease—a process referred to as *social contagion*.[12] For instance, people tend to gain weight if their friends and partners do. To work social contagion to your advantage, you can associate with people who eat well, exercise, balance work and play, treat others with kindness, cope with stress in positive ways, and refrain from substance abuse.

Diversity in our relationships stimulates personal growth and deepens empathy and compassion. One of the great opportunities of a college campus is learning about people from different backgrounds. Take advantage of that. Spending time with someone who seems foreign—whether the strangeness is political, religious, cultural, or otherwise—allows you to discover common ground and to understand disparities.

Furry Friends

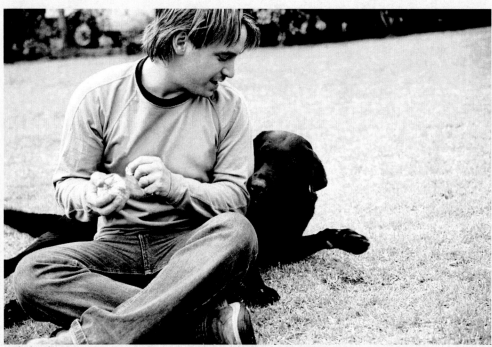

© *Thinkstock*

Humans can connect with other animal species. Studies show that companion animals provide us with social support and a buffer against loneliness.[13] The beneficial relationship between dogs and humans has attracted the most research attention, perhaps because most well-nurtured, domesticated dogs offer adoring acceptance and unconditional love to their humans. If only relationships between two people could be so simple. "If you feed me, walk me, and scratch behind my ears, you can count on me as your friend for life. You don't have to keep telling me you love me. I can tell that you do."

Cats, birds, reptiles, spiders, fish, rodents—all have their virtues. Dogs and horses both get us outside exercising, though fewer people are injured walking a dog than riding a horse. Successfully training animals can boost self-esteem. Petting friendly, furry animals buoys mood, lowers blood pressure, and improves arterial and immune function.[14],[15] Pets have therapeutic benefits for people with a variety of conditions.

On the other hand, pet ownership carries significant responsibilities. The more social the animal, the less well it tolerates being alone. And as with any profound attachment, grieving follows the loss of a beloved animal companion.

1.3 Factors That Foster Healthy Relationships

In addition to being a naturally sociable species, a number of things help us work and play well with others.

- **Find positive role models.** Parents, other caregivers, and siblings teach us how to relate to other people and how to give and receive love. If you grew up in a nurturing family, count yourself as lucky. If you didn't, you're not alone. Regardless of the quality of your early childhood experiences, you can take advantage of other opportunities to improve your social skills.

  In addition to allying yourself with caring people, you can learn from fictional characters in books, movies, theater, and television shows. Brain scans illustrate a significant overlap between the way we process fictional stories and the way we interpret real-life social interactions.[16] In essence, stories provide a way for us to study relationships and sharpen our social skills. Of course, fictional relationships do not substitute for face-to-face interactions.

- **Love and accept yourself.** Positive life experiences and self-acceptance help you build healthy *self-esteem*—a belief that you are worth something. A related concept is *self-concept*, your perception of who you are (e.g., a tall young man who plays Ultimate Frisbee, earns good grades, likes indie folk music, and collects Pez dispensers). Self-concept can take time to develop. It's not uncommon during adolescence to try on different personae and see how they fit.

- **Be yourself.** As famous author Oscar Wilde pointed out, "Everyone else is already taken." If you can relax into who you are, you'll put other people at ease.

- **Expect respect.** Tell yourself you deserve acceptance, respect, and attention.

- **Cultivate humor.** Try not to take yourself and every occurrence too seriously. Laugh. Look on the bright side. Watch comedy shows. Look up jokes online. Stay clear of jokes that demean people, including you.

- **Stay humble.** No one enjoys a braggart. Arrogance usually stems from an underlying insecurity. Let people discover what a remarkable person you are. Your good qualities will shine without the need for explanation.

- **Demonstrate an interest in others.** Ask questions, but don't interrogate or pry. As part of a college community, you're surrounded by interesting people—many of whom are eager to make new friends. Rather than prattle on about yourself, ask what the other person enjoys doing. You can apply this skill to interviews. Come with questions about the academic institution/workplace and the prospective employer.

- **Notice the good in others.** People like to be noticed. They also prefer hearing deserved praise to endless criticism. For example, a good teacher or parent will draw attention to a child's strengths, bolster weaknesses, and either ignore or gently discourage undesirable behavior. The same principle holds true when interacting with coworkers, friends, and lovers.

- **Share information, within reason.** Withholding self-disclosure thwarts the development of intimate relationships. On the other hand, you need to know you can trust someone before you divulge personal details. New acquaintances needn't hear your entire life story.

- **Practice gratitude.** If someone does you a kindness small or large, thank him or her. You'll both feel happier. Many times a verbal thank you will do. For bigger favors, written thanks count for much. Notice the effect of slipping a thank you note under the door of a friend. If one of your faculty taught a great course, wrote you a recommendation, or granted you an extension when you were ill, communicating your gratitude increases the odds you will be remembered in a positive light.

- **Apologize, when necessary.** It's important to own up to our mistakes. A sincere apology, while it can't undo an act, can help bridge the resultant rift. Follow with an effort to repair the damage and to avoid repeating the injurious behavior. Save the apologies for when you're at fault. Women have a tendency to apologize for things they have no control over and perhaps had nothing to do with.

- **Forgive.** When someone apologizes, accept it. Holding a grudge only hurts you. Forgiveness doesn't mean that you let someone wrong you repeatedly. That's a person you need to forgive and get out of your life.

- **Reciprocate.** Unless you want to discourage a relationship, return a potential friend's smiles, phone calls, texts, e-mails, invitations to events, and other kindnesses. It's not as though you're keeping track, but rather you are participating in a give-and-take relationship. The highest level of giving is when you don't expect anything back. However, in relationships, one-sided giving isn't sustainable or healthy.

- **Show you care.** *Empathy* means you understand how situations might make another person think and feel. The next step is offering your *sympathy*. With compassion and sensitivity, you support a friend going through a difficult time.

- **Learn to listen.** It's not uncommon to think more about what you want to say at the next break in the conversation rather than to pay attention to what the other person is saying. You might hear the person speaking but not actually listen. Concentrate. Use body language that shows you're paying attention. Sit up straight, lean slightly toward the person, and maintain eye contact. Avoid gazing out the window or checking out other people. Rather than interrupt, wait for the other person to finish. Ask clarifying questions. Give feedback. "It sounds like your telling me…" "That sounds wonderful." "That must have made you angry." If you're busy and distracted when someone is talking to you, it's fair to say, "I'd like to continue this conversation when I can really listen to you," then set a time to do just that.

- **Communicate clearly.** Active listening is one-half of effective communication. The other half is expressing your thoughts, emotions, needs, and desires. Body language is again important. Face the person and establish eye contact. To avoid looking guarded, relax your hands and arms. Get feedback from the other person's body language. If he or she looks confused, clarify. Rephrasing is also effective when the other person is upset. ("I think you're telling me that…" "How can we work that out?") If the person signals that he or she has stopped listening (looking away, fidgeting, yawning, slumping, texting), either he or she is rude or you have nattered on too long.

- **Learn to express difficult emotions.** Intimate relationships engender potent feelings. If a loved one disappoints or wrongs us, we hurt physically and emotionally. Intense emotions such as anger, jealousy, and grief can overwhelm reason. Sometimes it's better to cool off before speaking. Other times, you have to speak your mind even when you fear the other person's reaction. "I have herpes." "I need to be alone." If you need to confront another person about his or her objectionable actions, try using "I" statements, which are less threatening. For instance, "I feel insecure when you spend time with your ex" is less inflammatory than "You're cheating on me, aren't you?!" "I'm having a hard time finishing this project without your piece of it" versus "This is a group project and you've done nothing!"

Assess Yourself: Your Communication Skills

Interpersonal communications are essential to creating healthy relationships. Ask yourself the following questions. More checks in the "Always" or "Usually" columns indicate you're communicating effectively. If you have a lot of checks in "Sometimes" and "Rarely or Never," you might want to work on those particular skills.

	Always	Usually	Sometimes	Rarely or never
I make eye contact with people when I speak and listen.				
I am able to clearly and concisely convey my message.				
If I'm feeling emotional, I think before I open my mouth.				
I'm comfortable that I can politely but firmly assert my needs				
When someone has something to say to me, I give him or her my complete attention (which includes putting away my mobile phone).				
If I can't conveniently give someone my attention, I ask if we can talk sometime in the near future.				
When someone is speaking, I pay attention to his or her message rather than planning my next comment.				
When someone is talking, I refrain from "butting in."				
When someone is speaking, I make occasional, empathetic comments to show I'm listening.				
I ask questions that show I'm interested in what others do and think.				
I ask for clarification when I don't understand what someone means.				
I am aware of how my body language affects communication.				

Social Media and Your Health

The launch of MySpace in 2003 and Facebook in 2004 sparked a social revolution. Other networking services, including Twitter, quickly followed. Before then, people communicated via face-to-face interactions, telephone, e-mail, and text messages. But social media networks made it possible to connect with multitudes at once. Savvy political activists have used the new media to sway public opinion.

While social media have many merits, some people lose untold hours compulsively checking Facebook and Twitter—a desire that a recent study indicated was more difficult to resist than alcohol and cigarettes.[17] In essence, people can become addicted to social media. If you think that's true for you, set limits for the time you spend on these sites.

An entirely different matter has to do with the quality of electronic relationships. While they may help you initially connect and communicate with people, they can't substitute for real-time human interactions. Studies have shown that time communicating on the Internet often takes away from time spent actually socializing and sleeping.[18] People can paradoxically end up feeling lonelier and more at risk for depression.[19],[20]

Furthermore, there are risks associated with social networking sites. For one, people with ill intent can use them to troll for attractive, vulnerable youth. That's why you shouldn't accept friend requests from unknown people. Manage your profile settings to restrict access to content you only want friends to see. Do not provide personal information such as your address and phone number.

Think carefully about the image you project through the text and photos you send or display on social networking sites. It's unwise to post compromising photographs of you and your friends, especially when you tag individuals. Sexual predators and pornographers may make use of nude or seminude photos. Furthermore, admissions officers at academic institutions and potential employers might turn down your application based on your social media persona.

Electronic communications should never be used to demean, bully, harass, stalk, or slander another person. Such acts, regardless of whether they occur in cyberspace, are cruel, morally corrupt, and potentially punishable by law.

On a brighter note, social and other electronic media have successfully been used to provide health education; promote healthy behaviors; and help people lose weight, quit smoking, and become more physically active.

Etiquette for the Electronic Age

While face-to-face exchanges allow for richer interchanges, most modern humans now spend hours communicating via phone, e-mail, text, and social networking sites. Sometimes, however, people forget simple rules of etiquette. Here are a few tips:

1. Be respectful and polite. Words are impossible to take back, especially when written. You're creating an enduring record with your e-mail message. Furthermore, it's all too easy for your words to be forwarded to a larger audience.
2. Keep communications with faculty, employers, and business associates formal. Use titles, at least until the other person gives you permission to use his or her first name. Proofread. Leave out emoticons and slang.
3. Think carefully when deciding whether to click "reply" or "reply all" in response to a message. If your message is only intended for the eyes of a single person, you certainly don't want to broadcast it to the entire group.
4. Remember that the recipient of your message can't see your facial expressions. For that reason, the other person may miss the tone of a short text or e-mail, misinterpreting a joke as an insult.
5. If you're feeling strong emotions, consider journaling or writing a letter as a way to vent. Save the document, but don't send it. Wait at least 24 hours, reread it, and then reassess your decision to press "send." What do you hope to accomplish? How do you imagine the recipient will respond? Will sending the message do more harm than good? Strong feelings between people are usually better aired face-to-face.
6. A corollary to number five is the following: Have the courtesy to break up with someone face-to-face. If you're geographically separated, talk to the person on the telephone. It takes courage to break off relations in this way.

7. Sexting—sending sexual text or images via text message—is a very bad idea. This kind of activity has jeopardized reputations and ended careers. In many states, minors who send sexually explicit photos can be prosecuted for creating and distributing child pornography.[21]

8. Incoming text messages and phone calls are difficult to ignore. Turn off your phone when you're driving and attending meetings, lectures, and cultural events—anywhere that it might be dangerous or rude to respond.

1.4   How to Enrich Your Social Life

When you're a college student, you may find it difficult to balance work and social life. That balancing act becomes more challenging if you're also working and/or raising a child. Nevertheless, it's important to make time for friends, family, and lovers—but not so much that you fail academically or lose your job.

One way to get around time-management obstacles is to multitask judiciously. While simultaneously doing several things often generates stress, social interactions can prove an exception. For instance, you can exercise with a buddy. Even just walking with a friend accomplishes two objectives. Find things you can do with people. Maybe study groups work for you. If your living situation allows it, cook and eat with other people.

If you're interested in making new friends, you need to put yourself in situations where you'll meet like-minded people. Table 6.1 provides a few ideas.

TABLE 6.1   Making New Friends

Action	Example
Volunteer for an activity that requires a team effort.	Work on a political campaign, build nature trails, gather goods for a food bank, or write/edit for the college newspaper.
Learn a new skill.	Take a group exercise, music, art, or dance class.
Share a hobby.	Join a bird-watching, quilting, photography, book, singing, or cooking club.
Turn acquaintances into friends.	Invite likeable people you meet in the dorm, classroom, or library to do something safe and low-key. Go outside to throw a ball or Frisbee. Catch a movie. Meet for coffee, tea, or lunch. Wait until you know someone better before you plan a dinner date.
Walk your dog, if you have one.	Not only does the dog provide companionship, but other dog lovers may approach you.

KEY TAKEAWAYS

- Humans are social animals. Lack of positive social support contributes to a number of diseases and premature death.
- Social health can be applied to entire societies, communities, and individuals.
- Social skills begin in infancy but are built over a lifetime.
- Maslow's hierarchy of needs demonstrates that basic necessities must first be met before we can develop satisfying intimate relationships.
- Sternberg's triangular theory of love defines three dimensions that can exist in relationships: intimacy, passion, and commitment.
- Our social relationships have huge effects on psychological and physical health.
- Social contagion theory posits that thoughts, moods, and behaviors spread among social networks.

DISCUSSION QUESTIONS

1. When you were growing up, at whose house did your friends tend to hang out? What about the social environment made you want to be there?

2. If you visited more than one college, you probably picked up on the social health of each college community. What have you noticed about your campus that suggests a friendly, supportive atmosphere? You might comment about the ambiance of the student union and other gathering places, the social climate in the dorms, the kinds of literature posted on message boards, the way your instructors treat students, and so on.

3. The people we interact with affect our health. Thoughts, moods, and behaviors can spread like viruses among social networks.[22] For instance, happiness is catching. Overweight, substance use, exercise habits, sexual mores, and health-related phenomena can spread among friends and family. Scientists haven't yet determined how social "contagion" occurs. Theories include that social groups establish norms and behaviors. How have your interpersonal relationships at college affected your health?

4. Examine Figure 6.1 (Maslow's Hierarchy of Needs). Which needs have you met already? At what stage do you think you are now? Justify your assessment with examples. What do you need in your life to proceed to the next level?

5. Examine Figure 6.2 (Sternberg's Triangular Theory of Love). Think of three important people in your life and analyze those relationships based on the triangle.

6. Can social support sometimes negatively affect a person's health and well-being? Think of a past or present relationship wherein, although the person meant to help you, he or she actually did the opposite. If no one comes to mind, think of an interpersonal relationship you've witnessed (in real life or in the media) or read about. Describe the relationship and explain in what ways it either stunted personal growth or did outright harm.

7. Make two columns on a sheet of paper. In the left-hand column, list all of your attributes that make you a good friend. In the right-hand column, list any personality traits and behaviors that you think get in the way of making and keeping friends.

2. SEX AND GENDER: INFLUENCES ON HEALTH

LEARNING OBJECTIVES

1. Define sex and gender.
2. Identify key influences on the development of gender identity.
3. Explore ways in which gender stereotypes affect men's and women's health behaviors.
4. Analyze health disparities between men and women.

This section will explore the ways in which sex, gender, and sexual preferences influence social interactions and overall health. We'll start with a few definitions. **Sex** refers to the biological determination of male and female. There are two sex chromosomes. Males have one X and one Y chromosome. Females have two X chromosomes. The chromosome combination influences hormones secreted during intrauterine life, which in term determines whether reproductive structures develop into testes and a penis or ovaries, a vagina, and a uterus. Males have testes, which make sperm and testosterone. Females have ovaries, which make the eggs and the female hormones estrogen and progesterone.

sex

Biological determination as male or female; short for sexual activity.

Male hormones (androgens) thicken muscles and bones, deepen voices, add hair to the body, and eventually subtract it from the head. In men, the testes and adrenal glands produce androgens. Women's adrenal glands generate relatively small amounts of androgens. The main androgen is testosterone. In men, testosterone promotes the development and maintenance of male reproductive structures. In men and women, testosterone generates libido (sexual drive), increases aggressiveness, and strengthens bones and muscles.

Female hormones soften bodily contours. In women, estrogen stimulates development of the breasts and uterus and the maturation of eggs in the ovaries. It has a protective effect on the cardiovascular system and preserves bone mass. Estrogen and progesterone both affect the brain. Progesterone helps regulate monthly menstrual cycles, prepares the lining of the uterus for conception, and maintains pregnancy. Men make relatively small amounts of estrogen and progesterone.

Male or female sex is usually apparent at birth. Sometimes, however, genitals may appear ambiguous. The term *intersex* refers to a number of conditions that result in reproductive anatomy that's not typically male or female. For instance, a baby may be born with external genitalia that appear female but without a uterus and with testes rather than ovaries. A genetic test would demonstrate XY sex chromosomes rather than XX chromosomes. Treatment and gender assignment depend in part upon the reason for the female appearance.

gender

Roles, behaviors, attributes, and activities that society deems proper for men and women.

Gender has to do with culturally based characteristics of being male or female. Biology also influences our perception of gender. For instance, reproductive hormones affect brain development, mood, and behavior. Girls' brains mature more rapidly. They tend to talk sooner. Boys tend to be more physically active. Suppressing physical activity, as often happens in school, may more adversely affect boys.

Culture also defines gender. Parents, other significant adults, peers, and the media teach us how boys and girls are supposed to behave. Early in life, we develop our *gender identity*, our sense of what it means to be male or female. Most of us conform to gender roles congruent with religion, politics, ethnicity, and socioeconomic status. That's why being a woman or man in an American suburb differs from being a woman or man in, say, rural Afghanistan.

Most people learn to fit into socially acceptable gender roles. For *transgender* people, gender identity clashes with social expectations for their biological sex. Even for people who conform to traditional gender roles, rigid stereotypes may constrict personal expression.

Gender role conflict theory explains the ill effects that arise from a disparity between socially accepted gender roles and self-perception. Girls, boys, men, and women can all suffer psychological distress, shame, and restricted personal freedom. People who don't fit these stereotypes may be devalued.[23] Let's now examine how biological sex and gender roles affect health and well-being.

2.1 Masculinity and Health

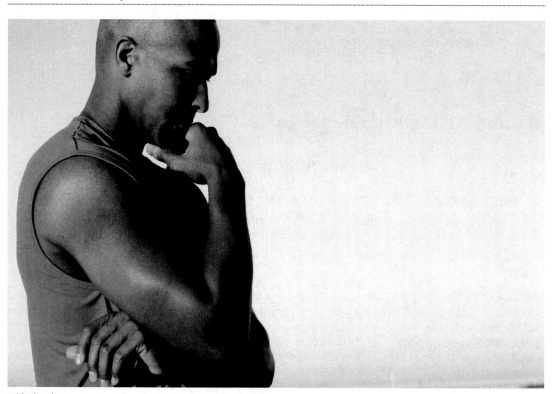

© *Thinkstock*

Whoever called women the weaker sex may have gotten it wrong. Women outlive men by an average of five years. During childhood, boys have more frequent and severe infectious illnesses than girls. As teens and young adults, they are more likely to die from accidental injuries, homicides, and suicides.[24] In adulthood, men visit doctors less often than women and have more chronic diseases such as heart disease and cancer. Paradoxically, men report better health than women.

How and why do men approach health differently than women? Early cultural influences provide clues. Starting in childhood, boys receive contradictory messages. On the one hand, health professionals encourage boys and men to seek help for their physical, psychological, emotional, and even spiritual struggles. On the other, authority figures (parents, teachers, coaches) may pressure them to become stoic, independent, and emotionally restrained—at least for "feminine" emotions like sadness, fear, or tenderness. Asking for help may be seen as a sign of weakness. Parents are also less likely to show affection toward their boys and more likely to dole out punishment.

Another problem is a relative lack of positive male role models. Nearly one-third of children live without their fathers.[25] Compare that figure to 1960, when only 1 in 10 kids lived in fatherless households. Single mothers may, by necessity, be absent as they work to make ends meet. Boys may be left to figure out what masculinity means in the absence of role models, relying instead on the media and gangs of other lost boys—influences that may only perpetuate the myth of rugged, aggressive, tough masculinity.

Harvard Medical School psychologist and author William Pollack, PhD, coined the term "boy code" to describe these gender stereotypes. Boys and men who dare to break the code may be ridiculed, punished, harassed, and socially isolated.[26]

Sometimes men who fear they're insufficiently masculine may overcompensate by engaging in activities such as carrying guns, abusing drugs and alcohol, gay-bashing, fighting, and bullying women.[27] Ironically, boys and men often view their male peers as more stereotypically masculine than themselves.[28] Guys tend to act more "manly" simply because they think that other guys feel more masculine, when in fact, they don't. These misperceptions perpetuate myths about masculinity.

Adherence to old-fashioned masculine stereotypes can mar academic performance, decreasing motivation and achievement.[29] It also facilitates a "player" mentality regarding sexuality, which can foster demeaning attitudes toward women, impair the ability to form intimate relationships, and increase the risk of sexually transmitted infections. Guys may also become preoccupied with becoming muscular. Feelings of anger and helplessness can also fuel risky behaviors, including suicide.

What's relevant to this chapter is how gender roles affect health behaviors. According to William Courtenay, PhD, author of *Dying to Be Men*, traditional attitudes about masculinity correlate with poor health behaviors such as smoking, drinking alcohol, taking illicit drugs, eating poorly, and having unprotected sex. Potential consequences of trying to conform include psychological stress and maladaptive coping patterns, anxiety, depression, and poor cardiovascular health.

A large Canadian study sheds some light on men's health in industrialized countries.[30] Compared to women, men were more likely to say they felt healthy, despite the fact they were more likely to die at younger ages. Pressure on men to be independent and emotionally reserved seems to fuel many of the disparities. The authors identified four main ways men respond differently from women.

1. Men tend to be more optimistic, which is generally an asset. However, men consistently overestimate the state of their health and may take naïve risks.

2. Men are less mindful of symptoms that may indicate a disease.

3. Men, particularly young men, tend to engage in more high-risk activities such as extreme sports, binge drinking, and drunk driving, hence their increased risk for unintentional injuries. Drinking and other risky activities can also make men vulnerable to violence, including homicide.

4. Men are more reluctant than women to let down their guard and seek help for personal concerns. They can ask a friend for help fixing a car but may balk at discussing intimate matters with peers, partners, and health care providers.

Of course, the ideal that guys should be square-jawed, tough, emotionally repressed, bronco-riding Marlboro men is neither accurate nor realistic. A real man is brave enough to experience the whole of life: the joy and suffering. He accepts his true nature and expresses his fears and sadness. He is kind and respectful to others. He takes care of his physical, emotional, mental, social, and spiritual health. He tries to do the right thing, no matter how hard it might be.

As a society, we've already begun moving toward broader concepts of masculinity. Recognition of the male approach to health can help men get the care they need. Promising changes have already taken place. For instance, more organizations are disseminating health care information at sports events, fitness centers, locker rooms, men's restrooms, truck stops, and other places men tend to gather. The Men's Network created National Men's Health Week, which coincides with Father's Day, to increase awareness that men need to take care of themselves. Famous athletes and other celebrities who have experienced health crises are acting as spokesmen for topics in men's health. For instance, cyclist Lance Armstrong had testicular cancer, which primarily affects young men. He became living proof that people with cancer and other health challenges could "live strong."

Video Clip 6.1

Men's Health Awareness Week
This KYTX news video contains facts about men's health and profiles men of various ages and discusses screening tests.

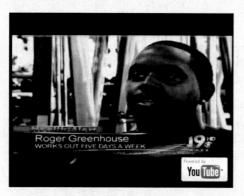

View the video online at: http://www.youtube.com/v/OyCrmXVadP4

2.2 Femininity and Health

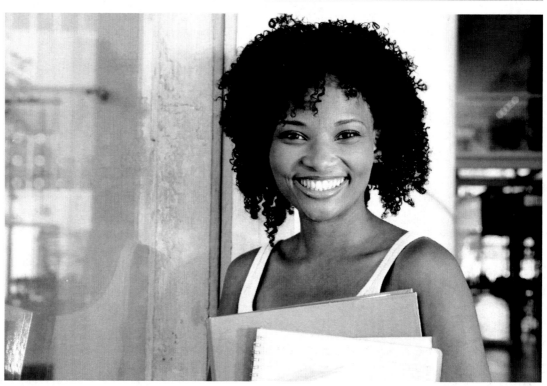

© *Thinkstock*

Starting in the womb, survival rates are better for females than males. The extra X chromosome in females provides a genetic advantage. The Y chromosome carries few genes. When males inherit a "bad" gene on their only X chromosome, the Y chromosome can't mask it with a "good" gene, as occurs in females. Furthermore, female hormones protect against certain conditions, such as cardiovascular disease.

Being a female in our culture carries certain advantages. Western society tolerates a greater range of emotional, stylistic, recreational, and, increasingly, vocational expressions. Women can more freely communicate joy, love, sadness, grief, and fear. They can wear a variety of clothing—without much fear of being ostracized.

On the other hand, parents may allow boys to express more aggressive, boisterous behavior than girls. ("Boys will be boys.") Bottled-up emotions such as anger seem to correlate with the development of depression,[31] eating disorders,[32] and other ills more prevalent among women.

Gender roles can have positive health effects. For instance, society once frowned on a woman lighting up in public and few women developed lung cancer. Shifts in attitudes led to an increase in women smokers and more cancer.

Like men, women may find themselves boxed in by rigid stereotypes. Myths such as "Girls aren't good at math and science" just don't hold water—though they can hold girls back. The truth is that girls now outperform boys academically. They dominate high school advanced-placement classes, including calculus. Among high school graduates in 2010, 74 percent of women went on to college versus 63 percent for men.[33] Of those students receiving a bachelor's degree, 58 percent are women.[34] Many of them go on to enroll in graduate programs. That's good news. Higher education correlates with greater financial security and better health. Women have more employment opportunities and have entered fields previously considered male. They serve in the military, hold political office, work as professional athletes, conduct orchestras, direct movies, run businesses, and practice law and medicine.

Nevertheless, women most commonly work as secretaries, nurses, teachers, cashiers, retails sales clerks, waitresses, and maids—all jobs traditionally considered female.[35] And they work for lower wages than men. These jobs typically come with many demands and little control. Recall from Chapter 3 that this combination is a recipe for stress overload. Although men are increasingly helping out with running a household and raising children, women still often feel responsible for much of the domestic duties, even if they work outside the home. Plus, women head the vast majority of single families.

When you compare the effect of sex and gender on health, an interesting paradox emerges. Women outlive men but experience more disease. They visit doctors more often, take more medicines, are more often hospitalized, and receive more diagnoses for acute and chronic diseases.[36]

Some female behaviors promote health and longevity. Women are less likely to drink heavily, smoke, use illicit drugs, become overweight, and behave recklessly. They more often get preventive dental and medical care.[37] When stressed, women tend to seek social support. Society sanctions their expression of emotional and physical affection. Much as women unashamedly ask for directions when lost, they call their health providers with questions or concerns about their health. Women's admittance of signs and symptoms of illness is less likely to be viewed as weakness.

One reason women engage with the health care system early is that many methods of female contraception require a prescription, which necessitates a physical exam. Pregnancy also sends women for routine check-ups. Men, who also deserve sexual health care, are less likely to visit the clinic about their sexual health.[38] For women, these regular interactions with health care professionals allow for advice about health promotion and earlier intervention when diseases develop.

Many of the differences between men and women create balance and delight in our lives. We can remodel dated gender roles that only limit and harm us and, at the same time, celebrate those positive differences. As the French say, "Vive la difference."

 Video Clip 6.2

Finding Balance in Gender Roles
This ABC news segment explores how shifts in the economy and culture have redefined gender roles.

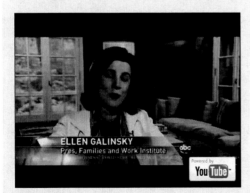

View the video online at: http://www.youtube.com/v/I51rxnKJRfk

Both biological sex and gender roles influence health-related behaviors and disease susceptibilities.

TABLE 6.2 Disparities in Men's and Women's Behaviors and Health

	Men	Women
Genetics	XY sex chromosomes	XX sex chromosomes
Average longevity	75.7	80.6
Health care visits	More likely to wait until symptoms become undeniable	More likely to access health care system when symptoms first arise
Overall health	Report better health	Experience more disease
Immune system	More frequent and severe infections, especially during childhood	Stronger immune system; more autoimmune disease
Sexually transmitted infections	Less likely to become infected after exposure	More vulnerable to infections and more at risk for complications such as infertility
Sleep	More at risk of obstructive sleep apnea	More at risk for insomnia
Stress	More likely to relieve stress with physical activity or become aggressive and hostile	More likely to seek out social support
Mental health	Attention deficit hyperactivity disorder (ADHD); more completed suicides	Depression and anxiety; more attempted suicides
Cardiovascular disease	Starts earlier	Atypical heart attack symptoms and more deaths
Headaches	Less frequent headaches; greater risk of cluster headaches	Tension headaches and migraines
Body composition	More lean body mass, with thicker muscles and bones; fat tends to accumulate in the belly	Relatively more body fat, with greater distribution over hips and thighs; more at risk for osteoporosis
Body image and eating disorders	More satisfied with appearance; more at risk for muscle dysmorphia (bigorexia)	More critical of appearance; more vulnerable to eating disorders (bulimia and anorexia nervosa)
Social interactions	Less comfortable in social settings; communications focus more on problem solving; prefer to share activities rather than innermost thoughts; value tenderness in long-term relationships	Smile more readily; lean forward and maintain eye contact when communicating; express more affection; more interested in talking about feelings and relationships
Tobacco use	More smoking and greater use of smokeless ("spit") tobacco	More vulnerable to lung cancer
Alcohol	More likely to abuse alcohol and become alcoholics	More sensitive to the effects of alcohol
Accidental injuries	Men are more likely to die at younger ages from accidental injuries	Less risk-taking behavior that might lead to injuries
Violence	More often the aggressors; more likely to die of homicides	More likely to become victims of gender-based violence

KEY TAKEAWAYS

- A man's health may be rooted in his ideologies of manhood. Research shows that the more a man identifies with traditional notions of masculinity, the less healthy he is likely to be—physically, socially, mentally (including academically), and emotionally.

- Redefining masculinity can promote men's health. One place to start is to understand that seeking help from others is a measure of courage and strength.

- Women exhibit certain behaviors that promote health. They are less likely to engage in risky behaviors and more likely to seek medical assistance when worrisome signs and symptoms arise.

3.   SEXUAL RELATIONSHIPS

LEARNING OBJECTIVES

1. Define sexual orientation and the main categories of sexual orientation.
2. Discuss the factors that influence romantic and sexual attraction.
3. Explore the characteristics of healthy and unhealthy relationships.

Sexual orientation dictates the types of romantic relationships we seek. The pattern of attraction becomes apparent early in life and remains stable. In other words, scientists regard sexual orientation not as a choice but as a condition programmed by biology and the environment, particularly the intrauterine environment.[39] **Heterosexual** people are sexually attracted to the opposite sex. **Homosexual** people feel sexual attraction for people of the same sex. The word *lesbian* refers to homosexual women, while gay can refer to both homosexual men and homosexual women. **Bisexual** describes sexual behavior in which an individual is attracted to both men and women. Regardless of sexual orientation, most people ultimately long for consummate love.

Heterosexuals form the dominant group. Unfortunately in our society, people with homosexual or bisexual preferences or who identify with the opposite gender (transgendered) are too often marginalized, discriminated against, harassed, and victimized. *Homophobia* means fear or hatred of homosexuals.

Decoding LGBTQIA

On your campus, there may be support groups for LBGTQIA students. Here's a glossary of what the letters stand for.

- **L** stands for lesbian, which refers to women (or people who self-identify as female) who are emotionally, sexually, or romantically attracted to other women.
- **G** stands for gay, which refers to men who are emotionally, sexually, or romantically attracted to other men.
- **B** stands for bisexual—people attracted to both sexes.
- **T** stands for transgender, referring to a person who self-identifies with the gender not matching biological sex. In other words, a person with XY sex chromosomes identifies with and may live as a woman. Gender identification is not the same as sexual orientation.
- **Q** stands for queer, a broad term that includes people with any non-normative sexual preference or gender identity.
- **I** stands for intersex, a condition in which the sexual anatomy doesn't quite fit the expected male or female anatomy.
- **A** stands for asexual, referring to people who are not sexually attracted to anyone.

For more information on terminology, visit http://sait.usc.edu/lgbt/education/lgbt-terminology.aspx.

sexual orientation

The direction of one's romantic interests toward people of the opposite sex, same sex, or both sexes.

heterosexual

Sexually attracted to people of the opposite sex.

homosexual

Sexually attracted to people of the same sex.

bisexual

Sexually attracted to people of both sexes.

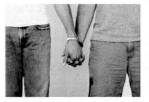

© *Thinkstock*

3.1　Laws of Attraction

A number of things influence our choice of sexual partners. Physical **proximity** is a big factor. We need to be near someone in order to get to know someone well enough to fall in love. Long-distance relationships are challenging, even when firmly established before the geographical separation.

Intimate partners often share many **similarities**. We often pick partners who resemble us physically and, more important, who share core values and interests and who validate our opinions. Strong couples may have a common life purpose. However, agreeing on everything and participating in the same activities can become boring, stifling, and sometimes competitive.

Because love is definitely not blind, **physical attraction** is key. Whether we're conscious of the fact or not, we seek out sexual partners with whom we could successfully sexually reproduce. Symmetrical features suggest good genetics. Glowing skin, bright eyes, and good muscle tone indicate robust health.

In a man, rugged good looks—the strong jaw, broad shoulders, narrow hips, and other features shaped by testosterone (as well as good genes and exercise)—indicate virility. Men are attracted to women with a waist-to-hip ratio of about 0.7. Women's breasts and hips are signs of functioning ovaries and, hence, fertility.

Men tend to be most stimulated by visual stimuli.[40] But senses other than sight influence attraction for both sexes. The sound of someone's voice can either soothe or grate. The way he or she touches you can calm, excite, or repel. The way a person smells can trigger desire or revulsion. Ill health produces odors that are less than sexually alluring. Men and women, when presented with shirts worn by the opposite sex, prefer the scent of healthy, symmetrical people.

Some of this perceptional processing occurs on a subconscious level, which helps to explain why a potential partner who is sufficiently smart, good-looking, accomplished, and otherwise compatible just doesn't light your fire.

Personality matters a great deal too. Men and women both may prefer partners who are kind, mature, dependable, smart, and sociable. Partners may also be looking for **economic security**. It's reassuring to have the resources for raising children, living comfortably, and retirement. Fidelity, which provides **emotional security**, is even more important. It's difficult to abandon yourself to a relationship (much less start a family) if you doubt your partner will stick around.

3.2　Types of Sexual Partnerships

Sexual relationships can vary in depth from no expectation of permanence to complete commitment.

Hooking up represents the most superficial form of sexual encounter—sex without romance. The duo may be friends, acquaintances, or strangers. Sexual activity can range from kissing to intercourse. Duration ranges from a "one-night stand" to multiple hookups with the same person. Alcohol and other intoxicating substances often catalyze these couplings. About 60 percent of college men and women have hookups involving oral, vaginal, or anal sex.[41]

By definition, casual sex lacks emotional investment. However, physical intimacy triggers the release of hormones related to bonding. That means that, despite your intentions to remain emotionally neutral, you may form an attachment to your partner. Risks include sexually transmitted infections (alcohol and spontaneity don't foster condom use) and feelings of regret, anxiety, and depression.

Dating does not have to involve sex. The overt goal is to do something fun together—catch a film, chat over coffee, visit a museum. Sex is often a covert objective. Traditionally, people initiated dating with acquaintances or friends. Recently, however, online dating sites such as Match.com have gained in popularity. While successful relationships can arise from such services, it makes sense to get to know someone in real time before you divulge many personal details. Regardless of whether you meet online or in the real world, it's safer to schedule an initial rendezvous in public places rather than in personal living spaces.

Cohabitation, or living together, has become exceedingly commonplace. According to US Census Bureau data, 7.5 million opposite-sex couples lived together in 2010, a 13 percent increase in a single year.[42] Young heterosexual couples may cohabitate because they're not yet ready to marry or as a prequel to marriage, although doing so doesn't increase the odds of a successful marriage. Older couples may cohabitate to avoid losing Social Security benefits. Homosexual couples living in states where same-sex marriage is not allowed have no other choice. Advantages of cohabitation include a sense of greater independence, fewer obligations, and, when compared to marriage, greater ease in dissolving the relationship. Disadvantages include feelings of insecurity and the absence of legal protections.

Another issue is children born outside of marriage to couples who live together and single women. In the United States, cohabitating couples break up at twice the rate of marriages. The significance is that many children live in single-parent households, nearly 90 percent of the time with their mothers. Overall, about 60 percent of women under age 30 are married when they give birth.[43] While over 90 percent of college-educated women marry before having children, single parenthood occurs much more commonly in less educated women. Children born outside of marriage to single mothers are at greater risk of living in poverty, performing poorly in school, and having emotional and behavioral problems.

Marriage remains a popular choice for committed couples. Over 70 percent of adults 25 to 44 years old have been married.[44] Since the 1950s, the age at first marriage has steadily risen to 28 for men and 26 for women. At any age, more people report having never married. Approximately 75 percent of first marriages make it to their tenth anniversary.[45] The 2009 divorce rate was 34 percent.[46]

In addition to the advantages of any devoted relationship (companionship, affection, emotional support, sexual satisfaction), marriage offers a certain degree of emotional and financial stability and legal rights. Married couples can file joint income tax returns (thereby reducing taxes paid), receive Social Security and disability benefits for spouses, receive insurance through a spouse's employer, more easily visit hospitalized spouses, and more.

As of this writing, same-sex marriage is allowed in California, Connecticut, Delaware, Iowa, Maryland, Maine, Massachusetts, Minnesota, New Hampshire, New York, Rhode Island, Vermont, Washington, and Washington, DC.[47] Until recently, couples in same-sex marriages were not entitled to the same legal benefits afforded married couples because the federal government did not recognize these relationships.[48]

However in 2013, the US Supreme Court ruled the Defense of Marriage Act, the law that had barred the federal government from recognizing same-sex marriages legalized by the states, as being unconstitutional.[49] This ruling means that in states allowing same-sex marriage, gay and lesbian married couples will be eligible for spousal and survivor benefits such as Social Security and Medicare.

Regardless of whether long-term couples are married or not, relationships require maintenance. You can't fall in love and expect the magic to effortlessly last. Periodic challenges test the strength of those bonds. On the other hand, a sturdy relationship acts like armor against life's slings and arrows.

Tips for Healthy Intimate Relationships

We don't receive user manuals when we embark on intimate relationships. We learn from watching other couples and by actively participating in our own relationships. Here are some strategies for growing strong bonds:

- **Learn to give and take.** Successful relationships with friends, family, and lovers all require reciprocity.
- **Keep communication lines open.** While we can infer another person's mental state, we can't mind read. If your partner's behavior puzzles you, ask what he or she is thinking. When your partner speaks, actively listen. When you speak, clearly articulate your thoughts and feelings. Keep the atmosphere warm and caring.
- **Make important decisions together.** Otherwise maintain balance in making decisions—even over seemingly small things like who plans the evening's events.
- **Be honest.** You need to disclose salient information about yourself. Some of it may be difficult but necessary. For instance, if you have a sexually transmitted infection, you must be able to tell your partner and take steps to protect you both. You also need to be honest with yourself. Sometimes we talk ourselves into acting in ways that don't fit us to please someone else. As Shakespeare wrote in *Hamlet*, "To thine own self be true."
- **Build trust.** The two of you won't feel free in the relationship without it. Intimacy requires removing your public "mask" and letting the other person see you at your most vulnerable.
- **Practice love and kindness.** Be sweet to one another. Help each other out.
- **Encourage the best for each other.** When you love someone, you want what's best for him or her. For instance, if one of you has an exam the next day, the other person might study too and encourage a reasonably early bedtime—as opposed to talking the other person into going to a late-night concert.
- **Give each other space.** Everyone needs time apart. You are, after all, two individuals. Trust, self-confidence, and concern for each other's well-being should allow for independence.
- **Find fun things to do together.** Routine is comfortable, but a little novelty keeps the relationship exciting. Try doing new things together. Go skating, fly kites, take a tango lesson, camp out, or cook an exotic meal together.

3.3   Signs That a Relationship Has Gone South

No one wants to end up in a relationship rife with neglect or abuse. Short of that, lesser evils sink relationships. Many times, the problem is simply that the two people want different things and a balance can't be found. One person wants a commitment; the other person isn't ready. One person enjoys lots of physical affection; the other is more reserved. One person wants to discuss the relationship; the other finds such analysis tedious. In many situations, it becomes like an elephant and a squirrel trying to balance a teeter-totter.

While every relationship is different, the following signs raise red flags:

- **Lack of reciprocity.** In healthy, reciprocal relationships, each partner gives and receives. A loving partner considers his or her partner's needs and wants and finds pleasure in meeting them. Each person also takes care of himself or herself. Normally, one person in a partnership tends to be more demonstrative and overtly nurturing than the other. However, when one does all the talking and the other does all the giving, guilt and resentment can surface.

- **Unequal commitment.** Expectations can differ about the seriousness of the relationship. The only way to clarify these expectations is to have an honest discussion. The more committed person will likely feel disappointed and insecure. The more circumspect person may feel guilty or skittish.

- **Disinterest.** The enchantment of infatuation fades quickly. Sometimes people find it easier to break up by drifting away rather than having an open, direct conversation. The latter takes more courage and maturity. Loss of interest can manifest as the following:

  - Persistent failure to call or text. Dwindling communication suggests the person's attention has drifted elsewhere.
  - Repeated or prolonged texting and phoning with someone else when you're together. A little is OK. A lot is rude and demonstrates a shift in priorities.
  - Roving eyes when you're trying to talk to him or her. You may also get the sense he or she doesn't listen to you.

- **Criticism and condescension.** These two unhealthy signs suggest one person feels superior to the other. Insecure people are often also hypercritical—no doubt a hangover of having critical parents. If one person wants to "fix" the other, the one who apparently needs improvement may feel compelled to adjust in order to hang onto the relationship. He or she may hesitate to speak or act in certain ways for fear of a correction. No one's perfect. But there's someone out there who will love you just as you are, someone you will love without renovation.

- **Dependence.** The person starts to feel like a drain on your time. He or she wants to be with you all the time and bridles when you wish to see your friends or family. If you try to pull away, he or she pleads, demands, or otherwise manipulates you.

- **Jealousy and possessiveness.** If you love someone, you can't help but feel threatened if another person seems to be vying for your beloved's attention. With unwarranted jealousy and possessiveness, one partner can scarcely make contact with a third party without kindling his or her partner's ire.

- **Distrust, doubt, and suspicion.** Intimate relationships falter without a foundation of mutual trust. If your partner has betrayed you, trust may be difficult or impossible to reestablish. If you're the one lying and cheating, you don't love and respect your partner.

- **Controlling behavior.** We can't help but influence the behavior of others. The problem comes if your significant other constantly gives you advice and, worse, wants to know where you are and what you're doing at all times. You may start to restrict your behaviors to fit your partner's expectations. Or you may rebel and move on.

- **Substance abuse and addiction.** Drug and alcohol problems adversely affect human relationships. One, the substance becomes more important than other people. Two, addictive substances alter behavior in ways that interfere with communication and intimacy.

- **Fighting.** Disagreements and misunderstandings occur in intimate relationships. The way partners resolve their differences distinguishes healthy from unhealthy relationships. In the former, two people discuss the matter as calmly as possible. They listen to one another and problem solve together. In the latter, people yell, threaten, interrupt, accuse, and call each other names. Even if they make up afterward, similar spats will recur.

- **Stonewalling.** This tactic involves rejection of open communication, at least on certain matters. You try to have a discussion with your partner and he or she walks or looks away, stalls, or refuses to answer. Ideally, when you speak, your partner hears you out and then responds. Sometimes partners stonewall as a response to nagging.

- **Sarcasm, hostility, scorn, and contempt.** You've entered a toxic relationship, one that's veered into verbal abuse. Even if your partner is sometimes kind, episodes of aggression hint of a greater violence. Time to get out as soon as possible. You deserve love and kindness.

- **Physical and sexual abuse.** Both are criminal acts. If you're the victim, call 911. If you're the aggressor, get your partner help, confess your actions, and seek immediate psychological treatment. Chapter 12 contains detailed information about gender-based violence.

If you have doubts about your relationship, discuss them with your partner. If you're afraid to do so, that tells you a lot. If your partner rejects your efforts to communicate, you've also learned something. If you're afraid to end the relationship, ask yourself why. Often we fear being alone. Or we like our partner's friends and hate the idea of perhaps losing them as well. Such fears don't justify perpetuating an unhealthy partnership. You will find someone better suited to you.

Assess Yourself: Relationships

Most people have a gut feeling about the soundness of their intimate relationships. Ask yourself the following questions:

- Do you generally feel happy and satisfied?
- When you're with the person, do you feel secure and relaxed?
- Do you feel appreciated and loved without feeling trapped?
- Do you share common interests?
- Do you feel free to spend time away from the other person?
- Are you comfortable speaking your mind without fear of rejection or criticism?
- Do you feel more or less equal to your partner?

If you can answer yes to all, congratulations! You likely have a healthy relationship.

3.4 When Relationships End

Intimacy, though life affirming, carries certain risks. Whether you're dating a classmate, a coworker, or someone within your social group, breaking up creates—at the very least—social awkwardness. In caring partnerships, it hurts regardless of whether you're the one ending the relationship. If you're still in love with the other person, the pain can feel unendurable. Perhaps we should not expect less.

Ending an intimate relationship gracefully takes skill and compassion. Simply changing your relationship status on Facebook is callous. The same goes for texting, e-mailing, or leaving a farewell voice message. Find a quiet time when the two of you can talk. Demonstrate respect and kindness. Give the other person a chance to express his or her anger and sorrow. Acknowledge your feelings.

Emotionally intimate relationships include friendships. The loss of a trusted friend can be just as traumatic as a breakup with a lover. The same care needs to be taken when friendships end. On the other hand, drifting away from acquaintances without explanation may be kinder than a blunt assessment of the reasons you couldn't possibly become intimate.

Mending a broken heart takes time. Most people need both solitude and supportive friendships. Allow yourself quiet times for reflection. Also let your friends know you need them. Talking about your feelings can help. Keep these other items in mind:

- **Take care of yourself.** Many of us have a tendency to do the opposite when in mourning. Eat well, exercise, and get enough sleep.

- **Do pleasurable activities.** Get a massage. Buy yourself flowers. Listen to music. Exercise. Go out dancing. Attend athletic and cultural events. Find healthy activities that bring you joy.

- **Forgive and forget.** These tasks are the hardest. Accomplishing them will help you heal. Holding a grudge won't.

- **Beware alcohol and boomerang relationships.** Alcohol won't drown your sorrows; it will mainly give you a hangover and a deepening sense of remorse. If you rebound into another relationship, you're likely doing it for the wrong reasons and may increase the odds of inflicting pain in the near future. Wait until you have healed, know what you want next time around (a very valuable lesson), and are ready to give again.

- **Monitor yourself for signs of depression.** Grieving is a normal response to the loss of love. For some people, the trauma of the breakup triggers a major depression. See Chapter 5 for warning signs. If you think you might be depressed, seek professional help.
- **Keep an open heart.** While a hasty reentry into romance isn't wise, neither is keeping everyone at a safe distance. You may think you're safer that way and have found a refuge from future loss and pain. In reality, you're cramping your soul, stymieing your personal growth, and denying yourself potential joy and love. When you are ready, opening your heart and making yourself vulnerable again may take courage. But it's worth it.

KEY TAKEAWAYS

- Sexual orientation becomes apparent early in life and exists along a continuum from heterosexual to homosexual.
- Several key factors influence whether or not we become romantically involved with someone, including physical proximity, physical attractiveness, and similarities that make you compatible.
- Sexual and romantic relationships span the gamut from hookups to marriage.
- Characteristics such as honesty, trust, fidelity, and open communications promote successful relationships.
- Attributes such as unequal commitment, lack of reciprocity, jealousy, and distrust undermine relationships.
- Ending a serious relationship is difficult. The resultant pain takes time to resolve.

DISCUSSION QUESTIONS

1. Think of a relationship that ended, leaving you feeling sad, betrayed, or angry. The person may have died, broken up with you, moved, or simply drifted away. Write a letter to that person. Explain how you felt and how you feel now. If you left important things unsaid, state them here.

2. Think of an important, positive relationship in your life. List all the ways this person makes your life more joyful, satisfying, and meaningful. How does this person show he or she cares? What do you do to positively contribute to the relationship?

3. Same-sex marriage is currently a topic of intense debate. What is your opinion? Defend it as best you can. See if you can find any evidence that same-sex couples are more or less successful at long-term partnership and more or less successful at parenting children. Is same-sex marriage legal in the state in which you live?

4. RECOMMENDED RESOURCES

4.1 Books

Courtenay W. *Dying to Be Men: Psychosocial, Environmental, and Biobehavioral Directions in Promoting the Health of Men and Boys*. New York, NY: Routledge; 2011.

Northrup C. *Women's Bodies, Women's Wisdom: Creating Physical and Emotional Health and Healing*. New York, NY: Random House; 2010.

4.2 Organizations and Websites

American Men's Studies Association. http://www.mensstudies.org.

Healthy Women. http://www.healthywomen.org.

MenEngage Global Alliance. http://www.menengage.org.

Men's Studies Press. http://www.mensstudies.com.

Men's Health Network. http://www.menshealthnetwork.org.

Men's Health Library. http://www.menshealthlibrary.org.

National Men's Health Week. http://www.menshealthweek.org.

National Organization for Women. http://www.now.org.

WebMD. http://men.webmd.com, http://women.webmd.com.

WomensHealth.gov. http://www.womenshealth.gov.

ENDNOTES

1. Social determinants of health: key concepts. World Health Organization. Available at: http://www.who.int/social_determinants/thecommission/finalreport/key_concepts/en/index.html. Accessed March 3, 2012.

2. Social determinants of health. Closing the gap in a generation—how? World Health Organization. Available at: http://www.who.int/social_determinants/thecommission/finalreport/closethegap_how/en/index1.html. Accessed March 3, 2012.

3. The index of social health. Institute for Innovation in Social Policy. Available at: http://iisp.vassar.edu/ish.html. Accessed March 3, 2012.

4. Infant mortality rate 2011. US Global Health Policy. Kaiser Family Foundation. Available at: http://www.globalhealthfacts.org/data/topic/map.aspx?ind=91. Accessed March 3, 2012.

5. Social connectedness and health survey. Mental Health America. May 2008. Available at: http://www.mentalhealthamerica.net/files/2008_MHM_Social_Connectedness_Survey_-_Executive_Summary.pdf. Accessed March 3, 2012.

6. Fisher HE, Aron A, Mashek MA, Haifang L, Brown LL. Defining the brain systems of lust, romantic attraction, and attachment. Arch Sex Behav. 2002;31(5):413–419.

7. Cacioppo JT, Hawkley LC. Social isolation and health, with an emphasis on underlying mechanisms. Perspect Biol Med. 2003;46(3 Suppl):S39–S52.

8. Levine MP. Loneliness and eating disorders. J Psychol. 2012;146(1–2):243–257.

9. Fothergill KE, Ensminger ME, Robertson J, et al. Effects of social integration on health: a prospective study of community engagement among African American women. Soc Sci Med. 2011;72:291–298.

10. Chen FS, Kumsta R, von Dawans B, Monakhov M, Ebstein RP, Heinrichs M. Common oxytocin receptor gene (OXTR) polymorphism and social support interact to reduce stress in humans. Proc Natl Acad Sci USA. 2011 Dec 13;108(50):19937–19942.

11. Emotional support and social support. The American Institute of Stress. Available at: http://www.stress.org/topic-emotional.htm. Accessed March 4, 2012.

12. Hill AL, Rand DG, Nowak MA, Christakis NA. Infectious disease modeling of social contagion in networks. PLoS Comput Biol. 2010 Nov 4;6(11):e1000968.

13. Krause-Parello CA. Pet ownership and older women: the relationships among loneliness, pet attachment support, human social support, and depressed mood. Geriatr Nurs. 2012 Feb 8. [In press.]

14. Arhant-Sudhir K, Arhant-Sudhir R, Sudhir K. Pet ownership and cardiovascular risk reduction: supporting evidence, conflicting data and underlying mechanisms. Clin Exp Pharmacol Physiol. 2011 Nov;38(11):734–738. doi:10.1111/j.1440-1681.2011.05583.x.

15. Charnetski CJ, Riggers S, Brennan FX. Effect of petting a dog on immune system function. Psychol Rep. 2004;95(3 Pt 2):1087–1091.

16. Mar RA. The neural bases of social cognition and story comprehension. Annu Rev Psychol. 2011;62:103–134. doi:10.1146/annurev-psych-120709-14546.

17. Hofmann W, Vohs KD, Baumeister RF. What people desire, feel conflicted about, and try to resist in everyday life. Psychol Sci. [In press.] Story reported at BGR.com and available at: http://www.bgr.com/2012/02/06/facebook-and-twitter-are-more-addictive-than-cigarettes-or-alcohol-study-finds. Accessed March 20, 2012.

18. Dixon K. Researchers link use of Internet, social isolation. Stanford Report. February 23, 2005. Available at: http://news.stanford.edu/news/2005/february23/internet-022305.html. Accessed March 20, 2012.

19. Kraut R, Lundmark R, Patterson M, et al. Internet paradox: a social technology that reduces social involvement and psychological well-being? Am Psychol. 1998;53(9):1017–1031.

20. van den Eijnden RJ, Meerkerk GJ, Vermulst AA, Spijkerman R, Engels RC. Online communication, compulsive Internet use, and psychosocial well-being among adolescents: a longitudinal study. Dev Psychol. 2008 May;44(3):655–665.

21. Klepper D. Teen sexting penalties may be relaxed by states. Huffington Post. June 6, 2011. Available at: http://www.huffingtonpost.com/2011/06/13/teen-sexting-penalties_n_875783.html. Accessed December 31, 2011.

22. Komaroff A. Social networks can affect weight, happiness. Harvard Health Blog. Available at: http://www.health.harvard.edu/blog. Accessed January 2, 2012.

23. O'Neil JM, Good GE, Holmes S. Fifteen years of theory and research on men's gender role conflict: new paradigms for empirical research. In: Levant R, Pollack W, ed. The New Psychology of Men. New York, NY: Basic Books; 1995.

24. Miniño AM. Mortality among teenagers aged 12–19 years: United States, 1999–2006. National Center for Health Statistics. Centers for Disease Control and Prevention. Available at: http://www.cdc.gov/nchs/fastats/deaths.htm. Accessed September 3, 2011.

25. Auge K. Fathers finding role in answer. The Denver Post. June 10, 2011:A1.

26. Pollack W. Real Boys: Rescuing Our Sons from the Myths of Boyhood. New York, NY: Random House; 1998.

27. Courtenay WH. Dying to Be Men: Psychosocial, Environmental, and Biobehavioral Directions in Promoting the Health of Men and Boys. New York, NY: Routledge Press; 2011.

28. Beatty A, Syzdek M, Bakkum A. The Saint John's Experience Project: challenging men's perceptions of normative gender role conflict. J Mens Stud. 2006;14(3):322–326.

29. Kahn J, Holmes J, Brett B. Concerns with men's academic motivation in higher education: an exploratory investigation of the role of masculinity. J Mens Stud. 2011;19:65–82.

30. Tremblay G. Quebec men's health: some important results—an explanatory model. In: Australasian Men's Health Forum. Debate and Invigorate: Challenges in Men's Health—7th National Men's Health Conference; October 3–5, 2007 Adelaide, South Australia.

31. Cheung RY, Park IJ. Anger suppression, interdependent self-construal, and depression among Asian American and European American college students. Cultur Divers Ethnic Minor Psychol. 2010 Oct;16(4):517–525.

32. Norwood SJ, Bowker A, Buchholz A, Henderson KA, Goldfield G, Flament MF. Self-silencing and anger regulation as predictors of disordered eating among adolescent females. Eat Behav. 2011 Apr;12(2):112–118.

33. College enrollment and work activity of 2010 high school graduates. Bureau of Labor Statistics. US Department of Labor. April 8, 2011. Available at: http://www.bls.gov/news.release/hsgec.nr0.htm. Accessed September 3, 2011.

34. Degrees conferred by sex and race. Fast Facts. Institute of Education Sciences. National Center for Education Statistics. Available at: http://nces.ed.gov/fastfacts/display.asp?id=72. Accessed May 28, 2013.

35. Quick stats on women workers, 2009. US Department of Labor. Available at: http://www.dol.gov/wb/stats/main.htm. Accessed September 3, 2011.

36. Verbrugge LM, Wingard DL. Sex differentials in health and mortality. Women Health. 1987;12(2):103–145.

37. Pinkhasov RM, Wong J, Kashanian J, Lee M, Samadi DB, Pinkhasov MM, Shabsigh R. Are men shortchanged on health? Perspective on health care utilization and health risk behavior in men and women in the United States. Int J Clin Pract. 2010 Mar;64(4):475–487.

38. Kalmuss D, Austrian K. Real men do…real men don't: young Latino and African American men's discourses regarding sexual health care utilization. Am J Mens Health. 2010 Sep;4(3):218–230.

39. Bao AM, Swaab DF. Sexual differentiation of the human brain: relation to gender identity, sexual orientation and neuropsychiatric disorders. Front Neuroendocrinol. 2011 Apr;32(2):214–226.

40. Fisher HE, Aron A, Mashek MA, Haifang L, Brown LL. Defining the brain systems of lust, romantic attraction, and attachment. Arch Sex Behav. 2002;31(5):413–419.

41. Gute G, Eshbaugh EM. Personality as a predictor of hooking up among college students. J Community Health Nurs. 2008 Jan–Mar;25(1):26–43.

42. Kreider RM. Increase in opposite-sex cohabiting couples from 2009 to 2010 in the Annual Social and Economic Supplement (ASES) to the Current Population Survey (CPS). US Bureau of Census. September 15, 2010. Available at: http://www.census.gov/population/www/socdemo/Inc-Opp-sex-2009-to-2010.pdf. Accessed March 20, 2012.

43. Deparle J, Tavernise S. For women under 30, most births occur outside marriage. New York Times. February 17, 2012. Available at: http://www.nytimes.com/2012/02/18/us/for-women-under-30-most-births-occur-outside-marriage.html?_r=1&scp=3&sq=jason%20deparle&st=cse. Accessed March 20, 2012.

44. Who marries and when? Age at first marriage in the United States: 2002. National Centers for Health Statistics. Centers for Disease Control and Prevention. Available at: http://www.cdc.gov/nchs/data/databriefs/db19.htm. Accessed March 20, 2012.

45. Kreider RM, Ellis R. Number, timing, and duration of marriages and divorces: 2009. US Census Bureau. May 2011. Available at: http://www.census.gov/prod/2011pubs/p70-125.pdf. Accessed March 20, 2012.

46. Births, marriages, divorces, and deaths: provisional data for 2009. National Vital Statistics Reports. Centers for Disease Control and Prevention. Available at: http://www.cdc.gov/nchs/data/nvsr/nvsr58/nvsr58_25.pdf. Accessed March 20, 2012.

47. Defining marriage: defense of marriage acts and same-sex marriage laws. National Conference of State Legislatures. February 24, 2012. Available at: http://www.ncsl.org/issues-research/human-services/same-sex-marriage-overview.aspx. Accessed May 28, 2013.

48. Marriage rights and benefits. Nolo Law for All. Available at: http://www.nolo.com/legal-encyclopedia/marriage-rights-benefits-30190.html. Accessed March 20, 2012.

49. Supreme Court DOMA decision rules federal same-sex marriage ban unconstitutional. Huffington Post. June 26, 2013. Available at http://www.huffingtonpost.com/2013/06/26/supreme-court-doma-decision_n_3454811.html. Accessed: July 12, 2013.

CHAPTER 7
Sexual and Reproductive Health

Sexual images are everywhere. Advertisers harness the power of sex to sell cars, appliances, and all kinds of sexless products. In the process we may lose sight of the importance of **sexual health** to overall health. According to the World Health Organization (WHO), "Sexual health is a state of physical, emotional, mental and social well-being in relation to sexuality; it is not merely the absence of disease, dysfunction or infirmity. Sexual health requires a positive and respectful approach to sexuality and sexual relationships, as well as the possibility of having pleasurable and safe sexual experiences, free of coercion, discrimination and violence."[1]

Sexuality is how you experience yourself as a sexual being and how you relate to others. Biology, culture, personality, values, beliefs, and attitudes shape your sexuality. Our families, communities, and society influence how we think about sex in general and express ourselves as sexual beings. Some of these messages may conflict. For instance, messages from the popular media may clash with the teachings of parents and religious figures. Eventually, you figure out your own point of view and become comfortable in body and mind.

Intimate sexual relationships can promote health and personal growth. They do, however, entail certain risks. Learning about sexual and reproductive health and applying that knowledge can minimize risks. This chapter will arm you with information about men's and women's reproductive health, sexual function, sexually transmitted infections, contraceptive options, pregnancy, and infertility.

An embrace should fill the heart as well as the arms.

- Hugh and Gail Prather, reverends

1. MEN'S SEXUAL HEALTH

LEARNING OBJECTIVES

1. Identify key anatomical structures in the male reproductive system.
2. Describe the diseases specific to men, including prevalence, risk factors, and potential effects on men's well-being.

FIGURE 7.1 Male Reproductive Anatomy

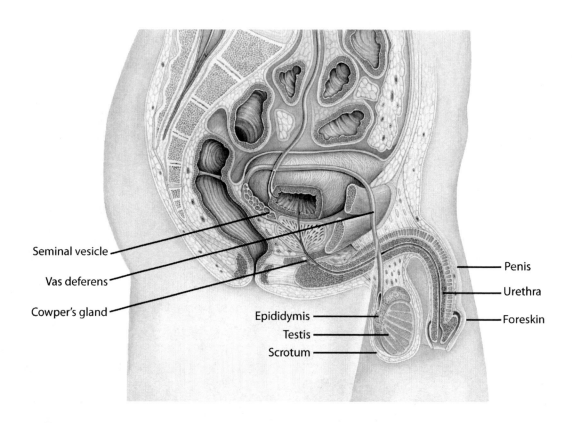

© *Thinkstock*

penis

Male external sexual organ; via the urethra, conveys urine and semen.

circumcision

Surgical removal of the foreskin, which normally covers the shaft of the penis.

testis

One of two male gonads; testes (plural) manufacture sperm and testosterone; also called testicles.

The most noticeable part of a man's reproductive system is the **penis**. The shaft is made of spongy tissue. When blood fills that tissue during sexual arousal, an erection occurs. The *urethra*, which carries urine and, during ejaculation, semen, runs down the middle and ends at the glans (head) of the penis.

The shaft of the penis may be covered by a *foreskin* (also called prepuce). Many American men are circumcised. **Circumcision** is a surgical procedure, usually performed soon after birth, that removes some or all of the foreskin. It's done for religious or cultural reasons rather than medical reasons. Because the health benefits are relatively small, the American Academy of Pediatrics does not recommend routine male circumcisions. Potential health benefits include a slightly reduced risk of infant urinary tract infections, penile cancer (which is very rare), and some sexually transmitted infections, including the acquisition and male-to-female transmission of human immunodeficiency virus (HIV).[2]

Within the sac of each *scrotum* lies the male gonad, the **testis**. The two testes make the male hormone *testosterone* and *sperm* (the male gamete or reproductive cell). Sperm and other fluids collect in a coiled tube at the top of each testis called the *epididymis*. The tube rising from the epididymis and snaking around to the back of the bladder is the *vas deferens*. Glands (the *seminal vesicles*, prostate, and *Cowper's gland*) contribute fluids that nourish and protect the sperm. This milky, sperm-laden fluid is called *semen*.

These organs rely on a healthy blood flow. That's why men should take steps to maintain arterial health. (For more on that topic, see Chapter 15.) Nerves and hormones control male reproductive functions.

Recall the discussion in Chapter 3 about the autonomic nervous system: The sympathetic nervous system has to do with the four Fs (flight, fight, fright, and fornication). It's responsible for ejaculation. The parasympathetic nervous system has to do with restful and restorative activities such as digesting food. It also causes the penis to become erect, due to its effects on local blood circulation.

Hormones from structures in the brain direct the testes to make sperm and testosterone. A rise in testosterone at puberty deepens the voice, causes hair to grow on the face, stimulates enlargement of the penis and testes, and matures the sperm. It also strengthens bones and muscles. While men make a lot more of it than women, *testosterone* contributes to sex drive (libido) in men and women.

Because it can cause problems, the **prostate** deserves more explanation. This walnut-sized gland encircles the urethra just below the bladder and between the scrota (plural of scrotum) and rectum. In addition to contributing fluid to the semen, the prostate—which contains muscular as well as glandular tissue—helps expel semen during ejaculation. Stimulation of the prostate can contribute to the sexual orgasm. Over 30 million men suffer from prostate conditions, including 230,000 diagnosed with prostate cancer each year.[3]

prostate

A gland surrounding the bladder neck and urethra in the male that contributes fluid to the semen.

1.1 Maladies in the Male Reproductive System

This section focuses on problems with the prostate gland and testes. A later section will address concerns about sexual function.

Prostatitis (prostate inflammation) is the most common prostate problem for men under 50. About half of adult men will be treated for it during their lifetime.[4] Bacteria can infect the prostate gland. The prostate is also susceptible to acute and chronic noninfectious inflammation, though the cause is poorly understood.

prostatitis

Inflammation of the prostate.

The symptoms of acute bacterial prostatitis include frequent and painful urination, pain in the lower back or behind the testicles, painful ejaculation, aching muscles, fever, chills, and fatigue. Chronic bacterial infection can occur without significant symptoms. Noninfectious prostatitis mainly causes pelvic pain, as well as pain with ejaculation and urination.

Health practitioners diagnose prostatitis based on the man's history, physical examination, and a urinalysis. Depending on the situation, blood tests and imaging studies such as an ultrasound may also be ordered.

Treatment of bacterial prostatitis centers on antibiotics. A recent study found improved success treating chronic bacterial prostatitis after combining an antibiotic with a supplement containing quercetin (an antioxidant substance found in many plants) and the herbs saw palmetto, nettles, and curcumin (the active ingredient in turmeric).[5] Noninfectious prostatitis is more challenging to manage. Some medications may relieve the pain as well as enlargement of the prostate. Physical therapy may also help.

Benign prostatic hyperplasia, also called benign prostatic hypertrophy (BPH), mainly affects older men. Noncancerous enlargement of the prostate encroaches on the urethra, decreasing the ability of urine to easily flow from the bladder. Consequently, symptoms include increased frequency and urgency of urination, nighttime urination, a weak urine stream, an inability to fully empty the bladder, and difficulty stopping and starting urination.

benign prostatic hyperplasia

The enlargement of the prostate, which can lead to compression of the urethra and obstruction of the flow of urine.

The prostate grows rapidly during puberty and then more slowly during middle age. Later in life, this enlargement picks up speed, mainly due to hormonal shifts. Although testosterone levels diminish, an enzyme that converts testosterone to dihydrotestosterone (DHT) becomes more active with age. DHT causes cells in the prostate to multiply. It's also responsible for male-pattern baldness. Levels of estrogen, which also stimulates prostate enlargement, rise with age.

FIGURE 7.2 Benign Prostatic
Hyperplasia

The left panel depicts a normal prostate. The right panel illustrates benign prostatic hyperplasia. Notice that an enlarged prostate pushes into the bladder and narrows the urethra, impeding urination.

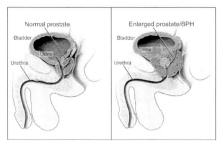

Source: National Cancer Institute. Benign prostatic hyperplasia. Available at: http://commons.wikimedia.org/ wiki/File:Benign_Prostatic_Hyperplasia_nci-vol-7137-300.jpg

andropause

A constellation of changes that occur in men after middle age, including decreased testosterone, purported to be analogous to menopause in women.

BPH is extremely common in older men. Approximately half of 50- to 60-year-old men develop BPH. Between ages 80 and 90, that proportion rises to nearly 90 percent.[6] Other risk factors for developing BPH include having a family history; having diabetes, obesity, high blood pressure, or heart disease; and consuming lots of carbohydrates and fats.[7] Traditional Asian diets are associated with a reduced likelihood of BPH and prostate cancer. These diets include regular consumption of soy and green tea, both of which contain substances that restrain prostate growth.[8]

Because symptoms of BPH can overlap with those of prostate cancer, it is important to consult a physician for an accurate diagnosis. Prescription medications can reduce prostate size and improve urine flow. Severe cases may require surgery. Some herbs may be helpful in cases of mild BPH. These include extracts of the African plant *pygeum*,[9] *saw palmetto*,[10],[11] and *nettle* root.[12] Reported side effects for these herbs are minor and rare.

Male Reproductive Cancers

Testicular cancer is the most common cancer to affect young men, though it can also manifest in older men. *Prostate cancer*, on the other hand, becomes more prevalent with advancing age. After skin cancer, it's the most commonly diagnosed cancer in men. *Penile cancer* is very rare. For more information, see Chapter 16.

Andropause

As men grow older, testosterone and growth hormones gradually decline. Normally, testosterone levels begin to drop at age 30 by approximately 10 percent every decade.[13] The resultant emotional and physical changes are referred to as **andropause**. Symptoms include generalized fatigue, decreased sex drive, erectile dysfunction, loss of physical agility, loss of muscle mass, problems with cognition and memory, and extreme moodiness and irritability. Conditions such as increased cardiovascular risks, osteoporosis, increased abdominal fat, varicose veins, and atrophy of the skin can also occur.

Lifestyle factors such as smoking, alcohol, and poor nutrition can harm the testes, leading to declines in testosterone levels.[14] They also interfere with erectile function. That's why it's important for men to establish good health habits early in life. Don't wait until irreversible damage has occurred.

Men who notice signs of andropause should meet with a health care professional for a thorough evaluation. A number of chronic diseases—diabetes, chronic renal failure, cirrhosis, anemia, and inflammatory conditions—can produce similar symptoms. Also, some medications can decrease testosterone.

KEY TAKEAWAYS

- A man's self-image and the way he presents himself in the world changes as he ages, especially as testosterone declines during andropause.
- Prostatitis may or may not be bacterial. It commonly affects younger men.
- Benign prostatic hyperplasia, a noncancerous enlargement of the prostate, becomes increasingly common with age and hinders urination.

DISCUSSION QUESTIONS

1. How might cultural beliefs about manhood interfere with a man's personal health, especially issues such as prostate issues, premature ejaculation, and andropause?
2. Describe some things that a guy could do to optimize the health of his prostate, using the information from this chapter as well as some of the additional resources listed in Section 6.

2. WOMEN'S SEXUAL HEALTH

LEARNING OBJECTIVES

1. Identify key female reproductive structures and name their functions.
2. Describe common female reproductive complaints and their management.

FIGURE 7.3 Female Reproductive Anatomy

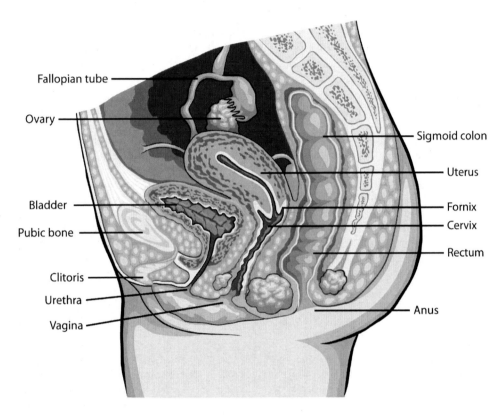

Source: Adapted from Sternberg E. Drawing of the female internal sexual anatomy. Available at: http://commons.wikimedia.org/wiki/

File:Female_reproductive_system_lateral.png.

Unlike a man, a woman's reproductive organs are secreted away in her pelvis. Only the external genitalia, also called the **vulva**, are readily visible. The *labia majora* (outer lips) and *labia minora* (inner lips) are folds of skin that drape over the other structures. The **clitoris** resides at the upper corner of the labia minora. Homologous to the penis, it's exquisitely sensitive and provides sexual pleasure. Just below it is the opening of the urethra, which is, technically, part of the urinary system. Below that the urethra is the entrance to the vagina, and below that the anus, the end of the gastrointestinal tract.

vulva

External female genitalia.

clitoris

Female organ homologous to the penis that contains spongy tissue and nerve endings, which make it sensitive to touch.

vagina

Muscular tubular structure that leads from the female external genitals to the uterus.

cervix

The opening of the uterus; located at the top of the vagina.

uterus

A hollow, muscular organ in which a fertilized egg develops; also called womb.

fallopian tube

One of two ducts through which mature ovum travels from the ovary to the uterus.

ovaries

Female gonads; contain eggs (ova) and manufacture estrogen and progesterone.

ovulation

Expulsion of a ripened ovum from the ovary midway through the menstrual cycle.

menses

The point in the menstrual cycle wherein estrogen and progesterone drop and the uterine lining is shed via the vagina.

The **vagina**, which sits behind the bladder, begins the internal genitalia. Menstrual flow exits here, and the penis enters during sexual intercourse. The vagina dead ends at the **cervix**, which is the lower part of the **uterus**, a hollow, muscular organ shaped like an upside-down pear. Two **fallopian tubes** branch from the top. Just outside their fingerlike ends lie the two **ovaries**, which are homologous to the testes. The ovaries make *ova* (eggs or female gametes) and the two female hormones, *estrogen* and *progesterone*. Women's adrenal glands (which sit like small party hats atop the kidneys) make male-like hormones, including small amounts of testosterone, which contributes to *libido* (sexual desire).

As in men, hormones from the woman's brain stimulate her ovaries' follicles (spherical arrangements of cells, each containing an ovum or egg). The follicles make estrogen. The hormone estrogen has many functions. During puberty, it causes the uterus to enlarge, the vagina to thicken, and breasts to develop. During each menstrual cycle, it thickens the endometrium, the lining of the uterus. Estrogen promotes healthy blood vessels, skin, and bones. Along with testosterone, it may contribute to the libido. The ovaries also make progesterone, which matures the lining of the uterus.

Between 10 and 14 days after the last menstrual period, one of the follicles extrudes its ovum—a process called **ovulation**. A woman may feel a brief, sharp pain in her low abdomen. The ovum is drawn inside the nearby fallopian tube. The ruptured follicle becomes a progesterone-making factory. Under the influence of estrogen and progesterone, the uterine lining thickens.

If the woman has recently had unprotected intercourse, the ovum, which lives for about 48 hours, may encounter sperm, which can survive about 5 days in a woman's reproductive tract. If a sperm penetrates the ovum, *fertilization* has occurred. This egg, fertilized or not, makes it way down the fallopian tube (pregnancy will be discussed further in Section 5). If the egg hasn't been fertilized, estrogen and progesterone levels fall and the uterine lining sloughs off and flows out the vagina, marking the onset of **menses**.

The well-orchestrated pattern of hormone fluctuations doesn't always work smoothly. Cycles can become irregular, absent, too frequent, too long, too light, too heavy, and accompanied by cramping and other bothersome symptoms. About the time a woman enters her sixth decade, the cessation of menses triggers another raft of symptoms. The rest of this section provides an overview of common complaints for women. Two generally female conditions are covered in other chapters—bladder infections (Chapter 14) and cancers of the breast, uterus, and ovary (Chapter 16).

2.1 Reproductive Years

Irregular or Absent Menses

Many women begin menstruating around age 12 and soon establish a rhythm, with each cycle lasting approximately 28 days. However, absent or irregular cycles are common—not a big surprise, considering the hormonal balancing act of a normal cycle. Lack of menstruation (**amenorrhea**) can be primary (fails to start by age 15) or secondary (after a normal start, menses cease for at least 3 months). Some women have sporadic menstrual flow due to irregular hormonal fluctuations. For instance, they may not ovulate, leading to inadequate progesterone production, which leads to irregular and often profuse bleeding.

A number of factors can disrupt the reproductive hormones, including excessive weight loss or gain, eating disorders, intense exercise, psychological stress,[15] illness, pregnancy, breast-feeding a baby, and the approach of menopause. Female athletes not uncommonly have delayed, irregular, and absent menstruation.[16] Being both underweight and overweight can contribute to irregular cycles.[17] Routinely skipping breakfast is associated with irregular menstrual cycles.[18] On the other hand, eating a healthy diet, managing stress, and getting enough sleep help promote normal cycles.

Another cause of menstrual irregularities is polycystic ovary syndrome, a condition of hormone imbalance that often involves a relative excess of male hormones. Other signs and symptoms include acne, facial hair, loss of hair from the scalp, difficulty becoming pregnant, and weight gain.

If you've missed a period and are sexually active, consider taking a pregnancy test. If it's positive, make a clinic appointment. Otherwise, it's wise to consult your health practitioner about persistently irregular or absent cycles. Normal levels of female hormones are important for maintaining reproductive, cardiovascular, and bone health. In the face of chronically low estrogen levels, bones demineralize.

Health professionals may prescribe hormonal contraceptives for absent, irregular, or painful menses. Preliminary research suggests extracts of chaste tree berries can help to regulate menstrual cycles.[19]

Menstrual cramps commonly afflict young women. A study of female university students in Mexico found that 64 percent had menstrual discomfort.[20] For 20 percent of them, the pain was severe. Many women missed classes because of it.

Discomfort, which can radiate from the pelvis to the lower back or thighs, often begins several hours before menstrual bleeding starts and continues for a day or two. As menses approach, a rise in

A woman is doing cobra pose, a yoga posture that may relieve menstrual cramps.

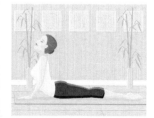

© *Thinkstock*

inflammatory chemicals causes the uterus to contract, which can hurt. Sometimes menstrual pain arises from an underlying condition such as an infection, uterine fibroids (noncancerous growths), or endometriosis (a condition in which uterine lining tissue takes root outside the uterus). If the pain is severe or prolonged, make an appointment with your practitioner.

The adage "time heals all" holds true; cramping often diminishes in women over age 24, but that's cold comfort if you hurt right now. Many women turn to over-the-counter nonsteroidal anti-inflammatory drugs such as ibuprofen (Advil, Motrin) and naproxen (Naprosyn, Aleve). If you do, do not exceed the recommended dosage.

Time-honored home remedies can also help. For instance, the application of heat—soaking in a warm bath, applying a hot water bottle or heating pad—improves blood flow and relaxes the uterus. Research supports this traditional practice.[21] Take care not to burn yourself. You can combine the heat with topical use of diluted essential oils. In a study of college women, an abdominal massage with one teaspoon of almond oil containing two drops of lavender, one drop of clary sage, and one drop of rose significantly reduced cramping.[22]

Another strategy is to drink warm tea made with herbs that relax the uterus and reduce inflammation. One study found that an extract of valerian root reduced menstrual cramps in young women.[23] Other traditional herbs include peppermint, lemon balm, catnip, cramp bark, ginger, wild yam, and dong quai.

Adequate intake of essential fatty acids correlates with a reduction in pain of all kinds, including the menstrual variety.[24] Sources of these "good fats" include cold-water fish (and fish oil supplements), borage oil, flaxseed oil, and evening primrose oil. Some studies have found success with magnesium supplements.[25]

Regular exercise can also reduce menstrual cramps.[26] A recent study showed that three yoga postures—cobra, cat-cow, and fish—practiced over two monthly cycles eased cramping in young women.[27] If you're interested, you can search for those poses on the Internet or try taking a yoga class. Acupuncture has been shown to relieve cramping.[28],[29] Nine out of 10 studies found acupressure (using fingers or other blunt objects to stimulate acupuncture points) effective.[30] If you do meet with a Chinese medicine practitioner, you might ask him or her to show you which points to stimulate.

Video Clip 7.1

Relieving Menstrual Cramps with Acupressure
This video shows how to stimulate one of the several acupressure points (spleen 6) shown to reduce menstrual cramps, a practice supported by research.[31] The correct point often feels a bit tender with pressure. That's OK. Do not stimulate this point (spleen 6) if you are pregnant; doing so may stimulate uterine contractions.

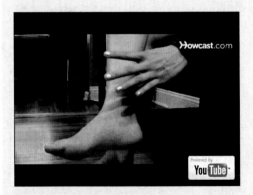

View the video online at: http://www.youtube.com/v/cBlOy4GL5R8

Premenstrual syndrome (PMS) is a cluster of recurrent symptoms that develop between the time of ovulation and the onset of menstruation. Symptoms can include fluid retention, abdominal bloating, headaches, breast tenderness, low back pain, constipation or diarrhea, fatigue, insomnia, sugar cravings, forgetfulness, irritability, decreased self-esteem, social withdrawal, anxiety, and mild depression. Many women develop symptoms around 10 days before their periods and feel instantly better with the onset of menstrual flow.

An estimated 80 percent of young women endure PMS during their reproductive years. While most women have mild symptoms, up to 8 percent report that severe PMS interferes with their routine activities.[32] Many of these women have **premenstrual dysphoric disorder** (PMDD), which is marked

premenstrual syndrome (PMS)

Symptoms such as bloating, breast tenderness, fatigue, and irritability that recur before the onset of menstruation.

by irritability, mood swings, depressed mood, and nervous tension during the days leading up to menstruation.

The cause of PMS remains a medical mystery, though monthly oscillations in reproductive hormones clearly contribute. Stress, overweight, and smoking correlate with more symptoms.[33],[34] Conventional practitioners may treat their patients with PMS with hormonal contraceptives (to smooth out the normal fluctuations in estrogen and progesterone) or antidepressants, given either continuously or only during the last two weeks of the monthly cycle. The latter is also used to treat PMDD. Diuretics may be prescribed to reduce fluid retention and breast tenderness.[35]

Healthy diet is, as always, important. Some women find they develop cravings for sweets and other unhealthy foods just before their periods. Try not to cave in to junk food cravings, which seem to worsen symptoms. Do eat enough. Low blood sugar (hypoglycemia) is thought to account for at least some PMS symptoms.[36] Watch out for caffeine and alcohol, which may also aggravate some of the symptoms.

Exercise can reduce PMS.[37] It also helps manage risk factors such as overweight and stress. Other stress-reducing techniques—yoga poses, breathing techniques, and meditation—can also help manage symptoms.[38] A recent analysis concluded that acupuncture produces promising results in women with PMS.[39]

Getting enough micronutrients from foods or dietary supplements may help. For instance, women consuming sufficient amounts of calcium, magnesium, vitamin D, B vitamins, and essential fatty acids in their diets are less likely to develop PMS.[40],[41],[42],[43],[44],[45] The best-researched herb for PMS is chaste tree.[46] A number of studies show that taking chaste tree berry extract daily over three cycles reduces PMS. Dosing depends on the product used.

Preliminary research also supports the use of St. John's wort extracts to manage PMS[47] and PMDD.[48],[49] The main drawbacks of St. John's wort are increased sun sensitivity and hastened breakdown of a number of medications, including hormonal contraceptives. The resultant reduction in the body's drug levels can undermine efficacy. In the case of hormonal contraceptives, pregnancy could occur.

Fibrocystic breasts affect many younger women, causing benign (noncancerous) lumps and/or discomfort. Fluctuations in reproductive hormones cause symptoms to become most noticeable just before menstrual periods. Wearing a supportive bra, reducing caffeine and dietary fat, consuming more essential fatty acids (particularly evening primrose oil), and taking anti-inflammatory medicines may help.[50],[51] Chaste tree berry extracts, taken all month long for at least three cycles, can reduce cyclic breast tenderness.[52] Oral contraceptives reduce symptoms for some women; others may notice worsened breast tenderness.

These lumps do not increase the risk of breast cancer. However, they may result in diagnostic tests to rule out cancer and make mammograms (low-dose X-rays of the breast) difficult to interpret. Normal breasts contain glands, fat, and fibrous (connective) tissue, all of which contribute to their texture. If you're a woman, examine your breasts at different times of the month to become familiar with their textural patterns. See your health practitioner if you notice changes in lumps or have other concerns.

2.2 Vaginal Infections (Vaginitis)

Vaginitis means inflammation of the vagina. Sometimes the term *vulvovaginitis* is used, referring to the fact that the vulva (labia and clitoris) are also involved. Sexual intercourse without sufficient lubrication can inflame the vagina. So can tampons and allergens and irritants in soaps, shower gels, bubble bath products, and vaginal sprays. Nevertheless, the term usually refers to infectious causes. Bacteria, viruses, protozoa, and fungi can all infect the vagina. This section addresses two types of vaginitis that can trouble women, even if they've never had sex. Then we will discuss those that are primarily sexually transmitted.

Bacterial Vaginosis

The most common vaginal infection during a woman's childbearing years, bacterial vaginosis (BV), is a frustrating condition characterized by an imbalance in the population of vaginal bacteria.[53] Rather than being primarily colonized with lactobacilli and other protective microorganisms, the vagina hosts pathogenic bacteria such as *Gardnerella vaginalis*. Having too few of the "good bacteria" and too many of the "bad bacteria" lead to telltale signs and symptoms.

The main sign of BV is a thin, grayish vaginal discharge with a fishy odor. Slight vaginal itching or burning with urination can occur. Some women have no symptoms at all. This infection can sometimes produce pelvic inflammatory disease, which is discussed next. BV during pregnancy can initiate premature labor.

Risk factors for developing BV include having a new sexual partner, multiple partners, douching (which disrupts the normal vaginal microbes), smoking, and having an intrauterine device (IUD).[54] However, women who have never had sexual intercourse can also get it. Having BV can increase a woman's risk of acquiring a sexually transmitted infection.[55]

Health care practitioners diagnose BV by examining vaginal fluid under a microscope. Antibiotic treatment usually involves metronidazole (Flagyl, given in pill form or as a vaginal gel) or clindamycin (Cleocin vaginal cream). Although these drugs sometimes cure the condition, recurrences are common. Sexual partners don't need to be treated.

Vaginal Yeast Infections

Yeast, which is a type of fungus, normally inhabits the vagina, though in smaller quantities than lactobacilli bacteria. An overgrowth of certain types of yeast, such as *Candida albicans*, produces *yeast vaginitis*, also called vaginal candidiasis. Usually the labia and clitoris are also inflamed. About 75 percent of women have at least one episode in their lifetime; 5 to 10 percent have recurrent attacks.[56]

A number of factors can create this imbalance: antibiotics (because they kill the "friendly" bacteria), douches and some vaginal "hygiene" sprays (because they can irritate the vagina and disrupt the microbial ecology), cancer chemotherapy and cortisone-like medications (because they depress immune function), diabetes mellitus (because yeast thrives in the presence of excess sugar), receptive oral sex (cunnilingus), pregnancy (because of hormonal shifts), and some contraceptives (contraceptive sponges, hormonal contraceptives, and intrauterine devices).

Symptoms include itching, burning, a thick white discharge, and discomfort during intercourse. Visual inspection and examining the discharge under a microscope confirms the diagnosis.

Health professionals usually treat the condition with a topical antifungal cream or possibly oral antifungal drugs. Boric acid suppositories have also been successfully used;[57] some products are available over the counter. Intravaginal boric acid, though generally safe, can cause a burning sensation.

Some natural medicine practitioners use *diluted* tea tree oil to manage vaginitis.[58],[59] Tea tree essential oil is antimicrobial against a number of organisms, including *Candida albicans*, herpes simplex virus 1 and 2, *Garnerella vaginalis* (a cause of BV),[60] and *Trichomonas vaginalis* (which causes trichomoniasis or "trich").[61] Local irritation and allergic reactions are possible. Tea tree essential oil is very strong and should only be applied externally; it can be toxic if ingested.

While some antifungal creams and other products are available over the counter, it's important first to get a professional diagnosis. Women correctly self-diagnose yeast vaginitis only about half the time. Other pathogens that don't respond to antifungal drugs—some with potentially serious complications—can cause similar symptoms or may coexist with the yeast overgrowth.

Preventing Vaginitis

Women troubled by recurrent bouts of BV or yeast vaginitis can avoid known, modifiable risk factors. Here are some strategies to try:

- Wear breathable underwear (no nylon), skirts, and looser pants.
- Use a hypoallergenic soap and rinse well with clear water. Avoid vaginal sprays and douches.
- Maintain good bathroom hygiene; always wipe front to back.
- Practice safe sex. While BV and yeast vaginitis can afflict virgins, sexual activity may spread the organisms.
- If you have diabetes, work with your health practitioner to control your blood sugar.
- Eat a healthy diet and avoid sweetened beverages, sweets and other refined carbohydrates, and alcoholic drinks (which contain carbohydrates). Include fermented foods such as plain yogurt, kefir, and kimchi (fermented cabbage). These foods contain probiotics, which promote the friendly bacteria in your body.
- Consider probiotic supplements. Some studies show that oral or intravaginal capsules or suppositories containing certain strains of lactobacilli (*Lactobacillus acidophilus, L. rhamnosus* GR-1, *L. fermentum* RC-14, *L. crispatus*, and *L. reuteri*) help reduce recurrences, with greater success for BV than candida vaginitis.[62],[63],[64]
- Stay in touch with your primary health practitioner. Get regular exams and screening tests. Get a diagnosis before using over-the-counter remedies.

2.3 Perimenopausal Years

menopause

The permanent cessation of menstrual periods; officially occurs 12 months after the last menstrual period.

Menopause is the point at which, for lack of estrogen and progesterone, monthly periods cease. Technically, it's defined as cessation of menses for 12 months. The average age of natural menopause is 51. Premature menopause can occur because of surgical removal of the ovaries, cancer treatment with chemotherapy or radiation therapy, some autoimmune disorders, and a number of hormone disorders. Sometimes there's a family history of premature menopause. Sometimes the cause is unknown.

Perimenopause is the transition leading up to menopause. It can last years. Menstrual cycles become irregular. Progesterone often wanes before estrogen, which can lead to more frequent, heavier periods. Some women also notice mood swings and more frequent headaches. As estrogen levels fall, many women experience hot flashes, which are sudden sensations of heat spreading over the body sometimes followed by sweating. Night sweats and other menopause-related changes can interrupt sleep. Concentration may waver. Vaginal tissues become thinner and drier. Sex drive can decline. The skin, mouth, and eyes may also become drier. Symptoms vary from one woman to the next. Some women sail easily through to menopause with few complaints, while others struggle during this transition.

In addition to physical complaints, menopause presents psychological challenges. It marks the end of the reproductive years. For women whose lives were defined by raising a family, the prospect of an "empty nest" may feel sad and lonely. Women who took pride in their lush, youthful beauty may feel dread and dismay as the elements, time, gravity, and their own biology age their features. For biological, social, and cultural reasons, depression can surface.[65] On the other hand, many women find this transition liberating. They may have more time to devote to careers, hobbies, travel, and friends.

osteoporosis

A condition marked by loss of bone mass and an increased risk of bone fractures.

Because estrogen benefits both the cardiovascular system and the bones, two long-term concerns for menopausal women are heart disease and osteoporosis. **Osteoporosis**, which means "porous bones," is a condition of severe bone loss. Although a woman's risk of heart disease mortality (death) climbs steadily with age, the incidence of osteoporosis rises sharply after menopause. While some people have genetic susceptibilities, healthy lifestyles go a long way toward preventing both conditions. See the sidebar "Preventing Osteoporosis".

Doctors used to recommend that all perimenopausal and menopausal women take hormone replacement therapy (HRT) with both estrogen and progesterone (the latter to counteract the risk of estrogen-stimulating uterine cancer). Then in 2002, a large study suggested that though HRT relieved perimenopausal symptoms and protected bones, it actually increased the risk of heart attack, stroke, and breast cancer.[66] Great consternation among health professionals and older women ensued. The study was criticized for several reasons, such as the fact that many of the women were older (postmenopausal) and all women took the medication. Conflicting findings about whether supplemental estrogen is good or bad for the cardiovascular system and brain have followed. While it seems clear that estrogen does increase breast cancer risk, the risk to any one woman appears to be small—unless she has a family or personal history. At this point, health practitioners should work with their female patients to identify the best options for managing bothersome symptoms and for keeping bones and blood vessels healthy.

Diet clearly affects bone and cardiovascular health and may also modulate short-term symptoms. Asian women, who consume more soy and veggies and fewer meats than the average American woman, reportedly have an easier transition into menopause and a lower risk of breast cancer. Soy and other legumes contain isoflavones, chemicals that have weak estrogen-like effects in the body. However, studies on soy's effectiveness during perimenopause have been inconclusive.[67]

A number of herbs may relieve some perimenopausal symptoms. The best researched is black cohosh, with the majority of studies on concentrated extracts producing positive results.[68] Black cohosh does not seem to pose a risk for uterine or breast cancer.[69] Other herbs with at least some positive research include red clover, St. John's wort, and maca.[70]

Preventing Osteoporosis

In osteoporosis, both protein and mineral are depleted, leaving bones fragile and easily fractured. More than 40 million Americans are affected.[71] About 1.5 million osteoporosis-related fractures happen each year, sending many older Americans to hospitals and nursing homes. While women are more at risk, men can get it too. Other risk factors include small body size, being Asian or Caucasian, a family history of the condition, eating disorders (particularly anorexia nervosa), poor diet, lack of exercise, smoking, and excessive alcohol and soda consumption. Some diseases (including diabetes) and drugs increase the risk.

We build bone into the third decade of our lives. After that, a steady loss begins, like sand slipping through an hourglass. Nevertheless, osteoporosis is not inevitable. Simple lifestyle habits can keep your bones strong. And prevention starts *now*. Whether you're a woman or a man, your goal should be to bank as much bone as possible when you're young. Past the third decade, you can still act to slow bone loss.

Physical activity is critical for preserving bone, strengthening muscles, and improving balance—all factors that help prevent falls and fractures. Choose weight-bearing exercises such as walking, jogging, jumping rope, dancing, climbing stairs, and strength training (working against the resistance of weights, elastic bands or tubes, or your own body weight).

Good diet is also critical. While much of the media focus on the consumption of milk and other dairy products, many Americans are either lactose intolerant or allergic to dairy. Consuming more vegetables and fruits can help maintain bone density.[72] Plants contain calcium, magnesium, protein, potassium, and other bone-friendly nutrients and tend to generate less calcium-leaching acid. It's also a good idea to avoid bone robbers such as soda and excessive amounts of alcohol. If you smoke, quit.

While calcium supplements can increase bone density, most studies fail to show significant protection against bone fractures. Worse, calcium supplements have been associated with an increased risk of heart attacks and kidney stones.[73],[74]

Among its other functions, vitamin D promotes calcium absorption from the intestines. Although ultraviolet light triggers vitamin D production in the skin, many people avoid exposure to the sun. Furthermore, few foods contain vitamin D. For those reasons, many experts recommend supplements: 600 international units (IU) a day for people 1 to 70, and 800 IU a day for those older than 70.

For more information, visit the National Osteoporosis Foundation online at http://www.nof.org.

KEY TAKEAWAYS

- The menstrual cycle is a complex process. Cycles can become irregular or absent or marked by pain and other uncomfortable physical and psychological symptoms. Lifestyle modifications, simple home remedies, and some dietary supplements can ease mild complaints. Significant changes in menstrual patterns and more severe symptoms deserve a medical evaluation.
- Two vaginal infections—bacterial vaginosis and vaginal candidiasis—can occur in women who are not sexually active.
- Perimenopause, the years leading up to menopause, can cause symptoms that disrupt a woman's life. A number of options—hormone replacement, other medications, lifestyle modifications, and some dietary supplements—help manage symptoms. The optimal choice depends on the individual woman.
- Two common chronic diseases for older women and men are cardiovascular disease and osteoporosis. Both can be largely prevented with avoidance of risks and adoption of healthy diet and regular exercise. Because both conditions take many years to develop, you should take steps now.

DISCUSSION QUESTIONS

1. What options are available to help a woman manage premenstrual syndrome?
2. Osteoporosis affects men and women, takes many years to develop, and causes no symptoms. What are you doing to protect your bones? What about risk factors? Do you smoke or drink a lot of alcohol or sodas? How might you change your behavior to avoid brittle bones and crippling fractures?

3. SEXUAL FUNCTION, SAFER SEX, AND CONTRACEPTION

3.1 The Sexual Response

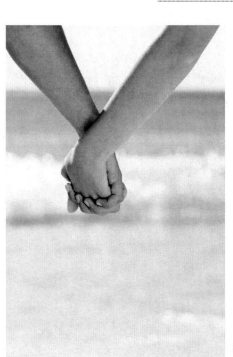

© *Thinkstock*

The normal sexual response follows a sequence of phases. However, the cycle can be interrupted at any point. (In other words, don't believe it if someone claims he or she can't stop.) The following phases occur with masturbation as well as sex with a partner.

The first phase is **excitement**. Something stimulates sexual arousal. Blood rushes to critical areas (though there's plenty remaining for your brain to function clearly). In men, the penis becomes engorged and erect. In women, the clitoris, labia, vagina, and nipples become flushed with blood. Vaginal lubrication increases. Skeletal muscles become more taut.

Next is the **plateau phase**, during which time responses in stage one steadily intensify. Phase three encompasses *orgasm*. In both sexes, the genital region is ground zero for a series of involuntary, rhythmic, pleasurable contractions. The contractions usually also propel semen from a man's urethra, a process called *ejaculation*. Women usually take longer reaching orgasm. Foreplay before penile-vaginal penetration can help women feel satisfied.

After the orgasm, the **resolution phase** marks a return to a relaxed state. The penis becomes flaccid. Men are more likely to fall asleep than women. They also enter a **refractory period** lasting minutes to hours, during which time they can't again reach orgasm and ejaculation. Women, on the other hand, can attain multiple organisms.

The sexual response slowly changes over an adult's life. Most healthy people continue to enjoy sex for decades. Older men and women often require more stimulation to enter the first phase. Vaginal secretions decrease after menopause, though over-the-counter lubricants can offset this effect. Older men tend to spend a longer time reaching orgasm and have more control of that event. Men's refractory periods also lengthen.

3.2 Challenges to Sexual Function

Both men and women can have less than satisfying sexual experiences. Some problems tend to resolve with time and practice. Some difficulties don't surface until later as a result of normal age changes or disease in other bodily systems. In men, erectile function is more obvious. Women can have sex without clitoral engorgement and orgasm, though the event may not be as fulfilling.

libido

Sexual desire.

In both men and women, **libido** (sexual desire) can drop. Possible contributing factors include stress, depression, anxiety, fatigue, illness, and certain medications (some antidepressants and drugs to reduce high blood pressure). Inhibited sexual desire can also be a long-standing state wherein the person has never been interested in sex or, after some event, lost interest. Low sex drive may only be a problem if the other partner's libido is friskier.

3.3 Sexual Dysfunction in Men

The most common male sexual problem, **premature ejaculation (PE)**, affects 20 to 30 percent of men. Experts define it as an inability to delay ejaculation more than a minute or so after vaginal penetration. As a consequence, the man feels increasingly frustrated, anxious, and distressed. Sexual self-confidence plummets and intimate relations may become strained.[75] Some men have PE for only a brief time; others have a lifelong problem.

Both biological and psychological factors contribute to PE. Biological problems include

- having a genetic predisposition to PE,
- penile hypersensitivity,
- a hyperexcitable ejaculatory reflex, and
- problems with the nerve chemical serotonin.[76]

Psychological factors include stress and anxiety. A vicious cycle can develop wherein anxiety causes PE, which in turn causes more anxiety. Recall that the stress response suppresses the parasympathetic nervous system activity (which is critical for getting an erection) and increases sympathetic nervous system activity (which causes ejaculation). That's why feeling stressed and anxious can produce both erectile dysfunction and premature ejaculation.

Many men with PE don't receive treatment, either because they're too embarrassed to discuss the subject or because their doctors don't ask about their sexual health. Treatment depends on the possible cause. When psychological factors underlie the problem, psychotherapy can facilitate a more positive mindset, reduce anxiety, and manage stress. Slow, deep breathing during sexual intercourse promotes the parasympathetic nervous system, which helps prolong an erection and postpone ejaculation.

Sexual therapy may help. For instance, it may be reassuring to learn that premature ejaculation is not uncommon with a new partner. Furthermore, sex is not all about intercourse. Using other means of stimulation, a man can bring his partner near to orgasm before penetration. That way it doesn't matter if ejaculation happens soon.[77] Also, with repeated orgasms, most men are able to last longer each time. Slowing one's rhythm or pausing can also delay ejaculation. So can wearing two condoms at once.

One drug treatment arose from the recognition that delayed orgasm was a common side effect among men and women taking antidepressants that raise the nerve chemical serotonin. Therefore, doctors may prescribe antidepressants. Research shows these drugs (particularly Paxil) can modestly prolong the time to ejaculation.[78] They do, however, have side effects such as nausea, fatigue, headache, agitation, and insomnia. Topical anesthetics are also used to desensitize the penis. When hypersensitivity is a problem, these agents lengthen the time to ejaculation without adversely affecting the sensation of that climax.[79]

The flipside of premature ejaculation is **delayed ejaculation**. As the name suggests, men require more than average sexual stimulation to achieve orgasm. Sometimes ejaculation doesn't occur at all. Intoxication with alcohol or illicit drugs and fatigue can temporarily impair ejaculation. Some medications, including some antidepressants, delay climax. Surgery and chronic ill health may also be to blame. So can psychological factors, including lack of attraction to one's sexual partner and emotional trauma. The treatment approach depends on the cause.

Erectile dysfunction (ED) is an ongoing inability to achieve or sustain an erection long enough for a man to satisfy himself and his partner. Occasional difficulty with erection is normal and may result from stress, anxiety, or excessive alcohol. Also called impotence, ED affects approximately 40 percent of men ages 40 to 70, and the risk of developing it increases with age.[80] Nevertheless, many older men continue to enjoy sex and can even father children.

As with premature ejaculation, erectile problems create mental stress. And once again, biological and psychological factors can cause it. In the case of ED, however, physical causes are more common and underlie about 80 percent of cases. One way to tell them apart is to find out whether erections occur in the night. If they do, daytime mental challenges are more likely to blame.

A common cause of ED is cardiovascular disease. In fact, ED may be the first sign a man has a condition like atherosclerosis (a disease in which fatty materials harden and narrow the arteries). Diabetes and tobacco use are also big problems, mainly because both accelerate arterial disease. Other causes include kidney disease, neurological disease, surgery and radiation treatment for prostate cancer, spinal cord injury, and certain prescription drugs. Men who wish to remain sexually active for many years should take care of their health now to avoid these chronic diseases.

Prolonged bicycling with a poorly fitting bike seat can potentially damage the arteries and nerves to the penis. Signs that your seat doesn't fit you properly are numbness, tingling, and pain in the area between anus and penis. On the other hand, physical activity, which promotes healthy arteries, improves erectile function.[81]

Psychological causes of ED include mental stress, anxiety, low self-esteem, and loss of interest in sex. Depression (and some of the drugs used to treat it) can both lead to and arise because of ED.

premature ejaculation (PE)

Ejaculation less than about one minute after penetration, inability to control ejaculation, and resulting negative personal consequences.

delayed ejaculation

A condition in which a man requires more than average sexual stimulation to achieve orgasm.

erectile dysfunction (ED)

The inability to achieve or maintain an erection long enough to engage in sexual intercourse. It was formerly known as impotence.

Proper treatment involves attempting to remedy the underlying cause. Drugs like Viagra and Cialis slow the breakdown of bodily chemicals that normally produce erections. They don't improve sexual performance in men without erectile problems. They can't be used with some medications and for people with certain diseases. Side effects include upset stomach, dizziness, diarrhea, flushing, headache, visual disturbances, and, less commonly, priapism (an erection that persists for more than four hours).

3.4 Sexual Dysfunction in Women

orgasmic dysfunction

The inability to reach orgasm despite sexual stimulation. More common in women.

Like men, women may have episodically or habitually depressed libido. They may not become easily aroused. The vagina doesn't secrete sufficient lubrication; the clitoris doesn't become engorged and more sensitive. Alternatively, women may become aroused but have difficulty reaching orgasm. Sometimes the problem is impatience on the part of the woman's partner. Or perhaps the woman feels worried, inhibited, fatigued, mentally preoccupied, not particularly attracted to her partner, uncomfortable, or unable to communicate her sexual needs. As with men, intoxication with illicit drugs or alcohol and some prescription medications interfere with the sexual response. The term **orgasmic dysfunction** (also called *anorgasmia*) is applied when women routinely can't climax, even with adequate stimulation.

Dyspareunia refers to painful intercourse. A common source is inadequate lubrication due to lack of attraction to one's partner, insufficient foreplay, insufficient estrogen (as occurs with menopause), medications such as antihistamines, anxiety, or fear. Other causes include scarring from surgery or childbirth, a poorly fitting diaphragm or cervical cap, reproductive or urinary tract inflammation/infection, uterine fibroids (noncancerous growths), ovarian cysts, and endometriosis (uterine lining tissue grows outside the uterus). Less often, *vaginismus*, a condition involving involuntary contraction of muscles in the pubic region, makes penile penetration painful. With all these conditions, the solution depends on the underlying cause. Women who have pain during intercourse should meet with their *gynecologist* (specialist in women's health) or family doctor.

3.5 Making Sex Safer

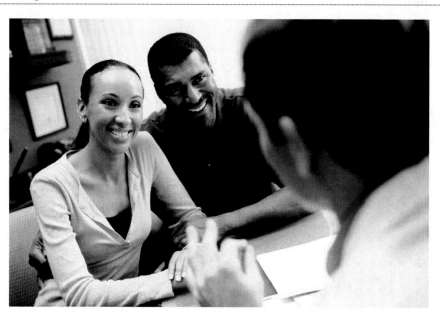

© *Thinkstock*

The two things most sexually active people hope to avoid are unintended pregnancies and sexually transmitted infections (also called sexually transmitted diseases or STDs). Couples need to work as a team. It takes two to share a sexual experience and to prevent undesirable consequences. Partners need to educate themselves, communicate clearly and openly, and use their chosen protective methods—each and every time they have sex.

abstinence

Complete avoidance of penile-vaginal sexual intercourse.

Because most people with STDs look and feel healthy, sexually active people can't reduce their risk to zero. Sometimes contraceptives fail. For these reasons, the only guaranteed strategy for preventing both infections and pregnancy is sexual **abstinence**. To avoid pregnancy, couples must refrain from penile-vaginal intercourse. To avoid STDs, couples must not share bodily fluids that could contain these microbes—vaginal secretions, semen, blood, and even breast milk. That means no oral, vaginal, or anal intercourse. Because of the nature of some viral infections, couples must also shun genital-to-genital contact.

Sexual abstinence is free and requires no prescription. It does, however, take iron willpower. Research indicates that abstinence-only-until-marriage education is not terribly successful.[82] Furthermore, it often supplants comprehensive sexual education, which has been shown to reduce teen pregnancy. If you choose to abstain from sex, consider carrying condoms or spermicide, just in case you change your mind.

Outercourse provides a way to avoid pregnancy and some STDs. It allows for any expression of sexual intimacy except inserting the penis into the vagina or anus. Outercourse practices that carry the risk of STDs include oral-genital sex and genital-to-genital contact. To reduce the risk, a condom can cover the penis during *fellatio* (oral stimulation of the penis). During *cunnilingus* (oral stimulation of the clitoris and vulva), a woman's external genitalia can be covered by a piece of plastic wrap or a dental dam, a rectangular piece of latex or silicone normally used in dentistry.

> **outercourse**
> Sexual stimulation that does not involve the penis penetrating the vagina. Some definitions also exclude anal intercourse.

As with total abstinence, willpower, commitment, and a high threshold for frustration are required. Carrying backup contraception could help avoid unfortunate consequences if resolve wilts in the heat of the moment.

Other tips for optimizing your sexual experiences are the following:

- **Be patient.** Wait until you're ready to have sex and have found a worthy, compatible, respectful partner.

- **Communicate with your partner.** Make sure you agree about sexual practices, methods for preventing STDs, and contraceptive options. Ask about his or her sexual history, including history of STDs and testing for these infections.

- **Limit your number of partners.** If possible, maintain a monogamous relationship with a partner whose screening tests indicate he or she has no STDs. That plan, while a good one, isn't bombproof. Some pathogens lack reliable, routine tests. Sometimes tests come back falsely negative.

- **Use a condom each and every time you have vaginal or anal intercourse**—no matter the results of STD tests. Male latex condoms reduce the risk of STD transmission and of pregnancy. Polyurethane condoms also offer protection, though they're more likely to slip and break. The female condom, which is made of nitrile, reduces STD transmission, but not as well as the latex condom for men.

- **Ensure adequate lubrication.** Natural lubrication may be enough. Otherwise, commercial products such as K-Y Jelly and Astroglide decrease the risk of a condom tearing and of tiny tears in mucous membranes, which both raise the risk of STD transmission. Do not use oil-based lubricants with latex condoms.

- **Avoid intoxication with drugs and alcohol**, which can lead to risky, unprotected sex. Inebriated people lose their inhibitions and good judgment. Impaired motor skills may interfere with proper condom use. Undesirable outcomes include STDs, pregnancy, bad feelings (guilt, shame, anger), and sexual assault.

- **Get vaccinated** against the human papillomavirus and hepatitis A and B.

- **Get tested.** Regular testing can detect infections even before symptoms develop. Early detection allows for early treatment, reduces the risk of complications, and prevents transmission to others. A more thorough discussion of STD testing appears in Section 4.

3.6 Contraceptive Options

Fortunately, sexually active heterosexual couples can choose from a wide range of contraceptives. The goal of all methods is to avoid **conception**, the moment at which a man's sperm fuses with a woman's ovum (egg) and the genetic material of both combines. This process, also called *fertilization*, occurs in one of the woman's fallopian tubes. These methods do not cause an abortion if pregnancy has already occurred.

> **conception**
> The union of sperm and egg; also called fertilization.

"Natural" methods rely on behaviors. They're free but require great discipline. These include abstinence, *coitus interruptus* (withdrawal or "pulling out"), and fertility awareness. None of them protect against STDs.

Barrier methods physically separate the sperm from a woman's reproductive tract and are relatively inexpensive. Examples include male and female condoms, diaphragms, cervical caps, and contraceptive sponges. Condoms also protect against STDs. Some barrier methods should be used with **spermicides**, products that contain nonoxynol-9, a chemical that impairs sperm. Condoms, spermicides, and the sponge are available over the counter. Other barrier methods require a physical exam and a prescription.

Hormonal methods, which are only available for women, also entail an examination and a prescription or a minor medical procedure. They use female hormones (estrogen and synthetic versions of progesterone called progestins or progestins only) to suppress ovulation, thin the uterine lining, and thicken cervical mucus. When used correctly, they're extremely effective. Most are rapidly reversible. They all reduce menstrual flow, thereby reducing the risk of iron-deficiency anemia. They also decrease menstrual cramping, acne, premenstrual syndrome (PMS), mood swings, ectopic pregnancy, ovarian cysts, and fibrocystic breasts. None protect against STDs. General side effects include breast tenderness, bloating, spotting (light bleeding between periods), depression, and headaches.

Intrauterine devices (IUDs) are small, T-shaped devices that sit inside the uterus. The "T" shape collapses, which allows a health professional to insert them through the narrow opening of the cervix. There are two main types: Mirena, which contains progestin and is effective for 5 to 7 years, and ParaGard, which contains copper and is effective for 10 to 12 years. Mirena prevents sperm from traveling to the fallopian tubes, thickens cervical mucus, and blocks ovulation. ParaGard works by preventing sperm from traveling to the fallopian tubes. Both IUDs require a significant initial expense but work for years. Neither protects against STDs.

Emergency contraception is available for women who wish to prevent pregnancy after unprotected intercourse. The copper IUD (ParaGard) can be inserted within five to eight days of unprotected intercourse. A more convenient option is progestin-containing emergency contraceptive pills (Plan B, Plan B One-Step, Next Choice). These must be taken within five days of unprotected intercourse. In 2013, this product became available as an over-the-counter medication (no prescription required). (ContraceptiveOptions.com has information on using oral contraceptives as emergency contraception.) A brand of emergency contraceptive pill called ella contains a chemical that modifies the action of progesterone. It requires an appointment with a health professional and a prescription. Progestin pills such as Plan B *do not cause an abortion*. Furthermore, physicians won't insert copper IUDs or prescribe ella until tests indicate the woman is not pregnant.

Male and female **sterilization** involve minor surgery, should be considered irreversible, and are best reserved for people certain they no longer wish to have children. Men receive a *vasectomy*. A physician makes a small incision on each side of the scrotum (above each testis) to interrupt the vas deferens, the tiny tube that carries sperm away from the testes toward the urethra. The procedure is brief, usually performed under local anesthesia, does not require hospitalization, and does not impair sexual function. Surgical reversal of a vasectomy is possible, though not always successful. Backup contraception necessary in first three months until tests confirm ejaculated semen contains no sperm.

There are three main methods of female sterilization, all of which should be considered permanent. All three interrupt the fallopian tubes, which normally conduct a woman's ovulated eggs to her uterus. The first is tubal ligation, in which a woman's fallopian tubes are surgically cut or blocked. The second is Essure. In a procedure lasting only minutes, the doctor inserts coils made of metal and fiber into the fallopian tubes. Once scar tissue forms, the tubes are blocked. The third method is Adiana, which involves using radiofrequency energy and an implant to block the fallopian tubes. Adiana and Essure procedures require no incision and occur in an outpatient setting with local anesthesia. Afterward, the couple should use three months of backup contraception. Sterilization methods do not protect against STDs.

Contraceptives are not effective unless used properly and consistently. That's why you need to choose a method you feel confident about using every time you have sexual intercourse. Consider the option that best fits your stage in life, your values, and your future plans. Keep in mind that, while most contraceptives carry some risks, they are minor compared with the risks associated with pregnancy.

Table 7.1 summarizes the most common contraceptive methods. Effectiveness is given for perfect use, meaning the method is used properly and consistently. In other words, a birth control pill is taken each day, the condom is placed before every intercourse and doesn't break, and so on. If a method is 90 percent effective, that means the failure rate is 10 percent. In other words, in a year, 10 out of 100 women will become pregnant. For further information, see the websites listed in Table 7.1. Another excellent resource is your college health clinic or other primary care provider. Most cities also have clinics that offer contraceptives services.

TABLE 7.1 Contraceptive Options

Contraceptive method	Description	Pros	Cons and cautions
"Natural" methods			
Abstinence	Outercourse: no vaginal or anal intercourse. Total abstinence: no sexual activity at all.	■ Free and safe. ■ Total abstinence eliminates the risk of STDs and pregnancy.	■ Some STDs can be transmitted during outercourse. Can be frustrating.
Coitus interruptus	Removing the penis from the vagina before ejaculation.	■ No semen enters the vagina.	■ Failure rate can be high. Pre-ejaculatory fluid contains a few sperm; it only takes one to fertilize an egg. ■ No protection against STDs. Not all men have this much control.
Fertility awareness	A woman tracks her menstrual cycles, noting signs of ovulation (slippery mucus, a sharp pain near the ovaries) and avoiding intercourse several days before and after.	■ No expense. ■ Requires no prescription.	■ Requires regular menstrual cycles and many days of abstinence (or use of backup contraception). ■ High failure rate—25 percent of women become pregnant in the first year. ■ No protection against STDs.
Barrier methods			
Male condom	A sheath that covers the penis. Available in latex and, for people with allergies, polyurethane.	■ 98 percent effective with perfect use. ■ Inexpensive and available over the counter. ■ Reduces the risk of STDs. ■ Men with premature ejaculations may last longer.	■ The condom can slip or tear. Decreases sensation to the penis; may be more difficult to maintain an erection.

Contraceptive method	Description	Pros	Cons and cautions
Female condom	A loose-fitting sheath of polyurethane or nitrile inserted into the vagina. It's closed at the end next to the cervix. A ring at either end holds it in place.	■ 95 percent effective with perfect use. ■ Available over the counter. ■ Reduces risk of STDs. ■ Women may like feeling in control. ■ Can be inserted up to eight hours before intercourse. ■ Rarely breaks.	■ During first year of use, failure rate can be as high as 21 percent. ■ More expensive than the male condom and not as widely available. ■ Should not be reused.
Diaphragm	A flexible dome-shaped latex or silicone device. After a tablespoon of spermicide is added to the inside and rim, it's inserted into the vagina to cover the cervix. Needs to be fitted by a health professional; requires a prescription.	■ Safe and 94 percent effective with proper, consistent use. ■ Can be inserted before sexual activity and left in place (without adding more spermicide) for up to 24 hours. ■ Gives women control.	■ Provides only partial protection against STDs; may protect against microbes that infect the cervix. ■ Must be left in place at least six hours after last intercourse. ■ Can increase the risk of urinary tract infections. ■ Slight increased risk of toxic shock syndrome, a rare but potentially fatal infectious condition.
Cervical cap (FemCap)	A silicone cup inserted into the vagina to cover the cervix. Smaller than a diaphragm. Also used with spermicide. Needs to fitted by a health professional.	■ Safe and fairly effective. ■ Convenient. ■ Can be inserted before sex.	■ Does not protect against STDs, aside from blocking the cervix. ■ 14 percent failure rate in women who have not given birth vaginally; 29 percent failure rate in those who have given birth. ■ Needs to be left in place 6 hours after last intercourse and should be removed within 48 hours. ■ Should not be used during menstruation.

Contraceptive method	Description	Pros	Cons and cautions
Contraceptive sponge (Today Sponge)	A round polyurethane foam impregnated with spermicide. It is inserted into the vagina to fit against the cervix. Must be left in place for six hours afterward.	■ With perfect use, about 91 percent effective. ■ Can be inserted up to 24 hours before intercourse. ■ Available over the counter in some drugstores and clinics, as well as online.	■ No STD protection. ■ Only 80 percent effective after vaginal delivery. ■ May irritate the vagina. ■ Should not be used during menstruation. ■ Must be removed within 30 hours because of a slight risk of toxic shock syndrome.
Spermicides			
Creams and gels; vaginal contraceptive film; foam; suppositories; Today Sponge	Products are usually inserted into the vagina 10 minutes before intercourse. Most spermicides must be reinserted before each vaginal intercourse.	■ Available over the counter. Relatively inexpensive. ■ Easy to use.	■ Not very effective. Used alone, 15 percent failure rate with perfect use; average failure rate of 29 percent. ■ Spermicides can irritate mucous membranes. ■ Does not protect against STDs. ■ May increase the risk of human immunodeficiency virus (HIV) transmission.
Hormonal methods			
Oral contraceptives	Most pills contain a combination of estrogen and progestin. Some contain only a progestin. Backup contraception (e.g., condoms) recommended for first month.	■ Extremely effective when no pills are missed. ■ Rapidly reversible. ■ Periods regular, predictable, and light. ■ Improve menstrual cramps, endometriosis pain, and polycystic ovary disease. ■ Does not seem to increase the risk of breast cancer.	■ No STD protection. ■ Side effects may include headaches, upset stomach, breast tenderness, mood changes, and fatigue. Spotting and depression more common with progestin-only pills. ■ Combination (estrogen + progestin) contraceptives increase the risk of blood clots, heart attack, and stroke, mainly in women who smoke or are over 35. ■ Not for use in women with migraine headaches (with auras), liver disease, high blood pressure, cancer, heart disease, or a history of stroke or blood clots. ■ Medications such as antibiotics and the herb St. John's wort can make the pill less effective.

Contraceptive method	Description	Pros	Cons and cautions
Skin patch (Ortho Evra)	A thin adhesive-backed patch that releases estrogen and progestin into the bloodstream. Replaced weekly for three weeks, followed by a patch-free week.	■ More than 99 percent effective with perfect use. ■ Convenient. ■ Similar benefits to oral contraceptives.	■ No STD protection. ■ Less effective in women who weigh more than 198 pounds. ■ Side effects include breast tenderness, headaches, mood changes, skin irritation at the patch site, blood clots, heart attack, and stroke. ■ Similar cautions as for oral contraceptives.
Vaginal ring (Nuvaring)	A flexible ring containing estrogen and progestin inserted into the vagina for three weeks, removed for one week (for menses), and then reinserted for another three weeks.	■ More than 99 percent effective if used as directed.	■ No STD protection. ■ Not recommended for women on bed rest. ■ Some women have breast tenderness and spotting between periods. ■ Can increase the risk of vaginal yeast infections. Should not be used with oil-based creams for yeast infections.
Implant (Implanon)	Matchstick-sized thin, flexible device inserted under the skin of the upper arm that slowly releases a progestin (etonogestrel).	■ 99 percent effective. ■ Can be left in place for up to three years. ■ Can be used when breast-feeding. ■ Periods usually become lighter and less frequent. ■ Effects rapidly reversible. ■ No estrogen-related side effects.	■ No STD protection. ■ Side effects include irregular bleeding and spotting between periods during the first year. Less often, scarring and discomfort at the insertion site, headache, nausea, breast tenderness, emotional instability, depression, and acne. ■ Costs $400–800 ($11–22/ month over 3 years).

Contraceptive method	Description	Pros	Cons and cautions
Injectable (Depo-Provera)	Progestin is injected into the arm, preventing pregnancy for three months.	■ About 99 percent effective. ■ Convenient. ■ No estrogen-related side effects.	■ No STD protection. ■ Requires return visits every three months for another injection. ■ Not rapidly reversible. ■ Irregular bleeding during the first months. ■ Can aggravate depression and cause weight gain, headaches, and breast tenderness. ■ May raise the risk of bone loss, especially with long-term use.
Intrauterine devices			
Copper IUD (ParaGard); Hormonal IUD (Mirena releases levonorgestrel, a synthetic form of progesterone)	A T-shaped device inserted by a health professional into a woman's uterus.	■ More than 99 percent effective. ■ Mirena decreases menstrual blood loss and reduces pain. ■ Long-lasting birth control that's cost effective over time. ■ May protect against uterine cancer.	■ No STD protection. ■ High initial cost to insert. ■ ParaGard can cause crampy pain and increased bleeding in the first months. Mirena can cause spotting in the first months. ■ Should not be used if the woman has an STD, pelvic inflammatory disease, or uterine cancer. ■ Mirena IUD is not recommended in women with liver disease or at risk for breast cancer. ■ Rarely, women are allergic to the copper in ParaGard. ■ Very rarely, the IUD perforates the uterine wall.
Emergency contraception	The copper IUD (ParaGard), inserted within five to eight days of unprotected intercourse. Progestin-containing emergency contraceptive pills (Plan B, Plan B One-Step, Next Choice). Must be taken within five days of unprotected intercourse.	■ Both methods effective in preventing pregnancy. ■ Pills like Plan B can be purchased in advance.	■ Emergency insertion of an IUD may not be convenient. ■ Some pharmacies do not carry emergency contraceptive pills. A pharmacist must be on duty. ■ "ella" requires an office visit and prescription. ■ Possible side effects of the pills: nausea, vomiting, breast tenderness, fatigue, and headache. Can cause the next period to come later or sooner.

Contraceptive method	Description	Pros	Cons and cautions
Sterilization	Male sterilization (vasectomy) involves minor surgery on the scrotum to cut both of the vas deferens.	■ Very effective for the remainder of one's reproductive years.	■ No STD protection. ■ Irreversible or not easily reversed. ■ Expensive, though may be covered by insurance. ■ Vasectomy and tubal ligation: pain and swelling after the surgery. Pain and cramping during the Adiana and Essure procedure. ■ In the rare occurrence of the severed fallopian tubes reconnecting, ectopic pregnancy is possible.

Source: The information in this table came from multiple resources, most notably Planned Parenthood (http://www.plannedparenthood.org) and Choices by Robert A Hatcher, MD, MPH, Sharon A. Rachel, MA, MPH, and Aimee M. Mohnihan, MSEd, CHES. (http://www.managingcontraception.com).

How to Use a Male Condom

Used properly and consistently, condoms reduce your risk of pregnancy and STDs. Here's how:

- Always carry a few but don't keep them in your back pocket. Sitting on them can tear the packet and damage the condom.
- Check the expiration date on the package. If the date has expired, don't use it.
- Gently open the packet at one end with your fingers, not your teeth.
- Before removing the condom from the packet, the responsible partner should remove rings and check that fingernails are short and smooth.
- Place the condom over the glans penis, pinch the tip of the condom to expel air, and then gently twist the tip to allow room for ejaculated semen.
- With one hand, hold the twisted tip. With the other, roll down the condom until it smoothly covers the shaft of the penis.
- Use the correct kind of lubricant. Oil-based products deteriorate latex. Water-based products are fine.
- Immediately after ejaculating, hold the base of the condom in place with one hand and withdraw. Carefully remove the condom, taking care not to spill semen. Wrap in a tissue and discard in a trash can.
- Use a fresh condom each time you have intercourse.
- Practice the procedure in nonsexual settings. You can use a cucumber or a banana.
- Keep a good supply of condoms so that you don't run out.

Note: Condoms are packaged with a little **spermicide**, which adds to the cost without significant increased efficacy. To make condoms more effective, additional spermicide (nonoxynol-9) can be used. However, it can increase the risk of female urinary tract infections and irritate mucous membranes, thereby increasing the risk of HIV transmission. It should not be used multiple times a day with vaginal sex and not at all with anal sex.[83]

- The sexual response follows along four phases: excitement/arousal, plateau, orgasmic, and resolution.
- Both men and women can suffer from low libido and difficulty achieving orgasm. A number of factors can contribute.
- Men, particularly young men, may have premature ejaculation (PE). Delayed ejaculation and erectile dysfunction more commonly affect older men. However, stress, anxiety, medications, alcohol, and illicit drugs impair sexual function at any age.
- Sexual intimacy carries physical risks such as pregnancy and sexually transmitted infections.
    - The only zero-risk strategy is abstinence.
    - Outercourse without intercourse sidesteps the issue of pregnancy, though exposure to some STDs is still possible.
    - With correct, consistent use, male and female condoms reduce the risk of pregnancy and many STDs.
    - Avoiding intoxication with drugs and alcohol, limiting the number of partners, and maintaining open communication all contribute to safer, healthier sex.
- Sexually active heterosexual couples have a number of options for preventing unwanted pregnancy. The goal is to find a method you feel comfortable with, one that you'll use each and every time you have sex.

DISCUSSION QUESTIONS

1. After an orgasm, can a man have another within the next couple of minutes? Explain how the situation is different or similar in women.
2. Compare and contrast premature ejaculation and erectile dysfunction, including their causes and effects.
3. Do couples engaging in outercourse still need to protect themselves against STDs? Why or why not?
4. Why is *coitus interruptus* (withdrawal) not a foolproof contraceptive method, even assuming the man does pull out before he ejaculates?
5. Implanon and Depo-Provera are both progesterone-only methods of birth control and have similar potential side effects. What is an important difference between these two methods if a problem such as depression should arise?

4. SEXUALLY TRANSMITTED INFECTIONS

LEARNING OBJECTIVES

1. **Identify risk factors for acquiring sexually transmitted infections.**
2. **Explain strategies for reducing the chances of acquiring sexually transmitted infections.**
3. **Explain tests for sexually transmitted infections.**
4. **Discuss the causes, signs and symptoms, and treatments for common sexually transmitted infections.**

Sexually transmitted diseases (STDs), or **sexually transmitted infections (STIs)**, can be acquired during any type of sexual activity—vaginal or anal intercourse, oral sex, or the use of contaminated sexual devices (vibrators, dildos). A number of bacteria, viruses, and protozoa cause these infections. In the United States, some 19 million new infections occur each year.[84] Although sexually active people of any age, sex, race, or sexual orientation can get them, several risk factors increase the chances.

- **Age.** Young adults 15 to 24 years old make up only a quarter of the sexually active population but develop half the annual STDs.[85] Teenage girls and young women are particularly vulnerable because their cervixes (the opening to the uterus) haven't completely matured.
- **Race.** African Americans carry a greater burden of STDs because of the prevalence of sexually transmitted pathogens within their community, poverty, reduced access to health care, and other factors.[86]
- **Sexual behaviors.** Having multiple sexual partners and engaging in anal intercourse greatly elevate risk.

sexually transmitted disease (STD)

Refers to infections transmitted primarily by sexual contact.

sexually transmitted infection (STI)

Refers to infections transmitted primarily by sexual contact.

- **Sexual orientation.** Men who have sex with men are at higher risk. Nevertheless, heterosexual men and women develop plenty of STDs.
- **Current genital health.** Having one STD injures the tissues, raising the vulnerability to infection by other pathogens. For instance, having an active genital herpes infection increases susceptibility to infection with HIV (human immunodeficiency virus).
- **Vaginal douching.** Depending on what's in the douching solution, this practice upsets the ecology of normal, protective vaginal microbes. It may also increase the risk of STDs[87] and pelvic inflammatory disease.[88]

There are many reasons to protect yourself from STDs. While most infections don't have lasting health impacts, a few can make you very ill and even threaten your life. Some infections produce few, if any, symptoms, allowing the microbes to be passed to sexual partners. In women, symptoms and signs of some bacterial infections may not develop until serious tissue damage has occurred. This damage may impair fertility. Viral STDs can be difficult to treat. One of them (human papillomavirus) can cause cancer. If a woman is pregnant, some STDs can adversely affect the developing fetus or infect the baby during the birth.

Which STD Tests Do You Need?

Often, we delay any tests that might bring news we'd rather not hear. Procrastination and avoidance postpone prompt treatment and may allow the spread of STDs to others. A number of factors determine which tests you need and how often to have them, including your age, sex, sexual orientation, sexual habits, and any symptoms you might have. The tissue tested—blood, urine, secretions swabbed from infected tissue (e.g., vaginal secretions)—depends on the particular pathogen. Some pathogens require routine screening because they often fail to cause symptoms or only do so once the infection has caused serious health problems. Test results are confidential.

- The Centers for Disease Control and Prevention (CDC) recommends all sexually active people between ages 13 and 64 have a yearly blood test for **human immunodeficiency virus (HIV)**. If you have other STDs, which puts you at risk of HIV infection, request an HIV test.
- Men who have sex with men, people who use intravenous drugs, and those who have another STD should have blood tests for **HIV**, **syphilis**, and **hepatitis**. People with lesions suggestive of syphilis should have those swabbed and tested.
- Sexually active women under age 26, older women at risk due to new or multiple partners, and men who have sex with men should have annual screening tests for **chlamydia** and **gonorrhea**.
- **Human papillomavirus (HPV)** testing isn't routinely done. Health practitioners usually test women with abnormal Pap tests (which check for abnormal cervical cells) for HPV because aggressive strains can lead to cancer. However, HPV testing is becoming a more routine part of a woman's annual exam.

If you notice any symptoms, however mild and vague, make a medical appointment right away. Warning signs include discharge from the vagina, penis, or anus; vaginal itching or burning; genital sores or bumps; pelvic discomfort with or without sex; and fever.

To find a testing site near you, visit the National HIV and STD Resources site (http://www.hivtest.org) or Get Tested Now (http://www.GYTNOW.org) and enter your zip code. You can also text your zip code to GYTNOW (498669). Most college health clinics offer low-cost, confidential services. Combine regular STD testing with annual physical exams.

4.1 Viral STDs

Human Immunodeficiency Virus and Acquired Immunodeficiency Syndrome

FIGURE 7.4 HIV in the United States

This graph shows the prevalence (number of people who have the disease) and incidence (new cases) of HIV in the United States between 1977 and 2006. The bad news is that prevalence has steadily risen. The good news is that prevention efforts have stabilized incidence.

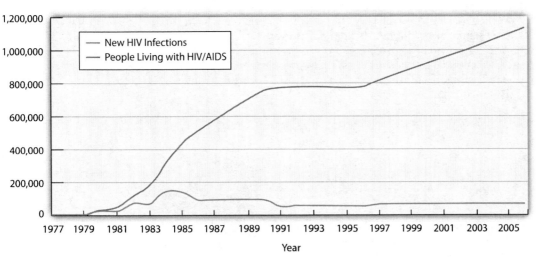

Source: Adapted from Centers for Disease Control and Prevention. Available at: http://www.cdc.gov/hiv/topics/surveillance/resources/factsheets/images/graph-lg.gif.

An estimated 33 million adults and children worldwide live with **human immunodeficiency virus (HIV)**.[89] More than two-thirds of them live in Sub-Saharan Africa. In the United States, about 1.2 million people carry HIV. Each year, 50,000 Americans learn they've become infected.[90] That rate has been stable for the last few years. However, between 2006 and 2009, new infections in young people ages 13 through 19 increased 21 percent, a rise driven mainly by men who have sex with men. Within that age group, the rate skyrocketed 48 percent among young black men who have sex with men.

Immediately after infection, the virus multiplies rapidly and levels in the blood soar. For a time, the immune system responds heroically to fight off the virus. This primary infection phase can produce a couple of weeks of flulike symptoms or no symptoms at all. The person is, however, very infectious. After that, the person enters a latent, symptom-free phase that can last anywhere from 2 to 20 years. He or she can still transmit the virus, though levels in tissue fluids aren't as high. During this time, the virus continues to chip away at the immune system.

The reason HIV infection can be so debilitating is that the virus infects helper T cells, as well as a few other immune cells that also express a surface protein called *CD4*. Helper T cells direct many aspects of immune system function. Their impairment greatly hinders the adaptive immune system.

If CD4 cells fall to a critical level, **acquired immunodeficiency syndrome (AIDS)** develops. The weakened immune system can no longer defend against pathogenic microorganisms. Even microbes harmless to healthy people can now cause *opportunistic infections*. Infections strike many bodily systems. People lose weight and develop swollen lymph nodes, chronic diarrhea, fatigue, headaches, fevers, and night sweats. The compromised immune system also raises the risk of cancer, including Kaposi's sarcoma, a normally rare cancer of lymph or blood vessels that causes purplish tumors on the skin. The disease can be fatal. Many children, particularly in areas such as Africa where drug treatment is inadequate, die or become orphans when AIDS kills their parents.

The virus is transmitted when infected blood, vaginal and cervical secretions, semen, or breast milk enter another person's body. People can acquire it through sexual intercourse (vaginal and anal), needle sharing, and transfusion of contaminated blood. Infected mothers can transmit the virus during the pregnancy and birth and when breast-feeding.

Casual contact does *not* transmit the virus. In other words, you can't get HIV from roommates, friends, or classmates—unless you're having sex or sharing needles with them. Unfortunately, needless fear of contagion has led to ostracizing of HIV-positive children and adults.

The highest risk groups are men who have sex with other men, female sex workers, and people who inject drugs. However, men and women in heterosexual relationships also get the disease. A break in skin or mucous membranes of the genital area allows the virus to enter the body. For that reason,

human immunodeficiency virus (HIV)

The virus that causes AIDS.

acquired immunodeficiency syndrome (AIDS)

A condition caused the human immunodeficiency virus, which weakens the immune system and leads to increased susceptibility to infections and certain cancers.

having another STD raises the risk of acquiring the virus and can also increase infectiousness. In 2009 in the United States, 12,860 teens and adults became HIV positive from heterosexual contact.[91]

To prevent spread of HIV, sexually active people should get regular tests, use condoms, refrain from sexual activity if another STD is present, and otherwise follow safe-sex practices. Recent research shows that some anti-HIV drugs can reduce transmission in at-risk populations, such as when one partner is HIV positive and the other isn't.[92] These medications can be used to prevent infection after known exposure and to block the mother-to-child transmission of HIV.[93] Furthermore, prompt treatment with antiviral drugs increases the odds of successfully fighting the infection.

The most commonly used HIV tests detect antibodies against HIV, not the virus itself. Most tests check for antibodies in the blood; some use saliva or urine. Rapid tests can provide answers in 20 minutes. A positive rapid test is followed by a confirmatory test that takes several days.

While virus levels rise quickly after infection, it takes between two to eight weeks to develop antibodies in significant quantities.[94] Sometimes tests aren't reliable until three to six months after exposure. After suspected or known exposure, a negative test within that three-month window is usually repeated. People who test positive should be counseled and referred to a provider with experience treating HIV. For more information, check out the National Institutes of Health website, AIDSinfo, at http://www.aidsinfo.nih.gov.

FIGURE 7.5 Main Symptoms of AIDS

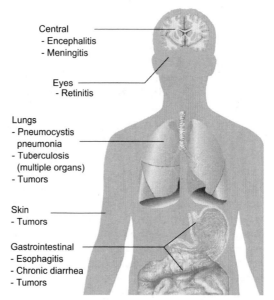

Source: Häggström M. 2008. Available at: http://commons.wikimedia.org/wiki/File:Symptoms_of_AIDS.png.

Human Papillomavirus

human papillomavirus (HPV)

A group of viruses that causes warts, including genital warts.

Extremely common, the **human papillomavirus (HPV)** infects skin and mucous membranes and can cause warts on the hands, feet, and genitals. More than 40 types of human papillomaviruses can infect the genital area, as well as the mouth, throat, anus, and rectum. These viruses are transmitted via genital, oral, anal, and genital-to-genital contact.

HPV is the most common STD. Because the virus doesn't always cause obvious lesions and many people aren't routinely screened, the exact prevalence and incidence are hard to pinpoint. The CDC estimates that 20 million Americans have current infections and that 6 million new cases occur each year. Over the course of a lifetime, at least half of the sexually active population acquires an HPV infection.[95]

Most people develop no obvious signs of infection because the immune system normally clears it. Sometimes the viruses cause warts—a small bump or groups of bumps—in the genital area and/or throat. Not all warts require treatment. If treatment is indicated, prescription creams can either destroy the warty tissue or stimulate the immune system to eradicate the virus. Failing that, doctors can freeze, electrocauterize (burn), laser, cut, or chemically remove the warts.

While the warts don't become cancerous, a few aggressive HPV strains can eventually lead to cancer of the vulva, vagina, penis, mouth, throat, cervix, anus, and rectum. People with immunodeficiency and those who smoke are at even greater risk for developing cancer.

HPV is now thought to cause nearly all cervical cancers. Because this disease causes no symptoms until the condition is advanced, women need regular screening with a Papanicolaou (Pap) test, a microscopic exam of cells swabbed from the cervix, plus or minus a DNA test for high-risk HPV strains.[96] Doctors often adopt a watch-and-wait policy for precancerous changes in cervical cells because they typically heal. If cancer develops and is caught early, a doctor removes the abnormal cells by freezing them, using an electric current, or through surgery. In that case, the prognosis is excellent. However, HPV can lead to advanced cancer, which can sometimes be fatal. That's why women need regular exams and screening tests.

HPV is also a major cause of mouth and throat cancer. Recent research reveals that nearly 7 percent of adolescents and adults have oral HPV infections, which may explain why rates of mouth and throat cancer have surged in recent years.[97]

Condoms reduce the risk of acquiring HPV—if the condom covers the infected tissue. Unfortunately, a person without visible lesions can still be contagious. While less aggressive strains often spontaneously resolve, others can linger for years. HPV testing is not routinely given to young men and women, because most sexually active people are exposed and the immune system usually clears the infection.

Two HPV vaccines are now available. Cervarix protects against two of the cancer-causing HPV strains (16 and 18); Gardasil guards against four (HPV 6, 11, 16, and 18). Three doses are recommended for girls and boys between the ages of 11 and 12, as well as for teens and young adults 13 to 26 years of age who haven't yet received the 3 doses. The vaccine is most effective when given before exposure.

Large clinical trials show the vaccines to be safe and effective at preventing these aggressive HPV strains.[98],[99],[100] A 2011 Australian study found that, since widespread vaccination programs began in 2007, the rate of precancerous cervical lesions in girls under 18 fell by nearly 50 percent.[101]

Herpes Simplex Virus

Herpes simplex virus (HSV) can be divided into two types: herpes simplex virus-1 (HSV-1) and herpes simplex virus-2 (HSV-2). Usually HSV-1 causes lesions on the mouth, and HSV-2 causes lesions on external genitalia. However, oral sex can infect both areas with both types of viruses. Chapter 14 covered oral herpes, commonly called "fever blisters" or "cold sores."

The virus infects mucous membranes and breaks in the skin. The immune system doesn't eradicate HSV. Instead, the virus becomes dormant in collections of nerve cells outside the spinal cord. Triggers such as stress, infection, and physical trauma (surgery, vigorous sexual intercourse) can reactivate the virus. Sunlight, heat, cold, and hormonal shifts can prompt recurrences of oral herpes.

Signs of infection include blisters and tender sores around the genitals or anus. The first outbreak may also produce fever, malaise, headache, muscle aches, burning with urination, and swollen lymph nodes in the groin. The lesions usually spontaneously resolve in about five days. Four or five outbreaks can occur in the first year. Afterward, reactivations usually decrease in frequency and intensity with time.

Because symptoms can be mild or absent, many people don't know they carry herpes. Furthermore, these very contagious viruses can be transmitted to sexual partners in the absence of symptoms or just before lesions develop. It's no wonder that more than 16 percent of Americans ages 14 to 49 have genital HSV-2.[102] Women are more commonly infected than men.[103]

Asymptomatic (symptomless) viral shedding is particularly problematic when pregnant women give birth, as infected newborns can become seriously ill. Most doctors recommend cesarean birth (via surgical incision in the abdomen) to women with symptoms or visible lesions. The majority of babies born to mothers positive for HSV-2 are born healthy.[104]

While no cure exists, some medications—Famvir (famciclovir), Valtrex (valacyclovir), and Zovirax (acyclovir)—can shorten the duration and severity of symptoms and help suppress reactivations.

You can reduce your risk of getting genital herpes by limiting your number of partners, always using a latex condom during sex, and refraining from sex altogether if a partner has active lesions. If you have genital herpes, inform your partners and refrain from sex if a tingling sensation heralds an outbreak or if you have active lesions.

Hepatitis Viruses

As discussed in Chapter 14, a number of agents can injure the liver and cause hepatitis, including the five types of hepatitis viruses—A, B, C, D, and E. Hepatitis B is readily transmitted with sexual intercourse. Less often, hepatitis C and D are sexually transmitted.[105] Hepatitis A is spread via a fecal-oral route, which means anal and oral sex with an infected partner can spread it. Vaccinations prevent

FIGURE 7.6 Human Papillomavirus

Human papillomavirus as seen with an electron micrograph.

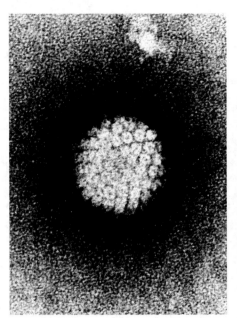

Source: *Laboratory of Tumor Virus. Human Papillomavirus (HPV). 1986. Available at: http://visualsonline.cancer.gov/details.cfm?imageid=2255.*

herpes simplex virus (HSV)

A virus that causes recurrent oral and genital lesions.

hepatitis A and B. Safer sexual practices are recommended. Avoiding contact with infected blood reduces the risk of hepatitis B, C, and D.

4.2　Bacterial STDs

Chlamydia

chlamydia

A bacterial STD transmitted by *Chlamydia trachomatis*.

According to the CDC, **chlamydia** is the most commonly reported, treatable STD in the United States, with nearly 1.25 million cases reported in 2009.[106] Because this infection often goes undiagnosed, the actual number of cases is probably higher.

The bacterium *Chlamydia trachomatis* can infect a man's urethra (the tube within the penis from which urine and semen exit) and a woman's cervix (a condition called cervicitis). Anal intercourse and oral sex can lead to infection of the rectum and throat, respectively. Young women shoulder most of the burden of this infection. Blacks are more commonly infected than other racial/ethnic groups.[107]

pelvic inflammatory disease (PID)

Infection of the structures in the female reproductive tract above the cervix.

The good news is that antibiotics cure chlamydia. The not-so-good news is that infections are often asymptomatic, particularly in women. Infected men and women can unwittingly spread it to other partners. Worse, in women, the infection can ascend to the lining of the uterus and fallopian tubes, a serious condition called **pelvic inflammatory disease (PID)**. An infected mother can pass the bacteria to her infant during vaginal delivery, leading to eye and respiratory infections.

When symptoms and signs occur, they're often mild and include burning with urination; discharge from the penis, anus, or vagina; and, less commonly, painful testes. Women may feel pain with intercourse or an ache in the lower abdomen.

Diagnosis is made after examination of swabs from the penis or cervix or from urine tests. If test results are positive, all sexual partners should be treated with antibiotics and remain abstinent until all the pills have been taken. Prompt treatment can prevent the development of PID.

 Video Clip 7.2

Chlamydia
This video provides facts about chlamydia infection.

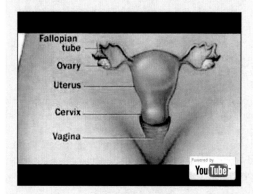

View the video online at: http://www.youtube.com/v/DRtt-zRgjbs

Gonorrhea

gonorrhea

A bacterial STD caused by *Neisseria gonorrhoeae*.

Like chlamydia, **gonorrhea** (also known as "the clap") is a bacterial infection that typically produces few symptoms and can lead to PID. In men and women, the bacterium *Neisseria gonorrhoeae* can infect the urethra, rectum, and throat. In women, infection can involve the cervix, uterus, and fallopian tubes. Although the rate of infection has steadily declined, gonorrhea remains a common STD, with 301,174 cases diagnosed in 2009.[108]

Infection is often asymptomatic in men and women. When symptoms do occur, they may not become obvious until a couple weeks after the infection begins. Men may have burning with urination, yellow-green discharge from the penis, and, less often, tender testes. Women may have discomfort with urination, vaginal bleeding unrelated to menstruation, and vaginal discharge. Rectal infections may cause pain with defecation and anal bleeding or discomfort. Throat infections may produce sore throat.

Complications include those associated with PID (see "Pelvic Inflammatory Disease") and also infection of a baby as it passes through an infected mother's vagina. Infection earlier in the pregnancy can trigger premature birth.[109] Antibiotics treat gonorrhea, although some strains have developed resistance to certain antibiotics.

Pelvic Inflammatory Disease

Pelvic inflammatory disease (PID) occurs when bacteria such as chlamydia and gonorrhea ascend from the vagina and cervix to infect the lining of the uterus and fallopian tubes and sometimes the ovaries and other nearby structures. While many people believe intrauterine devices (IUDs) raise the risk of PID, the actual risk is very low with current devices.[110] Furthermore, health practitioners typically screen for infections before inserting an IUD. Vaginal douching, a practice common among American women, is associated with PID and should be discouraged.[111]

Signs and symptoms range from mild to severe and include lower abdominal pain with and without intercourse, foul-smelling vaginal discharge, irregular menstrual bleeding, and fever. If you're a woman and suspect you might have PID, see your health practitioner right away.

Prompt treatment with antibiotics is important to reduce the risk of complications. The infection can cause scarring, which can lead to chronic pelvic pain, infertility, and ectopic pregnancy. *Ectopic* means the pregnancy occurs in an abnormal place. In that case, sperm successfully navigated the scarred fallopian tube to fertilize an egg, but the zygote (fertilized egg) gets stuck on its way to the uterus. It may start to grow inside the fallopian tube or the abdominal cavity. Either way, life-threatening internal hemorrhage (bleeding) can occur.

Video Clip 7.3

Pelvic Inflammatory Disease
This video explains how PID can develop, signs and symptoms, and potential complications.

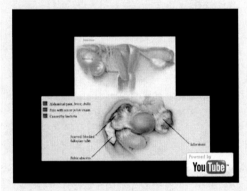

View the video online at: https://www.youtube.com/v/u1DcB8hIKvA

FIGURE 7.7
Syphilitic Chancre

A chancre—a painless ulcerated lesion—indicates primary syphilis. It occurs wherever the bacteria entered the body. This photo shows a chancre on the tongue.

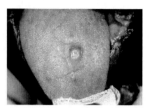

Source: CDC; Sumpter RE. ID# 12623. Public Health Image Library (PHIL). 1967. Available at: http://phil.cdc.gov/phil/details.asp.

syphilis

A bacterial STD caused by *Treponema pallidum*.

chancroid

An uncommon bacterial STD that causes painful ulcers on the genitals.

trichomoniasis

An STD caused by the protozoa *Trichomonas vaginalis*.

pubic lice

Caused by parasitic insects that attach themselves to hair and produce intense itching; also called crabs.

Syphilis

The "Great Pox" was once a sexual scourge responsible for deadly epidemics. Now imminently treatable, **syphilis** continues to infect many Americans. According to the CDC, more than 45,800 cases were reported in 2010.[112]

A spirochete (corkscrew-shaped) bacterium called *Treponema pallidum* causes syphilis. In the absence of treatment, the disease progresses through four stages. In the primary stage, a painless ulceration called a **chancre** appears wherever the bacteria entered the body. Usual sites are external genitalia and the vagina, anus, and rectum, as well as the breasts, lips, mouth, and fingers. These bacteria-packed lesions make this stage extremely contagious. The chancre heals within a couple of weeks.

Flu-like symptoms and a rash that usually involves the palms and soles usher in stage two (secondary syphilis), and then comes the asymptomatic latent phase, sometimes punctuated by recurrences of secondary syphilis. It can last years. The last stage is tertiary syphilis, which damages various organs, including the cardiovascular and nervous systems. Paralysis, dementia, and blindness can occur. Before the discovery of the antibiotic penicillin, many people died of the infection. And many people suffered through the toxicity of treatments with arsenic and mercury compounds.

Syphilis is transmitted by contact with the chancre. Also a pregnant woman can pass the bacteria to her fetus. In addition to blood tests, health care providers can examine material from the chancre under a special microscope. Ideally, it's treated in the early stages with an intramuscular injection of penicillin. The drug kills the bacteria but cannot repair damage done in later stages of the infection.

Chancroid

Caused by infection with the bacterium *Hemophilus ducreyi*, **chancroid** begins as a tender bump and then ulcerates (becomes an open sore). Unlike the chancres that appear in syphilis, these lesions are painful. The lesions can occur on the skin near the genitals, penis, anus, and mouth. Antibiotics treat the condition and are also recommended for sexual partners. Chancroid is rare in the United States but common in Africa and the Caribbean.

4.3   Sexually Transmitted Protozoa

Trichomoniasis

Unlike some of the other STDs, the trichomonas parasite (*Trichomonas vaginalis*) usually causes obvious symptoms in women: a profuse, foul-smelling vaginal discharge; genital irritation; and painful urination. **Trichomoniasis** can also precipitate premature birth in pregnant women. During birth, the baby can become infected. Men, on the other hand, usually have no symptoms and may unknowingly spread it to female partners.

Diagnosis is made by examining vaginal secretions under the microscope. The drug metronidazole (Flagyl) is given to both partners. Using condoms and practicing monogamy helps prevent this infection.

4.4   Sexually Transmitted Ectoparasites

Pubic Lice ("Crabs")

Pubic lice are tiny parasitic insects that attach themselves to pubic hair, as well as to facial hair, armpit hair, and chest hair. While sexual contact spreads pubic lice, you can also pick them up from infected clothing or bedding. The main symptom is intense itching. You can see the lice and their "nits" (eggs), which cling to the hair shafts, with the naked eye and even better with a magnifying glass.

The condition is treated with topical insecticides such as permethrin and pyrethrins. Some insecticide-containing lotions are available over the counter. All sexual contacts should be examined and, if carrying the lice, treated. Clothing, bedding, and towels should be washed in hot water and dried on high heat. The following website contains detailed instructions for treating pubic lice infestations: http://www.cdc.gov/parasites/lice/pubic/treatment.html. Because pubic lice can raise the risk of other STDs, people with lice should make an appointment with their health provider.

Scabies

A very contagious mite (*Sarcoptes scabei*) causes **scabies**. It results in an itchy rash, which is particularly intense at night. A rash of pimply bumps occurs in skin folds between the fingers, the groin, ankles, and wrists. Scratching can lead to further irritation and bacterial infection. Like pubic lice, sexual contact and other direct contact with infected skin, clothing, sheets, and bedding can spread the parasites. Treatment involves the topical use of prescription lotions or creams that kill scabies mites.

Coping with an STD

Most people are upset to learn they have an STD—particularly one that's impossible to eliminate (genital herpes) or has serious health consequences (HIV). People commonly feel depressed, anxious, and ashamed. If you develop an STD, know you are not alone. By the age of 25, one out of two people have had an STD.

The good news is that you can take steps to treat the infection and to avoid sharing the pathogen with your partners. Antimicrobial drugs cure bacterial STDs and the protozoa trichomonas. Even pathogens that can't be cured are treatable. Your sex life is not over.

It's normal to feel nervous to talk to your partner about STDs. If your partner had an STD, you'd want to know, right? Partners may also need to be tested and treated. Any partner worth his or her salt will be supportive. If he or she reacts with disgust, you might want to rethink that relationship.

Most centers that do STD testing also provide education and support for people and their partners. Check with your college's health center. Many colleges also have peer support groups. In addition, WebMD contains online support at http://exchanges.webmd.com/sexual-conditions-and-stds-exchange. On this page, you can find an STD slideshow with photographs and facts: http://www.webmd.com/sexual-conditions/ss/slideshow-std-pictures-and-facts.

Assess Your STD Risk

Being sexually active carries the risk of developing an STD. However, some behaviors further raise the stakes. Ask yourself the following questions. If you answered yes to any of them, take steps to protect yourself better. You're worth it.

Do you…

_____ ever have vaginal or anal sex without the protection of a condom?

_____ have multiple sexual partners?

_____ engage in serial monogamy but change partners frequently?

_____ have another STD or a tear or abrasion in the genital area?

_____ get drunk or use other substances that impair alertness, decision making, and judgment?

_____ use intravenous drugs?

KEY TAKEAWAYS

- The only way to avoid STDs completely is to abstain from sex. Otherwise, a number of strategies markedly reduce the risk of transmission among sexually active people.
- Many STDs cause few or no symptoms.
- Some STDs can cause serious complications.
- Regular testing and prompt treatment of infections are important for stopping the spread to intimate partners and preventing complications.

An enlarged view of a *Phthirus pubis*, more commonly known as the pubic or crab louse.

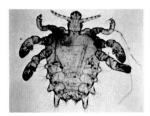

Source: World Health Organization. ID# 4077. Public Health Image Library (PHIL). 1975. Available at: http://phil.cdc.gov/phil/details.asp.

scabies

A contagious skin condition caused by mites that results in intense itching and irritation.

5. PREGNANCY AND INFERTILITY

LEARNING OBJECTIVES

1. Explain the process of pregnancy and the importance of healthy lifestyles and prenatal care for successful outcomes.
2. Review the facts about abortion.
3. Define infertility and identify key causes.

5.1 Pregnancy

This ultrasound image shows a developing fetus.

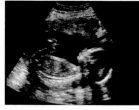

© Thinkstock

abortion

Termination of a pregnancy before the birth. A spontaneous abortion is a miscarriage. Medical (with medications) and surgical procedures are used to voluntarily end a pregnancy.

Finding out that you or your partner is pregnant can be exciting or distressing news. If both partners wanted a baby, life seems full of hope and happiness. However, nearly half of pregnancies in the United States are big surprises, with 3.2 million unintended pregnancies in 2006.[113] Unplanned pregnancies also happen disproportionately to women who are poor, less educated, black, cohabitating, or under age 25. Decreased public funding to family-planning clinics explains, at least in part, the rise in unintended pregnancies among the very women dependent upon these services.

Unintended pregnancy occurs for several reasons. Some couples, believing or hoping they won't get pregnant, don't use contraception. Intoxicated couples may forego contraceptives. Rapists seldom worry about birth control. Alternatively, mistakes happen—a pill or two is missed, the condom tears, and so on. Even when used consistently and correctly, contraceptives may fail. An astounding 44 percent of women become pregnant while using some form of contraception.[114]

Women who find themselves unexpectedly pregnant have three options: continue the pregnancy and keep the child, continue the pregnancy and give up the baby for adoption, or prematurely terminate the pregnancy with an **abortion**. Male partners may also be involved in this difficult decision-making process. The choices are particularly tough for single women and young couples who aren't physically, emotionally, or financially prepared to raise a child. Women's health clinics, counselors, and social workers can serve as resources for information about possible options.

Another factor to consider is that pregnancy and birth carry certain risks—more risks than are associated with contraceptives or abortion. Short-term discomforts include nausea and vomiting, backache, constipation, and fatigue. Some women develop diabetes during the pregnancy. Some develop preeclampsia, a condition of high blood pressure, water retention, and protein in the urine. The placenta can be in the wrong place, complicating the delivery. The delivery of the baby may not go smoothly, necessitating interventions such as a cesarean section (delivery of the baby through a surgical incision in the lower abdomen). The risks for mother and child tend to be higher with unintended childbearing, at times burdened with poverty, smoking, drinking, illicit drug use, delayed or absent prenatal care, and premature birth.

Before becoming a parent, it's wise to ask yourself serious questions about your motives and your resources. Do you want a baby because you think that will repair a handicapped relationship? Are you trying to escape loneliness or prove you're an adult? Is your relationship strong and committed enough for parenthood? If you're single, do you have support from family and friends? Would a pregnancy interfere with your education? Are you ready to take on 24-7 responsibility for another human being for the better part of two decades? Are you ready to give up much of your own independence? Can you afford to raise a child?

The Process of Conception and Pregnancy

Couples who wish to become pregnant need to pay extra attention to their health. Both partners should eat well and stay away from cigarette smoke, illicit drugs, and other toxic chemicals in the work or home environment. Men who drink alcohol should do so in moderation. Women should avoid alcohol altogether. Both partners should drink plenty of water from steel or glass containers. They should avoid food and beverage cans and plastic water bottles containing the hormone-disrupting chemical bisphen-ol A (BPA).

Women considering pregnancy should also meet with their primary care practitioners for a thorough medical history, physical exam, any recommended blood tests and screening tests for sexually transmitted diseases (STDs), and a discussion about the safety of any prescription or over-the-counter medications and dietary supplements. The doctor will also recommend a prenatal vitamin.

During the act of **fertilization**, the woman ovulates and a sperm fuses with the ovum (egg) in one of the fallopian tubes, forming a **zygote**. After five to seven days, the zygote has traveled down the tube to the uterus and burrowed into the uterine lining—a process called **implantation**. The inner layer of cells becomes the **embryo**, which, in few weeks, matures into a **fetus**. The outer layer of cells eventually forms part of the **placenta**, which provides nourishment to the developing fetus. The cells release chemicals that avert menstruation. Levels of a hormone called *HCG (human chorionic gonadotrophin)* may now be high enough in a woman's urine to turn the pregnancy test positive and to cause nausea.

After a positive pregnancy test, all the pillars of good health—sound nutrition, moderate physical activity, adequate sleep, stress management, social support, avoidance of toxins—become vitally important. In addition to staying away from tobacco, drugs, and alcohol, it's time for the woman to give up caffeine too.

Regular prenatal (before birth) check-ups are important. During those appointments, health practitioners monitor the growth of the fetus, check for the fetus's heart rate, and track things such as the woman's weight, pulse, blood pressure, blood sugar, and any abnormalities in the urine. An ultrasound can screen for obvious defects in the developing fetus. Depending on the mother's age and/or family history of genetic diseases, other screening tests may be recommended.

Pregnancy is divided into **trimesters** of roughly 3 months each, for a total of 40 weeks. The countdown starts with the first week after a woman's last period, even though conception didn't occur until about two weeks later.

During the **first trimester**, the embryo grows and organ systems start to develop. Around week 9, the embryonic, tadpole-like stage ends and the fetal stage begins. During these first 12 weeks, a pregnant woman may not initially look much different, though she may notice changes in appetite, nausea, and fatigue, a more acute sense of smell, and enlargement and tenderness of the breasts.

The first trimester is also the time when miscarriages, also called **spontaneous abortions**, tend to occur. Ten to 20 percent of known pregnancies end this way. The actual incidence is higher because many miscarriages occur so soon that the woman may not have realized she was pregnant. Causes include genetic defects, malformations of the developing embryo, abnormalities of the uterus or cervix, physical trauma, hormonal imbalances, infection, and other maternal illnesses. Most women who miscarry eventually successfully carry a pregnancy to term.

During the **second trimester**, the fetus grows from just over two inches in length to about nine inches. Organs continue to develop. By the end, the fetus can swallow, urinate, hear, and respond to familiar voices. The pregnant woman's breasts and belly continue to expand. The nipples and skin across her nose and cheeks may darken. About 18 weeks after conception (20 weeks after the last period—or the halfway point of the pregnancy), she feels the fetus move.

During the **third trimester**, the fetus grows rapidly. Bones and other organ systems finish developing. The fetus opens its eyes, starts to detect light, and, toward the end, starts "breathing" the fluid that surrounds it. The woman may start to feel physically uncomfortable, tired, and more than ready to birth the baby. As the fetus pushes under the diaphragm, it may feel harder to breathe and heartburn can occur. False labor contractions act as warm-up exercises for the real thing.

Labor and delivery mark the end of the pregnancy. Strong, regular contractions push the fetus, now usually head-down, out of the uterus through cervix, which dilates to accommodate the passage into the vagina. The process can be physically and emotionally challenging. Techniques learned in childbirth classes—breathing practices and calm focus—help. Anesthesia is available for women who want it and should not be viewed as failure or lack of courage.

The **postpartum (after-the-birth) period** extends for four to six weeks after the birth. During this time, the new family adjusts. The woman recovers from the birth of her baby. Ideally, the new mother is able to breast-feed the infant, which provides nutrition, antibodies, and other immune goodies. In addition to being better protected from infections, breast-fed babies seem to have enhanced intelligence quotients and reduced risk of eczema, obesity, diabetes, cardiovascular disease, and sudden

fertilization

The fusion of a sperm with an ovum (egg) to form a zygote. This process normally occurs within one of the woman's fallopian tubes. When assisted reproductive technologies are used to treat infertility, fertilization may occur outside the woman's body.

implantation

The attachment of the fertilized egg to the uterine lining at the beginning of pregnancy.

infant death syndrome (SIDS).[115] ,[116] It also protects the mother from type 2 diabetes, cardiovascular disease, and breast and ovarian cancer.[117]

During this time, emotions can range from exhilarating joy to sadness. Female hormones go on a rollercoaster ride. Plus, a first-time mother and her partner have to adjust to a big life change. A certain amount of "baby blues" is normal. The mother may feel a bit moody, overwhelmed, and irritable. Outright depression—with extreme sadness, tearfulness, loss of pleasure, feelings of guilt and worthlessness, sleep problems (unrelated to the newborn), and appetite changes—indicate it's time for professional help.

Postpartum depression strikes an estimated 20 percent of women.[118] Some experts prefer the term *perinatal (around-the-birth) depression*, because depression (and also anxiety) can begin during pregnancy. Contributing factors include genetic predisposition, previous depression, sleep deprivation, hormonal changes, life stress, marital dissatisfaction, single parenthood, unwanted pregnancy, depleted nutrients (essential fatty acids, vitamin D, B vitamins, calcium), and lack of social support. Treatment is vitally important to the well-being of mother and babe.

Though the topic isn't widely recognized, about 10 percent of men can become depressed during the pregnancy and after birth.[119] The rate may be even higher among men whose partners are struggling with postpartum depression.

For a week-by-week description of what happens during pregnancy, check out the Mayo Clinic website (http://www.mayoclinic.com/health/prenatal-care/PR00112). The site also has guidelines on nutrition and exercise, as well as information on general pregnancy health topics and childbirth classes.

postpartum depression

A mood disorder that occurs after the birth of the baby. Some specialists prefer the term "perinatal depression," which includes depression before and/or after the birth. While more common in women, depression and anxiety can also occur in expectant and new fathers.

Abortion

According to the Guttmacher Institute, a nonprofit organization dedicated to advancing sexual and reproductive health, 4 out of 10 unintended pregnancies end in abortion.[120] In the United States, about 60 percent of women requesting this procedure already have children. Nearly the same proportion of women are in their 20s. The majority are single and white. However, health disparities, including reduced access to contraceptives, make poor and minority women more vulnerable to unintended pregnancies and abortions. Ninety percent of abortions occur within the first trimester (first 12 weeks of pregnancy).

At this point, we need to define a few terms:

Spontaneous abortion, more commonly referred to as miscarriage, is much more common than most people realize. Fewer than 25 percent of fertilized eggs go on to become babies. Two-thirds of the time, the embryo is lost so soon the woman hasn't yet realized she's pregnant.[121]

Medical abortion uses pharmaceutical drugs rather than surgery to end the pregnancy. Although no anesthesia is required, a medical evaluation must first confirm that the pregnancy is not more than nine weeks along and has implanted within the uterus rather than ectopically (e.g., in the fallopian tubes). The woman then takes two medications. Mifepristone (also known as RU-486 and sold as Mifeprex) blocks progesterone, thereby thinning the uterine lining. It's given as a pill or as an injection. Two days later, the woman takes misoprostol (Cytotec), which is a synthetic version of prostaglandin E_1, a naturally occurring chemical that stimulates uterine contractions. A few hours later, vaginal bleeding and cramping begin. Other side effects can include nausea and diarrhea. The abortion is usually completed within a week.

Surgical abortion is quicker and requires fewer office visits but requires minor surgery and local anesthesia. Most of the time, suction curettage is used to remove the fetus and placenta. First the cervix is dilated. Next the doctor inserts a tube to suction out the tissues of pregnancy. The procedure lasts about 10 minutes. If the pregnancy has entered the second trimester, a doctor dilates the cervix and then uses instruments as well as suction to empty the uterus.

Medical and surgical abortions safely and effectively terminate pregnancy. Serious adverse reactions are rare. Women typically feel distress before the abortion and primarily relief afterward. Temporary sadness, guilt, and anger are also possible. Long-term mental health consequences normally don't occur in women without preexisting psychiatric disorders.[122]

On the other hand, illegal abortions are dangerous. Not long ago, the procedure was illegal in the United States. Women who don't wish to carry an unintended pregnancy to term sought "back-alley abortions" and other desperate measures. Many women died in the process from hemorrhage or infection. Many women around the world still do.

In 1973, the US Supreme Court ruled in Roe v. Wade that women had a constitutional right to abortion within the first six months of pregnancy. Deaths from unsafe abortions plummeted.[123]

While it may seem counterintuitive, abortion rates are actually higher in countries where abortions are illegal or severely restricted. For instance, in Latin America, where the procedure is illegal in most countries, there are about 32 abortions for every 1,000 women of childbearing age. In contrast, the rate in Western Europe, where abortion is legal and accessible, is 12 per 1,000.[124]

Nevertheless, in the United States, restrictions enacted at the state level have chipped away Roe v. Wade. Depending on what state a woman lives in, she has limited ability to obtain an abortion. Often no public funds can be used to pay for abortions. In many states, clinics that perform them cannot accept state or federal funds. Private insurance may not cover the procedure. Medicaid does not cover abortion, except in cases of rape or incest or when the woman's life is endangered. Some states require mandatory counseling, waiting periods, parental involvement (for minors), and other limitations.

    Video Clip 7.4

Abortion in the United States
This video contains facts about unintended pregnancies and abortion.

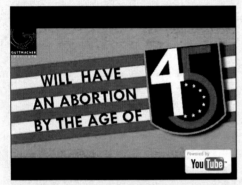

View the video online at: http://www.youtube.com/v/rY-bQ6UzhNl
Source: Guttmacher Institute (http://www.guttmacher.org).

Adoption

Another option for pregnant women who feel unready to become parents is to carry the pregnancy to term and then place the baby for adoption. Individuals and couples who are infertile or who have decided not to conceive their own children can then parent a nonbiological child. A finalized adoption is permanent; the biological parents forfeit their legal right to raise the child. The process requires maturity, courage, and compassion from all concerned. For that reason, professional counseling is recommended for anyone considering adoption.

There are two types of adoption: open and closed or confidential. The majority of adoptions are open, which means the biological and adopting parents know something about one another. They may simply share limited, written information or they may actually meet face-to-face. Biological parents may want to screen potential adoptive families to reassure themselves the infant is going to a good home. Adoptive parents may allow biological parents to remain in touch with the child, either directly or with the adoption agency mediating the interactions. Biological parents can then decide whether or not they wish to remain in contact. Children can have access to family and medical histories.

In a closed or confidential adoption, the birth and adoptive parents remain anonymous. While the adoptive parents do not receive private information about the biological parents, they can learn critical facts that affect how they need to care for the child. Biological parents can chose to provide contact information to the attorney, adoption agency, or national adoption registry. It is then up to the adoptive parents to decide whether to permit meetings between the child and the biological parents.

For more information about adoption, visit the Child Welfare Information Gateway (http://www.childwelfare.gov).

5.2 Infertility

Infertility is defined as the inability to conceive after 12 months of regular, unprotected intercourse. An estimated two million couples in the United States are infertile.[125] This problem is becoming more common as people delay childbearing in favor of establishing careers, finding a suitable life partner, and attaining financial security. The problem is more common among women. While men can father children into old age, women's fertility declines with age, particularly after age 35.[126]

Male infertility factors include low sperm count, poor sperm motility, blockages in the ducts that carry the sperm (usually due to infection or surgery), testosterone deficiency, and erectile dysfunction. Causes of infertility in women include reproductive hormone imbalances, polycystic ovary syndrome (ovarian dysfunction and hormonal imbalance), endometriosis, hypothyroidism (low thyroid hormone), blocked fallopian tubes, and anatomical abnormalities present since birth. Chronic pelvic inflammatory disease (PID) resulting in blocked fallopian tubes represents a common and largely preventable cause of infertility. In both men and women, tobacco smoke and other environmental toxins impair fertility. So does obesity.[127] Sometimes the cause of infertility can't be determined.

The first step for couples having trouble conceiving is meeting with a physician. Physical examinations and lab work can help determine possible causes of the infertility. Women can learn to gauge their fertile times by following their body temperature.

Couples with persistent infertility may elect to use **assisted reproductive technology**, artificial or partially artificial methods of achieving pregnancy. Medication may be used to stimulate ovulation. If the man is infertile, donor sperm may be placed in the woman's cervix or uterus, a process called *artificial insemination*.

In vitro fertilization (IVF) is a multistep process. After medications stimulate ovulation, mature eggs are extracted. In the lab, eggs and sperm are combined. After several days, one or two embryos are placed inside the woman's uterus. The success rate is about 30 to 40 percent.[128]

Acupuncture can sometimes help restore ovulation and also improve the success of IVF.[129] A few studies show that extracts of chaste tree berries may help restore fertility in women with irregular cycles[130],[131] and that maca and Asian ginseng may improve sperm counts and erectile function.[132],[133],[134],[135]

If the woman can't carry a child to term, some couples opt to engage a *surrogate mother*, who agrees to be inseminated by the man's sperm and, at the end of her pregnancy, surrenders the child to the couple. Some aspiring parents prefer to adopt a child.

KEY TAKEAWAYS

- Nearly half of pregnancies in the United States are unplanned. Many occur in couples using some form of contraception.
- Couples interested in becoming parents need to follow a healthy lifestyle. Ideally, women should meet with their primary care practitioners before becoming pregnant.
- Regular prenatal visits are important throughout the pregnancy.
- Abortion is an option for women who don't wish to remain pregnant. The vast majority of abortions in the United States occur during the first trimester. Women who don't want an abortion but also feel unable to raise a child may choose to give the newborn baby up for adoption.
- Some couples who want to become parents have difficulty conceiving. It's important for young people to protect their reproductive health by avoiding STDs, environmental toxins such as tobacco, and chronic, preventable diseases.

DISCUSSION QUESTIONS

1. When should couples wishing to conceive start cleaning up their lifestyles? Explain your answer.

2. What proportion of pregnancies are unplanned? What proportion of pregnant women had been using some form of contraception?

3. What should you be doing now to ensure your future fertility?

4. Abortion has become a controversial, political, and emotional issue in the United States. Some people say abortion should be outlawed, regardless of whether the woman has been raped. In August 2012, Missouri congressman Akin made a statement that "women who are victims of 'legitimate rape' rarely get pregnant." Medical specialists vehemently disagree.

   What is your opinion about the legality of abortion? Who do you think has the right to decide whether or not to end a woman's pregnancy: the woman, her doctor, the courts, or the legislature? What has most influenced your point of view—your parents, other authority figures (teachers, religious leaders), peers, or the media?

---

6. RECOMMENDED RESOURCES

6.1 Books

Anderson B. *Reproductive Health: Women and Men's Shared Responsibility*. Burlington, MA: Jones & Bartlett; 2004.

Hatcher RA, Nelson A, Zieman M, Darney P. *A Pocket Guide to Managing Contraception*. 5th ed. Atlanta, GA: Bridging the Gap Communications; 2002.

Hudson T. *Women's Encyclopedia of Natural Medicine: Alternative Therapies and Integrative Medicine for Total Health and Wellness*. 2nd ed. New York, NY: McGraw-Hill; 2007.

Lanou AJ, Castleman M. *Building Bone Vitality*. New York, NY: McGraw-Hill; 2009.

Norsigian J; Boston Women's Health Book Collective. *Our Bodies, Ourselves*. New York, NY: Touchstone; 2011.

Simon H. *The Harvard Medical School Guide to Men's Health: Lessons from the Harvard Men's Health Studies*. New York, NY: Free Press; 2004.

6.2 Websites

Bedsider. http://www.bedsider.org.

Division of STD Prevention, Centers for Disease Control and Prevention. http://www.cdc.gov/std.

Guttmacher Institute. http://www.guttmacher.org.

Managing Contraception. http://www.managingcontraception.com.

Pathfinders International. http://www.pathfind.org.

Planned Parenthood. http://www.plannedparenthood.org.

ENDNOTES

1. Sexual health. World Health Organization. Available at: http://www.who.int/topics/sexual_health/en. Accessed August 28, 2012.

2. Male circumcision and risk for HIV transmission and other health conditions: implications for the United States. Centers for Disease Control and Prevention. Available at: http://www.cdc.gov/hiv/resources/factsheets/circumcision.htm#ref5. Accessed September 19, 2011.

3. Centers for Disease Control and Prevention website. Available at: http://www.cdc.gov/cancer/prostate/statistics. Accessed September 21, 2011.

4. Men's prostate health. University of Tennessee Medical Center. Available at: http://www.utmedicalcenter.org/healthy-tips/68/mens-prostate-health. Accessed September 21, 2011.

5. Cai T, Mazzoli S, Bechi A, et al. Serenoa repens associated with Urtica dioica (ProstaMEV) and curcumin and quercitin (FlogMEV) extracts are able to improve the efficacy of prulifloxacin in bacterial prostatitis patients: results from a prospective randomised study. Int J Antimicrob Agents. 2009;33(6):549–553.

6. Lepor H. Pathophysiology, epidemiology, and natural history of benign prostatic hyperplasia. Rev Urol. 2004;6:3–10.

7. Nandeesha H. Benign prostatic hyperplasia: dietary and metabolic risk factors. Int Urol Nephrol. 2008;40(3):649–656.

8. Guess HA. Benign prostatic hyperplasia and prostate cancer. Epidemiol Rev. 2001;23(1):152–158.

9. Wilt T, Ishani A, Mac Donald R, Rutks I, Stark G. Pygeum africanum for benign prostatic hyperplasia. Cochrane Database Syst Rev. 2002;(1):CD001044.

10. Wilt T, Ishani A, Mac Donald R. Serenoa repens for benign prostatic hyperplasia. Cochrane Database Syst Rev. 2002;(3):CD001423.

11. Altavilla D, Bitto A, Polito F, et al. The combination of Serenoa repens, selenium and lycopene is more effective than Serenoa repens alone to prevent hormone dependent prostatic growth. J Urol. 2011 Oct;186(4):1524–1529.

12. Lopatkin N, Sivkov A, Schläfke S, Funk P, Medvedev A, Engelmann U. Efficacy and safety of a combination of Sabal and Urtica extract in lower urinary tract symptoms—long-term follow-up of a placebo-controlled, double-blind, multicenter trial. Int Urol Nephrol. 2007;39(4):1137–1146.

13. Tan RS. Perceptions of and risk factors for andropause. Arch Androl. 1999;43(2):97.

14. Vermeulen A. Environment, human reproduction and andropause. Environ Health Perspect. 1993;101:91–100.

15. Yamamoto K, Okazaki A, Sakamoto Y, Funatsu M. The relationship between premenstrual symptoms, menstrual pain, irregular menstrual cycles, and psychosocial stress among Japanese college students. J Physiol Anthropol. 2009;28(3):129–136.

16. Roupas ND, Georgopolos NA. Menstrual function in sports. Hormones (Athens). 2001;10(2):104–116. Available at: http://hormones.gr/preview.php?c_id=722. Accessed September 4, 2011.

17. Wei S, Schmidt MD, Dwyer T, Norman RJ, Venn AJ. Obesity and menstrual irregularity: associations with SHBG, testosterone, and insulin. Obesity (Silver Spring). 2009 May;17(5):1070–1076.

18. Fujiwara T, Sato N, Awaji H, Sakamoto H, Nakata R. Skipping breakfast adversely affects menstrual disorders in young college students. Int J Food Sci Nutr. 2009 May 26:1–9.

19. Milewicz A, Gejdel E, Sworen H, et al. Vitex agnus castus extract in the treatment of luteal phase defects due to latent hyperprolactinemia: results of a randomized placebo-controlled double-blind study. Arzneimittelforschung. 1993 Jul;43(7):752–756.

20. Ortiz MI. Primary dysmenorrhea among Mexican university students: prevalence, impact and treatment. Eur J Obstet Gynecol Reprod Biol. 2010 Sep;152(1):73–77.

21. Proctor ML, Farquhar CM. Dysmenorrhoea. Clin Evid. 2007 Mar 1;2007. pii:0813. Available at: http://www.ncbi.nlm.nih.gov/pmc/articles/PMC2943779/?tool=pubmed. Accessed August 31, 2011.

22. Han SH, Hur MH, Buckle J, Choi J, Lee MS. Effect of aromatherapy on symptoms of dysmenorrhea in college students: a randomized placebo-controlled clinical trial. J Altern Complement Med. 2006;12(6):535–541.

23. Mirabi P, Dolatian M, Mojab F, Majd HA. Effects of valerian on the severity and systemic manifestations of dysmenorrhea. Int J Gynaecol Obstet. 2011;115(3):285–288.

24. Tokuyama S, Nakamoto K. Unsaturated fatty acids and pain. Biol Pharm Bull. 2011;34(8):1174–1178.

25. Proctor ML, Murphy PA. Herbal and dietary therapies for primary and secondary dysmenorrhoea. Cochrane Database Syst Rev. 2001;(3):CD002124.

26. Brown J, Brown S. Exercise for dysmenorrhoea. Obstet Gynecol. 2010 Jul;116(1):186–187.

27. Rakhshaee Z. Effect of three yoga poses (cobra, cat and fish poses) in women with primary dysmenorrhea: a randomized clinical trial. J Pediatr Adolesc Gynecol. 2011 Aug;24(4):192–196.

28. Bu YQ, Du GZ, Chen SZ. Clinical study on the treatment of primary dysmenorrhea with preconditioning acupuncture. Chin J Integr Med. 2011 Mar;17(3):224–227.

29. Witt CM, Reinhold T, Brinkhaus B, Roll S, Jena S, Willich SN. Acupuncture in patients with dysmenorrhea: a randomized study on clinical effectiveness and cost-effectiveness in usual care. Am J Obstet Gynecol. 2008 Feb;198(2):166.e1–8.

30. Lee EJ, Frazier SK. The efficacy of acupressure for symptom management: a systematic review. J Pain Symptom Manage. 2011 Apr 29 [Epub ahead of print].

31. Gharloghi S, Torkzahrani S, Akbarzadeh AR, Heshmat R. The effects of acupressure on severity of primary dysmenorrhea. Patient Prefer Adherence. 2012;6:137–142.

32. Cunningham J, Yonkers KA, O'Brien S, Eriksson E. Update on research and treatment of premenstrual dysphoric disorder. Harv Rev Psychiatry. 2009;17(2):120–137.

33. Bertone-Johnson ER, Hankinson SE, Willett WC, Johnson SR, Manson JE. Adiposity and the development of premenstrual syndrome. J Womens Health. 2010 Nov;19(11):1955–1962.

34. Bertone-Johnson ER, Hankinson SE, Johnson SR, Manson JE. Cigarette smoking and the development of premenstrual syndrome. Am J Epidemiol. 2008 Oct 15;168(8):938–945.

35. Dickerson LM, Mazyck PJ, Hunter MH. Premenstrual syndrome. Am Fam Physician. 2003 Apr 15;67(8):1743–1752. Available at: http://www.aafp.org/afp/2003/0415/p1743.html. Accessed September 2, 2011.

36. Low Dog, T. Premenstrual syndrome. In: Rakel D, ed. Integrative Medicine. Philadelphia, PA: Saunders/Elsevier; 2007:601–611.

37. Daley A. Exercise and premenstrual symptomatology: a comprehensive review. J Womens Health. 2009 Jun;18(6):895–899.

38. Dvivedi J, Dvivedi S, Mahajan KK, Mittal S, Singhal A. Effect of "61-points relaxation technique" on stress parameters in premenstrual syndrome. Indian J Physiol Pharmacol. 2008 Jan–Mar;52(1):69–76.

39. Kim SY, Park HJ, Lee H, Lee H. Acupuncture for premenstrual syndrome: a systematic review and meta-analysis of randomised controlled trials. BJOG. 2011 Jul;118(8):899–915. doi:10.1111/j.1471-0528.2011.02994.x.

40. Bertone-Johnson ER, Hankinson SE, Bendich A, Johnson SR, Willett WC, Manson JE. Calcium and vitamin D intake and risk of incident premenstrual syndrome. Arch Intern Med. 2005 Jun 13;165(11):1246–1252.

41. Thys-Jacobs S, Starkey P, Bernstein D, Tian J. Calcium carbonate and the premenstrual syndrome: effects on premenstrual and menstrual symptoms. Premenstrual Syndrome Study Group. Am J Obstet Gynecol. 1998;179:444–452.

42. De Souza MC, Walker AF, Robinson PA, Bolland K. A synergistic effect of a daily supplement for 1 month of 200 mg magnesium plus 50 mg vitamin B6 for the relief of anxiety-related premenstrual symptoms: a randomized, double-blind, crossover study. J Womens Health Gend Based Med. 2000;9:131–139.

43. Wyatt KM, Dimmock PW, Jones PW, Shaughn O'Brien PM. Efficacy of vitamin B-6 in the treatment of premenstrual syndrome: systematic review. BMJ. 1999 May 22;318(7195):1375–1381.

44. Chocano-Bedoya PO, Manson JE, Hankinson SE, et al. Dietary B vitamin intake and incident premenstrual syndrome. Am J Clin Nutr. 2011 May;93(5):1080–1086.

45. Rocha Filho EA, Lima JC, Pinho Neto JS, Montarroyos U. Essential fatty acids for premenstrual syndrome and their effect on prolactin and total cholesterol levels: a randomized, double blind, placebo-controlled study. Reprod Health. 2011 Jan 17;8(1):2. Available at: http://www.ncbi.nlm.nih.gov/pmc/articles/PMC3033240/?tool=pubmed. Accessed September 2, 2011.

46. Dante G, Facchinetti F. Herbal treatments for alleviating premenstrual symptoms: a systematic review. J Psychosom Obstet Gynaecol. 2011 Mar;32(1):42–51.

47. Canning S, Waterman M, Orsi N, Ayres J, Simpson N, Dye L. The efficacy of Hypericum perforatum (St John's wort) for the treatment of premenstrual syndrome: a randomized, double-blind, placebo-controlled trial. CNS Drugs. 2010 Mar 1;24(3):207–225. doi:10.2165/11530120-000000000-00000.

48. Huang KL, Tsai SJ. St. John's wort (Hypericum perforatum) as a treatment for premenstrual dysphoric disorder: case report. Int J Psychiatry Med. 2003;33(3):295–297.

49. van Die MD, Bone KM, Burger HG, Reece JE, Teede HJ. Effects of a combination of Hypericum perforatum and Vitex agnus-castus on PMS-like symptoms in late-perimenopausal women: findings from a subpopulation analysis. J Altern Complement Med. 2009 Sep;15(9):1045–1048.

50. Norlock FE. Benign breast pain in women: a practical approach to evaluation and treatment. J Am Med Womens Assoc. 2002 spring;57(2):85–90.

51. Pruthi S, Wahner-Roedler DL, Torkelson CJ, Cha SS, Thicke LS, Hazelton JH, Bauer BA. Vitamin E and evening primrose oil for management of cyclical mastalgia: a randomized pilot study. Altern Med Rev. 2010 Apr;15(1):59–67.

52. Halaska M, Beles P, Gorkow C, Sieder C. Treatment 25 of cyclical mastalgia with a solution containing a Vitex agnus castus extract: results of a placebo-controlled double-blind study. Breast. 1999;8:175–181.

53. Bacterial vaginosis: CDC fact sheet. Centers for Disease Control and Prevention. Available at: http://www.cdc.gov/STD/bv/STDFact-Bacterial-Vaginosis.htm. Accessed August 11, 2011.

54. Wilson J. Managing recurrent bacterial vaginosis. Sex Transm Infect. 2004;80:8–11. Available at: http://www.ncbi.nlm.nih.gov/pmc/articles/PMC1758381/?tool=pubmed. Accessed July 6, 2011.

55. Allsworth JE, Lewis VA, Peipert JF. Viral sexually transmitted infections and bacterial vaginosis: 2001–2004 National Health and Nutrition Examination Survey data. Sex Transm Dis. 2008 Sep;35(9):791–796.

56. Mårdh PA, Rodrigues AG, Genç M, Novikova N, Martinez-de-Oliveira J, Guaschino S. Facts and myths on recurrent vulvovaginal candidosis—a review on epidemiology, clinical manifestations, diagnosis, pathogenesis and therapy. Int J STD AIDS. 2002 Aug;13(8):522–539.

57. Iavazzo C, Gkegkes ID, Zarkada IM, Falagas ME. Boric Acid for recurrent vulvovaginal candidiasis: the clinical evidence. J Womens Health. 2011 Aug;20(8):1245–1255.

58. Hudson T. *Women's Encyclopedia of Natural Medicine: Alternative Therapies and Integrative Medicine for Total Health and Wellness.* 2nd ed. New York, NY: McGraw-Hill; 2007.

59. Pena EF. Melaleuca alternifolia oil: its use for trichomonal vaginitis and other vaginal infections. *Obstet Gynecol.* 1962 Jun;19:793–795.

60. Hammer KA, Carson CF, Riley TV. In vitro susceptibilities of lactobacilli and organisms associated with bacterial vaginosis to Melaleuca alternifolia (tea tree) oil. *Antimicrob Agents Chemother.* 1999 Jan;43(1):196.

61. Carson CF, Hammer KA, Riley TV. Melaleuca alternifolia (Tea Tree) oil: a review of antimicrobial and other medicinal properties. *Clin Microbiol Rev.* 2006 Jan;19(1):50–62. Available at: http://www.ncbi.nlm.nih.gov/pmc/articles/PMC1360273/?tool=pubmed. Accessed August 29, 2011.

62. Barrons R, Tassone D. Use of Lactobacillus probiotics for bacterial genitourinary infections in women: a review. *Clin Ther.* 2008;30(3):453–468.

63. Reid G, Dols J, Miller W. Targeting the vaginal microbiota with probiotics as a means to counteract infections. *Curr Opin Clin Nutr Metab Care.* 2009 Nov;12(6):583–587.

64. Abad CL, Safdar N. The role of lactobacillus probiotics in the treatment or prevention of urogenital infections—a systematic review. *J Chemother.* 2009 Jun;21(3):243–252.

65. Rubinow DR, Girdler SS. Hormones, heart disease, and health: individualized medicine versus throwing the baby out with the bathwater. *Depress Anxiety.* 2011 Jun;28(6):E1–E15. doi:10.1002/da.20833.

66. Women's Health Initiative Investigators. Risks and benefits of estrogen plus progestin in healthy postmenopausal women: principal results from the Women's Health Initiative randomized controlled trial. *JAMA* 2002;288:321–333.

67. Huntley AL, Ernst E. Soy for the treatment of perimenopausal symptoms—a systematic review. *Maturitas.* 2004 Jan 20;47(1):1–9.

68. Wuttke W, Seidlova-Wuttke D, Gorkow C. The *Cimicifuga* preparation BNO 1055 vs. conjugated estrogens in a double-blind placebo-controlled study: effects on menopause symptoms and bone markers. *Maturitas.* 2003;44 Suppl 1:S67–S77.

69. Low Dog T, Powel KL, Weisman SM. Critical evaluation of the safety of *Cimicifuga racemosa* in menopause symptom relief. *Menopause.* 2003;10(4):299–313.

70. Lee MS, Shin BC, Yang EJ, Lim HJ, Ernst E. Maca (Lepidium meyenii) for treatment of menopausal symptoms: a systematic review. *Maturitas.* 2011 Aug 12 [Epub ahead of print].

71. What is osteoporosis? Fast facts. National Institutes of Health. Osteoporosis and Related Bone Diseases National Resource Center. January 2011. Available at: http://www.niams.nih.gov/Health_Info/Bone/Osteoporosis/osteoporosis_ff.asp. Accessed September 4, 2011.

72. Prynne CJ, Mishra GD, O'Connell MA, et al. Fruit and vegetable intakes and bone mineral status: a cross-sectional study in 5 age and sex cohorts. *Am J Clin Nutr.* 2006;83:1420–1428.

73. Bolland MJ, Avenell A, Baron JA, et al. Effect of calcium supplements on risk of myocardial infarction and cardiovascular events: meta-analysis. *BMJ.* 2010. doi:10.1136/bmj.c3691. Available at: http://www.bmj.com.

74. Jackson RD, LaCroix AZ, Gass M, et al. Calcium plus vitamin D supplementation and the risk of fractures. *N Engl J Med.* 2006;354:669–683.

75. Melnik T, Glina S, Rodrigues OMJ. Psychological intervention for premature ejaculation. *Nat Rev Urol.* 2009;6(9):501–508.

76. Linton KD, Wylie KR. Recent advances in the treatment of premature ejaculation. *Drug Des Dev Ther.* 2010 Feb 18;4:1–6. Available at: http://www.ncbi.nlm.nih.gov/pmc/articles/PMC2846147/?tool=pubmed. Accessed September 21, 2011.

77. Valeo T. Overcoming ejaculation problems. WebMD. Available at: http://men.webmd.com/guide/overcoming-ejaculation-problems. Accessed September 21, 2011.

78. Waldinger MD, Zwinderman AH, Schweitzer DH, Olivier B. Relevance of methodological design for the interpretation of efficacy of drug treatment of premature ejaculation: a systematic review and meta-analysis. *Int J Impot Res.* 2004;16:369–381.

79. Morales A. A review of the current status of topical treatments for premature ejaculation. *BJU Int.* 2007;100(3):493.

80. Douglass MA, Lin JC. Erectile dysfunction and premature ejaculation: underlying causes and available treatments. *Formulary.* 2010;45(1):17.

81. La Vignera S, Condorelli R, Vicari E, D'Agata R, Calogero A. Physical activity and erectile dysfunction in middle-aged men: a brief review. *J Androl.* 2011 May 19. Available at: http://www.andrologyjournal.org/cgi/rapidpdf/jandrol.111.013649v1. Accessed October 2, 2011.

82. Ott MA, Santelli JS. Abstinence and abstinence-only education. *Curr Opin Obstet Gynecol.* 2007 Oct;19(5):446–452.

83. Food and Drug Administration, Health & Human Services. Over-the-counter vaginal contraceptive and spermicide drug products containing nonoxynol 9; required labeling. Final rule. *Fed Regist.* 2007;72(243):71769–71785.

84. Weinstock H, Berman S, Cates W Jr. Sexually transmitted diseases among American youth: incidence and prevalence estimates, 2000. *Perspect Sex Reprod Health.* 2004;36(1):6–10.

85. Weinstock H, Berman S, Cates W Jr. Sexually transmitted diseases among American youth: incidence and prevalence estimates, 2000. *Perspect Sex Reprod Health.* 2004;36(1):6–10.

86. Aral SO, Adimora AA, Fenton KA. Understanding and responding to disparities in HIV and other sexually transmitted infections in African Americans. *Lancet.* 2008;372(9635):337–340.

87. Low N, Chersich MF, Schmidlin K, et al. Intravaginal practices, bacterial vaginosis, and HIV infection in women: individual participant data meta-analysis. *PLoS Med.* 2011 Feb 15;8(2):e1000416.

88. Foxman B, Aral SO, Holmes KK. Interrelationships among douching practices, risky sexual practices, and history of self-reported sexually transmitted diseases in an urban population. *Sex Transm Dis.* 1998 Feb;25(2):90–99.

89. HIV and AIDS estimates and data, 2007 and 2001. 2008 Report on the Global AIDS Epidemic. World Health Organization. Available at: http://www.who.int/hiv/data/en. Accessed September 5, 2011.

90. Prejean J, Song R, Hernandez A, et al. Estimated HIV incidence in the United States, 2006–2009. *PLoS ONE.* 2011;6(3):e17502.

91. HIV surveillance report: diagnoses of HIV infection and AIDS in the United States and dependent areas, 2009. Centers for Disease Control and Prevention. Available at: http://www.cdc.gov/hiv/topics/surveillance/basic.htm#hivest. Accessed September 5, 2011.

92. Anglemyer A, Rutherford GW, Baggaley RC, Egger M, Siegfried N. Antiretroviral therapy for prevention of HIV transmission in HIV-discordant couples. *Cochrane Database Syst Rev.* 2011 Aug 10;(8):CD009153.

93. Coffie PA, Kanhon SK, Touré H, et al. Nevirapine for the prevention of mother-to-child transmission of HIV: a nation-wide coverage survey in Côte d'Ivoire. *J Acquir Immune Defic Syndr.* 2011 Jul;57 Suppl 1:S3–S8.

94. HIV testing basics for consumers. Centers for Disease Control and Prevention. Available at: http://www.cdc.gov/hiv/topics/testing/resources/qa/index.htm. Accessed September 5, 2011.

95. Genital HPV infection: CDC fact sheet. Centers for Disease Control and Prevention. 2009. Available at: http://www.cdc.gov/std/hpv/stdfact-hpv.htm. Accessed August 22, 2011.

96. Rebolj M, Lynge E, Bonde J. Human papillomavirus testing and genotyping in cervical screening. *Expert Rev Anticancer Ther.* 2011 Jul;11(7):1025–1033.

97. Gillison ML, Broutian T, Pickard RK, et al. Prevalence of oral HPV infection in the United States, 2009–2010. *JAMA.* 2012 Feb 15;307(7):693–703.

98. Muñoz N, Manalastas R Jr, Pitisuttithum P, et al. Safety, immunogenicity, and efficacy of quadrivalent human papillomavirus (types 6, 11, 16, 18) recombinant vaccine in women aged 24–45 years: a randomised, double-blind trial. *Lancet.* 2009 Jun 6;373(9679):1949–1957.

99. Castellsagué X, Muñoz N, Pitisuttithum P, et al. End-of-study safety, immunogenicity, and efficacy of quadrivalent HPV (types 6, 11, 16, 18) recombinant vaccine in adult women 24–45 years of age. *Br J Cancer.* 2011 Jun 28;105(1):28–37. doi:10.1038/bjc.2011.185. Available at: http://www.ncbi.nlm.nih.gov/pmc/articles/PMC3137403/?tool=pubmed. Accessed August 22, 2011.

100. Giuliano AR, Palefsky JM, Goldstone S, et al. Efficacy of quadrivalent HPV vaccine against HPV Infection and disease in males. *N Engl J Med.* 2011 Feb 3;364(5):401–411.

101. Brotherton JML, Fridman M, May CL, et al. Early effect of the HPV vaccination programme on cervical abnormalities in Victoria, Australia: an ecological study. *Lancet.* 2011;377:2085–2092.

102. Genital herpes: CDC fact sheet. Centers for Disease Control and Prevention. Available at: http://www.cdc.gov/std/Herpes/STDFact-Herpes.htm. Accessed August 24, 2011.

103. Xu F, Sternberg MR, Kottiri BJ, et al. Trends in herpes simplex virus type 1 and type 2 seroprevalence in the United States. *JAMA.* 2006;296:964–973.

104. Kriebs JM. Understanding herpes simplex virus: transmission, diagnosis, and considerations in pregnancy management. *J Midwifery Womens Health.* 2008;53(3):202–208. doi:10.1016/j.jmwh.2008.01.010.

105. Brook MG. Sexually acquired hepatitis. *Sex Transm Infect.* 2002 Aug;78(4):235–240. Available at: http://www.ncbi.nlm.nih.gov/pmc/articles/PMC1744490/?tool=pubmed. Accessed August 27, 2011.

106. Chlamydia: CDC fact sheet. Centers for Disease Control and Prevention. Available at: http://www.cdc.gov/STD/chlamydia/STDFact-Chlamydia.htm. Accessed August 11, 2011.

107. 2008 sexually transmitted diseases surveillance: national profile. Centers for Disease Control and Prevention. Available at: http://www.cdc.gov/std/stats08/toc.htm. Accessed July 03, 2013.

108. 2009 sexually transmitted diseases surveillance: gonorrhea. Centers for Disease Control and Prevention. Available at: http://www.cdc.gov/std/stats09/gonorrhea.htm. Accessed August 27, 2011.

109. Johnson HL, Ghanem KG, Zenilman JM, Erbelding EJ. Sexually transmitted infections and adverse pregnancy outcomes among women attending inner city public sexually transmitted diseases clinics. *Sex Transm Dis.* 2011 Mar;38(3):167–171.

110. Stanback J, Shelton JD. Pelvic inflammatory disease attributable to the IUD: modeling risk in West Africa. *Contraception.* 2008 Apr;77(4):227–229.

111. Cottrell BH. An updated review of evidence to discourage douching. *MCN Am J Matern Child Nurs.* 2010 Mar–Apr;35(2):102–107.

112. Cases of sexually transmitted diseases reported by state health departments and rates per 100,000 population, United States, 1941–2010. 2010 sexually transmitted diseases surveillance. Centers for Disease Control and Prevention. Available at: http://www.cdc.gov/std/stats10/tables/1.htm. Accessed March 20, 2012.

113. Finer LB and Zolna MR. Unintended pregnancy in the United States: incidence and disparities, 2006. *Contraception.* 2011. doi:10.1016/j.contraception.2011.07.013.

114. Jones RK, Darroch JE, Henshaw SK. Contraceptive use among U.S. women having abortions in 2000–2001. *Perspect Sex Reprod Health.* 2002;34(6):294–303. Available at: http://www.guttmacher.org/pubs/journals/3429402.html. Accessed September 12, 2011.

115. Smithers L, McIntyre E. The impact of breastfeeding—translating recent evidence for practice. *Aust Fam Physician*. 2010 Oct;39(10):757–760. Available at: http://www.racgp.org.au/afp/201010/39421. Accessed September 9, 2011.

116. Hauck FR, Thompson JM, Tanabe KO, Moon RY, Vennemann MM. Breastfeeding and reduced risk of sudden infant death syndrome: a meta-analysis. *Pediatrics*. 2011 Jul;128(1):103–110.

117. Gouveri E, Papanas N, Hatzitolios AI, Maltezos E. Breastfeeding and diabetes. *Curr Diabetes Rev*. 2011 Mar;7(2):135–142.

118. Gavin NI, Gaynes BN, Lohr KN, Meltzer-Brody S, Gartlehner G, Swinson T. Perinatal depression: a systematic review of prevalence and incidence. *Obstet Gynecol*. 2005 Nov;106(5 Pt 1):1071–1083.

119. Paulson JF, Bazemore SD. Prenatal and postpartum depression in fathers and its association with maternal depression: a meta-analysis. *JAMA*. 2010;303(19):1961–1969.

120. An overview of abortion in the United States. Guttmacher Institute. Available at: http://www.guttmacher.org/media/presskits/2008/01/12/abortionoverview.html. Accessed September 25, 2011.

121. Boklage CE. The survival probability of human conceptions from fertilization to term. *Int J Fertil*. 1990;35:75–94.

122. Charles VE, Polis CB, Sridhara SK, Blum RW. Abortion and long-term mental health outcomes: a systematic review of the evidence. *Contraception*. 2008 Dec;78(6):436–450.

123. Wind R. Long-term decline in abortions has stalled; medication abortion becoming more common. Guttmacher Institute. January 11, 2011. Available at: http://www.guttmacher.org/media/nr/2011/01/11/index.html. Accessed September 25, 2011.

124. Sedgh G, Singh S, Shah IH, Ahman E, Henshaw SK, Bankole A. Induced abortion: incidence and trends worldwide from 1995 to 2008. *Lancet*. 2012 Feb 18;379(9816):625–632.

125. Chandra A, Martinez GM, Mosher WD, Abma JC, Jones J. Fertility, family planning, and reproductive health of U.S. women: data from the 2002 National Survey of Family Growth. *Vital Health Stat*. 2005;23:1–160.

126. Quinn F. We're having trouble conceiving. *Aust Fam Physician*. 2005;34(3):107–110.

127. Macaluos M, Wright-Schnapp TJ, Chandra A, et al. A public health focus on infertility prevention, detection, and management. Centers for Disease Control and Prevention. Available at: http://www.cdc.gov/reproductivehealth/Infertility/Whitepaper-PG1.htm. Accessed October 3, 2011.

128. McLachlan RI. Management of the infertile couple. *Aust Fam Physician*. 2005;34(3):111–117.

129. Huang DM, Huang GY, Lu FE, Stefan D, Andreas N, Robert G. Acupuncture for infertility: is it an effective therapy? *Chin J Integr Med*. 2011 May;17(5):386–395.

130. Westphal LM, Polan ML, Trant AS. Double-blind, placebo-controlled study of Fertilityblend: a nutritional supplement for improving fertility in women. *Clin Exp Obstet Gynecol*. 2006;33(4):205–208.

131. Gerhard II, Patek A, Monga B, Blank A, Gorkow C. Mastodynon(R) for female infertility. *Forsch Komplementarmed*. 1998;5(6):272–278.

132. Shin BC, Lee MS, Yang EJ, Lim HS, Ernst E. Maca (L. meyenii) for improving sexual function: a systematic review. *BMC Complement Altern Med*. 2010 Aug 6;10:44. Available at: http://www.ncbi.nlm.nih.gov/pmc/articles/PMC2928177/?tool=pubmed. Accessed September 4, 2011.

133. Chen JC, Chen LD, Tsauer W, Tsai CC, Chen BC, Chen YJ. Effects of Ginsenoside Rb2 and Rc on inferior human sperm motility in vitro. *Am J Chin Med*. 2001;29(1):155–160.

134. Hong B, Ji YH, Hong JH, et al. A double-blind crossover study evaluating the efficacy of Korean red ginseng in patients with erectile dysfunction: a preliminary report. *J Urol*. 2002;168:2070–2073.

135. Choi HK, Jung GW, Moon KH, et al. Clinical study of SS-Cream in patients with lifelong premature ejaculation. *Urology*. 2000;55:257–261.

CHAPTER 8
Nutrition: Eating Right for Life

After years of eating, you might think we would all be nutrition experts. We should know what to eat and when and how much. It should be simple. It certainly used to be. Our ancestors harvested wild plants and cultivated others. They hunted game. Families prepared and ate meals at home.

Then food became mass produced. Agriculture shifted from family-run businesses to industrial operations. Food was processed and packaged and delivered to stores. It became a lucrative industry, one based on profit rather than health. Fast-food restaurants sprang up, offering meals that were quick, cheap, tasty, and, all too often, detrimental to our health. We lost our connection to the earth. We started to rely on the food industry, nutrition scientists, and the media to tell us what to eat. Ironically, we became fatter and sicker.

Food is about more than human survival or even the pursuit of human health. What and how we eat defines culture and personal identity. Likewise, our culture also shapes our eating habits. When we "break bread together," we strengthen social bonds. Good food appeals to the senses. It's beautiful, aromatic, tasty, and healthy. It should be as good for the environment as it is for our bodies.

To that end, this chapter will provide basic information on nutrition and tips on eating patterns that support vibrant health. We'll also discuss initiatives to combat food insecurity, support sustainable agricultural practices, and make good food available to all.

Eat food. Not too much. Mostly plants.

- Michael Pollan, In Defense of Food

1. NUTRITION BASICS

LEARNING OBJECTIVES

1. Understand basic caloric requirements.
2. For each of the four macronutrients, explain their function, daily requirements, dietary sources, and the health consequences of deficiency and excess.
3. Define micronutrients, vitamins, and minerals.
4. List the water-soluble and fat-soluble vitamins.
5. Discuss other healthy substances found in plants and animals.

Nutrition has at least two meanings. One, it's a biological process whereby organisms take in nutrients and assimilate them into their tissues. Two, nutrition also refers to the scientific study of food and how it sustains our bodies and influences our health. *Diet* comes from the Greek word "diaita," which means "way of life." The word broadly refers to the foods a person usually consumes. For too many people, "diet" suggests restricted calories and deprivation of favorite foods. In the ideal, your diet comprises a group of foods that promote your health—a diet you can sustain.

A basic understanding of nutrition is important because diet is a major determinant of health. Both the type of foods you eat and the way in which they're prepared matter. Eat too much and too little of various substances in food and your health will fail.

The expression "You are what you eat" is true. It takes us back to the first definition of nutrition. These biologic processes seem no less than miraculous. Toss back a handful of nuts and dried fruit, chew, swallow, digest. The stomach churns like a cement mixer. The mush moves into the small intestine, where most nutrients are absorbed. Throw in bile and enzymes and—presto!—big molecules break down into molecules small enough to slip into the bloodstream. From there, they end up where they're needed to build bones, muscles, hormone-gushing glands, and crackling neurons. Amazing, yes?

FIGURE 8.1 The Digestive System

Digestion starts in your mouth, where your teeth grind food and salivary glands add enzymes to start breaking down starch into sugar. Your tongue propels the bolus of food to the back of your throat. Swallowing sends it down the esophagus and into the stomach, where acids, enzymes, and muscular contractions further break down food chemicals. Next, food moves into the small intestine where, with additions from the liver (bile) and pancreas (enzymes), nutrients fragment into particles small enough to slip into the bloodstream—a process called absorption. The function of the large intestine (colon) is to absorb water and some salts and vitamins. This remaining solid waste collects in the rectum until it's defecated (evacuated via the anus).

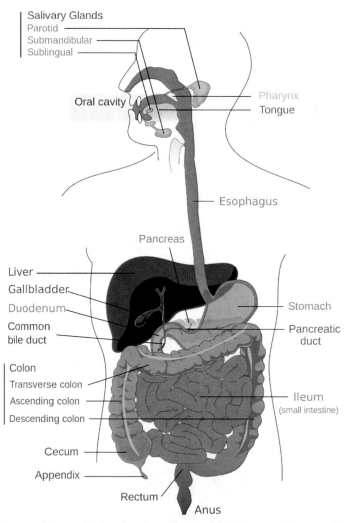

Source: Ruiz Villarreal M. Diagram of a human digestive system. Gaspar JA, ed. 2006. Available at: http://commons.wikimedia.org/wiki/ File:Digestive_system_diagram_edit.svg.

Food sustains us because it provides energy and essential nutrients. Food energy is measured in **kilocalories**. One kilocalorie is the energy needed to raise the temperature of one kilogram (2.2 pounds) of water 1°C (1.8°F). Technically, 1 kilocalorie contains 1,000 calories. However, people commonly use the word "calorie" to refer to a kilocalorie. For the rest of this chapter, we'll use calorie in this way.

A person's caloric requirements depends on several factors, most notably body size, body composition (the relative amounts of different types of tissues), and level of physical activity. A sedentary person requires about 13 calories per pound of body weight.[1] For instance, a 125-pound office worker who gets little exercise needs about 1,625 calories a day. However, if she's moderately active, her energy requirements rise to 2,000 calories a day.

Age and sex can also affect caloric requirements. Men generally have relatively more lean body mass (e.g., muscle and bones) than women. Older people tend to lose lean body mass relative to fat, although regular physical exercise counters the trend. Because muscle requires more calories to maintain than fat, caloric requirements decline with loss of lean body mass.

Conditions such as being pregnant and nursing a baby increase energy requirements. Some diseases—infectious diseases, cancer, hyperthyroidism, heart failure—increase caloric demands. As you can see, estimates for caloric requirements are just that—estimates.

In addition to calories, your body requires two main kinds of **nutrients** (food components): macronutrients and micronutrients. **Macronutrients** are substances required in relatively large amounts for growth and maintenance of basic bodily functions. **Micronutrients** are dietary elements needed in small amounts, such as vitamins and minerals.

1.1 Macronutrients

Technically, the macronutrients are carbohydrates, proteins, and fats. However, because water is also required in large quantities, it's usually included in the discussion. You need all these nutrients. Be wary of fads promoting one macronutrient and demonizing another.

Water

If you think of the things you can't live without, water and air should float to the top. After six minutes without oxygen, brain cells start to die. Depending on the conditions, humans can survive only about three to five days without water. In contrast, humans can go about a month without eating.

Water composes up to 60 percent of an adult's body. Because muscle holds much more water than fat, more muscular people contain more water, pound for pound, than less brawny people.

Water has numerous bodily functions. It

- provides a solvent for *electrolytes* (mineral salts that dissolve in bodily fluids);
- moistens mucous membranes in tissues such as the mouth, eyes, respiratory tract, and digestive tract;
- lubricates joints;
- regulates body temperature;
- provides a medium for moving blood cells and chemicals through the vascular and lymphatic systems;
- flushes waste products from the kidneys and liver; and
- participates (along with its dissolved electrolytes) in the regulation of nerve impulses and muscle contractions.

Dietary sources of water include beverages, soups, and many foods, particularly fresh fruits and vegetables. You may have heard that caffeinated and alcoholic beverages aren't good hydration beverages. That's because caffeine and alcohol both act as *diuretics* (agents that increase water lost in urine). In the case of caffeine, the effect is relatively weak, particularly in people accustomed to caffeine.

You lose water through your urine, perspiration, bowel movements, and with every breath you exhale. So how do you stay hydrated? Eat fresh produce and drink when you're thirsty. Individual needs vary. The following factors increase water requirements: ambient heat, body temperature, humidity (more body water is lost in arid climates), and physical activity.

For years, health experts hounded people to drink at least eight 8-ounce glasses (about 1.9 liters) of fluid a day, mainly in the form of water. The Institute of Medicine sets the adequate intake for men at 3.7 liters (about 4 quarts, or 15 cups) and for women at 2.7 liters a day (about 3 quarts, or 11 cups) a day.[2]

However, you don't really need to track your water intake. Most of the time, thirst is a good guide. Exceptions are the very young (who can't yet fetch themselves a glass of water) and the very old (whose thirst mechanisms weaken). If you exercise, run a fever, nurse a baby, or have diarrhea or vomiting, you'll need extra fluids. Some chronic illnesses (e.g., diabetes, kidney disease, cystic fibrosis) also increase water demands.

If you're getting enough to drink, your bowel movements are relatively soft (especially if you consume enough fiber) and you urinate several times a day (and the urine is pale yellow). If you don't drink quite enough water, you may develop constipation and headaches.

macronutrients

Substances required in relatively large amounts for growth and maintenance of basic bodily functions; they include water, carbohydrates, proteins, and fats.

micronutrients

Dietary elements needed in small amounts, such as vitamins and minerals.

dehydration

Abnormal depletion of body fluids.

water intoxication

Hyperhydration or water poisoning; can lead to hyponatremia.

Abnormal depletion of body fluids is called **dehydration**. Signs and symptoms include dry mouth and lips, scanty urine output (usually dark), no tears, listlessness, sunken eyes, and tenting of the skin (when you pinch a flap it stays up rather than snapping back into place). Furthermore, as the volume of fluid in the vascular system contracts, blood pressure falls and the heart beats faster.

Water intoxication (also called *hyperhydration*) is the reverse situation. For instance, if you exercise hard for long periods of time, excessive amounts of water will dilute the sodium in your blood, producing a condition called *hyponatremia*. Low levels of the electrolyte can lead to vomiting, headache, confusion, muscle cramps, seizures, and even coma. Most people don't need to worry about water intoxication, which is very rare. After moderate exercise, drink water and eat a snack. If you embark on a prolonged workout and won't be able to eat food (which replaces lost electrolytes), drink a sports beverage. If you've been vomiting, sip soup broth (which contains sodium chloride, better known as table salt). Keep bouillon cubes (dehydrated broth) on hand; mix one with one cup of hot water as needed.

Most of the time, plain old tap water is your best hydration fluid. It's cheap and calorie free. Though fruit juices, sports drinks, and sodas contain plenty of water, they're also high in sugar (unless they're artificially sweetened).

Why Bottled Water Isn't Better

Around the world, 780 million people lack access to clean water and 3.4 million die each year from water-related illness.[3] In the United States, we have the luxury of clean running water. The Environmental Protection Agency regulates the quality of municipal water; the Food and Drug Administration oversees bottled water.

According to the public interest organization Food & Water Watch, nearly half of bottled water products contain tap water.[4] Many bottled water companies don't disclose their source or their water quality tests. A 2008 test by the Environmental Working Group found that 10 popular brands of bottled water contained 38 chemical pollutants. Basically, you're paying good money for tap water that may be contaminated.

In addition, an enormous amount of energy (oil) goes into the production and distribution of plastic water bottles—enough oil to fuel 1.5 million cars for a year.[5] Production and transportation also generate pollution. Few bottles are recycled. Most clog trash cans, landfills, and waterways. Plus, some of the chemicals from plastics adversely affect health.

In a nutshell, bottled water is expensive, bad for the environment, and no safer than tap water. What can you do? Buy a safe, refillable water bottle made of metal or glass. (If you use plastic, look for a label promising it's free of the hormone-disrupting chemical bisphenol A [BPA].) Fill it up from the tap. Carry it with you. Wash and dry it at the end of each day. If you're hosting an event, encourage participants to bring their own bottles. Or sell (or give away) water bottles to benefit your organization.

To start a Take Back the Tap movement on your college campus, visit the Food & Water Watch website (http://www.foodandwaterwatch.org/water/take-back-the-tap/students). Also, check out the video "The Story of Bottled Water" at http://www.foodandwaterwatch.org/water/bottled.

Carbohydrates

Carbohydrates in your diet provide energy—specifically, four calories per gram. Two other macronutrients (protein and fat) also supply energy, just not as efficiently and quickly. The nervous system is fussy about using carbohydrates (glucose, specifically) as its energy source. During intense exercise, the muscles also require carbohydrates.

simple carbohydrates

Carbohydrates composed of one sugar (monosaccharides) or two linked sugar units (disaccharides); also called simple sugars.

complex carbohydrates

Carbohydrates composed of three or more sugars linked together; also called polysaccharides.

There are two major dietary carbohydrates: simple and complex. **Simple carbohydrates** are made from either one sugar (*monosaccharide*) or two sugar units linked together (*disaccharides*). **Complex carbohydrates**, also called **polysaccharides**, are made of three or more sugars linked together.

The typical American diet tends to be overloaded in simple carbohydrates. Common food sources include fruits and fruit juices (which contain the monosaccharide fructose), milk (which contains the disaccharide lactose), and table sugar (the disaccharide sucrose, which is glucose and fructose hooked together). Sucrose shows up in sweetened drinks, baked goods, and even condiments (barbeque sauce, marinades, salad dressings). The main sugar in maple syrup is sucrose. Honey contains glucose and fructose. Beer and some vegetables contain the disaccharide maltose, which is two glucose molecules linked together.

Why Is Beer Fattening?

Speaking of beer, in the creation of all alcoholic drinks, the fermentation process breaks down sugars and releases ethanol. Though it's not an essential nutrient, ethanol does provide energy (about 7 calories per gram). In fact, a recent study found that alcoholic beverages rival sodas and other sweetened drinks as a course of "empty" calories (foods providing calories but few nutrients). The average adult consumes 100 calories a day from alcoholic beverages. Of course, many adults don't drink. Typical drinkers consume more than 300 calories a day from alcohol—about 15 percent of total calories.[6] A simple way to cut calories is to drink less (or no) alcohol.

Complex carbohydrates can be divided into three categories: starch, fiber, and glycogen. The body can break down (metabolize) starches from plants into simple sugars for absorption into the blood stream. **Fiber**, on the other hand, is indigestible plant polysaccharides. **Glycogen** is the body's storage form for the monosaccharide glucose. The main storage depots for glycogen are muscles and the liver. When the body needs more glucose, the liver breaks down glycogen, releasing glucose into the bloodstream.

fiber

Indigestible polysaccharides found in plants.

Foods rich in starch include grains (rice, wheat, corn, barley, oats), root vegetables (especially potatoes), and legumes. Most Americans consume starches such as potatoes (especially chips and french fries), pasta, bread, crackers, and other baked goods.

Even though it's indigestible, fiber is important for health. It creates bulk in the intestinal tract, which, if consumed with sufficient water, improves bowel regularity. Diets high in refined grains (and consequently low in fiber) can lead to constipation, which in turn raises the risk for hemorrhoids (swollen veins in the rectum and anus) and diverticulosis (a condition in which small pouches protrude from the large intestine). On the other hand, diets rich in fiber are associated with a reduced risk of cardiovascular disease, heart disease, diabetes, and some cancers. Also, fiber-rich foods require more chewing and linger in the intestinal tract, which makes you feel full and helps with weight management. Although the Academy of Nutrition and Dietetics recommends a daily intake of 25 to 38 grams, most people consume about 15 grams.[7]

There are two types of fiber, both of which come from plants. **Insoluble fiber** doesn't dissolve in water and passes through the intestinal tract unaltered. Sources include whole grains such as whole wheat, brown rice, bulgur, and couscous. The bran (outer layers of grain cereals) contains the insoluble fiber. Refining the grain removes this exterior. That's why most health authorities recommend that people choose whole grains over refined grains. In addition to fiber, whole grains contain vitamins, minerals, and healthy oils.

Another source of insoluble fiber is cellulose, a component of plant cell walls. Good sources include carrots, lentils, dark-green leafy vegetables, broccoli, cabbage, cucumbers, summer squashes, and celery. (Leave the skin on to get the insoluble fiber from carrots, cucumbers, and squashes like zucchini. The flesh under the skin contains soluble fiber.)

Many fruits contain soluble and insoluble fiber. An apple, for instance, holds its insoluble fiber in the skin. The tiny seeds in many berries, as well as sunflower and pumpkin seeds, contain insoluble fiber. So do the skins of almonds and peanuts. Unbuttered popcorn (which contains corn bran) is low in calories and high in insoluble fiber.

On the other hand, **soluble fiber** dissolves in water to form a gel, which slows digestion and enhances feelings of satiety. Bacteria that normally inhabit the intestinal tract ferment the gel. Soluble fiber helps reduce cholesterol and slows the absorption of glucose into the bloodstream. Sources include oats, barley, beans, flaxseed, psyllium seed (the husk), nuts, broccoli, carrots, apples, oranges, pears, strawberries, and blueberries.

Excluding fiber, carbohydrates are broken down in the intestinal tract and absorbed as monosaccharides (single, simple sugars). After the liver finishes its work, glucose is the primary monosaccharide circulating in the bloodstream. Cells either break down glucose for energy or store it as glycogen (chiefly in the liver) or fat (mainly in the fat cells).

The complexity of carbohydrates in your diet affects how quickly blood glucose rises after a meal. In response to blood glucose, the pancreas releases the hormone *insulin*. Insulin moves glucose inside cells, where it's either burned for energy or stored as glycogen or fat.

Glycemic index (GI) is a measurement of food's effect on blood glucose. Foods that cause a rapid rise in glucose are referred to as having a high GI. Examples of such foods include table sugar, corn and maple syrup, candy, white bread, other baked goods, sodas, juices, and other sweetened drinks.

High-GI foods have three main problems. One, most contain few nutrients, hence the term "empty calories." An occasional dessert is fine. However, if you're eating a lot of energy-dense (high-calorie), nutritionally poor foods, you can become malnourished and overweight. Two, a spike in blood glucose is often followed by a crash that leaves you feeling fatigued. Three, repeated spikes in glucose eventually tax the ability of insulin to move glucose into cells.

Foods relatively low on the GI scale cause a more gradual rise in blood glucose. More nutritionally complex foods tend to have a lower glycemic index. An apple has a lower glycemic index than a cookie.

Fiber and the complexity of the carbohydrate lower the glycemic index. That's why bran cereal's glycemic index is about half that of puffed rice or corn flakes. For the same reason, legumes (peas, beans, lentils) are lower on the glycemic index.

However, the glycemic index ranking system isn't simple. The exact GI of a meal depends on the other foods consumed with the carbohydrates. For instance, fat in a meal slows glucose absorption from carbohydrates. Other factors come into play too. The riper the fruit, the higher its GI. And some starchy foods—namely, potatoes and white bread—rank high on the GI scale.

A good takeaway message is to get your carbohydrates from foods that are unprocessed (fruits and vegetables) or only minimally processed (whole oats and other unrefined grains). Also, if you're going to eat a high-GI food, combine it with protein and fat. An everyday example is spreading peanut butter on a piece of whole-wheat bread.

Recommended Carbohydrate Intake

The Food and Nutrition Board of the Institute of Medicine has established recommendations for macronutrients called **Acceptable Macronutrient Distribution Ranges** (AMDRs). The AMDR indicates the relative proportion of a macronutrient in your total daily energy intake that reduces your risk of chronic diseases. The AMDR for carbohydrates is 45 to 65 percent of your daily calories.[8] These carbohydrates should include 25 grams a day of fiber for women and 38 grams a day for men. You can accomplish that goal by selecting carbohydrates found naturally in fruits, vegetables, and whole (unrefined) grains and restricting foods high in refined carbohydrates and added sugar.

Read food labels. If you're buying bread, look for whole wheat and other whole grains. "Wheat flour" means refined wheat, not whole wheat. (Better yet, instead of a processed food like bread, consume whole grains such as rice, millet, oats, and amaranth.) Another thing you'll learn from food labels is that many processed foods have added sugars. Examples include all bakery items (including bread), sodas, juices, sports beverages, energy drinks, sweetened yogurt, salad dressings, ketchup, barbeque sauce, other marinades, desserts, candy, and breakfast cereals.

Most Americans don't have to worry about becoming deficient in carbohydrates. That said, if you don't consume enough carbohydrates, your blood glucose could fall. *Hypoglycemia* is a condition of abnormally low blood glucose. Symptoms include sweating, tremors, hunger, elevated heart rate, nervousness, and light-headedness. However, you can derive energy from fat and protein. If you deplete carbohydrate stores (glycogen) in the body, you start to break down your fat stores (a good thing if you would like to reduce body fat). Metabolism of fats releases acidic chemicals called ketones, which cause a fruity-smelling breath.

High-Fructose Corn Syrup: A Sweetener That Sours Health

Corn, as you might have noticed, is sweet. The corn is milled to make cornstarch, which is processed to yield corn syrup. Corn syrup is primarily glucose. Further enzymatic processing converts about half of the glucose into fructose, which tastes sweeter than glucose. High-fructose corn syrup (HFCS) tastes similar to table sugar (the disaccharide sucrose, which is made of glucose and fructose).

Because our government subsidizes corn, it's cheap. Processed-food manufacturers increasingly began using HFCS rather than sucrose from beets or sugar cane. Over the past four decades, consumption of HFCS has soared. The prevalence of overweight and obesity has also reached epidemic proportions. New research shows that whereas glucose quiets the brain's appetite centers, fructose does not.[9] In fact, it seems to promote food intake. While you can't pin the blame on HFCS alone, it's clear that sodas and other sweetened snack foods are a major source of calories. Furthermore, aside from sugar, these calories are largely devoid of nutrients.

In addition to promoting obesity, long-term and excessive consumption fructose has been linked to elevated triglycerides (a blood fat associated with cardiovascular disease), type 2 diabetes mellitus, nonalcoholic fatty liver disease (a disease characterized by abnormal deposition of fat in the liver), and cellular aging.[10] Because fructose isn't well absorbed from the intestine, it can also cause bloating, gas, discomfort, and diarrhea.

Paying attention to food labels can help you avoid added sugars. If the first ingredient is sugar or HFCS, put it back on the shelf. Increased media coverage of the potential ill effects of HFCS has inspired some processed-food manufacturers to advertise that their products are sweetened with sugar. Keep in mind that sugar (sucrose) in excess isn't good for you either. Try instead to make the switch to unsweetened beverages (water, tea, coffee) and real foods (fruits, vegetables, fish, eggs, dairy, and meat).

Protein

Dietary protein provides us with the raw materials for the body's structural components—bones, teeth, tendons (fasten muscle to bone), and ligaments (hold bones together). Two proteins, collagen and elastin, give many tissues (including your skin) their strength and resiliency. Enzymes, which speed chemical reactions, and some hormones are made of protein. Some neurotransmitters (chemicals involved in nerve communications) are derived from **amino acids**, the building blocks of proteins. The immune system's antibodies are made of protein. Like carbohydrates, the energy content of dietary protein is four calories per gram.

Proteins are made up of amino acids. When you consume protein, your digestive system breaks it down into amino acids for absorption. Of the 20 amino acids, 9 are *essential*, meaning the body can't make them. Our bodies can manufacture the other 11 amino acids, which is why they're called nonessential amino acids. Some foods supply **complete proteins**, meaning they contain all 9 essential amino acids. Animal foods—meat, fish, poultry, pork, eggs, and dairy (milk, yogurt, cheese)—are sources of complete proteins.

Individual vegetables, fruits, and grains contain less than a full deck of essential amino acids. However, if you combine plant foods, you get what you need. **Complementary proteins** are two or more incomplete protein sources that, combined, supply all the essential amino acids. Traditional cuisines commonly contain complementary protein pairings such as a legume with a grain, which provides a complete protein. Examples include beans and rice, beans and corn, lentils and rice, peanut butter and bread, and tofu (from soybeans) with vegetables and rice. Nuts and seeds also contain protein. Previously, people thought you had to consume complementary proteins in the same meal. It turns out that eating them the same day is sufficient.

Recommended Protein Intake

The AMDR for protein is 10 to 35 percent of daily calories. More precisely, the minimum daily protein intake required is 0.8 grams per kilogram (2.2 pounds). If you weigh 154 pounds (70 kilograms), you need at least 56 grams of protein. Because of their greater muscle mass, men usually need more than women (an average of 56 grams per day versus 46 grams per day for women).

Because protein is needed for tissue repair, requirements can rise after surgery or other trauma. Protein needs are also higher for children, teens, and women who are pregnant or breast-feeding, and athletes.[11] (Note that consuming extra protein won't bulk up your muscles; only exercise can do that.)

If you consult Table 8.1, you'll see that you could meet minimum protein requirements if you had a cup of yogurt (plus or minus fruit and a topping of granola) for breakfast, a cup of beans at lunch, and a three-ounce serving of meat for dinner. By the way, a three-ounce serving of meat is about the size of a deck of cards.

TABLE 8.1   Protein Content of Selected Foods

3 ounces of lean fish, poultry, or meat	21 grams
1 cup cottage cheese	26 grams
1 cup cooked quinoa (a seed)	18 grams
1 cup cooked black beans	15 grams
1 cup of yogurt	11 grams
1 cup of milk or soymilk	8 grams
half cup of firm tofu (4 ounces)	10 grams
1 large, cooked egg	6 grams
1 ounce (24 nuts) almonds	6 grams
1 tablespoon peanut butter	4 grams
1 tablespoon grated parmesan cheese	2 grams

Source: Protein content of selected foods per common measure. USDA National Nutrient Database for Standard Reference, Release 18. Available at: http://www.ars.usda.gov/Services/docs.htm?docid=13747. Accessed November 5, 2012.

Many people worry that they're not getting enough protein. However, most Americans meet or exceed daily protein requirements—even vegans, who consume no animal foods, including dairy and eggs. Excessive protein is mainly a problem for people with kidney disease. If the diet is high in proteins and very low in carbohydrates, body fat is broken down for energy, releasing ketones. Signs of protein deficiency include fatigue, weakness, muscle loss, brittle nails, hair loss, poorly healing wounds, low immune function, and edema (excess fluid in the tissues).

Fat

Of all the macronutrients, fats are the most energy dense. Each gram packs nine calories—more than double the caloric content of protein and carbohydrates. Dietary fat helps you absorb fat-soluble vitamins (A, D, E) and other fat-soluble plant chemicals, adds flavor and "mouth feel" to food, and promotes satiety. Which would satisfy your hunger better? A cup of plain salad greens, or the same greens dressed with a teaspoon or two of oil and vinegar? Once in the body, fats contribute to cell membranes (the thin barrier separating the inside of your cells from the outside). About 60 percent of the brain's dry weight is fat. Fat stores cushion bones and internal organs, fill out the face, insulate you from the cold, and lubricate your skin and hair.

When calorie intake exceeds immediate needs, the surplus is stored as fat—regardless of macronutrients consumed. Strictly speaking, it's not dietary fat that adds body fat but rather an excess of calories from all macronutrients. There are two main storage depots: under the skin (*subcutaneous fat*) and within the abdomen (*visceral fat*). As discussed in Chapter 10, an excess of visceral fat has detrimental effects on health.

Because dietary fat is calorically dense, a little goes a long way. The key is consuming relatively more of the "good fats." The type of fat you eat determines the type of lipid in your cell membranes, nervous system, and blood.

A bit of chemistry illustrates the differences among dietary fats, or as they're more properly called, **lipids**. Lipids are oily or waxy substances that don't dissolve into water. They include fats, fatty acids, and cholesterol.

Cholesterol has a ring structure and occurs in animal tissue. (Plant foods and vegetable oils contain only small amounts of cholesterol.) Our livers manufacture plenty of cholesterol. It's used to form cell membranes; bile acids (which help with digestion of dietary fat); vitamin D; and hormones such as testosterone, estrogen, and progesterone. Chapter 15 discusses cholesterol's health effects in more detail.

Examine Figure 8.2 and find the chemical structure for glycerol. This three-carbon molecule serves as a backbone to which fatty acids attach to form a fat. A monoglyceride contains one fatty acid; a diglyceride contains two; and a **triglyceride** contains three. Animals, humans included, store fats as triglycerides. Most of the fats we eat are triglycerides.

Fats are further distinguished by the type of **fatty acids** they contain. Fatty acids contain chains of carbon molecules. Fatty acids vary by the following three factors: (1) chain length (number of carbon atoms), (2) the "saturation" of the bonds (the number of hydrogen atoms binding to each carbon), and (3) the shape of the molecule. Based on length, fatty acids are categorized into short-chain (fewer than 6 carbon atoms), medium-chain (6 to 12 carbons), and long-chain (13 or more carbons) fatty acids.

Turn your attention back to Figure 8.2. Fatty acids can be broken into two main categories: saturated and unsaturated. The top figure shows an example of a **saturated fatty acid** (SFA). Each carbon has four bonds (noted by the straight lines extending at 90 degrees from the carbon). The letter C stands for carbon, H stands for hydrogen, and O stands for oxygen. Each carbon is "saturated" with the maximum number of bonds to hydrogen and carbon atoms. There are no double bonds between carbon atoms as there are in unsaturated fatty acids.

Unsaturated fatty acids are fatty acids that can absorb additional hydrogen atoms. They are subdivided into monounsaturated and polyunsaturated. The right-hand figure in the second row depicts a **monounsaturated fatty acid** (MUFA). The double line (called a double bond) means the bond is "unsaturated." Since there's only one, it's a MUFA. A **polyunsaturated fatty acid** (PUFA) contains more than one double bond and, therefore, fewer hydrogen atoms binding to the carbons. Double bonds create kinks in the chain, thus changing the shape. More double bonds lead to a more fluid molecule. The orientation of the hydrogen atoms also affects the configuration of the molecule.

Each type of fatty acid has distinctive characteristics and effects on health. A complicating factor in discussing the dietary sources is that most foods, whether animal or vegetable, contain more than one type of fatty acid. In the case of animals, the fatty acid profile depends on the animal's diet. The dietary sources listed are examples of foods that are relatively high in a particular fatty acid.

---

lipids

Oily or waxy substances that don't dissolve into water; include fats, fatty acids, and cholesterol.

triglyceride

A molecule consisting of three fatty acids attached to glycerol; the most common type of dietary fat and the storage form of body fat in all animals.

saturated fatty acid

A fatty acid whose carbon chain cannot accept additional hydrogen atoms.

unsaturated fatty acid

A fatty acid whose carbon chain can accept additional hydrogen atoms.

monounsaturated fatty acid

A fatty acid whose carbon chain contains one double bond, allowing it to accept one additional hydrogen atom.

polyunsaturated fatty acid

A fatty acid whose carbon chain contains two or more double bonds, allowing it to accept additional hydrogen atoms.

FIGURE 8.2   The Chemistry of Lipids

This figure provides the chemical structure of a saturated fatty acid, monounsaturated fatty acid, and glycerol (the backbone for triglycerides). In those structures, the letter C stands for a carbon, H stands for a hydrogen atom, and O stands for oxygen. In the shorthand structure of the monounsaturated fatty acid, most of the carbon and hydrogen atoms aren't labeled. The bends in the long tail indicate where carbons would be.

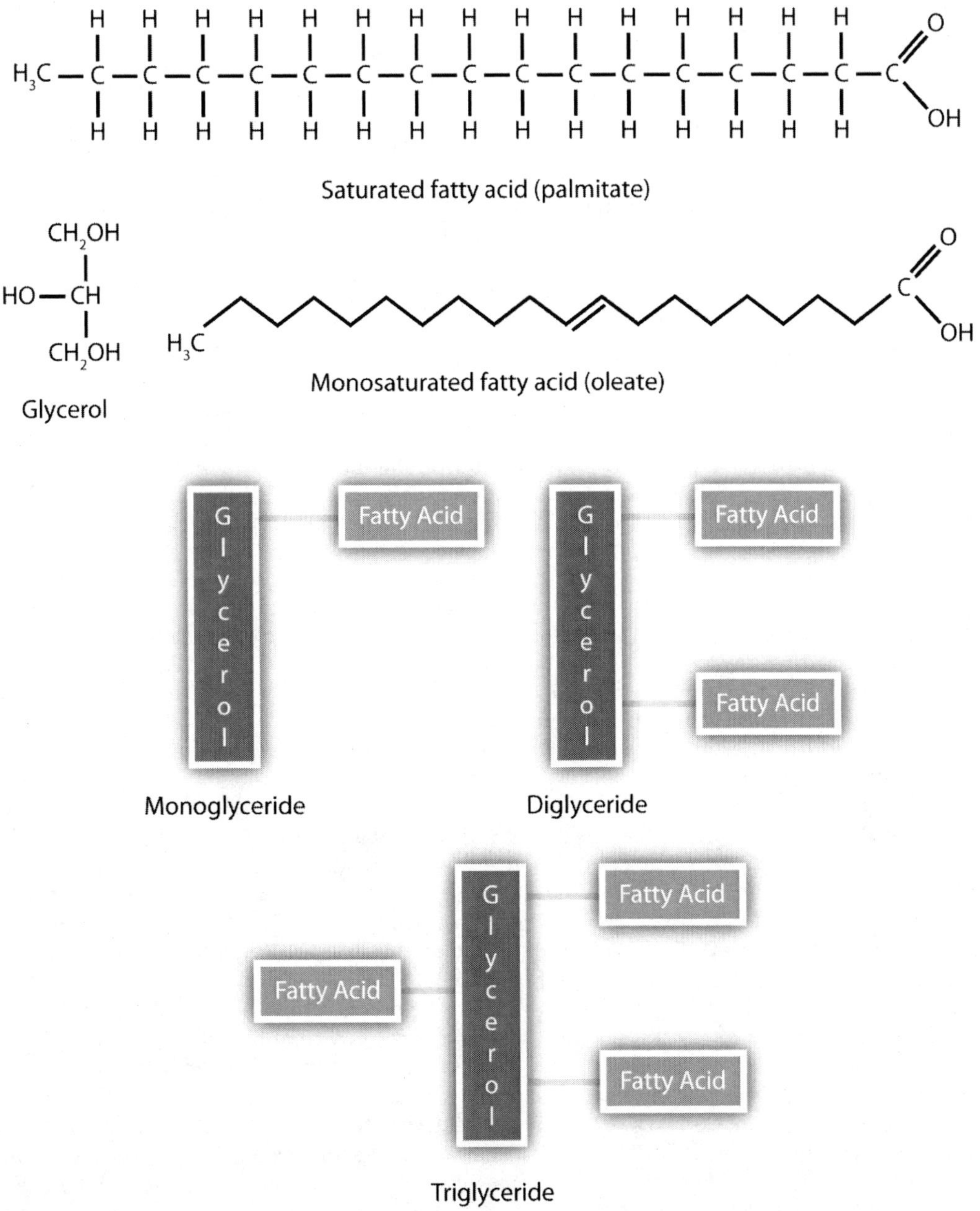

Saturated fatty acid (palmitate)

Glycerol

Monosaturated fatty acid (oleate)

Monoglyceride

Diglyceride

Triglyceride

Source: Adapted from Boumphreyfr. Structure of fats. 2009. Available at: http://commons.wikimedia.org/wiki/File:Fats1.png.

Saturated Fatty Acids (SFAs)

SFAs are solid at room temperature. All animal foods contain SFAs. That list includes beef fat, pork fat (lard), butter, whole-fat milk and cheese, and cream cheese. Lean poultry is fairly low in saturated fat. Some plant foods—coconut oil and coconut milk, palm oil, cocoa butter, macadamia nuts, and avocado—also contain significant amounts of SFAs.

For years, doctors advised patients at risk for cardiovascular disease to avoid SFAs. Recent research has challenged that dogma. It seems that refined carbohydrates (high glycemic index foods) pose a greater cardiovascular disease risk. Study results show that SFAs either have no effect on low-density lipoprotein (LDL) cholesterol (the "bad" cholesterol) or that SFAs increase LDL cholesterol but also increase high-density lipoprotein (HDL) cholesterol (the "good" cholesterol).[12] High levels of LDL cholesterol raise the risk of *atherosclerosis*, a disease characterized by the deposit of fatty material within the artery walls. In contrast, HDL cholesterol lowers the risk.

Monounsaturated Fatty Acids (MUFAs)

MUFAs are liquid at room temperature but become solid or semisolid in the refrigerator. Sources include olives, avocados, macadamia nuts, hazelnuts, almonds, pistachios, and peanuts. Avocados and olive oil are excellent sources of MUFAs. Other oils relatively high in MUFAs are high-oleic safflower oil, canola oil, and peanut oil. While whole milk products, butter, and red meats contain MUFAs, the proportion of saturated fat is higher.

The research on health benefits of MUFAs, which usually uses olive oil, demonstrates a reduction of LDL cholesterol, particularly when MUFAs replaces SFAs.[13] MUFAs such as olive oil reduce inflammation, blood pressure, and blood clotting—all of which protect against heart disease. Olive oil also improves blood sugar control, which reduces the risk of type 2 diabetes. These benefits may be related to other constituents in olive oil, namely health-promoting plant chemicals called polyphenols. These polyphenols also have antioxidant and anticancer effects. Commercial processing refines the oil and simultaneously lowers the polyphenol concentration. Extra virgin olive oil (obtained from the first pressing of the olives) preserves more of the polyphenols.

Polyunsaturated Fatty Acids (PUFAs)

Liquid at room temperature, PUFAs are the most flexible of the fatty acids. The upside is that they become incorporated into cell membranes, keeping these structures more flexible. The downside is that PUFAs are more vulnerable to oxidation (going rancid). Sources include nuts, seeds, fish, algae, and leafy greens.

PUFAs lower LDL cholesterol and HDL cholesterol. Put another way, both the good and the bad cholesterol types go down. While that sounds like a wash, the end result is that PUFAs may reduce the risk of atherosclerosis when they replace SFAs. However, the potential benefit depends on the type of PUFA.

PUFAs are subdivided into **omega-3 fatty acids** and **omega-6 fatty acids**. The difference has to do with the placement of double bonds (unsaturated bonds) within the fatty acid chain. Two polyunsaturated fatty acids—*alpha-linolenic acid*, an omega-3 fatty acid, and *linoleic acid*, an omega-6 fatty acid—are *essential*, meaning our bodies can't manufacture them.

As noted, PUFAs are less stable than SFAs. When they oxidize, they generate oxidative stress and inflammation in the body. Omega-6 fatty acids seem to be particularly problematic. For example, recent research shows that substituting omega-6 fatty acids (safflower oil and margarine made from that oil) for saturated fatty acids in people with cardiovascular disease actually increased the risk of death.[14]

On the other hand, omega-3 fatty acids are anti-inflammatory and have multiple health benefits. That's particularly true for the long-chain omega-3 fatty acids eicosapentaenoic acid (EPA) and docosahexaenoic acid (DHA). EPA and DHA are essential for nervous system development, growth, and maintenance. Low levels are associated with inflammatory conditions, cardiovascular disease, reduced cognitive (mental) function, and some psychological disorders (attention deficit hyperactivity disorder, depression, bipolar disorder, and schizophrenia).[15]

Higher consumption of foods rich in omega-3 fatty acids, especially fish, correlates with protection from cardiovascular disease, stroke, arthritis, and *osteoporosis* (a condition of thin, fragile bones). A 2012 study found that supplementation with EPA and DHA improved working memory in young adults.[16] Omega-3 fatty acids may also benefit people with asthma.[17]

Dietary sources of omega-6 fatty acids (linoleic acid and others) include sunflower, safflower, corn, soybean, and evening primrose oils. Sources of omega-3 fatty acids are algae (e.g., seaweed), fish, fish oil, flaxseeds, hempseeds, chia seeds, walnuts, rapeseeds (canola), and some green vegetables (spinach, kale, Brussels sprouts). Plants contain the omega-3 fatty acid alpha-linolenic acid (ALA). To a limited extent, our bodies convert ALA to EPA and DHA. Seafood is naturally high in EPA and DHA, which is one reason experts recommend eating it a couple times a week. Particularly good sources are fatty fish such as herring, kipper, mackerel, sardines, salmon, and trout.

Trans Fatty Acids (TFAs)

As mentioned, PUFAs lack the stability of more saturated fats. A manmade process called *hydrogenation* forces hydrogen atoms to saturate or partially saturate the carbon atoms in PUFAs. The end result is **hydrogenated fats**. Hydrogenation makes PUFAs more solid at room temperature and extends shelf life. Many processed foods (cookies, crackers, cakes, etc.) contain hydrogenated or partially hydrogenated fats.

Hydrogenation also changes the shape of the fatty acid. In nature, hydrogen atoms are mainly located on the same side of the double bonds in unsaturated fatty acids, a configuration referred to as "cis." Partial hydrogenation causes the remaining double bonds to take a "trans" configuration, with hydrogen atoms attached on opposite sides of each double bond. That's why they're called **trans fatty acids** (TFAs, often shortened to "trans fats"). (TFAs also occur naturally in limited amounts in beef, lamb, and dairy products. Most of the trans fats in your diet, however, come from hydrogenation.)

The trans configuration makes fatty acids more rigid, similar to SFAs. Trans and saturated fatty acids indirectly raise LDL cholesterol (associated with heart disease risk). In addition, trans fatty acids oxidize LDL cholesterol (making them more dangerous), lower HDL cholesterol (which protects the arteries), and make platelets stickier (and therefore more likely to clot within a blood vessel). For a time, doctors recommended patients at risk for heart disease eat stick margarine (a trans fat) rather than butter. Subsequent research showed that margarine was worse for health.

trans fatty acid

A fatty acid formed by hydrogenation (a manmade process that forces hydrogen atoms to saturate double bonds in unsaturated fatty acids); also referred to as hydrogenated fats.

Types of Fatty Acids

1. Saturated fatty acids (SFAs)

2. Unsaturated fatty acids

   a. Monounsaturated fatty acids (MUFAs)

   b. Polyunsaturated fatty acids (PUFAs)

   - Omega-6 fatty acids (e.g., linoleic acid)
   - Omega-3 fatty acids (e.g., alpha-linolenic acid, eicosapentaenoic acid [EPA], docosahexaenoic acid [DHA])

Recommended Fat Intake

The AMDR for dietary fat is between 20 and 35 percent of daily calories.[18] Of that total, the AMDR for omega-6 PUFAs is 5 to 10 percent; for omega-3 PUFAs it's 0.6 to 1.2 percent. That works out to about 17 grams a day for PUFAs. You can get that much in a mere 3 to 4 teaspoons of oil.

At this point, the dietary guidelines for lipids become complicated. Few Americans consume too little fat. A greater issue is consuming the wrong types of fats—too few omega-3 fatty acids and too many omega-6 fatty acids, saturated fats, and trans fats. Humans evolved on a diet with an omega-6 to omega-3 ratio of 1:1. A healthy ratio ranges from one to four times more omega-6 fatty acids than omega-3 fatty acids.

However, changes in the food industry (e.g., the boom in processed foods and grain-fed beef) skewed the ratio to between 10:1 and 25:1 and also increased SFA and TFA.[19] That shift has undesirable health consequences. While omega-3 fatty acids are anti-inflammatory and required for proper nervous system function, omega-6 fatty acids, SFAs, and TFAs are proinflammatory (thereby raising the risk of multiple chronic diseases). High levels of TFAs most definitely worsen human health. Finally, excessive intake of any kind of fat promotes overweight and obesity.

The takeaway message is to avoid trans (hydrogenated) fats, eat limited amounts of saturated fats and cholesterol (both of which are found primarily in animal foods), and choose monounsaturated fats and omega-3 polyunsaturated fats.

Tips for Choosing Fats Wisely

- Limit intake of baked goods such as cakes, pies, cookies, and crackers. Hydrogenated fats are often used in their production. Pay attention to ingredients listed on the label. Keep in mind that, even if the fat used is relatively healthy, these processed foods don't have much nutritional value. Be wary when labels advertise "low fat." Such products are often high in refined carbohydrates, especially sugar.

- Avoid or restrict fried foods. Even if the cooking oils aren't hydrogenated, high heat oxidizes unsaturated fatty acids, which, when consumed, increases free radicals in your body.[20] Plus, fried foods are high in calories and often low in nutritional value.

- Restrict saturated fat. Choose nonfat dairy products. Select lean cuts of meat and cut away visible fat (which is all saturated fat) before cooking. Pass up bacon, bologna, salami, pepperoni, and other preserved and fatty meats.

- When sautéing foods, use fats that are liquid at room temperature (monounsaturated and polyunsaturated fats). In salad dressings, go with olive oil and vinegar, or make the oil portion a 50-50 blend of olive.

- Boost your omega-3 fatty acid intake. Eat fish a couple times a week. (During pregnancy, it's especially important to avoid shark, swordfish, king mackerel, and tilefish, which contain high levels of mercury.) For the oil portion of salad dressing, try blending olive oil with flaxseed oil (which provides omega-3 fatty acids but can't be heated). Sprinkle omega-3-containing seeds (flax, chia, hemp) over food.

You Are What *You Eat* Eats

A recently sighted bumper sticker with that saying made me think of beef. The original North Americans ate bison, elk, and deer, all of which ate grass. When cattle were introduced to the continent, these animals also ate grass. Grazing cattle, goats, and sheep makes good use of land that doesn't easily support crops and fertilizes the grasslands. It's a sustainable system.

Over the last 50 years, agricultural practices have changed dramatically. Factory farms, large-scale confined animal-feeding operations, involve crowding animals into feedlots (or, for many animals, cages), where they eat corn, soy, and other grains. Cattle and other ruminants (cud-chewing animals) don't digest grains very well. But because of government subsidies, grains such as genetically modified corn and soy are cheap and plentiful. In cattle, grains create marbling: fatty deposits within the meat. Marbling adds flavor.

However, grain-fed beef contains lower amounts of omega-3 fatty acids but more total fat, with higher SFAs, MUFAs, and trans fatty acids.[21] Cholesterol is also slightly higher, though it's still on par with pork and poultry. In comparison, grass-fed beef is leaner with relatively more omega-3 fatty acids, including health-promoting long-chain omega-3s and conjugated linoleic acid (a PUFA with health benefits).[22] ,[23] And although it still contains saturated fatty acids, the profile of those fats differs from grain-fed beef. Specifically, it contains a lower proportion of the saturated fatty acids that increase blood cholesterol levels. Grass feeding also increases several vitamins and other compounds that act as antioxidants in the body.[24] Pastured dairy cows produce milk higher in omega-3s and vitamin E.[25]

The same principle applies for other animals—bison, elk, sheep, goats, and chickens. In general, so-called factory farming increases overall fat content and the amount of unhealthy fats and depresses healthier fat levels. For instance, eggs from hens allowed to forage in pastures have higher omega-3s than hens deprived of greens.[26] The meat is also higher in omega-3s.[27] ,[28]

Factory farms also increase the risk of infectious diseases and pollute air, water, and soil. The cramped, dirty conditions that restrict natural behaviors stress the animals. On the other hand, ranchers and farmers who allow their animals to forage are also less likely to give them growth-promoting hormones, antibiotics, and other additives—all of which end up in you when you eat them.

TABLE 8.2 Summary of Macronutrients

Name	Chief functions	Energy content and recommended intake	Dietary sources	Deficiency	Excess
Water	Provides the fluid content for saliva, urine, blood, mucus, tears, joint fluid, and the fluid inside and outside of cells.	0 calories per gram 2.7 liters a day, women 3.7 liters a day, men	Water, other beverages, fresh fruits and vegetables. Meat and cheese contain fewer amounts.	Dehydration: headache, muscle cramps, decreased output of dark urine, no tears, dry mouth and skin, tenting of skin, sunken eyes, low blood pressure	Water intoxication and hyponatremia
Carbohydrate	Supplies energy for daily activities. Fiber provides bulk to maintain intestinal health and improves control of blood levels of glucose and cholesterol.	4 calories per gram 45–65 percent of daily calories	Plant foods (grains, fruits, vegetables), milk (lactose), table sugar (sucrose), candy, sweetened beverages	Hunger and possibly low blood glucose. (You can, however, derive energy from other nutrients.) Prolonged deficiency causes you to break down fat stores. Low fiber causes constipation.	Elevated blood glucose
Protein	Needed to build bones, teeth, tendons, ligaments, and other connective tissues. Used to make enzymes, some hormones, and some neurotransmitters.	4 calories per gram 10–35 percent of daily calories	Animal foods (meat, seafood, eggs, dairy), legumes (beans, peas, lentils, peanuts), nuts, seeds	Fatigue, weakness, muscle and bone loss, brittle nails, hair loss, poorly healing wounds, low immune function, and edema (excess fluid in the tissues)	Can cause problems for people with kidney disease
Fat	Energy source. Important for absorption of fat-soluble vitamins. Polyunsaturated fats have other health benefits. Needed to create cell membranes, for communication between cells, and for normal skin function.	9 calories per gram 20–35 percent of daily calories—less than 10 percent from saturated fat	Animal foods (saturated fats in butter, dairy, and meats; omega-3 fatty acids in fish). Mono- and polyunsaturated fats in plants oils, including nuts. Baked goods may contain any kind of fats, including trans fats (which should be avoided).	Poor absorption of fat-soluble vitamins, dry skin and hair	Cardiovascular disease (trans fatty acids)

1.2 Micronutrients

Micronutrients, nutrients required in small amounts, include vitamins and minerals. Vitamins are organic (carbon-containing) molecules. Minerals are inorganic molecules, which means they lack carbon atoms.

Vitamins

Vitamins are divided into those that dissolve into water and those that dissolve into fat.

Water-Soluble Vitamins

The water-soluble vitamins are vitamin C and the B-complex vitamins. As the name suggests, these vitamins dissolve into water compartments of the body: blood plasma and the fluid inside and outside of cells. When you consume them, they move readily from the small intestine into the blood stream. If you ingest more than you need, the excess is excreted in the urine. That significance is twofold. One, you need to consume these vitamins daily. Two, there's a relatively low chance of toxicity from taking too much.

Vitamin C has gone down in history as the vitamin that prevents scurvy, a condition marked by bleeding gums, bruising easily, poorly healing wounds, and weakness. Long ago, sailors who embarked on long voyages developed scurvy. The British earned the nickname "limeys" because they brought limes and lemons on board to prevent the disease.

Citrus fruits are, of course, an excellent source of vitamin C. But all fresh fruits and vegetables contain vitamin C. Our bodies need vitamin C to manufacture collagen, a protein that provides structure in skin, blood vessels, and other connective tissues (bones, tendons, ligaments, teeth).

Vitamin C is also an **antioxidant**, a substance that inhibits oxidation (see the sidebar "Combating Oxidation and Inflammation"). It regenerates vitamin E, a fat-soluble antioxidant. And it contributes to immune system function.

Some people advocate "megadosing" (taking much more than required) vitamin C to prevent or treat the common cold. The research, however, suggests that doing so is not that helpful. Furthermore, high doses (over 2,000 milligrams a day) can cause nausea and diarrhea. Men only need about 90 milligrams a day and women need about 75 milligrams a day. Smokers, who subject themselves to additional oxidative stress, need to increase their vitamin C intake to 120 milligrams a day. Also, because of the role of vitamin C in wound healing, requirements rise after traumatic injuries, burns, and surgery.

Normally, you can get your daily requirement for vitamin C in foods. For instance, a cup of chopped, raw, red or green pepper contains 149 milligrams. One orange contains 130 milligrams. A cup of cooked broccoli contains 156 milligrams.[29]

The **B vitamins** include thiamin (vitamin B1), riboflavin (vitamin B2), vitamin B6, vitamin B12, folate, niacin, biotin, and pantothenic acid. Their various functions include assisting in the metabolism (chemical processing of) macronutrients, formation of blood, synthesis of DNA, and normal function of the nervous system.

Food sources also vary, depending on the particular B vitamin. Sources include animal flesh (shellfish, fish, beef, pork, poultry), eggs, dairy, grains, enriched breads and cereals, legumes, and nuts. In addition, green leafy vegetables, oranges, asparagus, and yeast contain folate. A wholesome diet should provide plenty of B vitamins.

Megadosing single B vitamins is generally not recommended, as doing so can disrupt the balance of the B vitamins. That said, a woman's folate requirements rise from 400 micrograms a day to 600 micrograms a day during pregnancy and 500 micrograms a day while breast-feeding. The food supply (particularly cereals) is fortified with folate to meet that need. Many doctors recommend their pregnant patients take prenatal vitamins, which contain an array of vitamins and minerals.

antioxidant

A substance such as vitamin C and vitamin E that inhibits oxidation.

Combating Oxidation and Inflammation

Oxidation and inflammation accelerate aging and underlie most chronic human diseases. The trouble starts with *free radicals*, atoms or groups of atoms with unpaired electrons. All atoms contain negatively charged particles called electrons. An even number of electrons keeps the atom stable. To stabilize themselves, free radicals steal electrons from other molecules, which can create a chain reaction of tissue-damaging electron raiding. *Oxidation* is a loss of electrons. Free radicals cause what's called *oxidative stress*.

Everyday examples of oxidation are rancid butter, rusted iron, and browning apple slices. The same process causes lipids, proteins, and DNA in our bodies to become damaged. Over the long haul, the risk rises for diseases such as cardiovascular disease, diabetes, cancer, arthritis, cataracts, Parkinson's disease, and Alzheimer's disease.[30]

Normal metabolic processes—breaking down, using, and storing nutrients—generate free radicals. So do other chemical reactions in the body. Your immune system, in the process of fighting infections, produces oxidative stress. Other factors that fan the oxidative fire include extreme exercise, fever, high blood sugar (as happens in diabetes), pollution (especially tobacco smoke), ultraviolet light, drugs, and consumption of trans fatty acids and fried foods.[31]

Oxidation and inflammation go hand in hand. Inflammation is a protective tissue response to injury. Immune system chemicals cause tissue to become reddened, hot, swollen, and tender. Inflammation generates free radicals; free radicals activate inflammatory chemicals.

A host of compounds protect against the twin scourges of oxidation and inflammation. Our bodies manufacture **antioxidants**. They inhibit oxidation by donating an electron to free radicals and other reactive chemicals. Examples include melatonin, glutathione, and superoxide dismutase. Levels decline with age and may otherwise be insufficient to meet demands. Eating a healthy diet ensures production of these natural antioxidants.

We also consume dietary antioxidants. While animal food contains antioxidants, your richest sources are plants. Because they can't seek shelter, plants make chemicals to counter challenges such as bombardment with ultraviolet light. These chemicals include vitamin C, vitamin E, selenium, carotenoids, and flavonoids. Because carotenoids and flavonoids act as plant pigments, you can easily recognize foods rich in them by their bright colors.

Fat-Soluble Vitamins

The fat-soluble vitamins are vitamins A, D, E, and K. Because these vitamins don't dissolve in water, you need to consume fat with them to move them from your intestines into the blood stream, where they float within protein carriers. If you consume more than you need, the surplus is stored in the liver and fat. If you habitually consume too much—a problem more commonly associated with vitamin supplements than with foods—fat-soluble vitamins accumulate and cause toxicity symptoms.

Vitamin A is required in adequate amounts for normal cellular division, vision, bone growth, immune function, and reproduction. It maintains the skin and the mucous membranes lining the intestinal, respiratory, and urinary tracts. Food sources include egg yolk, beef liver, chicken liver, and whole-fat dairy (or fortified nonfat dairy). Acquiring vitamin A from foods is safe. Taking vitamin A supplements, however, is risky. Excessive amounts can cause toxicity. Symptoms include loss of appetite, fatigue, blurred vision, bone and joint pain, hair loss, gastrointestinal upset, birth defects (if a woman is pregnant), and liver and nervous system damage.

Vitamin D is unique. In the presence of ultraviolet light, our skin manufactures it from cholesterol. Increased skin pigmentation and sunscreen impair this process. Unless you live relatively near the equator, the weaker sunlight of winter months isn't intense enough to stimulate the skin's vitamin D production. Furthermore, few foods contain vitamin D. They include fatty fish (sardines, mackerel, salmon), cod liver oil, and fortified cow's milk and soymilk. Butter and eggs contain smaller amounts.

Because vitamin D is needed for intestinal absorption of calcium, deficiency of vitamin D causes loss of bone mass. Vitamin D deficiency in children causes *rickets*, which manifests as bone deformities (bowed legs, knocked knees, knobs on the ribs, abnormal spinal curvature).

More recently, scientists have recognized that vitamin D has many more functions than optimizing calcium levels. Vitamin D insufficiency is common.[32] Low levels can lead to muscle weakness, falls, and bone fractures and have been linked to a higher risk of cardiovascular disease, some cancers, infections, asthma, autoimmune disorders, depression, diabetes, reduced fertility, and Alzheimer's-type dementia.[33] ,[34] ,[35] ,[36] In light of this new awareness of vitamin D, the Institute of Medicine increased the recommended daily allowance for children and adults to 600 international units (IU) and 800 IU for people over the age of 70.[37]

To get enough vitamin D, many experts now recommend exposing bare skin to the sun for 5 to 30 minutes between 10 a.m. and 3 p.m. at least twice a week during the spring, summer, and fall.[38] The darker your skin, the longer your exposure time should be. After you finish, apply sunscreen, cover up, or move into the shade.

Vitamin E exists in eight different forms called tocopherols. All have powerful antioxidant activity. The most active is alpha-tocopherol. Because vitamin E is fat soluble, it counters oxidation in the body's lipids. Whole foods normally contain a blend of tocopherols. In addition to protecting us from oxidative damage, vitamin E protects the eyes, brain, and cardiovascular system. It enhances immune function and may reduce the risk of some cancers. Food sources include plant oils (safflower, sunflower, canola, soybean), seeds, nuts, wheat germ, and fortified cereals.

Vitamin K is required for the production of proteins involved in blood clotting. Deficiency can lead to easy bruising and excessive bleeding. Food sources include dark-green leafy vegetables (kale, collard greens, turnip greens, spinach, dandelion greens), lettuce, broccoli, cabbage, and Brussels sprouts.

Minerals

These inorganic elements come from the earth. Living organisms don't make them. Plants pull minerals into their roots. Animals obtain minerals by eating plants, algae, fungi (mushrooms, yeast), and other animals and by drinking water.

We require minerals to provide structure to bones and other connective tissues and to regulate numerous chemical processes. **Major minerals** are those we need in amounts greater than 100 milligrams a day. They include calcium, magnesium, sodium, chloride, potassium, phosphorus, and sulfur. **Trace**

minerals are needed in much smaller amounts. They include iron, iodine, zinc, selenium, copper, manganese, chromium, fluoride, and molybdenum.

Rather than discuss all the minerals, we'll focus on major minerals that may be deficient in the diet and one trace mineral—iron.

Calcium is the most abundant mineral in the body. Among its many functions, calcium is required for blood clotting, nerve signaling, muscle contractions, and the formation of teeth and bones.

Bones represent a reservoir for calcium. Hormones tightly regulate blood levels of calcium. If levels rise, calcium is added to bone. If blood levels fall, calcium is released from the bone. Chronic calcium deficiency can lead to osteoporosis (brittle bones).

The two keys to strong bones are adequate intake of bone-friendly minerals, particularly calcium, and regular weight-bearing exercise. The big question is which foods maintain bone. Advertisements (e.g., the "Got Milk?" campaign) have created the impression that everyone should drink milk. However, many Americans are allergic to cow's milk or lack the intestinal enzyme that digests milk sugar (a condition called *lactose intolerance*). Many people of Asian, African, and South American descent are lactose intolerant.

Furthermore, consumption of milk and other dairy products doesn't seem to reduce bone fracture rates.[39],[40] Nevertheless, for many Americans, dairy is a significant source of calcium and vitamin D, both of which are critical for bone health.

Interestingly, a 2012 study found that vegan diets (no animal foods) correlate with a slower rate of bone loss than diets that include dairy and other animal foods.[41] Fruits, vegetables, seeds, and nuts contain calcium and other bone-essential nutrients, including vitamin K and minerals such as potassium, magnesium, and boron. These foods also generate less acidity, which is relevant because calcium is removed from bone to buffer acidity. A prominent bone robber in America is carbonated soft drinks because the acidity and high phosphorus content lead to loss of calcium from bone.

The recommended calcium intake for adults is 1,000 milligrams a day.[42] The intake increases to 1,200 milligrams a day in women over age 50 and also for men over age 70. If you eat well, you ought to be able to satisfy those requirements from food. Food sources include dairy, dark-green leafy vegetables, sardines (with the bones), green cabbage, Chinese cabbage, broccoli, cauliflower, dried figs, and sesame seeds. One cup of low-fat plain yogurt contains 415 milligrams of calcium. A cup of cooked kale contains 250 milligrams of calcium.

Like calcium, **magnesium** also contributes to the structure of bone. It's also a critical cofactor in many enzyme systems. Low blood levels can cause muscle cramping, weakness, irritability, and confusion. Prolonged deficiency is associated with heart disease, high blood pressure, type 2 diabetes, migraine headache, asthma, osteoporosis, and other chronic conditions. Nearly half of Americans consume less than the required amount.[43] Women need 265 milligrams a day; men need 350 milligrams a day. Food sources are green leafy vegetables, whole grains, seeds, nuts, beans, and seafood.

Sodium, **chloride**, **phosphorus**, and **potassium** help maintain fluid and acid-base balance. These mineral salts dissolve in water to become *electrolytes*. Sodium and potassium also participate in nerve impulses and muscle contraction. Phosphorus is part of bone's mineral complex. Sodium chloride (salt) is abundant in foods (both naturally and as an additive). Unless you're exercising hard in the heat, you're not likely to run low. Americans also consume more phosphorus than is necessary. Milk, meats, dairy, and soft drinks are rich in it.

Potassium is abundant in fresh fruits and vegetables. People who take diuretics to reduce blood pressure, have uncontrolled diabetes, and have prolonged vomiting and diarrhea (including from laxative abuse) can become deficient. Low blood levels can lead to decreased appetite, weakness, confusion, and irregular heart rate.

Iron is important for the creation of hemoglobin and myoglobin. Hemoglobin carries oxygen within red blood cells. Myoglobin stores oxygen in muscle cells. Deficiency causes anemia (reduced numbers of red blood cells in the blood) and weakness. Because of iron loss with menstruation and increased needs during pregnancy, requirements are higher in women under age 50 (18 milligrams a day) than for men (8 milligrams a day). But it's still a trace element. You don't need much. Food sources include meat, poultry, fish, enriched grains, dark leafy vegetables, dried fruit, and legumes. Most people don't need iron supplements. That's good because they cause constipation. Exceeding recommended intakes can lead to toxicity with nausea; diarrhea; and damage to the heart, central nervous system, liver, and kidney.

1.3   Other Substances in Food

In addition to water, macronutrients, and micronutrients, foods contain a multitude of other chemicals. Most of them originate from plants. Being rooted to the ground, plants generate **phytochemicals** (phyto = plant) to defend against predators, ultraviolet light, and other threats. Over the past several decades, nutrition scientists have focused their research on individual phytochemicals with potential benefits for human health.

The plant chemicals listed here periodically make headline news. However, keep in mind that any one plant is chemically diverse. When you consider that humans consume a variety of plant and animal foods, the chemical complexity grows exponentially. That said, the following chemicals benefit the plants that make them and the humans who consume them. By consuming a variety of colorful plants, you'll get them all.

Carotenoids are a group of over 600 compounds that act as natural plant pigments. Many plants contain provitamin A *carotenoids*, substances the body can convert to vitamin A. They include alpha-carotene, beta-carotene, and beta-cryptoxanthin. Other common carotenoids include lycopene and lutein. In addition to benefits associated with vitamin A, carotenoids are antioxidant, protect the skin from ultraviolet radiation (sunlight), maintain eye health, and enhance immune function. Some also guard against certain cancers. Orange, deep-yellow, and dark-green fruits and vegetables are rich in carotenoids. Examples include mango, cantaloupe, tomatoes, carrots, and spinach.

Polyphenols are another large family of phytochemicals. Within that class are **flavonoids**, also called bioflavonoids. Flavonoids also contribute to the color of plants. Some cause deep red, blue, and purple hues such as those in berries, red grapes, and cherries. Others occur in citrus fruits, onions, garlic, dark chocolate, coffee, and tea (green and, in lesser quantities, black tea). Flavonoids are antioxidant and anti-inflammatory. Some protect structural proteins and promote cardiovascular health. Some inhibit cancer.

Sulfur-containing compounds in plants also have health benefits. Cruciferous vegetables (cabbage, broccoli, cauliflower, kale, Brussels sprouts) contain chemicals such as indole-3-carbinol that have anti-cancer effects. Sulfur-containing chemicals in garlic and onions promote immune health, inhibit some disease-causing microorganisms, reduce the risk of cardiovascular disease, and guard against cancer.

Phytoestrogens are chemicals that mimic the body's estrogen. However, their effect is weaker. They may ease hot flashes accompanying menopause (the cessation of menstruation) and protect the cardiovascular system. Because phytoestrogens compete with the body's estrogen, they may protect against cancers associated with estrogen excess such as breast and uterine cancer. The effect seems to hold true when phytoestrogens (particularly soy) are consumed early in life. Lab studies have raised concerns about the safety of phytoestrogenic foods in older women and women at risk for breast cancer. However, studies in women have not revealed such a risk.[44] Food sources include legumes (especially soybeans and products made from them), flaxseeds, sesame seeds, and pomegranate seeds.

phytochemicals

Nonnutritive chemicals made by plants that provide health benefits to humans (and other animals) who eat them.

How Much of a Nutrient Is Enough?

Now that you know about the macronutrients and micronutrients, you may want to calculate how much you need each day. The Institute of Medicine's Food and Nutrition Board establishes guidelines for recommended dietary intakes for nutrients. The **Dietary Reference Intakes** (DRIs) provide guidance for how much of a nutrient you need to stay healthy. DRI is an umbrella term that, for most nutrients, includes the following four values.

The **Recommended Dietary Allowance** (RDA) is specific about the daily dose of a nutrient sufficient to meet the needs of healthy people of a particular gender and age group.

Adequate Intake (AI) provides an estimate of adequate nutrient intake based on observations and experiments. This term is used when the ideal amount isn't precisely known.

The **Tolerable Upper Intake Level** (UL) sets a maximum safe level of consumption. It's the highest intake level that's unlikely to cause harm.

Estimated Average Requirements (EAR) defines the amount of a nutrient sufficient for the needs for half of all people of a particular gender and age. The RDA is sufficient for nearly all healthy people of a particular gender and age group.

As noted earlier, the DRI for macronutrients is the **Acceptable Macronutrient Distribution Range** (AMDR), a range of intakes for any given macronutrient that's sufficient to maintain health.

The **Estimated Energy Requirement** indicates the average energy (calorie) intake to maintain energy balance. If you're in energy balance, your weight stays the same. If your energy balance is negative, you lose weight. If it's positive, you gain weight. Energy gained from food and energy lost from physical activity influence energy balance. For more information on energy balance, see Chapter 10.

The United States Food and Drug Administration (FDA) uses **Daily Values**, a simpler standard, for its food and dietary supplement labels. Nutrients are represented as a proportion of the recommended intake, assuming a 2,000-calorie diet (the energy intake for a 150-pound sedentary person).

To find DRI values for macronutrients and micronutrients, go to the Institute of Medicine's website at http://www.iom.edu/Global/ Search.aspx?q=DRi&output=xml_no_dtd&client=iom_frontend&site=iom&proxyreload=1.

The US Department of Agriculture (USDA) provides an interactive DRI glossary at http://fnic.nal.usda.gov/ interactive-dri-glossary.

KEY TAKEAWAYS

Food is chemically complex. Nutrients are broken into macronutrients (water, carbohydrates, protein, and fat) and micronutrients (vitamins and minerals).

- Carbohydrates provide energy (four calories per gram) and should make up between 45 and 65 percent of your daily calories. Healthy sources include fruits, vegetables, and whole grains. These foods will provide simple and complex carbohydrates, including fiber. Restrict foods high in refined carbohydrates and added sugars.

- Proteins provide building blocks for structural components of our bodies, as well as enzymes, antibodies, and neurotransmitters. The energy contained in protein is four calories per gram. Between 10 and 35 percent of your daily calories should come from protein. Animal foods provide complete proteins. Plant foods are incomplete proteins. Combining some vegetables and grains completes the number of essential amino acids.

- Fats are lipids, a chemical family that also includes cholesterol. We consume most of our fats as triglycerides, which are made of a glycerol molecule and three fatty acids. The number of carbons, saturation of the carbons, and shape of the fatty acids determine its properties and actions in the body.

  - Fatty acids can be divided into saturated and unsaturated. Saturated fatty acids come mainly from animal foods. Unsaturated fats are either monounsaturated or polyunsaturated. Omega-3 fatty acids are a type of polyunsaturated fatty acid with notable health benefits.

  - Most trans fatty acids are formed through hydrogenation, a process in which hydrogen atoms are added to polyunsaturated fatty acids. Trans fatty acids can negatively affect human health. In particular, they raise the risk of cardiovascular disease.

- Micronutrients can be divided into vitamins (organic molecules) and minerals (inorganic molecules). Vitamins are further divided into water-soluble and fat-soluble vitamins. Major minerals are needed in larger amounts than trace minerals.

- Plants contain other healthy substances such as carotenoids and flavonoids.

- The Institute of Medicine's Food and Nutrition Board establishes Dietary Reference Intakes (DRIs), guidelines for recommended dietary intakes for nutrients.

DISCUSSION QUESTIONS

1. A 50-year-old woman has recently received a diagnosis of diverticulosis, a condition in which pouches bulge outward from the wall of the large intestine. This woman is also overweight and often constipated. Her blood cholesterol and fasting blood sugar levels are at the upper limits of normal. In what way might diet account for all of her health problems? What dietary changes would you recommend?

2. Go to this webpage at the Institute of Medicine: http://www.iom.edu/Activities/Nutrition/SummaryDRIs/ DRI-Tables.aspx. Click on "Table: Estimated Average Requirement Values." How much protein do you need? (To calculate your weight in kilograms, divide your weight in pounds by 2.2.)

3. What type of fat has no health benefits and may actually harm health? What foods do you eat that contain these fats? How could you change your diet to avoid this type of fat and eat more healthy fats?

4. Again, go to http://www.iom.edu/Activities/Nutrition/SummaryDRIs/DRI-Tables.aspx. Click on "Table: DRI Values Summary." How much calcium should you consume each day? Now visit this USDA webpage: http://ods.od.nih.gov/factsheets/Calcium-HealthProfessional. List the foods you could eat at breakfast, lunch, and dinner that would provide your daily requirements for calcium.

2. HEALTHY EATING

LEARNING OBJECTIVES

1. Identify food patterns that promote health.
2. Review government guidelines on serving sizes.
3. Learn to read food labels.

2.1 The Rise of the Western Diet

Now that you know the nutrition basics, it's time to move on to choosing a diet that promotes your health and tastes good. Food patterns are much more important to human health than individual macro- and micronutrients. Some diets support vibrant health and longevity; others ultimately foster illness.

Unfortunately, the way most Americans eat falls into the latter category. The "Western" diet—high in refined grains, sugar, grain-fed meat, and artificial ingredients and low in fruits and vegetables—is associated with obesity and the top causes of death: heart disease, stroke, cancer, and diabetes.

On the other hand, people who follow traditional diets have a lower incidence of these chronic conditions. This association holds true despite the fact that traditional diets vary widely around the globe, from the vegetable-based Asian diet to the animal-based Inuit diet. Furthermore, many immigrants to the United States develop these "Western" diseases within a generation. Admittedly, other factors such as increased psychological stress, reduced physical activity, and smoking could contribute to the disease burden.

The fact remains that diet is a powerful contributor to health. Humans do better when they eat real food rather than factory-made, highly processed goods.

How did we veer into such unhealthy eating habits? For one, large-scale agriculture made food cheaper and more available. Government subsidies of corn, soy, and wheat promoted monocropping (growing the same crop on the same land year after year). Unfortunately, monocropping depletes the soil (increasing reliance on synthetic fertilizers) and reduces plant diversity. Also, the resultant surplus of grains ends up in animal feed (including for ruminants who sicken on such a diet) and in processed foods. If you read food labels, you'll have a hard time finding items devoid of wheat, corn, soy, or rice.

Mass production of baked goods meant that items that previously took a long time to prepare (e.g., cake) could be eaten every day. Added sugars, salts, and fats made foods irresistible. We consumed more synthetic chemicals by way of artificial colors, tastes, and preservatives. Chemicals used in plastic containers and the epoxy linings in cans leached into our food. We took in the antibiotics and growth hormones given to animals.

Another thing that changed was the way in which we viewed food. Traditional rituals around food withered. We have become impatient and time pressured. Why sit at a restaurant over a leisurely meal when you could drive up to a window; receive an inexpensive burger, fries, and soda; and wolf it all down while driving? Portion sizes became super sized, and so did we.

Energy bars and energy drinks began to act as meal substitutes. Advertisements suggested that processed foods (and even water) with added vitamins, minerals, and phytochemicals could make us healthier—though they often do the opposite. We started to snack continuously, often alone, and at almost every place but the dinner table. Home-cooked meals shared with family and friends now seem almost quaint.

Meanwhile, access to fresh food became a luxury. In the recent past, consumers could save money by buying fruits and vegetables. However, the cost of those foods has climbed faster than the rate of inflation.[45] Now if you're poor in America, you may not have the means to buy nutritious food or even to grow your own garden. You may not live near a store that sells fresh food. Your best option for the next meal may take the form of an inexpensive burger at the fast-food stand or a package of donuts at the "convenience store."

So how do we turn back the clock? We demand real food. We go out of our way to find it. We prepare it ourselves. We shun processed food. The tide has already started to turn. We'll close this section with proof of these changes.

FIGURE 8.3

What will you put on your plate?

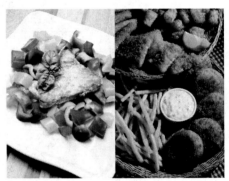

© Thinkstock

Video Clip 8.1

The Food Industry
In part one of this video series, Michael Pollan discusses the impact of the food industry on public and environmental health. He also examines the deception behind advertising campaigns and advocates a commonsense approach to eating. Although the food industry is powerful, the choices you make count. Unhealthy processed foods can't persist unless people buy them.

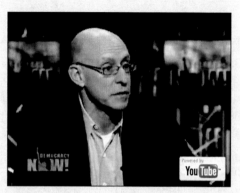

View the video online at: http://www.youtube.com/v/UWl5dobSZ1Y

2.2 Choosing Food Wisely

Now that we've established the pitfalls of the Western diet, the question is, what should you eat? The short answer is, real food. More specifically, eat plenty of vegetables and moderate amounts of seafood, meat, eggs, fruits, dairy, and grains. You don't need to weigh and measure and count out grams and calories. You generally don't need dietary supplements, because plants and animals contain an array of nutrients, fiber, and other beneficial substances.

The healthiest people on earth simply eat, and they eat simply. Their meals come from fresh, local foods with an emphasis on plant foods. Vegetables are nutritionally dense without being energy dense (high in calories). The energy in plants goes up as you go from leaves, to roots (carrots, sweet potatoes), to fruits, and, finally, to nuts and seeds. Grains are the least nutritionally dense. (From a botanical standpoint, legumes [peas, beans, peanuts] and grains [wheat, rice, barley, corn, oats] are fruits containing a single seed. Quinoa, which is eaten as a grain, is a seed.) Seafoods and grass-fed meats are also packed with nutrients.

If you eat a variety of real foods (versus highly processed foods), you'll instinctively satisfy your nutrient requirements. Even small children possess an inner compass that guides food choices. Around 1939, a Chicago pediatrician named Clara Davis carried out a famous experiment about toddlers' ability to self-select a balanced diet.[46] These little ones had access to a banquet of 33 foods. Without any adult intervention, the toddlers ate what they wanted. While any given meal wasn't nutritionally balanced, over the long term these kid-selected diets were wholesome. The trick is that kids were offered a variety of foods—none of it processed.

If the experiment were conducted with today's Western smorgasbord, it would fail. Highly processed food with added sugar and fat perverts appetite, even in toddlers and nonhuman animals. Give a laboratory rat high-fat, high-sugar treats and it will gorge itself into obesity and ignore the blander, healthier kibble.[47] The same thing happens to us.

Over the years, the United States Department of Agriculture (USDA) has created a series of symbols for healthy eating. The latest is MyPlate, which replaces the somewhat confusing food pyramids of the past. This graphic provides a practical, visual guideline that requires no weighing and measuring. The plate is divided into four unequal quadrants that correspond to the major food groups. The main idea is that vegetables and fruits should occupy half of your plate. On the other half, grains (mostly whole grains) take up more than a quarter and protein (from meat, poultry, fish, eggs, beans, peas, or nuts) fills in the gap. The cup contains a dairy product. However, as we'll discuss, some people either can't digest milk or prefer not to eat dairy. Because they're not considered a food group, fats don't show up on the plate. These should be used sparingly.

To learn more about MyPlate and USDA guidelines, go to http://www.choosemyplate.gov. You'll find sample menus and recipes, tips for healthy eating on a tight budget and when dining out, and more.

Another helpful concept is servings. For most Americans, the challenge is eating more plant foods and fewer animal foods and, especially, junk foods. Each day, most adults need two-and-a-half cups of vegetables (equivalent to five servings) and two cups of fruit (about four servings).[48] To satisfy that recommendation, you need to consume fruits or vegetables at every meal. If you're hungry for a snack, grab a piece of fruit or a vegetable and pair it with another food group. For instance, you might spread peanut butter on celery (topping it with raisins for "ants on a log") or chop an apple and add a dollop of plain yogurt and a sprinkle of chopped walnuts. Additionally, many experts recommend two servings of fish a week.

Here are some examples of servings of major food groups:

FIGURE 8.4 MyPlate

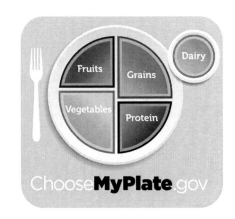

Source: USDA/ChooseMyPlate.gov. Available at: http://www.choosemyplate.gov.

- 1 serving of vegetables = ½ cup cooked or 1 cup raw vegetables or 6 ounces vegetable juice[49]
- 1 serving of fruit = 1 medium fruit (an apple or orange), 1 cup chopped or canned fruit, or 6 ounces fruit juice
- 1 serving of meat, fish, or poultry = 3 ounces (about the size of a deck of cards)
- 1 serving of grain = 1 slice of bread or ½ cup cooked rice (or other grain), pasta, potatoes, or breakfast cereal
- 1 serving of dairy = 8-ounces milk or yogurt or 1½ ounces cheese (4 cubes or 2 slices)
- 1 serving of nuts = 1 ounce = just under ¼ cup
- 1 serving of fat = 1 teaspoon butter or oil

For visual images of portion sizes, check out the pocket guide from the National Heart, Lung, and Blood Institute (http://hp2010.nhlbihin.net/portion/servingcard7.pdf) or WebMD's interactive tool (http://www.webmd.com/diet/healthtool-portion-size-plate).

Identifying Processed Foods

The words "processed food" keep coming up in this chapter. But what exactly is it? Clearly, if you pluck raspberries from a bush and pop them into your mouth, the only process going on is digestion. However, we process much of what we eat. In our own kitchens, we wash, peel, chop, cook, freeze, can, blend, or marinate. To extract a plant's oil, the plant part must be pressed. Grains are milled. Foods such as yogurt and sauerkraut require bacterial fermentation. That sort of minimal processing is fine and even desirable.

The words "processed food" suggest a higher level of manipulation, a transition from food to supermarket product. Whole grains become paler, refined grains (e.g., whole-wheat flour versus white flour). Salt, sugar, fat, and synthetic chemicals (preservatives and artificial flavors, colors, and sweeteners) might be added. The product is then boxed, bagged, canned, or jarred. It might need to be refrigerated or frozen. In addition to the energy involved in creating the product, more fossil fuels are consumed to transport the item and stock it in stores. You'll also hear the term "junk food," which refers to items such as sodas, baked goods, chips, and candy that provide "empty calories" (lots of calories and few nutrients).

Whole foods are those that resemble the plant or animal from which they came. They include fresh fruits and vegetables; whole grains; eggs; and fresh or frozen seafood, poultry, and meat. Dairy products (milk, yogurt, cheese, butter) also make the list of real foods. Deli meats (especially hot dogs), however, are highly processed. With a few exceptions (e.g., nuts, seeds, whole grains, and honey), you find most of these real foods along the periphery of a supermarket and farmers' markets.

Here are some ways to identify highly processed foods (so you can avoid them).

- It is stocked in the middle of the store.
- It was made in a factory.
- It contains added sugar, salt, and fat.
- The ingredients list is long and contains things you don't recognize as food and don't know how to pronounce.
- It comes in a package.
- It is stocked in a convenience store or vending machine.
- You've seen it advertised on television and in magazines.

Assess Yourself: Does Your Diet Contain Processed Foods?

It's hard to give up anything if you don't have something better to take its place. The first step is to identify the processed foods in your diet.

To that end, draw a line down the middle of a piece of paper. Keep a diary of what you eat for two days. If the food was real (recognizably from a plant or animal and minimally processed), record it in the left-hand column. If it was processed, write it in the right-hand column. Note the times you ate the food and the serving size. You may get insights into when you're particularly vulnerable to snacking on junk foods.

Now take out a fresh piece of paper. Again, create two columns. In the left-hand column, list the processed foods you regularly eat. In the right-hand column, list the whole food you might eat instead. Here's an example.

Processed foods	Whole-food alternatives
Commercial breakfast cereal	Fruit and yogurt, eggs, oatmeal (made from rolled or steel-cut oats)
Barbeque-flavored corn chips	Carrots, almonds, celery with peanut butter, homemade popcorn
Soda, sports drinks	Water, sparkling water with a splash of juice
Energy drinks	Tea, coffee (these are minimally processed and you can consume them without sugar)

Now that you've made your list, pick at least one substitution you can start making now. Compare how you feel after eating the processed food versus the real food.

2.3 Plant-Based Diets

omnivore

An animal (human or not) that consumes plant and animal foods.

vegetarian

A person (or other animal) who only eats food originating from plants.

The human diet varies widely in the ratio of plant food to animal food. Most people are **omnivores**, eating both plant and animal foods. Some people shun, to various extents, animal foods. According to a 2012 survey, 4 percent of American adults are **vegetarians**, meaning they eat no meat, poultry, or fish.[50] Another 43 percent eat one or more vegetarian meals a week. Included in the category of *vegetarian* are lacto-ovo (or ovo-lacto) vegetarians, who eat eggs and dairy, and vegans, who consume no animal foods.

People may become vegetarians for a variety of reasons: moral, environmental, religious, cultural, and medical. Research indicates that vegetarian diets, and also diets high in plants and relatively low in animal foods, confer protection against obesity, some cancers,[51] and diabetes.[52] However, if you love meat, know that the main problem is a diet high in grain-fed meats and low in vegetables. Rather than making meat the main attraction, try the approach used in traditional Asian diets. Use half the portion size you normally select, slice it, and sauté it with fresh vegetables.

Most people question whether vegetarians get all the essential nutrients. The answer is a qualified yes. As long as a person consumes a variety of plant foods—fruits, vegetables, whole grains, nuts, and seeds—he or she will obtain necessary nutrients, as well as an abundance of fiber, antioxidants, and other phytochemicals. On the other hand, a diet founded on pasta, tortillas, bread, and cheese will likely lead to nutrient deficiencies and excess body fat.

The micronutrient of greatest concern is vitamin B12, which is required to form red blood cells, build proteins, and maintain nerve tissue. Ovo-lacto vegetarians can obtain this vitamin from dairy and eggs. For strict vegetarians, B12-fortified commercial cereals, rice and soy beverages, veggie burgers, and nutritional yeast can suffice.[53]

The Academy of Nutrition and Dietetics maintains a website on vegetarian nutrition at http://vegetariannutrition.net. There you can find detailed information, recipes, and strategies for transitioning to a plant-based diet. You can find other vegetarian diet tips on the USDA Choosemyplate.gov website (http://www.choosemyplate.gov/healthy-eating-tips/tips-for-vegetarian.html).

2.4 Reading Food Labels

The Food and Drug Administration (FDA) requires that processed foods bear labels. Ingredients are listed in order of predominance by weight. If sugar appears in the top three entries, the product packs empty calories. Sugar may also be called powdered sugar, brown sugar, sucrose, fructose, dextrose, honey, molasses, fruit nectar, corn syrup, high-fructose corn syrup, cane syrup, rice syrup, malt syrup, or maple syrup. The ingredients list alerts you to chemical additives (e.g., synthetic dyes, flavors, and preservatives) and the types of fat. If you see "hydrogenated fat" or "trans fat," consider returning the box to the shelf.

FIGURE 8.5 Nutrition Facts

Which ingredients does this macaroni and cheese product contain that you ought to avoid or restrict in your diet? What do you think about the sodium content? Did you know that more than 75 percent of the salt you consume comes from processed and restaurant foods?[54]

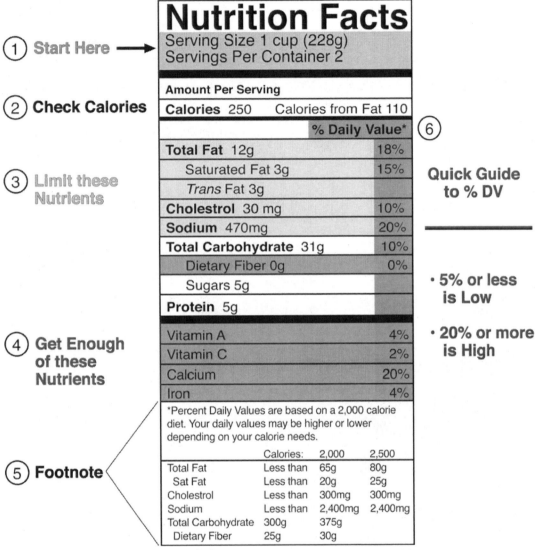

Source: Trounce/USDA. 2008. Available at: http://commons.wikimedia.org/wiki/File:US_Nutritional_Fact_Label_2.svg.

The nutrition facts label gives you yet more valuable information, as you can see in Figure 8.5. Note that the serving size may be smaller than the amount contained in the box, bag, or bottle—or the amount you put into your mouth. The daily values are expressed as a percentage of a daily energy intake of 2,000 calories.

Organic Foods

Package labels about the relative purity of food can be confusing. For instance, the word "natural" doesn't mean much. According to the USDA, "natural" meat or poultry means it does not contain artificial ingredients or added color and has been only "minimally processed."[55] On processed food, it suggests an absence of synthetic chemicals but may contain genetically modified organisms and other things not exactly natural.

organic food

Plants grown without the use of synthetic pesticides, fertilizers, sewage sludge, ionizing radiation, or genetic modifications; animals that aren't fed nontherapeutic antibiotics and growth hormones.

The USDA certifies **organic foods**. Organic crops are grown without the use of synthetic pesticides, fertilizers, sewage sludge, ionizing radiation, or genetic modifications; animals aren't fed non-therapeutic antibiotics and growth hormones. To ensure compliance, specially trained government agents periodically inspect farms and industries that process food.

However, the single word "organic" doesn't necessarily mean that all the ingredients are organic, unless the package only contains a single ingredient such as a fruit, vegetable, or animal product. The seal "USDA Organic" ensures that the food is 95 percent organic. On a multi-ingredient processed food, the statement "100 percent organic" means what it says. The statement "Made with Organic Ingredients" indicates that at least 70 percent of the ingredients are organic and that no ingredients came from genetically modified organisms. If fewer than 70 percent of a product's ingredients are organic, the front of the package can't state "organic," but side panels can list organically produced ingredients.

Whether or not organic agriculture improves the nutritional quality of food is controversial.[56] ,[57] Nevertheless, farming and ranching practices can indeed alter the nutrient content of plants and animals. Organic agriculture reduces the environmental impact on water, soil, and air. When you choose organic foods, you also lower the load of potentially toxic chemicals entering your body.

Granted, organic foods can be more expensive, though they're increasingly becoming more cost competitive. If your budget is limited, focus on organic meats, eggs, and dairy. Here's the reason: Chemicals such as pesticides concentrate in animal fat. Furthermore, eating conventionally grown produce is better than shying away from fruits and vegetables out of concerns for chemical contamination.

According to the Environmental Working Group, 12 conventionally grown crops (the "Dirty Dozen") are particularly high in pesticides: apples, celery, bell peppers, peaches, strawberries, imported nectarines, grapes, spinach, lettuce, cucumbers, blueberries, and potatoes.[58] Green beans and dark-green leafy vegetables may also be contaminated. If you can afford it, choose organic versions of these foods.

 Video Clip 8.2

Food Rules

Award-winning journalist Michael Pollan relays the key principles from the illustrated edition of *Food Rules: An Eaters Manual.*

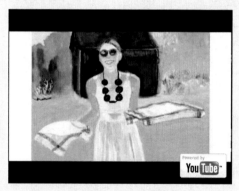

View the video online at: http://www.youtube.com/v/fugCMaPp0mY

Eating Well in College

College can present some unique dietary challenges. You may be on a tight budget and may not have access to a kitchen. If you cook your own food, you control whether the ingredients are fresh and organic. Choose cooking methods that preserve nutrients and minimize exposure to highly heated fats. Flavor food with health-promoting culinary herbs and spices rather than salt and sugar. If you can't cook, you still have ways to eat well.

- If you eat in a cafeteria in your dorm, start at the salad bar. Go with an oil-and-vinegar dressing. Progress next to vegetables and then grains and lean meats. Keep a mental image of a serving size and don't heap more on your plate. If it's breakfast, look for fresh fruit, eggs, and plain oatmeal.
- Limit foods that are fried, sugary (including fruit juices), and made with refined grains.
- Eat only when you're hungry and stop when you aren't.

- If you need a snack, keep it real. Eat some kind of whole food—an apple, carrot, a quarter cup of nuts. Keep such foods on hand in your room and in your backpack. That way chips and cookies will tempt you less.

- If you're on a tight budget, buy food that's fresh, local, well prepared, and high in nutrients. Fruits and vegetables (especially if they're bought when in season) are less expensive than seafood and meats, but you don't need much animal food in your diet. Skip relatively expensive "convenience" foods—precut vegetables, frozen dinners, instant grains. Limit yourself to reasonable portions. Make tap water (it's free!) your main beverage. Save money by skipping processed foods, expensive cheeses, and fancy espresso drinks.

- Request nutritional analyses of menu items at fast-food restaurants so that you can make informed choices. Turn down the supersized fries and sodas—no matter how inexpensive. You may save yourself expensive medical procedures down the line.

2.5   Do You Need Dietary Supplements?

In Chapter 2, you learned about dietary supplements. The list of products classified as ingredients in these supplements included vitamins, minerals, amino acids, and botanicals (medicinal plants, algae, and fungi).[59] Most supermarkets and pharmacies stock shelves of supplements. Health magazines usually display advertisements for them, and articles often recommend you take them. The question is, should you? The answer is, usually not, but it depends. If most people don't need supplements, why are we bombarded with information about them?

As mentioned earlier, nutrition has become a reductionist science. Researchers have focused more on the impacts on human health of individual macronutrients, micronutrients, and phytochemicals. Less attention has been paid to dietary patterns—mainly because there's little financial gain in telling people to eat more fruits and vegetables. There is, however, money to be made in selling expensive dietary supplements.

Research on various vitamins and minerals also generates media buzz. (After all, how many times can the media report on the benefits of a whole-foods diet?) At any given time, there's usually a "hot" supplement. Americans, being of the mind that more is better, gobble up the stuff.

There are several problems with this tactic.

1. Food is more than the sum of its individual ingredients. It's chemically complex. Scientists haven't yet identified all the chemicals in edible plants. Some may promote health effects; some may buffer the potential side effects of other chemicals.

2. The media often put the cart in front of the horse, trumpeting the benefits of a single chemical before it's been thoroughly researched. Sometimes a first study looks promising, but subsequent studies fail to show benefit or uncover adverse effects.

3. Taking large amounts of a single nutrient can unbalance other chemicals.

4. People may mistakenly assume that supplements will compensate for lousy diet, smoking, stressing, undersleeping, and other health-depleting lifestyle habits. They don't.

5. Supplements aren't cheap. Save your money for high-quality food instead.

If you eat a whole-foods diet, you generally ingest plenty of the required nutrients and you run little risk of exceeding tolerated doses of micronutrients. That said, some health experts recommend a multivitamin, particularly for people who can't eat well. Health practitioners also recommend prenatal vitamins for pregnant and nursing women. And people with certain diseases, as well as those at risk for certain diseases, may have increased demands for particular nutrients. Before you supplement, seek the advice of your doctor or a registered dietitian.

KEY TAKEAWAYS

- The shift from small farms to large-scale agriculture and food processing created an abundance of inexpensive food. Unfortunately, many of these practices harmed the environment and human health.
- For good nutrition, eat real food: unprocessed fruits, vegetables, and meats. Let fruits and vegetables make up at least 50 percent of every meal.
- Reading food labels can help consumers make educated food choices.

3. FOOD SAFETY

LEARNING OBJECTIVES

1. Distinguish between food allergies and intolerances.
2. Learn how you can protect yourself from foodborne illnesses.
3. Examine safety issues regarding food additives, genetic modification of crops and animals, and food irradiation.

3.1 Food Allergies and Sensitivities

food allergy

An abnormal immune system response to harmless foods.

Chapter 13 discusses allergies. In the case of **food allergies**, the immune system becomes hypersensitive, responding to proteins in foods as though they posed a threat of bodily harm. In this way, our immune systems make us feel ill, and for no good reason.

Between 1997 and 2007, the prevalence of food allergies rose by 18 percent.[60] Up to 8 percent of American children and 3 to 4 percent of adults have allergic reactions to foods, many of which are severe.[61] Scientists aren't sure why. Theories include a decline in microbial exposure early in life (which matures the immune system), changes in infant feeding schedules, antibiotics (which alter the natural microbes colonizing the intestines), agricultural and food-processing practices, and insufficiency of certain dietary micronutrients.[62]

Food allergies are usually identified with blood tests and skin tests. Eight foods account for most food allergies: cow's milk, soy, wheat, eggs, peanuts, tree nuts (e.g., almonds, walnuts, pecans, cashews), shellfish, and some fish. Symptoms can occur immediately or not surface for a couple of days. They include nausea, stomach pain, and diarrhea, as well as hives, respiratory congestion, and dizziness.

In some people food allergies can trigger *anaphylaxis*, an extreme and life-threatening allergic reaction. Signs include swelling of the lips and mouth, hoarseness, difficulty breathing, wheezing, rapid heart rate, low blood pressure, confusion, and collapse.[63] Emergency treatment is needed. People with known severe allergies can inject themselves with epinephrine and head to the emergency room if symptoms persist.

food intolerance

Adverse response to food that doesn't directly involve the immune system.

Unlike food allergies, **food intolerances** (also called food sensitivities) don't directly involve the immune system. Many times the problem lies with the digestive system's inability to digest food. For example, *lactose intolerance* arises from insufficiency of the enzyme lactase, which is needed to digest milk sugar. In the case of food allergy, the immune system reacts to milk protein.

Food intolerances cause nausea, gas, bloating, diarrhea, and headache—but no respiratory distress. Whereas a tiny amount of allergen can cause food allergies, it takes larger amounts and/or frequent exposures to elicit symptoms of intolerance.[64]

Elimination diets can identify foods a person doesn't tolerate well. The protocol usually involves eliminating suspect foods from the diet for two weeks. Potential offenders are then reintroduced slowly over a period of weeks. People with true food allergies should not try reintroducing problem foods without medical supervision.

Celiac disease is a genetically linked autoimmune disorder, a condition in which the immune system attacks normal tissue. Consumption of *gluten*, a protein found in wheat (including spelt and kamut), barley, and rye, triggers the immune to attack the lining of the small intestine.

Symptoms include abdominal bloating and pain; nausea; vomiting; diarrhea; weight loss; poor growth in children; and pale, foul-smelling stool. Health consequences extend beyond gastrointestinal upset. Damage to the small intestine impairs absorption of nutrients. Resultant problems include fatigue, bone and joint pain, arthritis, bone loss (which can progress to osteoporosis), anemia, numbness and tingling in the hands and feet, seizures, absent menstrual periods, infertility, skin rash, anxiety, and depression.

Diagnosis entails blood tests and examination of tissue from the small intestine. The main treatment is a lifelong avoidance of foods containing gluten. Complete elimination of gluten takes vigilance. In addition to the grains listed, less obvious sources include processed foods (even if they don't list any gluten-containing ingredients), medications, dietary supplements, and even lip balms.[65] For more information, see the list on the National Digestive Diseases Information Clearinghouse (http://digestive.niddk.nih.gov/ddiseases/pubs/celiac).

celiac disease

A genetically linked autoimmune condition triggered by gluten, a protein found in many grains.

3.2 Foodborne Illnesses

People often use the words "food poisoning" to refer to foodborne illnesses. These conditions are caused by contamination of food and beverages with microorganisms (most often bacteria) or toxins produced by bacteria. These may carry viruses such as hepatitis A and rotavirus, protozoa such as giardia, and helminths (parasitic worms). Other culprits include metals, mushroom toxins, and shellfish contaminated with phytoplankton.

You're probably heard of "mad cow disease," officially known as bovine spongiform encephalopathy (which translates to spongy brain disease in cattle). It's caused by infectious agents called *prions*. In Chapter 14, you'll learn more about these microscopic protein particles. Humans can become infected when they eat meat contaminated with brain and spinal cord tissue. (Cooking, by the way, doesn't destroy prions.) Fortunately, occurrences are exceedingly rare.

Bacterial contamination of food, on the other hand, is common. In December 2010, the Centers for Disease Control and Prevention (CDC) announced that the incidence of foodborne illnesses had dropped from 76 million cases in 1999 to 48 million cases estimated for 2011.[66] That's great news. However, out of 15 percent of Americans sickened by disease-causing microbes in food, about 128,000 of them wind up in the hospital and 3,000 die. The key culprits are bacteria such as salmonella, shigella, toxin-forming *Escherichia coli* (E. coli), and campylobacter.

A major source of foodborne microbes is factory farms, where animals live and die in each other's excrement. Contamination of conventionally produced fruits (melons) and vegetables (spinach and scallions) has also led to outbreaks of food poisoning. Furthermore, ingredients in our meals come from around the world, including places with less strict food safety requirements. Crops may be irrigated with tainted water, fertilized with fresh animal manure, and handled by people who failed to wash their hands after using the bathroom. Fortunately, the Food Safety Modernization Act of 2010 enhanced the Food and Drug Administration's authority to regulate food safety and the CDC's surveillance and investigation of foodborne infection outbreaks.

Depending on the microbe, foodborne illness usually begins one to two days after exposure. The main symptoms are diarrhea, nausea, and vomiting. Others include fever, loss of appetite, headache, and abdominal cramps. Fever and blood in stool indicate serious infection. See Chapter 14 for information about coping with gastrointestinal infections.

FIGURE 8.6
Factory Farming

Factory farms are large-scale operations where animals are concentrated and confined. This image depicts the warehouse-like building in which pigs are raised until they reach slaughter weight.

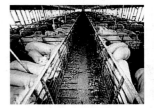

Source: Environmental Protection Agency. Hog confinement barn interior, slatted floor. Available at: http://commons.wikimedia.org/wiki/File:Hog_confinement_barn_interior.jpg

Reduce Your Risk of Foodborne Illness

Bacteria reproduce rapidly in the presence of nutrients and hospitable temperatures. Don't make it easy for them. Animal foods—meat, fish, poultry, dairy, and eggs—are the most common foods to contain bacteria. However, we cook these foods, whereas we may not subject contaminated fruits and vegetables to bacteria-killing heat. Once contaminated, almost any food can support a thriving bacterial colony. The following practices can reduce your risk of foodborne illness:

- Wash your hands with soap and water. Wash after using the toilet and before and after handling food. Failure to do so transmits a broad spectrum of microorganisms.
- Rinse produce under the tap. You can scrub firmer vegetables and fruits with a vegetable brush.

- Use separate cutting boards, knives, and other utensils for raw animal foods. In other words, don't cut raw chicken with the same knife you used to slice an apple—not without first sanitizing the knife.
- Thoroughly cook meat, poultry, pork, fish, and eggs. If cookie dough contains raw eggs, refrain from nibbling until the cookies emerge from the oven.
- Store perishable food in the refrigerator. Don't leave it sitting around.
- Scrub utensils, dishes, and cutting boards with hot, soapy water. Either air dry or use a clean dish towel. Wash the dish towel often.
- Sanitize surfaces that contact raw eggs, meats, and seafood, as well as surfaces contaminated by someone with an infection. For a simple disinfection solution, mix one teaspoon of chlorine bleach with one quart water.
- Don't share utensils and glasses.
- In the United States, tap water is generally safe to drink and may be cleaner than commercially bottled water. Public water fountains, however, can become contaminated. Improperly cleaned water coolers can too.
- Reusable water bottles are a great way to reduce waste. Just be sure to clean the bottle thoroughly with soap and water at the end of each day and allow to air dry.
- If you're camping, filter your drinking water with a device designed to eliminate microbes.
- If you're traveling outside the country, check with a health care authority about food and water safety. A good resource is the CDC's website on traveler's health (http://wwwnc.cdc.gov/travel/page/safe-food-water.htm). If the municipal water isn't safe, drink purified, bottled water. Avoid raw fruits and vegetables, unless they have a peel or rind you can remove.

3.3   Chemical Contamination of Food and Food Additives

The list of chemicals in our foods is long. Many of them aren't considered food additives, because they weren't added during the manufacturing process. For instance, water and soil can be contaminated with industrial chemicals and heavy metals. Plants pull chemicals into their roots. Pesticides form a residue on plants (which you can wash off) and may become incorporated into fruits and vegetables.

Animals, humans included, ingest chemical residues on and in plants. Many of these chemicals concentrate in animal fat. That means the higher you eat on the food chain, the bigger your dose will likely be. (Humans are high on the food chain because they eat animals, including those that eat smaller animals. Sharks, which eat other fish and sea mammals, are likewise high in this hierarchy.)

Processed foods typically contain food additives. Manufacturers may add vitamins, minerals, and even medicinal plants thought to have health benefits. Salt and sugar provide flavor but may also be used to inhibit microbes. Preservatives extend shelf life by discouraging microbial growth and oxidation. Sodium nitrate is used to preserve meats such as bacon, hot dogs, and luncheon meat. Sulfites preserve fruit and vegetable color. Artificial colors, flavors, and sweeteners are supposed to enhance aesthetic appeal. Flavor enhancers include chemicals such as monosodium glutamate (MSG). The Food and Drug Administration (FDA) requires that all ingredients, including additives, be listed on the food label.

People may be sensitive or allergic to additives, particularly sulfites and MSG. For instance, those substances can trigger migraines in sensitive individuals.

Antibiotic Overuse in Farm Animals

Food animals routinely receive antibiotics. In fact, about 80 percent of antimicrobial drugs sold in this country end up in animals.[67] Rather than being reserved to treat bacterial infections, the medications are added to feed to promote the animals' growth and prevent infections due to unsanitary, crowded conditions rampant in confined animal feeding operations, better known as "factory farms."

A big problem is that overuse of antibiotics leads to antibiotic resistance. That means that humans who acquire bacterial infections may find themselves without an effective antibiotic. These illnesses include food poisoning. Animal foods can be contaminated with antibiotic-resistant strains of bacteria such as salmonella and E. coli. Scientists have begun to pressure the FDA and the US Congress to regulate antibiotic use in agriculture.[68] Currently, the FDA has asked but not required the animal pharmaceutical industry to stop selling antibiotics for nontherapeutic uses.

Genetically Modified Foods

Gardeners and farmers have tinkered with the genes of plants for millennia. They hybridized plants to increase vigor and productivity. They planted seeds from the crops they liked and eradicated the "weeds." Ranchers selectively bred animals.

Of course, plant hybridization and animal husbandry are in a different ballpark from the process referred to as **genetic modification** (GM), in which an organism's genes are deleted or others inserted. The donated genes may come from entirely different species, not to mention different kingdoms (plant genes inserted into animals and vice versa). The resultant plant or animal is called a **genetically modified organism** (GMO).

The intent is usually honorable. If you genetically modify a crop to be resistant to weeds or insects or drought, you reduce your need for environmentally unfriendly practices (pesticides and excessive water consumption). Many crops are engineered to be resistant to the herbicides applied to eliminate weeds. (Note that many so-called weeds are edible and even medicinal.) Plants can be engineered to have brighter colors and contain additional vitamins and minerals. And why not seek to increase crop yield and nutrient value in the face of global food insecurity, especially in areas hit by malnutrition and famine?

However, the use of GM crops also has problems. For instance, if a crop becomes contaminated with pollen from GM plants, that farmer can no longer claim his or her crop is organic. Also the companies patenting the altered genes have sued the farmers. Scientists have genetically engineered some crops to produce sterile seeds, which inhibits spread of the plant, but also requires the farmer to buy new seed each year from large companies.

Another problem is that GM fosters monocropping, which reduces plant diversity. Diversity is important for several reasons. You know the saying "Don't put all our eggs in one basket." If you're growing only one crop and an insect devours it all or it succumbs to a flood or any other calamity, you're out of luck. If you grow a variety of plant foods, chances are some will survive. The plant gene pool is richer, as are the nutrients provided through consumption of a host of plants. Rotating crops can naturally restore nutrients in soil, decreasing the need for fertilizers.

Since their introduction in the 1990s, there's been a surge in the adoption of genetically modified crops. According to the US Department of Agriculture (USDA), just less than 90 percent of corn and almost all the soy grown in this country is genetically modified.[69] Cotton is also largely GM. The tinkering doesn't stop with plants. Biotechnology firms have also genetically modified hogs and salmon.[70] Some experts believe that the impact on human health and the environment has not been adequately studied. They have also called for mandatory labeling so that consumers at least know whether they're buying GMOs.

Irradiated Foods

Another practice that, on its face, sounds concerning is food irradiation. Low doses of radiation can control disease-causing bacteria, mold, and parasites and extend the shelf life of fresh foods. Nutrients aren't significantly altered, though some vitamin levels may be reduced in irradiated meat, and the food isn't radioactive.[71] The rays simply travel through the food and do not linger. Foods most commonly subjected to radiation are dried herbs and spices, meat, pork, and poultry. Fruits, vegetables, and wheat flour may also be irradiated. The FDA requires that irradiated foods display the "radura" logo, which appears in Figure 8.7.

FIGURE 8.7

The radura symbol appears on irradiated food.

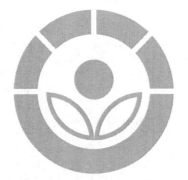

Source: US Department of Agriculture, Food Safety and Inspection Service. Available at: http://commons.wikimedia.org/wiki/File:Radura-Symbol.svg.

genetic modification

Human manipulation of organisms' genetic material.

genetically modified organism

An organism resulting from human manipulation of its genetic material.

4. COMBATING HUNGER AND MALNUTRITION

LEARNING OBJECTIVES

1. Discuss food insecurity and ways you can reduce food waste.
2. Examine positive signs of transformation in the production, preparation, and enjoyment of food.
3. Discuss the environmental impact of consumer food choices.

food insecurity

A reduced ability to access and utilize food.

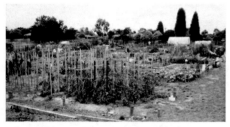

A community garden in Melbourne, Australia.

Source: HelloMojo. Community garden, Melbourne, Australia. 2007. Available at: http://en.wikipedia.org/wiki/File:Community_Garden,_Melbourne,_Australia.jpg.

With junk food now available in most public places, our relationship with food has become a bit less straightforward. Some of us have the means to acquire food but overindulge in unhealthy choices. Others may experience **food insecurity**, a reduced ability to access and utilize food.

The World Health Organization (WHO) describes three criteria for food security: (1) consistently sufficient quantities of food; (2) resources to ensure adequate access to nutritious foods; and (3) the knowledge about nutrition basics, clean water, and basic sanitation required to use food.[72]

In the United States, many people face unemployment and poverty, which restrict their ability to acquire food. Poorer neighborhoods often lack grocery stores. People living in these "food deserts" may lack the means to travel to a grocery store. Their best option might be an inexpensive hot dog at the fast-food stand or a package of cookies. In the developing world, even those shabby selections may not exist.

Unfortunately, a growing number of people suffer food insecurity, unreliable access to sufficient quantity and quality of food. According to the UN Food and Agriculture Organization (FAO), 1 out of 8 people—about 870 million—go hungry each day.[73] About a billion people are chronically undernourished. More than twice that number is deficient in various important nutrients.[74]

In the United States, the economic crisis has pushed more people into poverty and, hence, hunger. A 2010 survey found that 14.5 percent (17.2 million) households suffered food insecurity.[75] In nearly 4 million households, children at times went hungry.

Food-assistance programs provide a safety net for many Americans. The Supplemental Nutrition Assistance Program (formerly known as the Food Stamp Program) is the largest. The Special Supplemental Nutrition Program for Women, Infants, and Children (WIC) serves at-risk, low-income women, infants, and children under age five. In 2011, WIC provided assistance to nine million women and children a month, including half of American infants.[76] School breakfast and afterschool meal programs continue to grow. President Obama has pledged to maintain these programs. Budget projections anticipate that, as the economy bounces back, fewer people will require assistance.[77]

However, world hunger is expected to worsen because the world's population continues to grow, intensive agriculture and deforestation have depleted soil, and global warming has expanded areas too arid to support crops. The WHO notes that, while enough food is currently produced, distribution to those who most need it remains a problem. It isn't yet clear how globalization will impact food insecurity in developing countries.[78]

Another problem that needs to be addressed is food waste. The FAO estimates the yearly food waste tally at 1.3 billion tons. The annual loss in the United States is about 33 million tons. About 40 percent of food produced in America isn't eaten.[79] Reducing food loss by 15 percent annually could feed another 25 million people.

At home and abroad, some organizations are working to reduce food waste. Many retail vendors (grocery stores, restaurants) discard edible food. Some organizations distribute that food to homeless shelters and food kitchens. For example, the Boulder Food Rescue (http://www.boulderfoodrescue.org) delivers food in bicycle-pulled carts. Concrete Jungle (http://www.concrete-jungle.org) harvests Atlanta's "neglected produce" (e.g., apples no one would otherwise eat) and donates it to homeless shelters and food banks. Individuals can also contribute by refraining from buying, cooking, and serving more perishable food than can be used.

Activists have also started community gardens in low-income urban neighborhoods. Large greenhouse gardens can provide food year round. For an example, check out GrowHaus, which is in Denver, Colorado (http://www.thegrowhaus.com/about).

College campuses are getting on board with planting crops to provide educational opportunities and food relief. Take, for instance, the Yale Farm, part of Yale University's Sustainable Food Project (http://www.yale.edu/sustainablefood/farm.html). Participants learn about production and distribution of food that's economically and environmentally sustainable.

 Video Clip 8.3

A Place at the Table
This video is the trailer for the documentary film *A Place at the Table*, about food insecurity in America. The film's website provides the means for you to get involved and end hunger in this country. Check out http://www.takepart.com/place-at-the-table.

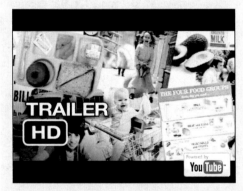

View the video online at: http://www.youtube.com/v/DKOiT1vY7v0

Reducing Food Waste: What You Can Do

Disposing of wasted food consumes even more energy. Plus, food rotting in landfills releases methane, a powerful greenhouse gas that contributes to global warming. Here are some simple ways you can help.

- **Shop smart.** Buy only as much as you can eat before it goes bad. Plan your menu for the next few days and bring a shopping list to the store. Don't give in to impulses or special deals.
- **Buy minimally packaged food.** Doing so reduces the cost to produce food, your cost at the checkout stand, and the environmental burden associated with packaging.
- **Embrace imperfections.** Produce doesn't have to be perfect. A blemish or two won't undermine the nutritional content.
- **Use up what's in the fridge.** The Internet abounds with recipe websites. If you find yourself with too much of, say, rutabaga, find a recipe that will help you put it to use.

- **Freeze for later.** Have leftovers but no chance to eat them? Freeze for a rainy day. You can also freeze fresh produce in freezer bags. (Alternatively, leftovers can be fed to chickens or a pig.)
- **Order small plates at restaurants.** You can always order more. The same goes for cafeteria lines. You don't need to try everything. Make up your mind on what you want and don't be tempted to heap more on your plate. If you arrive famished, you may overestimate how much you can put away. Alternatively, request a to-go box to package the remains to eat later.
- **Compost discards.** Doing so will enrich your garden and reduce landfill overloads. To learn more, go to http://howtocompost.org.
- **Get involved.** Donate unspoiled food to soup kitchens and food banks. Find out whether your campus has programs for rounding up food from campus dining halls and delivering it to food banks. Find out if any local organizations rescue and redistribute food to hungry people. Volunteer at a soup kitchen.
- **Plant seeds for the needy.** If your campus lacks a community garden, perhaps you're the right person to get one started.

Source: Adapted from "Your Scraps Add Up: Reducing Food Waste Can Save Money and Resources." National Resources Defense Council website. Available at: http://www.nrdc.org/living/eatingwell/files/foodwaste_2pgr.pdf.

4.1   Positive Changes in the Food Industry

Increasingly, activists have promoted a return to our roots. They offer to reinvent the food system in America and beyond. Small organic farms have cropped up. Farmers' markets stocked with local produce, meat, eggs, and flowers attract throngs. Even mainstream supermarkets stock organic food.

Organizations like Slow Food work to counter the fast-food culture. This international grassroots movement seeks to make good, clean food available to everyone. Educational projects teach children and adults about where their food comes from. The goal is to help people appreciate food and take responsibility for the impact of their choices. The concept is antithetical to fast food: good food takes time to grow, prepare, and properly enjoy. It's beautiful, smells good, and tastes delightful. It nourishes us without harming the planet. Slow Food advocates for farmers and cooks who produce wholesome food. The organization supports biodiversity (preserving a variety of plant and animal species) and celebrates cultural diversity.

Farmers' markets represent a manifestation of these values. Between 1970 and 2011, the number of farmers' markets increased twenty-fold.[80] That couldn't have happened without the public's support. What's to like about farmers' markets? The farmers who sell at community markets operate smaller operations. They tend to grow their plants in ways that better conserve soil. For instance, rather than monocrop, they rotate the plants grown in any given area. Animals are more likely to be treated humanely.

Check out local markets. Ask questions. Are the fruits and vegetables organic? Were the animals allowed to range? How are the animals housed? Were they given antibiotics and hormones to stimulate growth?

Buying directly from farmers who adopt sustainable, responsible practices helps them stay in business. An increase in regional food production creates jobs. Buying locally reduces the energy costs of processing, packaging, and shipping foods long distances. Buying from local farmers and ranchers reduces energy costs from shipping.

You benefit too. The food is fresh. People who shop at farmers' markets tend to buy more fruits and vegetables than those who only shop at supermarkets. That means you might eat better. It also provides an opportunity to get outside, walk, and meet people in your community.

Another way you can get involved is to join a CSA, which stands for community-supported agriculture. The economic model is radically different from the traditional supermarket. A group of people pledge their support to a farm. At the start of the season, each member buys a subscription, which entitles him or her to a weekly box of fresh produce. In this way, small farmers have the funds to invest in the spring harvest, promoting agricultural methods that are economically and environmentally sustainable.

Video Clip 8.4

Community-Supported Agriculture
This video explains how a CSA functions.

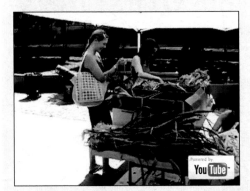

View the video online at: http://www.youtube.com/v/rcR2J63_44c

 Video Clip 8.5

Sustainably Produced Local Food
Emory University's Sustainable Food Initiative discusses initiatives to promote sustainable local food
production and biodiversity.

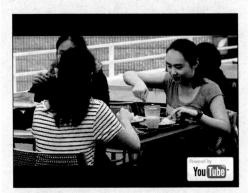

View the video online at: http://www.youtube.com/v/IWVourjphj4
Source: Emory University.

KEY TAKEAWAYS

- Food insecurity is a pressing concern around the world.
- People have the power to transform the way we grow, prepare, and eat food. Hopeful signs abound.
- Consumers can make food choices that lessen the negative impact on the environment.

DISCUSSION QUESTIONS

1. For the next day, keep notes about the food waste in your everyday life. What are your ideas for reducing food waste?
2. Keep a record of the foods and beverages you consume that come in packages. If you do your own grocery shopping, pay attention to where the food comes from. What steps could you take immediately to reduce the negative environmental impact of your food choices?

5. RECOMMENDED RESOURCES

5.1 Books

Pollan M. *Food Rules: An Eater's Manual*. New York, NY: Penguin Press; 2011.

Pollan M. *In Defense of Food: An Eater's Manifesto*. New York, NY: Penguin Press; 2008.

Pollan M. *The Omnivore's Dilemma: A Natural History of Four Meals*. New York, NY: Penguin Press; 2006.

Schlosser E. *Fast Food Nation: The Dark Side of the All-American Meal*. New York, NY: Houghton Mifflin Harcourt; 2001.

5.2 Organizations and Websites

Academy of Nutrition and Dietetics (formerly American Dietetics Association). http://www.eatright.org.

Alternative Farming Systems Information Center. National Agricultural Library. US Department of Agriculture. http://www.nal.usda.gov/afsic/pubs/csa/csa.shtml.

Centers for Disease Control and Prevention, Nutrition for Everyone. http://www.cdc.gov/nutrition/everyone/index.html.

Food and Agriculture Organization of the United Nations. http://www.fao.org.

Food and Nutrition Center, National Agriculture Library, US Department of Agriculture. http://fnic.nal.usda.gov.

Food & Water Watch. http://www.foodandwaterwatch.org.

Food Research and Action Center. http://www.frac.org.

Hunger in America: 2012 United States Hunger and Poverty Facts. http://www.worldhunger.org/articles/Learn/us_hunger_facts.htm.

Office of Dietary Supplements, National Institutes of Health. http://ods.od.nih.gov.

Save Food. http://www.save-food.org.

Slow Food International. http://www.slowfood.com.

Slow Food USA. http://www.slowfoodusa.org.

US Department of Agriculture. http://www.usda.gov.

Vegetarian Nutrition, Academy of Nutrition and Dietetics. http://vegetariannutrition.net.

World Hunger. http://www.worldhunger.org.

5.3 Movies

Food, Inc. (2008) is a documentary film that investigates corporate-controlled agriculture in America.

A Place at the Table (2012) is a documentary film about hunger in the United States.

Super Size Me (2004) is a documentary of what happens when independent filmmaker Morgan Spurlock eats only McDonald's food for 30 consecutive days.

5.4 Videos

Food Rules for Healthy People and Planet (2010). In this video (produced by the Royal Society for the encouragement of Arts, Manufactures and Commerce), Michael Pollan discusses food choices that promote the health of humans and the environment. http://www.youtube.com/watch?v=c31cAdYUvT8.

In Defense of Food with Michael Pollan (2008). In this University of California, Santa Barbara, video, Michael Pollan discusses using ecology and tradition to inform the way we eat. 55 minutes. http://www.youtube.com/watch?v=sBr_i1mH_08&feature=relmfu.

Michael Pollan: The Omnivore's Dilemma (2006). In this lecture, filmed at the University of California, Davis, UC Berkeley journalism professor and award-winning author Michael Pollan explores the ecology of eating. 59 minutes. http://www.youtube.com/watch?v=kFpjskn3_Pc.

ENDNOTES

1. Good nutrition: should guidelines differ for men and women? Harvard Medical School Family Health Guide. Harvard Health Publications. Available at: http://www.health.harvard.edu/fhg/updates/update0906b.shtml. Accessed November 2, 2012.

2. Dietary reference intakes: electrolytes and water. Institute of Medicine. Available at: http://www.iom.edu/Global/News%20Announcements/~/media/442A08B899F44DF9AAD083D86164C75B.ashx. Accessed June 5, 2013.

3. Water facts. Water.org. Available at: http://water.org/water-crisis/water-facts/water. Accessed November 3, 2012.

4. Bottled water: illusions of purity. Food & Water Watch. Available at: http://www.foodandwaterwatch.org/water/bottled/bottled-water-illusions-of-purity. Accessed July 3, 2013.

5. Bottled water costs consumers and the environment. Food & Water Watch. Available at: http://www.foodandwaterwatch.org/water/bottled/bottled-water-bad-for-people-and-the-environment. Accessed November 3, 2012.

6. Nielsen LJ, Kit BK, Fakhouri T, Ogden C. Calories Consumed from Alcoholic Beverages by US Adults, 2007–2010. Centers for Disease Control and Prevention; 2012. NCHS Data Brief, no. 110. Available at: http://www.cdc.gov/nchs/data/databriefs/db110.pdf. Accessed November 15, 2012.

7. Hanaway PJ. Irritable bowel syndrome. In: Rakel D, ed. Integrative Medicine. 2nd ed. Philadelphia, PA: Elsevier; 2007:465.

8. Dietary reference intakes: macronutrients. Institute of Medicine. Available at: http://www.iom.edu/Global/News%20Announcements/~/media/C5CD2DD7840544979A549EC47E56A02B.ashx. Accessed November 11, 2012.

9. Page KA, Chan O, Jagriti A, et al. Effects of fructose versus glucose on regional cerebral blood flow in brain regions involved with appetite and reward pathways. JAMA. 2013;309(1):63–70.

10. Gaby AR. Adverse effects of dietary fructose. Alternat Med Rev. 2005;10(4):294–306.

11. Evans WJ. Protein nutrition, exercise and aging. J Am Coll Nutr. 2004 Dec;23 Suppl 6:601S–609S.

12. Baum SJ, Kris-Etherton PM, Willett WC, et al. Fatty acids in cardiovascular health and disease: a comprehensive update. J Clin Lipidol. 2012 May;6(3):216–234.

13. Baum SJ, Kris-Etherton PM, Willett WC, et al. Fatty acids in cardiovascular health and disease: a comprehensive update. J Clin Lipidol. 2012 May;6(3):216–234.

14. Ramsden CE, Zamora D, Leelarthaepin B, et al. Use of dietary linoleic acid for secondary prevention of coronary heart disease and death: evaluation of recovered data from the Sydney Diet Heart Study and updated meta-analysis. BMJ. 2013 Feb 4;346:e8707. doi:10.1136/bmj.e8707.

15. Simopoulos AP. Evolutionary aspects of diet: the omega-6/omega-3 ratio and the brain. Mol Neurobiol. 2011;44(2):203–215.

16. Narendran R, Frankle WG, Mason NS, Muldoon MF, Moghaddam B. Improved working memory but no effect on striatal vesicular monoamine transporter type 2 after omega-3 polyunsaturated fatty acid supplementation. PLoS One. 2012;7(10):e46832. doi:10.1371/journal.pone.0046832.

17. Baum SJ, Kris-Etherton PM, Willett WC, et al. Fatty acids in cardiovascular health and disease: a comprehensive update. J Clin Lipidol. 2012 May;6(3):216–234.

18. Dietary reference intakes: macronutrients. Institute of Medicine. Available at: http://www.iom.edu/Global/News%20Announcements/~/media/C5CD2DD7840544979A549EC47E56A02B.ashx. Accessed November 11, 2012.

19. Simopoulos AP. Omega-3 fatty acids in health and disease and in growth and development. Am J Clin Nutr. 1991 Sep;54(3):438–463.

20. Ringsels R, Elder K. Biological effects of frying oils mediated by the activation of peroxisome proliferator-activated receptors (PRAR). Frying oils—nutritional aspects. The AOCS Lipid Library. Available at: http://lipidlibrary.aocs.org/frying/n-ppar/index.htm. Accessed November 13, 2012.

21. Daley AD, Abbott A, Doyle PS, Nader GA, Larson S. A review of fatty acid profiles and antioxidant content in grass-fed and grain-fed beef. Nutr J. 2010;9:10. Available at: http://www.ncbi.nlm.nih.gov/pmc/articles/PMC2846864. Accessed November 15, 2012.

22. Ponnampalam EN, Mann NJ, Sinclair AJ. Effect of feeding systems on omega-3 fatty acids, conjugated linoleic acid and trans fatty acids in Australian beef cuts: potential impact on human health. Asia Pac J Clin Nutr. 2006;15(1):21–29.

23. Dilzer A, Park Y. Implication of conjugated linoleic acid (CLA) in human health. Crit Rev Food Sci Nutr. 2012;52(6):488–513.

24. Daley CA, Abbott A, Doyle PS, Nader GA, Larson S. A review of fatty acid profiles and antioxidant content in grass-fed and grain-fed beef. Nutr J. 2010;9:10. Available at: http://www.ncbi.nlm.nih.gov/pmc/articles/PMC2846864. Accessed November 13, 2012.

25. Leiber F, Kreuzer M, Nigg D, Wettstein HR, Scheeder MR. A study on the causes for the elevated n-3 fatty acids in cows' milk of alpine origin. Lipids. 2005 Feb;40(2):191–202.

26. Lopez-Bote CJ, Sanz Arias AI, Rey A, et al. Effect of free-range feeding on omega-3 fatty acids and alpha-tocopherol content and oxidative stability of eggs. Anim Feed Sci Technol. 1998;72:33–40.

27. Ponte PI, Alves SP, Bessa RJ, et al. Influence of pasture intake on the fatty acid composition, and cholesterol, tocopherols, and tocotrienols content in meat from free-range broilers. Poult Sci. 2008;87(1):80–88.

28. Sun T, Liu Z, Qin L, Long R. Meat fatty acid and cholesterol level of free-range broilers fed on grasshoppers on alpine rangeland in the Tibetan Plateau. J Sci Food Agric. 2012 Aug 30;92(11):2239–2243. doi:10.1002/jsfa.5609.

29. USDA national nutrient database for standard reference, release 17. National Agriculture Library. US Department of Agriculture. Available at: http://www.nal.usda.gov/fnic/foodcomp/Data/SR17/wtrank/sr17a401.pdf. Accessed November 16, 2012.

30. Online resources for disorders caused by oxidative stress. Oxidative Stress Resource. Available at: http://www.oxidativestressresource.org. Accessed January 22, 2012.

31. Sivanandham V. Free radicals in health and diseases. Pharmacologyonline. 2011;1:1062–1077. Available at: http://www.unisa.it/uploads/4978/101.velavan.pdf. Accessed January 23, 2013.

32. Zittermann A. The estimated benefits of vitamin D for Germany. Mol Nutr Food Res. 2010;54(8):1164–1171.

33. Hewison M. Vitamin D and immune function: an overview. Proc Nutr Soc. 2012;71(1):50–61.

34. Tiosano D, Gepstein V. Vitamin D action: lessons learned from hereditary 1, 25-dihydroxyvitamin-D-resistant rickets patients. Curr Opin Endocrinol Diabetes Obes. 2012 Dec;19(6):452–459. doi:10.1097/MED.0b013e32835a3415.

35. Lerchbaum E, Obermayer-Pietsch B. Vitamin D and fertility: a systematic review. Eur J Endocrinol. 2012 May;166(5):765–778.

36. Balion C, Griffith LE, Strifler L, et al. Vitamin D, cognition, and dementia: a systematic review and meta-analysis. Neurology. 2012;79(13):1397–1405.

37. Dietary reference intakes for calcium and vitamin D. Report brief. Institute of Medicine. November 30, 2010. Available at: http://www.iom.edu/Reports/2010/Dietary-Reference-Intakes-for-Calcium-and-Vitamin-D/Report-Brief.aspx. Accessed November 16, 2012.

38. Dietary supplement fact sheet: Vitamin D. Office of Dietary Supplements. National Institutes of Health. Available at: http://ods.od.nih.gov/factsheets/VitaminD-HealthProfessional. Accessed January 23, 2013.

39. Frassetto LA, Todd KM, Morris RC Jr, Sebastian A. Worldwide incidence of hip fracture in elderly women: relation to consumption of animal and vegetable foods. J Gerontol A Biol Sci Med Sci. 2000 Oct;55(10):M585–M592.

40. Lanou AJ. Should dairy be recommended as part of a healthy vegetarian diet? Counterpoint. Am J Clin Nutr. 2009 May;89(5):1638S–1642S.

41. Ho-Pham LT, Vu BQ, Lai TQ, Nguyen ND, Nguyen TV. Vegetarianism, bone loss, fracture and vitamin D: a longitudinal study in Asian vegans and non-vegans. Eur J Clin Nutr. 2012 Jan;66(1):75–82. doi:10.1038/ejcn.2011.131.

42. Dietary supplement fact sheet: calcium. Office of Dietary Supplements. National Institutes of Health. Available at: http://ods.od.nih.gov/factsheets/Calcium-HealthProfessional. Accessed January 23, 2013.

43. Rosanoff A, Weaver CM, Rude RK. Suboptimal magnesium status in the United States: are the health consequences underestimated? Nutr Rev. 2012 Mar;70(3):153–164. doi:10.1111/j.1753-4887.2011.00465.x.

44. Messina MJ, Loprinzi CL. Soy for breast cancer survivors: a critical review of the literature. J Nutr. 2001 Nov;131 Suppl 11:3095S–108S.

45. Can you afford to eat right? Tufts University Health & Nutrition Letter. May 2008. Available at: http://www.tuftshealthletter.com/ShowArticle.aspx?rowId=545. Accessed November 30, 2012.

46. Strauss S, Clara M. Davis and the wisdom of letting children choose their own diets. CMAJ. 2006;175(10):1199–1201. Available at: http://www.ncbi.nlm.nih.gov/pmc/articles/PMC1626509. Accessed November 2, 2012.

47. DiLeone RJ, Taylor JR, Picciotto MR. The drive to eat: comparisons and distinctions between mechanisms of food reward and drug addiction. Nat Neurosci. 2012;15(10):1330–1335. doi:10.1038/nn.3202.

48. Everyday eating for a healthier you. Academy of Nutrition and Dietetics. Available at: http://www.eatright.org/search.aspx?search=servings%20fruits%20and%20vegetables. Accessed November 28, 2012.

49. Thompson JL, Manore MM, Vaughan LA. The Science of Nutrition. San Francisco, CA: Pearson; 2008:398.

50. Stahler C. How often do Americans eat vegetarian meals? How many adults in the US are vegetarian? The Vegetarian Resource Group Blog. May 18, 2012. Available at: http://www.vrg.org/blog/2012/05/18/how-often-do-americans-eat-vegetarian-meals-and-how-many-adults-in-the-u-s-are-vegetarian. Accessed June 6, 2013.

51. Tantamango-Bartley Y, Jaceldo-Siegl K, Fan J, Fraser G. Vegetarian diets and the incidence of cancer in a low-risk population. Cancer Epidemiol Biomarkers Prev. 2012 Nov 20 [Epub ahead of print].

52. Tonstad S, Stewart K, Oda K, Batech M, Herring RP, Fraser GE. Vegetarian diets and incidence of diabetes in the Adventist Health Study-2. Nutr Metab Cardiovasc Dis. 2011 Oct 7 [Epub ahead of print].

53. Vitamin B12 in vegetarian diets. Vegetarian nutrition. American Dietetic Association. Available at: http://vegetariannutrition.net/docs/B12-Vegetarian-Nutrition.pdf. Accessed November 28, 2012.

54. Nutrition facts label programs and materials. Food and Drug Administration. Available at: http://www.fda.gov/Food/ResourcesForYou/Consumers/NFLPM/default.htm. Accessed November 25, 2012.

55. Meat and poultry labeling terms. Fact sheets. US Department of Agriculture. Available at: http://www.fsis.usda.gov/FACTSheets/Meat_&_Poultry_Labeling_Terms/index.asp#14. Accessed November 25, 2012.

56. Sousa AA, Azevedo E, Lima EE, Silva AP. Organic foods and human health: a study of controversies. *Rev Panam Salud Publica*. 2012 Jun;31(6):513–517.

57. Smith-Spangler C, Brandeau ML, Hunter GE, et al. Are organic foods safer or healthier than conventional alternatives? A systematic review. *Ann Intern Med*. 2012 Sep 4;157(5):348–366. doi:10.7326/0003-4819-157-5-201209040-00007.

58. EWG's 2012 shopper's guide to pesticides in produce. Environmental Working Group. Available at: http://www.ewg.org/foodnews/summary. Accessed November 13, 2012.

59. What is a dietary supplement? Food and Drug Administration. Available at: http://www.fda.gov/Food/DietarySupplements/default.htm#what_is. Accessed November 25, 2012.

60. Branum AM, Lukacs SL. Food allergy among children in the United States. *Pediatrics*. 2009;124:1549–1555.

61. Gupta RS, Springston BA, Warrier MR, et al. The prevalence, severity, and distribution of childhood food allergy in the United States. *Pediatrics*. 2011 Jul;128(1):e9–17. doi:10.1542/peds.2011–0204.

62. Leonard SA. Food allergy: what you need to know. *Medscape Today*. November 15, 2010. Available at: http://www.medscape.com/viewarticle/732184. Accessed June 12, 2011.

63. Anaphylactic reactions. *The Merck Manual Home Health Handbook*. Online version. Whitehouse Station, NJ: Merck Sharp & Dohme Corp. (a subsidiary of Merck & Co.); 2010. Available at: http://www.merckmanuals.com/home/sec16/ch185/ch185i.html. Accessed June 3, 2011.

64. Is it a food allergy or intolerance? Allergies Health Center. WebMD. Available at: http://www.webmd.com/allergies/foods-allergy-intolerance. Accessed June 3, 2011.

65. Celiac disease. National Digestive Diseases Information Clearinghouse. Available at: http://digestive.niddk.nih.gov/ddiseases/pubs/celiac. Accessed November 21, 2012.

66. Osterholm MT. Foodborne disease in 2011—the rest of the story. *N Engl J Med*. 2011;364(10):889–891.

67. McVeigh K. Scientists: overuse of antibiotics in animal agriculture endangers humans. *The Guardian*. Sept. 19, 2012. Available at: http://www.guardian.co.uk/science/2012/sep/19/scientists-antibiotics-animal-agriculture. Accessed November 13, 2012.

68. Prescription for trouble: using antibiotics to fatten livestock. Union of Concerned Scientists. Available at: http://www.ucsusa.org/food_and_agriculture/our-failing-food-system/industrial-agriculture/prescription-for-trouble.html. Accessed November 13, 2012.

69. Recent trends in GE adoption. US Department of Agriculture. Available at: http://www.ers.usda.gov/data-products/adoption-of-genetically-engineered-crops-in-the-us/recent-trends-in-ge-adoption.aspx. Accessed November 29, 2012.

70. Genetically engineered food: an overview. Food & Water Watch. Available at: http://www.foodandwaterwatch.org/reports/genetically-engineered-food. Accessed November 29, 2012.

71. Keener KM. To zap or not to zap. Department of Food Science, Food Irradiation. FSR 98-13. North Carolina State University. Available at: http://www.ces.ncsu.edu/depts/foodsci/ext/pubs/irradiation.pdf. Accessed November 29, 2012.

72. Food security. World Health Organization. Available at: http://www.who.int/trade/glossary/story028/en. Accessed November 30, 2012.

73. The state of food insecurity in the world 2012. Food and Agriculture Organization of the United Nations. Available at: http://www.fao.org/infographics/pdf/FAO-infographic-SOFI-2012-en.pdf. Accessed November 1, 2012.

74. Barrett CB. Measure food insecurity. *Science*. 2010;327(5967):825–828. doi:10/1126/science.1182768.

75. Coleman-Jensen A, Nord M, Andrews M, Carlson S. Household food security in the United States in 2010. Economic Research Report No. (ERR-125). September 2011. USDA Economic Research Service. Available at: http://www.ers.usda.gov/publications/err-economic-research-report/err125.aspx. Accessed November 1, 2012.

76. WIC program. Food & nutrition assistance. USDA Economic Research Service. Available at: http://www.ers.usda.gov/topics/food-nutrition-assistance/wic-program.aspx. Accessed November 30, 2012.

77. Fiscal year 2013. Food Research and Action Center. Available at: http://frac.org/leg-act-center/budget-and-appropriations/budget-analysis. Accessed November 30, 2012.

78. Food security. World Health Organization. Available at: http://www.who.int/trade/glossary/story028/en. Accessed November 30, 2012.

79. Wasted: how America is losing up to 40 percent of its food from farm to fork to landfill. Natural Resources Defense Council. Available at: http://www.nrdc.org/food/wasted-food.asp. Accessed November 1, 2012.

80. Market forces: creating jobs through public investment in local and regional food systems. Union of Concerned Scientists. Available at: http://www.ucsusa.org/food_and_agriculture/solutions/expand-healthy-food-access/market-forces.html. Accessed November 13, 2012.

CHAPTER 9
Physical Fitness

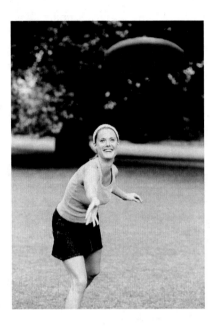

© Thinkstock

Explorers such as Juan Ponce de Léon searched for the legendary Fountain of Youth. We mortals can't live forever, but we do have the means to improve current well-being and ensure healthy aging. Our best tool is physical activity. Our bodies are designed to move. Exercise maintains the infrastructure; sedentary lifestyles dismantle it. Bones thin and muscles weaken; fat takes up the slack. As the late fitness guru Jack LaLanne famously said, "The only way you can hurt your body is if you don't use it."[1]

This chapter reviews physical activity guides, the many benefits of exercise, and the perils of sedentary lifestyles. You'll find tips on incorporating physical activity into your life—no matter how busy and penny-pinched you are. You'll learn how to choose equipment, start and stick with an exercise plan, and avoid injury.

1. FITNESS BASICS

LEARNING OBJECTIVES

1. Define physical activity, exercise, and physical fitness.
2. Identify and define the components of health-related fitness.
3. Describe the Federal government's guidelines for physical activity.
4. Compare and contrast health benefits associated with aerobic exercise, resistance training, and flexibility training.
5. Calculate your target heart rate for aerobic exercise.
6. Define skill-related components of fitness.

The sad fact is that few Americans take time to exercise. Among people 18 and older, just over one-third engage in some kind of regular leisure-time physical activity; one-third are sometimes physically active; and another third do no physical activity outside of work.[2] About 55 percent of adults never exercise vigorously; a mere 13 percent do so five times a week or more.

Geographic, economic, racial, and gender disparities exist. The least active parts of the country are also the poorest—the South and Appalachia (Alabama, Louisiana, Mississippi, Kentucky, Oklahoma, and Tennessee).[3] Whites and Asians/Pacific Islanders tend to be more active than Hispanics and blacks.[4]

Boys are more active than girls. However, even children aren't getting enough exercise. Our government recommends that children and teens engage in moderate physical activity at least 60 minutes a day. Yet most states don't require school recess, and only about half have laws requiring the recommended minimum for school physical education.[5]

FIGURE 9.1 Participation in Physical Activity

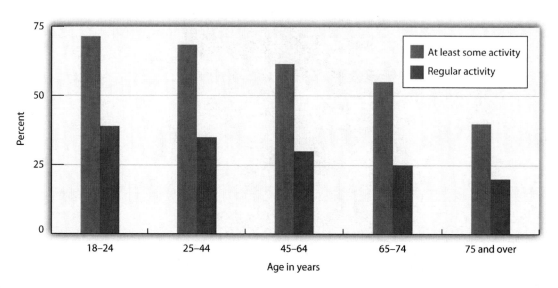

You may have noticed that I've been using *physical activity* and *exercise* interchangeably. However, their meanings differ slightly. **Physical activity** means any movement of skeletal muscles requiring extra energy. (Skeletal muscles are those that move your body and maintain your posture when sitting or standing.) **Exercise** is any type of physical activity designed to improve health and physical fitness. More regimented and planned than physical activity, exercise usually involves repetitive actions. For instance, vacuuming your room is a physical activity, but you probably wouldn't vacuum daily to keep fit.

Another key term is **physical fitness**, which generally means a person has the capacity to perform a variety of physical activities. A fit individual possesses health, overall well-being, vitality, and energy. More specifically, physical fitness refers to particular attributes: a lean physique, a strong heart and lungs, sturdy bones and muscles, and skills such as agility, balance, and speed.[6]

1.1 Components of Health-Related Fitness

There are two main fitness categories. *Skill-related* physical fitness includes agility, balance, coordination, speed, and quick reactions. Such skills might enable you to play a rousing game of tennis. Fitness that more generally improves health is called **health-related physical fitness**. Its five components are body composition, cardiovascular fitness, muscular endurance, muscular strength, and flexibility. The US Department of Health and Human Services (HHS) has established recommendations for each of the components of health-related fitness.

physical activity

Any bodily movement produced by skeletal muscles and requiring an energy expenditure beyond resting.

exercise

Structured, planned, and repetitive physical activity that improves health and physical fitness.

physical fitness

The body's ability to function efficiently during physical activities. Fitness can be general for overall health, as well as specific to a particular activity.

health-related physical fitness

Consists of those components of physical fitness that contribute to good health: body composition, cardiovascular fitness, muscular endurance, muscular strength, and flexibility.

Body Composition

Body composition is the proportion of fat to lean tissue (muscle, bone, organs, and water). **Fat-free mass** is another name for lean tissue. While fat has useful functions such as storing extra calories, too much fat correlates with conditions such as diabetes and heart disease.

In Chapter 10, we discuss different methods for measuring body composition. A commonly used estimate of body fat is **body mass index (BMI)**. The formula for determining it is as follows:

$$BMI = \text{weight in kilograms} \,/\, \text{height in meters squared}$$

or

$$BMI = \text{weight in pounds}/(\text{height in inches})^2 \text{x} 703$$

Alternatively, you can go to the online BMI calculator provided by the Centers for Disease Control and Prevention (CDC) at http://www.cdc.gov/healthyweight/assessing/bmi/adult_bmi/english_bmi_calculator/bmi_calculator.html.

BMI, while useful, tells only part of the story. Two people with the same BMI may not have the same body composition. For instance, a football linebacker and sedentary computer programmer might both stand 6 feet tall and weigh 200 pounds. Both have a BMI of 27, which is in the overweight range. The more muscular football player, however, carries less fat.

Physical activity improves body composition in two ways. One, if caloric intake is held constant, fat is lost. Two, regular exercise increases muscle and bone mass. Additionally, after a person has successfully lost unhealthy weight, continued exercise helps prevent regain of unhealthy abdominal fat.[7]

Cardiorespiratory Fitness

The cardiovascular system includes the heart and blood vessels (arteries, veins, and the tiny capillaries). Add in the lungs and you get the cardiorespiratory system. The respiratory system's job is to inhale oxygen-rich air and exhale carbon dioxide and other gaseous waste products. The cardiovascular system's job is to deliver oxygen and nutrients to cells all over the body and to return carbon dioxide and other waste products to the lungs.

Cardiorespiratory fitness is the ability of the cardiovascular and respiratory systems to deliver oxygen and nutrients to muscles during sustained activity. **Aerobic exercise** or "cardio" improves this type of fitness. The American College of Sports Medicine (ACSM) defines aerobic exercise as "any activity that uses large muscle groups in a continuous, rhythmical fashion, and that is relatively easy to maintain at a consistent intensity."[8] Examples include brisk walking, jogging, swimming, cross-country skiing, cycling, dancing, and pushing a lawn mower.

These exercises are sufficiently vigorous to increase the need for oxygen—without surpassing the ability of the respiratory and cardiovascular systems to supply it. In response, heart and breathing rates increase. During aerobic exercise, large muscle groups have to work for a sustained period.

How do you know your exercise is aerobic? Your respiratory and heart rate rise such that you can carry on a brief conversation but have trouble singing. In fact, heart rate is used to gauge the intensity of aerobic exercise. The sidebar "Calculating Your Target Heart Rate" explains how to calculate your target heart rate for moderate or vigorous aerobic exercise. Brisk walking, cycling over flat terrain, and doubles tennis count as moderate exercise; running, cycling up a steep hill, and singles tennis count as vigorous exercise. For more examples of moderate-intensity versus vigorous-intensity activities, go to the following page on the World Health Organization's website: http://www.who.int/dietphysicalactivity/physical_activity_intensity/en/index.html.

If you begin gasping for air, you've entered the realm of **anaerobic exercise**. Anaerobic means "without oxygen." It's hard to sustain that kind of exercise, and you're more likely to feel sore afterward. Sprinting and lifting heavy weights represent types of anaerobic exercise.

The HHS recommends that adults participate in at least 2.5 hours of moderately intense aerobic exercise or 1.25 hours of vigorously intense aerobic exercise each week. Usually, the total weekly time is distributed over two or three days. Each exercise period can be as short as 10 minutes. Who doesn't have time for a 10-minute brisk walk or bike ride?

The overall accumulation of exercise is what's important, not the length or intensity of any single event. If you can't fit in a couple of hours of aerobic exercise each week, don't despair and don't give up. Even getting half the recommended amount has significant benefits and decreases your risk of chronic illnesses such as heart disease.

One of the many benefits of regular cardiorespiratory exercise is an increase in **VO$_2$ max**, your body's efficiency at using oxygen. A more precise definition is the rate of oxygen utilization per kilogram (2.2 pounds) body weight per minute during maximal exercise. Basically, the lungs, heart, and arteries get better at delivering oxygen to muscles, which excel at extracting oxygen from the blood. The

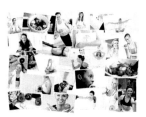

© *Thinkstock*

body composition

Proportion of fat to lean tissue.

fat-free mass

The cumulative mass of all body tissues except fat tissue.

body mass index (BMI)

Body weight in kilograms divided by height in meters squared, or weight in pounds times 703 divided by height in inches squared.

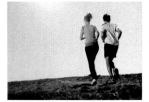

© *Thinkstock*

cardiorespiratory fitness

The ability of the heart and lungs to work efficiently during sustained exercise bouts.

aerobic exercise

Exercises using large muscle groups that increase heart rate and breathing rate for a sustained time period.

anaerobic exercise

Short bursts of exercise that last fewer than three minutes.

net result is that your capacity for sustained, vigorous exercise rises. Long hikes and bike rides with friends become pleasurable rather than arduous.

Calculating Your Target Heart Rate

In cardiorespiratory exercise, the goal is to elevate your heart rate. Your maximum heart rate is a function of your age. To calculate yours, subtract your age from 220. However, you don't need to push your heart to its limits. Benefits occur at a target heart rate range of 50 to 85 percent of your maximum heart rate. Moderate-intensity aerobic exercise is in the 50 percent to 70 percent zone; vigorous-intensity exercise occurs in the 70 percent to 85 percent zone.

To figure out your target heart rate range for moderate-intensity aerobic exercise, multiply your maximum heart rate by 0.50, then multiply it by 0.70. For example, if you're 20 years old, you calculate it as follows:

$$(220-20) \times 0.50 = 200 \times 0.50 = 100$$

$$(220-20) \times 0.70 = 200 \times 0.70 = 140$$

That means your heart rate should be between 100 and 140 beats per minute. If you want to push yourself into vigorous activity, your heart rate should be between 140 and 170 (200×0.85) beats per minute.

Muscular Strength and Endurance

Regular physical activity promotes muscular strength and endurance.

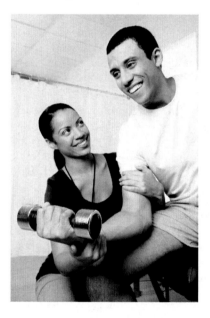

© *Thinkstock*

muscular strength

The ability of skeletal muscle tissue to contract in order to move or hold against resistance.

resistance training

Activity that voluntarily recruits motor units in order to enhance muscular strength and/or endurance.

Muscular strength is the muscle's capacity to generate force to move against resistance. Resistance is anything that a muscle needs to overcome in order to contract. The greater your muscular strength, the less effort it takes to perform physical work. It's what allows you to jump with joy, scramble into an upper bunk, and hoist a backpack of books.

To build muscular strength, you need to do **resistance training**. The goal is to load the muscles with more weight than they're accustomed to by using weight machines, free weights (dumbbells), elastic bands, or rubber tubes. Lifting everyday objects—jugs of milk, bricks, and textbooks—counts too. You can also work against your own body weight by doing exercises such as push-ups, sit-ups, standing calf raises, squats, and lunges—all activities that fit nicely into a study break. Pull-ups, which require grasping an overhead bar and lifting your body weight off the ground, recruits more muscles than simple bicep curls.

For people with access to a gym, weight machines offer a couple advantages. One, they stabilize your body in proper form in order to avoid potential injury as you perform the movement. Two, you usually don't need a personal trainer to figure out how to use them. If you have doubts, ask a gym attendant. It's also wise to get advice about reasonable settings for weights on these machines and the number of repetitions recommended.

On the other hand, free weights and resistance bands may require initial training about correct usage. The advantage is that they also require balance and control. You add the challenge of working out while standing on inflatable cushions or half-dome-shaped objects called BOSU balls. Doing so recruits muscles in your torso (which builds core strength); the balance required also trains the nervous system. Before you begin, ask a professional to teach you proper techniques so you don't get hurt. Your college gym may provide personal trainers for free or at reasonable fees.

Resistance exercises build strength by causing tiny tears in muscle cells. The body's repair process adds more muscle tissue. While you don't grow extra muscle cells, each exercised muscle cell thickens—a process called **hypertrophy**.

Resistance training for the major muscle groups is recommended two to three days each week.[9] Training for one to two days a week maintains an established strength level; three or more days a week increases strength. Alternate days to allow for a rest day between resistance-training sessions.

Before each session, warm up for five minutes. For instance, you can walk and swing your arms. Start with a weight or resistance band that permits 10 consecutive flexions and extensions. Each time you perform the same movement, it is called a "rep"—short for repetition. Each series of reps is called a "set." A typical protocol is 2 to 3 sets of 10 reps each, resting a minute between each set.

Over a week's time, you should work all the major muscle groups: arms (forearm, biceps, triceps), shoulders, back, abdominals, buttocks, and legs (the calves, the quadriceps on the front of the thigh, and the hamstrings on the back of the thigh). Training all these groups promotes balance and good posture, protects surrounding joints, and reduces the risk of injury.

If your goal is to maintain muscle tone, choose a resistance that allows you to perform 12 to 15 reps. If your goal is to build muscle mass, choose a weight that allows for the completion of 8 to 10 reps. The last couple of reps in a set should feel challenging but not cause you to lose proper form. Once a routine seems fairly effortless, steadily increase the resistance, rather than increasing the number of reps or sets. Doing the latter builds endurance.

Muscular endurance is a muscle's capacity to contract and generate force for extended periods of time. Improving your muscular endurance allows you to perform a physical activity for a longer period. Endurance makes it possible to summit a mountain, run a marathon, swim the English Channel, and dance for an entire concert.

To build muscular endurance, you complete a greater number of repetitions and sets against lighter resistance. A reasonable goal is 3 to 5 sets of 10 to 15 repetitions. Separate sets by about 1 to 2 minutes. Assuming your body weight isn't changing, you can gain endurance by steadily increasing the number of times you do activities such as push-ups and lunges. You also gain endurance during aerobic exercises by steadily lengthening the distance you walk, jog, climb stairs, swim, cycle, ski, or row.

hypertrophy

Enlargement of an organ or tissue due to an increase in the size of component cells. Regularly exercised muscles hypertrophy.

muscular endurance

The ability of skeletal muscle to contract and create tension repeatedly for a sustained period of time.

Core Strength

In the past 10 years, the importance of core strength has finally gotten the attention that it deserves. Core strength entails having strength and endurance in the torso muscles. These core muscles are located in your abdomen, sides, back, and buttocks.

Core strength maintains good posture, promotes balance and stability, improves overall sports performance, and prevents and helps rehabilitate back injuries. While core strengthening can be a multifaceted process, anyone can be taught to safely and effectively strengthen these muscles. Some common exercises used today to improve core strength are push-ups, holding a plank pose, and doing abdominal exercises with medicine balls.

Because people often don't maintain proper form during sit-ups and crunches, other abdominal exercises are often recommended. A straightforward exercise that strengthens a number of core muscles, particularly the abdominals, is holding a low plank, also called a forearm plank. Here's how. Drop onto your knees and lay your forearms on the ground so that they form the number 11. (For a bit more support, you can clasp your hands, while keeping your elbows under your shoulders.) Push onto your toes and straighten your legs. Your buttocks should neither sag nor poke up higher than your shoulders. Keep your head and neck in the same neutral position as if you were standing. In other words, look like a plank of wood. Hold the position for 20 seconds or more. Rest 30 seconds and repeat at least three times. A more advanced version is to balance your forearms on a small exercise ball.

If your college has a gym with athletic trainers, ask for instruction on core-strength training or enroll in a class. Some exercise programs, such as Pilates, focus on core strength.

Flexibility

flexibility

The ability of a joint to move through its range of motion.

Flexibility is the ability of joints to move through their full range of motion. Joints are places where the ends of bones come together. Muscle and connective tissue hold the structure together; suppleness in both tissue types allows the joint to move freely.

Stretching exercises help maintain and improve flexibility. For years, the popular belief was that stretching before athletic activity prevented muscle soreness and injury and improved performance.[10] However, studies show benefits to be small or nonexistent. Add this notion to the dustbin of exercise myths.

Nevertheless, flexibility is important. It helps overcome the stiffness inherent in exercises such as running. It also helps counteract the declining range of motion that often accompanies advancing age. Stretching exercises help manage arthritis and low back pain[11] and can reduce musculoskeletal injuries in the workplace.[12] If you're flexible, you'll move more freely and easily. You'll have better balance and agility. You'll glide across the dance floor and be able to do "the limbo" at parties. If you maintain that limberness, you may never need to ask someone else to tie your shoes for you.

FIGURE 9.2

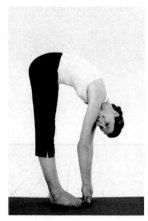

© *Thinkstock*

You don't want to stretch cold muscles. Instead, warm up by using major muscle groups in your legs, backs, and arms. For instance, you can do jumping jacks and jog in place. Stretch at the end of every workout. Stretching exercises are either static or dynamic.

Static stretching entails slowly moving to the point of resistance, then holding the position for about 20 to 60 seconds. An example of a static stretch is to stand with your spine erect. Lean your torso down with your fingers pointing toward your toes. Let your head drop, releasing any tension in your neck, and keep a slight bend in your knees. If you're very flexible, your palms may reach the floor. People with tighter hamstrings may not be able to reach much past their knees. That's okay. You're stretching your spine and the backs of your legs. Plus, your flexibility will improve with practice. Maintain a slow, steady breathing rate while you hold the stretch. See Figure 9.2.

A similar stretch is to sit on the ground with one leg straight ahead of you and the other bent to the side with your foot toward your groin. With a straight spine, hinge forward at the hips. Grasp the foot, ankle, shin, or knee (whatever is available to you) of that straightened leg. If you can reach your foot, pull it gently toward you to stretch your calf and ankle. Hold. Switch legs and repeat. See Figure 9.3.

FIGURE 9.3

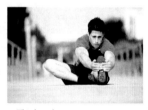

© *Thinkstock*

Dynamic stretching involves moving a joint through its range of motion in a slow and controlled fashion—no bouncing or jerking motions. You're doing a dynamic stretch when you swing your leg or circle your arms. Many athletic activities involve moving certain joints through their range of motion. Think of a tennis player serving, a swimmer doing the butterfly, a ballet dancer kicking a leg into the air, or a gymnast landing a handstand in the splits.

Recommendations are to stretch at least two to three times a week. Ideally, you'll stretch every day. Systematically, address all the major muscle groups and joints—fingers, wrists, arms, shoulders, neck, back, legs, ankles, toes. Flexibility exercises make for nice study breaks. They also can become part of a soothing bedtime ritual.

Most fitness classes and athletic teams add stretching to their routines. Yoga, as practiced in the West, focuses on the physical poses (*asanas*), which combine static stretching, strength, mental focus, and breathing exercises. Pilates combines stretching with working against resistance using a person's own body weight or special equipment. Tai chi, which is adapted from a Chinese martial art, involves flowing movements that build flexibility, coordination, and physical and mental balance.

1.2 Basic Training Principles

overload

Stressing a body system (e.g., the muscles) such that it adapts to a new, higher level of strength or fitness. Progressive overload refers to gradual increases over time in intensity, frequency, or duration.

In order to improve any type of fitness, you must consistently increase the physical demands on your body. The principle of progressive **overload** comes in here. Overload entails stressing a body system (e.g., the muscles) such that it adapts to a new, higher level of strength or fitness. The word "progressive" means that the overload steadily increases to make further fitness gains. You start an exercise routine beyond your current baseline activity level. Soon, that becomes your new normal. To become more fit, you gradually increase the demands.

The principle of progressive overload applies to all the components of health-related fitness. To gain cardiovascular fitness, you might jog a bit farther or a bit faster each week. To build bigger muscles, you gradually increase the resistance while doing the same number of repetitions and sets. For better endurance, you perform the activity for longer and longer periods. To become more flexible, you gently, regularly move your joints.

Set reasonable goals. The trick is to start slowly and gradually increase the demands you're placing on your body. In this way, the body responds by getting stronger. If you impatiently force your muscles to take on too much for too long, the resultant pain and inflammation can make you regret your rash behavior and may discourage further attempts. If you pay attention, you'll know when you're ready to move forward. For example, you've been doing 3 sets of 10 repetitions of bicep curls using 5-pound free weights. At the point at which you realize you could easily do more repetitions, switch to 7- or 8-- pound weights. When that becomes easy, try the 10-pound weights.

Workouts are often built using the **FITT** acronym, which stands for frequency, intensity, time, and type. You can continue to overload the system by increasing any of the first three variables.

- *Frequency* is how often you do the activity. Recommendations are for three to five days of cardiorespiratory exercise, two to three days of resistance training, and two to three days minimum of stretching.

- *Intensity* reflects how hard you exercise. Earlier you learned that your heart rate provides a good estimate of cardiorespiratory exercise intensity. When you increase the weight you move against, you augment your resistance training—the principle of progressive overload. When you stretch a bit farther, you gain flexibility.

- *Time* refers to how long you do the activity. If you're doing resistance training or aerobic exercise longer, you're building endurance. Ideally, you can find at least 20 minutes a day to exercise. The HHS recommends a minimum of 150 minutes over a week.

- *Type* has to do with the kind of exercise. Varying the type provides a means for avoiding monotony and overuse injury and for addressing different fitness components. You might practice yoga and Pilates for strength and flexibility, lift weights for your resistance training, and row for your cardiorespiratory training.

Maintaining physical fitness is a lifelong process. If you stop training, you lose strength, endurance, and, to some extent, flexibility. This concept is known as **reversibility**. Those hypertrophied muscles begin to atrophy. Unstimulated bones start to thin. If you've ever had an arm or leg in a cast for a few weeks, you probably noticed that when the cast came off, that extremity was now skinnier than the other. Unfortunately, those changes begin sooner than we'd like. That's why doctors are much less likely to recommend bed rest and hospital staff roust patients out of bed and onto their feet as soon as possible.

Another training principle is **specificity**. Echoing the "type" in the FITT acronym, particular activities may only benefit certain components of health-related fitness and only the muscle groups worked. Flexibility training doesn't improve cardiorespiratory fitness. Bicep curls will strengthen the flexor muscles in your upper arm but won't improve strength in your legs and torso. The goal is to address all components of health-related fitness and gain strength, endurance, and flexibility in all the major muscle groups. If you do, you can freely and easily skip, carry groceries, shovel snow, and stow a small suitcase in the overhead bin in an airplane.

reversibility

Fitness gained through physical activity is lost with disuse.

specificity

The training principle that the body only responds to the particular demands placed upon it. The effects of any one activity depend on the muscles exercised.

Training Videos

Physical activity has so much value in maintaining health, preventing illness, and managing disease that the American College of Sports Medicine and the American Medical Association joined forces to create Exercise is Medicine. This organization provides tools for health care providers and the general public that promote physical activity, including the group guidelines for assessing health and potential risk factors for exercise, identifying barriers to exercise, mapping your goals, creating an exercise schedule, and learning simple exercises to address the various aspects of health-related fitness.

You can find all of these tools by visiting http://www.myexerciseplan.com/assessment. Scroll down the page to find short videos on aerobic exercises, strength training, and flexibility.

You can also find helpful information including videos on the Centers for Disease Control and Prevention website at http://www.cdc.gov/physicalactivity/everyone/guidelines/adults.html.

TABLE 9.1 Physical Activity Guidelines

Type of activity	Recommended schedule
Cardiorespiratory (aerobic) exercise	At least 150 minutes each week (30 minutes, 5 days a week) at moderate intensity or 75 minutes at vigorous intensity (15 to 25 minutes, 3 to 5 days a week)
Resistance training	Work out all major muscle groups 2 times a week with at least 1 rest day between
Flexibility training	Stretch at least 2 to 3 days a week
Note: For more information on government guidelines, go to http://www.health.gov/paguidelines. Also check out the MyActivity Pyramid created by the University of Missouri, available at http://extension.missouri.edu/p/n388.	

1.3 Skill-Related Fitness

Skill-related fitness encompasses all aspects of health-related fitness with the addition of power, speed, agility, stability, coordination, and rapid reaction times. Usually, you're developing skills needed for a particular activity—tennis, lacrosse, rock-climbing, hip-hop. You train those abilities as you would any other, usually by participating in a program geared for that activity. Proficiency in some activities may require years of practice. Ideally, you're having fun along the way. You don't have to be a pro to enjoy a game of touch football, intramural soccer, or dancing to your favorite band.

Fitness Myths and Facts

Myths abound. Some lead to self-defeating ideas about fitness. Test yourself. Are the following statements facts or myths? Answers follow.

1. *If you can't exercise hard an hour a day, you may as well not bother.*
2. *You must get your recommended daily exercise in one block of time.*
3. *Exercise is dangerous for people with disabilities or chronic illnesses.*
4. *Past a certain age, it's too late to start exercising.*
5. *If you don't exercise, your muscles turn to fat.*
6. *If you want a "six pack," you need to do a lot of sit-ups.*
7. *Running will ruin your knees.*

Answers:

1. **Myth.** Some activity is better than none. Benefits begin as soon as you get off the couch. For instance, even brisk walking markedly improves heart health. One study found that women who walked reduced their cardiovascular disease risk as much as women who exercised more vigorously. Women in both groups who exercised 2.5 hours a week (about 20 minutes a day) cut their risk of vascular calamities such as heart attacks and strokes by 30 percent.[13]

2. **Myth.** While Federal guidelines recommend adults get at least 30 minutes of moderate activity most days of the week, you can break that time into 10-minute increments. A brisk walk across campus to your next class counts, as does doing calisthenics while watching your favorite show.

3. **Myth.** Physical activity benefits everybody, no matter his or her current state of health. Nevertheless, it's a good idea to get medical clearance from a doctor, who may recommend developing an exercise plan with a physical therapist or certified personal trainer.

Video Clip 9.1
No More Wheelchairs
This inspirational music video features a number of physically disabled athletes.

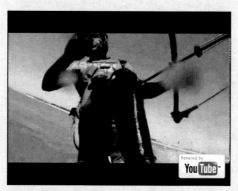

View the video online at: http://www.youtube.com/v/SbqE655OlTg

4. **Myth.** Exercise benefits people of any age. Unfortunately, Americans often move less (and weigh more) with each passing year.[14] Yet it's never too early or too late to begin. Start now. Make it a habit. Young people who exercise tend to remain physically active,[15] which promotes healthy aging.

Video Clip 9.2
100-Year-Old Man Running Marathon
Fauja Singh began running at age 89 after tragically losing his wife and child. On October 16, 2011, 100-year-old Mr. Singh completed the Toronto Marathon, breaking a world record.

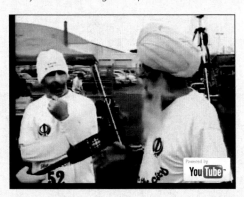

View the video online at: http://www.youtube.com/v/U0mKdo2-Gfc

5. **Myth.** Fat and muscle are two different types of tissue. They don't interchange any more than straw turns into gold. Such things only happen in fairy tales. Here's what does happen: You only have a certain number of individual muscle cells. Unexercised muscles become thinner; exercised muscles thicken. If you diminish your level of physical activity without changing your diet, extra calories are stored as fat.

6. **Myth.** Abdominal exercises can thicken individual muscle fibers but don't melt the layer of fat between skin and muscle. To lose that padding, you must burn more calories than you consume. As discussed in the sidebar "Core Strength", sit-ups and crunches (truncated sit-ups) are not the only abdominal exercises.

7. **Myth.** In otherwise healthy people who have good form, moderate running doesn't seem to raise the risk of knee arthritis.[16] Actually, obesity is much harder on knees and other joints. However, high-intensity running, particularly when combined with spinning and twisting movements, may lead to arthritis. Sports that increase the odds of arthritis include soccer (knees), football (knees and neck), baseball pitching (elbows), and gymnastics (spine).[17] Even once arthritis develops, proper exercises that maintain the strength of supporting muscle actually improve the outcome. If an activity produces persistent pain, stop and get a doctor's evaluation.

KEY TAKEAWAYS

- Health-related physical fitness promotes health and well-being and prevents injury and a number of illnesses.
- Health-related fitness encompasses cardiorespiratory fitness, muscular strength, muscular endurance, and flexibility.
- You can improve cardiorespiratory fitness with as little as 30 minutes per day of moderate-intensity physical activity; this 30 minutes can be divided into 10-minute periods of time.
- Resistance training does NOT have to take place in a gym. Your own body weight provides resistance in exercises like push-ups, squats, and lunges, which can be done anywhere.
- Some physical activities also require particular skills, such as power, speed, agility, stability, coordination, and rapid reaction times.
- In order to improve any component of fitness, you must progressively overload that system. Inactivity soon reverses fitness gains you have made. That's why daily activity is so important.

2. THE IMPACT OF PHYSICAL ACTIVITY ON YOUR HEALTH

LEARNING OBJECTIVES

1. Establish human history in the context of physical activity.
2. Identify the health risks of physical inactivity.
3. Discuss the role of physical activity in the aging process.
4. Discuss the health benefits of regular physical activity.
5. Explore the dangers of compulsive overexercising.

A Brief History of Human Physical Activity

Then and Now: Hunter-Gatherers to Passive Observers

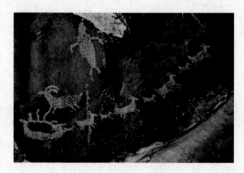

© *Thinkstock*

Our ancestors were physically active. They hunted fish and game, gathered plants and insects to eat and wood to burn, and handcrafted their lodgings, tools, and clothes. Agriculture took root a mere 8,000 years ago. In the era before tractors and all-terrain vehicles, farming and ranching required a lot of manual labor.

During the 18th century, the Industrial Revolution began to, well, revolutionize the way humans lived. Soon, machines mass produced goods and transported us. People migrated from the countryside into burgeoning towns. Despite problems inherent in pollution and crowding, living standards rose. Post–World War II prosperity spawned suburbs and lengthened commutes. Increasingly, automobiles took people where they needed to go; televisions and movie theaters provided endless entertainment. People began to sit more—at home, at school, and at work.

For multiple reasons, kids began to spend more and more time indoors. One study showed that, between 1981 and 2003, kids spent progressively more time at school, studying, and engaging with electronic devices and less time being physically active.[18] Specifically, the time spent being physically active dropped from 6.5 hours to 4.5 hours a week. A 2005 report from the Kaiser Family Foundation found that nonschool use of media (television, videos, computers, movies, and print) had increased to 6.5 hours a day, or 44.5 hours a week[19] —the same amount of time as a full-time job. We have allowed electronic devices to hypnotize us into immobility.

This shift toward sedentary lifestyles is a relatively recent phenomenon. Our genome (genetic information) evolved over thousands of years of physical activity. Perhaps because inactivity runs counter to this genetic disposition, it promotes a host of common chronic conditions. The solution? Move!

2.1   The Hazards of Sedentary Lifestyles

If you thought a life of leisure reduced bodily wear and tear, think again. The "use it or lose it" principle applies to most bodily systems. Physical activity maintains structure and function. Disuse leads to decline.

- **Inactivity kills.** It is one of the most important predictors of chronic illness and premature death. Physical inactivity and being overweight or obese tie as the second leading preventable causes of death, just behind tobacco smoking and high blood pressure, which share the number-one spot.[20] In 2005, physical inactivity was responsible for nearly 1 in 10 deaths, or approximately 200,000 deaths, in America.

  A 14-year study from the American Cancer Society found that, compared to people who sat fewer than three hours a day, women glued to their chairs for six hours or more were 34 percent more likely to die.[21] Women who also got little recreational activity were twice as likely to die. The risk was lower for men.

- **Inactivity leads to physical frailty.** You can separate bodily processes into two camps: *catabolic* (tearing down) and *anabolic* (building). In catabolism, complex molecules (proteins, complex carbohydrates, and fats) are broken down into simple molecules (amino acids, glucose, glycerol, and fatty acids) your cells can use as fuel. This process helps keep you alive during prolonged fasting.

  In anabolism, those same chemical reactions run backward, allowing storage of small molecules as protein, fat, and the starchy compound glycogen. Hormones such as insulin, testosterone, estrogen, and growth hormone drive these processes. Moderate exercise combined with good nutrition generally promotes anabolic processes and building muscles and bones.

  Perhaps because your genome evolved with lots of physical activity, your body interprets inactivity as an anomaly[22] and responds as though you must endure a prolonged fast—even if you have plenty to eat. Ancient genetic mechanisms dismantle your energy stores and flood your bloodstream with amino acids, fats, and sugar. Meanwhile, an ample diet elevates the same nutrients.

  Also, unstimulated bones begin to dissolve. Moderate bone loss is called *osteopenia*; severe loss is called **osteoporosis**. In the face of inactivity, muscle cells shrink, a process called **atrophy**. With advancing age, muscle cells are lost as well, resulting in a state of diminished muscle mass and strength called **sarcopenia**. Everyday activities like cleaning, cooking, climbing stairs, and getting up from a chair become difficult. Falls become more likely, which raises the risk of painful, debilitating bone fractures.

- **Inactivity raises the risk of chronic conditions.** Compared to their exercising peers, inactive people aged 30 to 69 increase their risk of heart attack by nearly 100 percent, colon cancer by 80 percent, type 2 diabetes by 76 percent, and stroke by 72 percent. In women, breast cancer risk rises 56 percent.[23] Obesity and depression also become more likely. Recall from Chapter 1 that these are the very conditions that are so common in the United States.

- **Inactivity is expensive.** If you were concerned about the price of a pair of running shoes, consider the costs of sitting around, which raises the risk of many chronic conditions—conditions that become increasingly expensive to treat. One analysis showed that physical inactivity, combined with overweight and obesity, accounted for 27 percent of national health care charges.[24] A portion of our taxpayer dollars foots the bill.

osteoporosis

Means "porous bone"; a significant loss of bone mass that greatly raises the risk of bone fractures (broken bones).

atrophy

Wasting away of tissue. For example, without physical activity, muscles atrophy.

sarcopenia

Age-related loss of muscle mass and strength.

2.2   The Benefits of Physical Activity

While unused muscles atrophy and bones demineralize, physical activity does the opposite—muscles and bones thicken, joints gain flexibility, and the heart and lungs work more efficiently. Moving proves to your body that you're still alive and that maintenance is a worthwhile investment. If you place consistent physical demands on your body, it generally rises to the occasion. Here are some examples of improved function in many bodily systems.

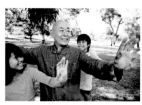

© Thinkstock

basal metabolic rate (BMR)

The rate at which the body uses energy (as defined by calories burned) to maintain normal bodily functions.

- **Muscular system.** Each major muscle is composed of bundles of parallel muscle fibers (cells). As mentioned, regular exercise doesn't increase the number of muscle cells, but rather their size. It stimulates synthesis and repair of skeletal muscle protein.[25] Other cellular components increase: energy molecules, enzymes, and mitochondria (structures that generate the energy molecule ATP). Enhanced blood supply brings more oxygen and nutrients to muscles, which also become more efficient at extracting oxygen from the blood. The net result is greater speed and endurance and hastened recovery times.

- **Skeletal system.** Flexibility training improves the range of motion at joints. Two types of exercise add bone mass: weight-bearing exercises (jumping, skipping rope, running, walking, climbing stairs) and resistance training.

    Bone mass rises during childhood and adolescence and peaks in the third decade of life. Good nutrition and ample exercise ensure optimal peak bone mass. After that, bone density declines, a process that accelerates with declines in hormones such as estrogen and testosterone in older age. Nevertheless, bone-stimulating activities retard the loss of bone, thereby reducing the risk of osteoporosis.

- **Cardiovascular and respiratory systems.** Cardiorespiratory training conditions the heart, blood vessels, and lungs. Because a strong heart works more efficiently, resting heart rate and blood pressure decline. Circulation improves. Blood is less likely to clot within blood vessels. Blood lipids are favorably altered; triglycerides and low-density lipoprotein (LDL, or "lousy") cholesterol decline and high-density lipoprotein (HDL) cholesterol rises.[26],[27] All of those changes protect against conditions such as high blood pressure, atherosclerosis (arterial disease), heart attacks, and strokes.

- **Nervous system.** Exercise increases circulation of blood to the brain and elevates growth factors that protect nerve cells and promote their ability to interconnect and repair themselves. It also regulates neurotransmitters, the chemicals nerve cells use to communicate. Exercise stimulates repair and helps regenerate injured or severed nerves. For those and other reasons, regular physical activity improves mood, attention, learning, and memory.[28],[29] Aerobic exercise seems to reduce the risk of Alzheimer's disease and vascular dementia, the two most common causes of dementia (loss of memory, reasoning, and other brain changes).[30]

- **Immune system.** This system protects you from cancer and infection. Whereas prolonged, intense, stress-inducing exercise can suppress the immune system, moderate exercise positively modifies it and may reduce the risk and severity of developing colds and other respiratory infections.[31]

- **Hormonal system.** Glands manufacture regulatory chemicals called hormones and secrete them into the blood. For instance, the pancreas produces insulin, which regulates the amount of glucose (sugar) in your blood. In diabetes, which is discussed in detail in Chapter 15, either the pancreas doesn't make enough insulin or, more commonly, cells become resistant to its action. Either way, blood sugar rises to unhealthy levels. Inactivity is among the health behaviors that foster insulin resistance. On the other hand, regular exercise makes cells more sensitive to insulin. It also increases growth hormone,[32] which stimulates growth and cellular reproduction and regeneration. These two anabolic (building) hormones help maintain muscle and bone.

- **Digestive system.** Sedentary lifestyles, as well as low intake of dietary fiber and fluids, correlate with constipation. Reversing those lifestyle factors can relieve the problem.[33] Physical activity has also been shown to improve symptoms of irritable bowel syndrome,[34] a common disorder marked by abdominal discomfort, bloating, gas, diarrhea, and constipation.

- **Metabolism and weight management.** While metabolism isn't an organ system, it involves several organ systems and affects every cell in the body. It's defined as an organism's life-sustaining chemical reactions. **Metabolic rate** is the energy expenditure over a given period of time. The resultant released heat is measured in calories. A calorie—technically speaking, a kilocalorie—is the amount of energy needed to raise the temperature of one kilogram of water by 1°C. **Basal metabolic rate (BMR)** is the number of calories burned during resting conditions.

    Exercise burns calories. It raises your metabolic rate during the workout and for some period of time afterward. Regular exercise adds muscle, which is much more metabolically active (burns more calories) than fat. For that reason, regular exercise elevates BMR. It's as though your engine is idling faster. Physical activity prevents and remedies unhealthy body fat, provides the caloric leeway to consume recommended nutrients, and often motivates healthy food choices.

- **Prevention of chronic diseases.** All those improvements in bodily systems act to protect against cardiovascular disease, high blood pressure, obesity, diabetes, stroke, and some cancers.[35] Authors of an article published in the *Journal of Applied Physiology* put it this way: "Indeed, with the possible exception of diet modification, we know of no single intervention with greater promise than physical exercise to reduce the risk of virtually all chronic diseases simultaneously."[36]

- **Existing chronic diseases get better.** That said, people with chronic diseases should get clearance from their doctors before heading to the gym. For some conditions, working with a physical therapist or athletic trainer is also advised.

- **Greater longevity.** Longevity studies have identified places such as Okinawa, Japan, and Sardinia, Italy, where people tend to live particularly long lives. Not surprisingly, these elders are physically active and continue to garden, walk, cycle, dance, and so forth. A study of people age 65 found that physical activity strongly predicted successful aging as defined by health and well-being seven years later.[37]

When researchers analyzed activity levels of adults ages 18 and up, they found that those who followed federal guidelines for physical activity, particularly for aerobic exercise, reduced their risk of dying by 25 to 35 percent.[38] The association was strongest in people with chronic conditions. Numerous other studies have found similar results. An ideal combination is being physically active and having a lean body composition.[39]

 Video Clip 9.3

Exercise Reverses Aspects of Aging
This video relays key findings from a 2007 study that showed elders who underwent a six-month resistance-training program gained strength and reversed some age-associated changes within skeletal muscles.[40]

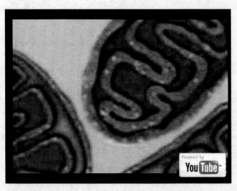

View the video online at: http://www.youtube.com/v/6-rm9cKSsk8

- **Heightened energy and vitality.** A chief reason for feeling more energetic is that exercise conditions the cardiovascular system, thus improving the efficiency of the delivery of oxygen and nutrients to your cells. Muscles also become better at extracting oxygen from the blood.

- **Better nighttime sleep.** If you're physically active during the day, you'll be ready for sleep. However, experts recommend avoiding nighttime workouts, which can be stimulating and interfere with falling asleep. Stretching and mild exercise can be done anytime.

- **Release of tension and stress.** Moderate, enjoyable exercise reduces stress. It provides an outlet for frustration and helps you slip into the present moment, a state where distractions fade away and you're acutely aware of yourself and the world around you.

- **Improved mood and well-being.** Mastering a skill makes you feel better about yourself. It enhances self-esteem and self-efficacy, the sense that you can succeed. Plus, exercise tends to make us look and feel healthier, which also enhance feelings of self-worth. Also rigorous exercise temporarily bumps up *endorphins*, the body's natural pain killers, and other feel-good brain chemicals such as dopamine and serotonin—all substances implicated in the "runner's high." Although moderate exercise can have antianxiety and antidepressant effects,[41] people with persistent symptoms should make an appointment with a mental health expert.

- **Better social and reproductive health.** If your exercise routine involves other people—team sports, dancing, yoga, kickboxing—you expand your circle of friends. Even if it doesn't, even if you prefer solo activities, your social life may well improve because you feel happier, healthier, and more confident. Furthermore, a healthy delivery of blood to your reproductive organs averts sexual dysfunction. Exercise may also decrease menstrual cramping[42] and premenstrual syndrome.[43]

- **Heightened spiritual health.** For many people, exercise provides a means of spiritual expression or a vehicle for engaging with the present moment. Some people feel uplifted by the meditation and community of a yoga or tai chi class. But any group activity can provide a sense of community. Outdoor activities such as jogging, hiking, fishing, canoeing, cycling, surfing, and skiing can deepen your connection to nature.

- **Improved financial outlook.** Being physically active goes a long way toward preventing costly chronic diseases. Furthermore, higher physical activity during adolescence correlates with higher educational attainment and socioeconomic status.[44]

  Video Clip 9.4

UN Side Event on Physical Activity and Noncommunicable Diseases
Worldwide, three out of every five people die of noncommunicable diseases such as diabetes and heart disease. In 2011, the United Nations held a meeting to focus on associated problems and possible solutions. Prominent among those solutions is heightened physical activity, which both prevents and remedies chronic conditions. This short video clip captures statements from leading experts.

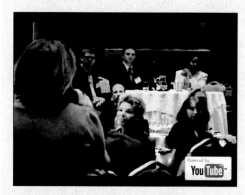

View the video online at: http://www.youtube.com/v/Dw3WC9nbfU4

The Dallas Bed Rest Study

Would you sign up for a study that required you to stay in bed? During finals week, such an opportunity might have a certain allure, especially if money was involved. Such a study began way back in 1966 at Dallas's Southwestern Medical School.[45] The volunteers were five healthy college men, two of whom were athletes. Researchers measured various aspects of cardiorespiratory fitness three times: at the start of the study, after three weeks of strict bed rest, and after a 54-day intensive training period.

The results showed that bed rest quickly deconditioned them. Overall body weight remained the same, but lean body mass decreased. Cardiorespiratory fitness measurements such as VO_2 max plummeted. Fortunately, the training period returned the athletes to their baseline measurements and improved the fitness of the other three guys.

The story gets more interesting. Thirty years later, the researchers tracked down the five volunteers.[46] Now in their early 50s, the men had gained weight, mainly as fat with few changes in fat-free mass. VO_2 max and maximum heart rate had fallen. While three decades had undermined their cardiovascular fitness, the deterioration was not as marked as after three weeks in bed. Astonishingly, six months of endurance training bumped VO_2 max to the baseline levels of the original experiment. Basically, the training program reversed the three-decade loss in aerobic power.

The persistent researchers also did a 40-year follow-up.[47] Cardiovascular fitness had declined at a more rapid rate, with overall VO_2 max descending to a level comparable to the end of the bed rest four decades earlier. However, the loss of aerobic fitness varied greatly. For instance, serious illness such as cancer eroded fitness. On the other hand, the men who continued to exercise lost much less ground.

Take-home messages: (1) Inactivity can rapidly decondition you and degrade cardiovascular fitness faster than several decades of normal aging. (2) Training can bring a sedentary middle-aged person back to a youthful level of fitness. (3) Aging eventually, inevitably erodes some aspects of physical fitness. (4) Physical activity retards this age-related decline.

2.3   Too Much of a Good Thing

As mentioned earlier, exercise generally relieves stress and promotes fat-free mass (i.e., more muscle and bone). On the other hand, prolonged, intense exercise counts as a physical stressor. Chronic stress elevates the catabolic hormone cortisol, which tends to dismantle fat-free mass. Chronic stress can also impair normal reproductive function.[48]

On the other hand, for most professional and recreational athletes, the exercise-induced hormonal changes tend to be positive. Negative hormonal alterations such as upward blips in cortisol are fleeting. Even marathon runners recover a couple of days after competing. For most intense athletic endeavors, recovery is within hours.

Nevertheless, women—particularly those engaged in sports that stress thinness such as running, dance, and gymnastics—can develop the **female athlete triad**. The three abnormalities are disordered eating, amenorrhea (no menstrual periods), and osteoporosis (bone loss).

Both men and women can become engaged in **compulsive exercise**. Exercise ceases to be a freely chosen, mainly pleasurable activity and becomes an urgent chore. It's done despite illness and inclement weather. It's done at the expense of social, academic, and work obligations. If the person can't exercise, he or she feels guilt and anxiety.

Compulsive exercise can accompany body image disorders such as anorexia nervosa, bulimia nervosa, and bigorexia (also called muscle dysmorphia). Chapter 10 discusses these disorders in detail.

How do you know if you have a problem? A preoccupation with exercise and personal appearance takes over your life. You feel dissatisfied with your body, moody, distressed, anxious, and possibly depressed. Perhaps you use substances that jeopardize your health because you believe they'll make you look better. If you have any doubt, call your doctor for a consultation right away. Professional treatment is essential.

female athlete triad

A syndrome that includes disordered eating, irregular or absent menstrual cycles, and osteoporosis.

compulsive exercise

Excessive exercise, usually with obsessive preoccupation with fitness, building muscles, and/or losing weight; may accompany body image disturbances such as bigorexia, anorexia nervosa, and bulimia disorders.

KEY TAKEAWAYS

- Throughout most of human history, we have been physically active during much of our waking hours. Sedentary lifestyles have become common over only the past few decades.
- Inactivity reduces longevity, increases the risk of common chronic conditions, worsens mental health, and promotes age-associated frailty.
- Physical activity benefits many bodily systems, promotes healthy aging, improves metabolism, prevents common chronic diseases, and enhances overall well-being.
- Gains made from physical activity are lost with prolonged inactivity.
- Extreme amounts of exercise can activate the stress response. Compulsive exercise can accompany body image disorders.

DISCUSSION QUESTIONS

1. Reflect on your childhood, and answer these questions: Did you grow up in a city, suburban neighborhood, or rural area? How did you commute to school? What kinds of physical activities did you do as a kid? How has the way you grew up influenced your current activity level?

2. Health insurance companies often raise premiums for individuals who smoke. Do you think they should also raise premiums for sedentary clients? Would the situation differ if employers instead rewarded physically active employees with reduced insurance premiums? Defend your opinions.

3. Discuss the diseases sedentary people (including young people) become progressively more vulnerable to as they age.

4. To get an idea of how various exercise types and levels of intensity burn calories, go to WebMD (http://www.webmd.com/diet/healthtool-fitness-calorie-counter). Pick five activities you are likely to do. For each, record the intensity, duration, and estimated calories.

5. Your roommate played soccer in high school. Now his or her main physical activity is walking to and from classes. Your roommate tells you his or her muscles will maintain a memory for sports, providing as proof the fact that his or her weight hasn't changed this past year. What do you think? How might your roommate's body composition have changed, even if weight has remained constant? What other components of your roommate's health-related fitness may have changed?

6. A few months ago, a female friend took up running and weight lifting. She seems to exercise all the time. She tells you she feels "weird" if she can't exercise. You notice that she's becoming very thin. When you ask how she's feeling, she says she's tired and her menstrual periods have stopped. What do you think could be going on?

3. YOUR EXERCISE PLAN

LEARNING OBJECTIVES

1. Analyze your personality and lifestyle to create an exercise plan that meets recommended guidelines.
2. Learn how to select proper equipment for your activities.
3. Identify basic measures to enhance recovery from exercise.
4. Examine the effectiveness and safety of supplements marketed to enhance athletic performance.
5. Discuss proper management of sports-related injuries.

3.1 Getting Started and Sticking with It

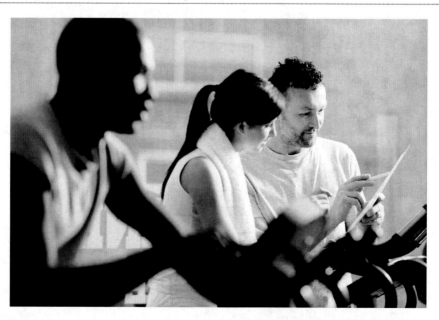

© Thinkstock

A number of factors can determine your fitness success. If you can find a routine that works for you, you'll soon start to feel so good that you won't want to quit. You'll move from intending to exercise, to doing it, to feeling like you can't live without it. Complete the following to-do list to start down the path to lifelong fitness.

1. List the types of physical activities you enjoy. If you don't like it, you won't keep doing it. Do you prefer the camaraderie of team sports and group classes or the solitude of walking, jogging, or cycling? Do you favor a fast-paced sport such as squash or more meditative movements such as tai chi? Do you enjoy novelty or repetition? Would you rather exercise indoors or outdoors? With music or in silence? Is expense a consideration?

2. Identify reasonable fitness goals. Do you want to have more energy, reduce your risk of disease, age more gracefully, fit back into the jeans you "outgrew," or train for an event such as a 5K, a ski trip, or a mountain trek? Base your goals on modest improvements over your current fitness level. Write down your goals and post the list somewhere you can see it.

3. List the changes you think you need to make to meet your goals. For instance, if you want to become better at doing push-ups, you will need to do push-ups—starting with a few reps and sets and working up. If you want to learn to play tennis, signing up for a class is a good start.

4. Create an exercise plan and post it on the wall alongside your goals. Consider your schedule and rhythms. Early-morning workouts, though they can kick-start the day, won't appeal to night owls. Some people prefer to dispel afternoon lethargy (or pent-up tension) with physical activity. Also consider whether you need to break your exercise time into smaller chunks of 10 to 20 minutes or can instead complete it within a 30- to 60-minute block. See the sidebar "Sample One-Week Exercise Plan".

5. Identify barriers to exercising. Here are some examples:

    a. "I don't have enough time." Would you rather schedule time to exercise or time to visit the doctor? All you need is 10 consecutive minutes. Any amount is better than nothing. Small lifestyle modifications can add up. Take the stairs, not the elevator. Park your car farther from your destination and walk. Commute by foot or bike. Tear yourself away from Facebook to do a few resistance exercises. Take a study break to throw a Frisbee with your roommate. Exercise is Medicine has an exercise time finder (http://www.myexerciseplan.com/assessment/).

    b. "I'm too tired." Exercise will ultimately give you more energy. Plus your sleep may become more efficient, which will help you feel more rested.

    c. "I don't look good in workout clothes." Most people are too self-centered to notice others. Plus, you'll look healthier if you exercise.

    d. "I'm going to make a fool of myself." Again, most people aren't paying attention to you. Maybe they'll actually encourage you. Plus, how are you going to improve if you don't start?

    e. "Exercise is painful and difficult." It shouldn't be, not if you gradually build the intensity and duration of your activities. When you need to, take a break. Pain is not a sign of weakness leaving your body but rather a warning that tissue damage might be occurring. Ask a personal trainer or the class instructor whether your technique is correct. If pain persists, consult your doctor.

    f. "I have a chronic illness." For most conditions, the risks of remaining sedentary exceed those associated with physical activity. If you have a serious condition, meet with your doctor. He or she may recommend you start out by working with a physical therapist or certified personal trainer.

    g. "I can't afford a gym membership or the gear." Physical activity can happen anytime, anywhere. You can walk, run, skip, jump rope, dance, practice yoga, cycle, hula hoop, climb rocks, shovel snow, and rake leaves. You can play tag, Frisbee, tennis, baseball, football, basketball, or volleyball. You can find exercise routines on YouTube and do them in your room. Remember that regular exercise prevents expensive chronic diseases.

    h. "My family and friends don't exercise." Join a class and make additional friends who will support your exercise program. Having at least one exercise buddy creates motivation and accountability. If the old friends distract you, ask yourself what kind of "friend" would want to jeopardize your health.

6. Get expert advice. If you join an exercise class, the instructor ought to be able to guide you. If you're unfamiliar with the gym equipment, ask the attendant on duty. Better yet, if you're new to exercising, enlist the services of a certified personal trainer (CPT). Your college physical education program most likely has a CPT available to help you get started. City recreation centers

also offer a wealth of information, support, and instruction in everything from group fitness classes to one-on-one personal training sessions.

7. Start slowly and build strength and endurance gradually to avoid discouragement and injury. Rome wasn't built in a day.

8. Consider finding a workout and accountability partner. You may be less likely to let down your friend than yourself. The two of you can share struggles and successes. You'll feel more motivated and committed.

9. Bring water and healthy snacks with you when you work out. That will help avoid dehydration and "bonking" because you're famished. It also helps to wear comfortable clothes and any protective gear relevant to the activity.

10. Chart your progress. Otherwise, you may not notice your steady improvement. Take photographs of yourself now in as little clothing as possible. Using a tape measure, determine the diameter of your waist, chest, biceps, thighs, and calves. Record these measurements, along with your weight and resting heart rate. (With regular aerobic exercise, your resting pulse should decline and it should fall back to baseline more quickly after exercise.) Write down how you feel physically, mentally, and emotionally. Track items relevant to your goals—distance run, number of push-ups, repetitions of weights lifted, level of flexibility. Every 30 days, take another round of photos, measurements, and goal assessments.

You can use this progress chart to track your progress or create one that better fits your goals. You can either check off the things you did or record the time, distance, and number of repetitions. You can also use icons to represent your overall state of being (happy, sleepy, sad, angry).

TABLE 9.2 Progress Chart

Goals/outcomes	MON	TUES	WED	THUR	FRI	SAT	SUN
Aerobic exercise							
Resistance training							
Flexibility training							
Weight (check no more than weekly)							
Overall state of being							
Note: If you have a smartphone or iPad, you might consider downloading fitness apps such as miCoach, Fleetly, B.iCycle, Workout Trainer, iMapMyFitness, RunKeeper Pro, and MyFitnessPal.							

11. Allow for setbacks. Everyone has them. You may develop a cough, pull a muscle, need to finish writing a paper, or decide you'd rather watch a movie or take a nap. Stay mentally flexible and optimistic. If you check off the boxes in your exercise plan, you'll see that, overall, you're making progress.

12. Pat yourself on the back. Regular exercise carries inherent rewards. You'll feel happier, stronger, and more flexible, agile, confident, and attractive. You'll sleep and learn better. However, you may want to set tangible rewards once you meet particular goals. Maybe you treat yourself to a new phone app, a sports watch, jeans, concert tickets, or a healthy meal with friends.

Sample One-Week Exercise Plan

The ideal workout routine should have some variability, such that, over the course of a week, you work in cardiorespiratory, resistance, endurance, and flexibility training. You can also vary the ways in which you build these skills. For instance, you may cross-train with a mixture of jogging, swimming, and cycling to increase several components of health-related fitness. In this way, you're less likely to become bored or injured.

The following outline of workouts for one week includes five moderately intense workouts and two recovery days. These workouts can be completed in about an hour. If you have less time, adjust the schedule.

For every workout, begin with a light warm-up to prepare your body for the demands about to be placed on it. Perform the workout. After strenuous activity, cool down and stretch. For instance, if you go for a run, cool down by walking around the block, then stretch for six to eight minutes.

- **Monday:** Upper-body resistance training. Shoulders, chest, back, and arms. Three sets of 8 to 10 reps. End with 5 minutes abdominal exercise.
- **Tuesday:** Cardio workout. 20 to 60 minutes within target heart rate zone.
- **Wednesday:** Recovery day. Gentle exercise is okay.

- **Thursday:** Lower-body resistance training. Squats, lunges, calf raises, and abdominal exercises. Three sets of 8 to 10 reps.
- **Friday:** High-intensity interval training. Mixed aerobic and anaerobic exercise for 16 to 20 minutes, as follows: Starting on the minute, do 20 seconds at an easy pace, the next 20 seconds at moderate intensity, and the last 20 seconds at highest intensity. Try running in place, jumping jacks, squat jumps, leg kicks, and boxing punches.
- **Saturday:** Total body and cardio combined. Perform the following in any order and any number of groupings as quickly as possible: four sets of 15 reps each of push-ups, pull-ups, sit-ups, rows, bicep curls, triceps exercises, and squats.
- **Sunday:** Active recovery day. Yoga, Pilates, or an extended stretching session for at least 30 minutes.

3.2   Choosing Equipment and Exercising Safely

Now that you have decided to begin an exercise program, you need to educate yourself about proper equipment, protect yourself from injury, and respond appropriately should injury occur. You need clothing that moves with you, wicks away moisture, and keeps you at a comfortable temperature.

Dressing in layers carries all-season advantages. Even when exercising outdoors in warmer weather, a thin top layer and hat can protect your skin from excessive ultraviolet radiation. In cooler weather, you'll need more layers to keep you warm. Wool and polypropylene both wick away moisture (though wool tends not to smell as foul—a bonus if you're planning a backcountry ski trip over many hours or days). Look for inner layers and socks made of either material. Down provides insulation in very cold weather. You may also need a shell to block wind or a waterproof but breathable outer layer. As exercise raises your core temperature, you can remove layers to decrease sweating. Wet clothes can later make you feel chilled. In any season, sunglasses with UV protection will shield you from the wind and minimize the risk of developing eye damage.

Unless you're performing an activity in your bare feet (e.g., swimming, yoga, some types of dance), you need comfortable footwear. In some circles, barefoot running and running in thin-soled, flexible shoes are popular. Proponents argue that we humans have run barefoot for thousands of years. Furthermore, feet that are barely or lightly shod tend to land on the forefoot, roll more gently to the heel, and then push off again from the forefoot. They claim that stiffer, more padded running shoes encourage us to strike with the heel, then roll to the forefoot, which increases repetitive stress injuries. Detractors claim that barefoot and minimalist running actually raise the risk of injuries. A recent review of studies on the subject did find that barefoot running produces differences in gait.[49] However, the authors couldn't find evidence to confirm or refute benefits in performance and reductions in injuries.

Now let's address equipment. If you don't have access to a gym, you can do resistance training against your own body weight. A number of low-cost items can provide variety and progressive resistance. Examples include exercise balls, jump ropes, elastic bands, and tubes. Pedometers can help you track your steps and find out how close you come to the recommended 10,000 steps a day. Some watches have a stopwatch function and heart rate monitor. You can find exercise equipment at sporting-goods stores, discount retailers, and numerous Internet sites.

Safety Equipment

Here is a list of simple measures that can reduce your risk of accidental injury:

Cycling

- Wear a properly fitted helmet to protect from possible skull fractures.
- Use gloves to protect the hands if you fall.
- Wear padded cycling shorts for a much more comfortable ride.
- Get a comfortable bike seat. Make sure it does not compress the arteries and nerves. Numbness or tingling with longer rides is a warning sign. Long-term compression can compromise erectile function. Ask for advice at a cycling shop.
- If riding in the dark, wear reflective clothing and make sure you have proper lights/reflectors for the bicycle.
- Follow all traffic rules: stop at stop signs and red lights, yield to pedestrians, ride single file, and use hand signals to indicate turns.

Skiing and snowboarding

- Wear proper outerwear: waterproof coats and pants are essential. Dress in layers.
- Wear a helmet, waterproof and nonconstricting gloves, and properly fitting boots.
- Wear wrist guards for snowboarding.
- Always ski or ride in control—avoid excessive speed.

Skateboarding or rollerblading

- Wear a helmet and wrist, knee, and elbow guards.

Water sports

- Use life vests, also called personal flotation devices (except for swimming and surfing in competent swimmers).
- Wear helmets for sports like kayaking.
- Never drink alcohol while operating a boat or jet ski.

Team sports

- Wear appropriate footwear for the playing surface.
- Use a properly fitted mouth guard; face guards for sports like lacrosse, field hockey, and ice hockey; and shin guards for sports such as soccer, rugby, hockey, and cricket.
- Wear appropriate padding and helmets for high-contact sports.

Recovery from Vigorous Exercise

The exercise recovery period is the time that your body adjusts and adapts to the demands of the exercise session, the time when your muscle tissues hypertrophy and become stronger.[50] A quicker recovery allows you to resume exercising sooner—something of vital importance to elite and professional athletes. For example, professional cyclists on the Tour de France must ride their bicycles for about 100 to 120 miles each day for 21 days—with only 2 rest days. In order to perform at an optimum level, their bodies need to take advantage of every moment off the bikes.

Even those of us who participate in fitness activities simply to stay healthy and have fun must also allow our bodies to recover between exercise bouts. Some of the recovery process has to do with replacing water lost during exercise. Every tissue in your body contains water. You lose water throughout the day—in urine, bowel movements, exhalations, and sweat. When you exercise, you lose even more because you're breathing harder and sweating more. The more vigorous the workout, the more water leaves your body. Exercising in an arid and/or hot environment further drives up the deficit.

The question is, what kind of hydration fluid do you need? If you're not exercising very hard or for very long, water will do. Physical activity does deplete energy molecules (glucose) and electrolytes (salts and minerals such as sodium chloride, potassium, and calcium). However, you can replace these by eating a meal after you finish your workout. A snack beforehand can help sustain energy during the workout.

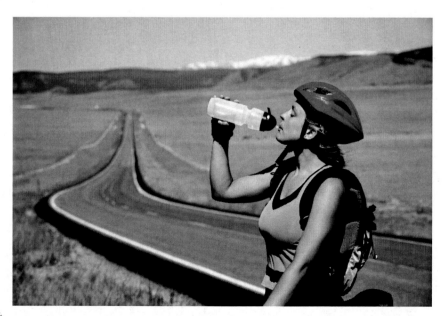

© *Thinkstock*

Sports drinks have gained popularity with elite athletes and the general public. They contain electrolytes and carbohydrates, mainly in the form of high-fructose corn syrup. Americans generally consume too many simple carbohydrates. Fructose, which sweetens many beverages and other foods these days, seems to be particularly bad for human health. Studies link habitual consumption with overweight and obesity, enhanced appetite, increased fat in the abdomen, liver disease, high blood pressure, and decreased sensitivity to insulin (which raises the risk of diabetes).[51] However, for athletes, the benefit of fructose in sports drinks is that it enhances the movement of fluid from the small intestine into the bloodstream.[52] The salt in these beverages also stimulates thirst, which helps ensure water is adequately replaced.

If you're exercising hard for an hour, drink a fluid that provides some carbohydrates. A normal diet will replace salt and other electrolytes. Broth-based soups and tomato juice are both good sodium sources. If you're exercising for longer periods, a sports drink makes sense. In fact, carbohydrate-electrolyte beverages enhance performance more than water during prolonged exercise.[53]

Make sure you're hydrated before you begin to exercise. Drink a couple of eight-ounce glasses two or three hours before you begin and another glass about a quarter hour before the exercise session. Depending upon the intensity of the exercise, drink eight ounces every 10 to 15 minutes. Don't wait until you're thirsty. At that point, you're already behind and catching up becomes difficult.

Dehydration impairs both physical and mental performance. Loss of fluid and electrolytes seems to increase the likelihood that fatigued muscles will cramp. Signs that you've become dehydrated are urinating less (and producing a darker urine) and losing weight after an exercise session. That lost poundage came from fluid, not fat. Replace fluids as soon as possible. Caffeinated soda, coffee, and alcoholic drinks do not count because they stimulate urination.

Your exercised muscles also need time to recover. Immediately after you finish exercising, do some gentle stretches, which will help your muscles maintain their normal anatomical length. Another method to help muscles recuperate is called *active recovery*, which entails exercising at a lower intensity level following a more strenuous bout. It has been shown to speed the rate at which muscles eliminate the waste products that accumulate during intense exertion.[54] Here are some examples. After sprinting for a certain distance, you walk to "cool down" and recover. After a session of resistance training, you can do several repetitions at very low resistance. Or, if you run a 5K or play a rollicking game of Ultimate Frisbee, you can take a brisk walk afterward.

There's a lot of hype around sports supplements. While some supplements may have some benefits, some have marginal to no effects, and some can be dangerous. Their use is generally discouraged, especially in young people.

TABLE 9.3 Supplements and Athletic Performance

Name of supplement	What it is	Effectiveness	Safety
Creatine (also known as creatine pyruvate and creatine monohydrate)	A naturally occurring compound formed in protein metabolism. People take this substance by mouth in hopes of increasing muscle mass. It increases an energy molecule called phosphocreatine in skeletal muscle.	Some research supports the use of this supplement for increasing muscle mass and performance during some types of exercise, such as intense resistance training. Other types of sport performance may not be enhanced.	Taken within recommended dosage guidelines, this supplement appears to be safe. High doses may adversely affect the liver, kidneys, and heart.
Whey protein	Whey is the liquid remaining after curdled milk is strained. Whey protein is protein isolated from whey. People use it for a variety of purposes, including to improve athletic performance.	Positive effects on muscle size and strength when combined with strength training. May enhance recovery from heavy exercise.	Likely safe within recommended dosage guidelines. High doses can cause nausea, bloating, cramps, and loose stools. Can contain the milk sugar lactose; avoid if you're lactose intolerant.
Chromium (also known as chromium picolinate)	This trace element is mainly used to improve blood sugar control. Some people use it in hopes of increasing muscle mass and decreasing fat.	Supplements do not seem to significantly enhance strength or muscle mass.	Generally safe within recommended dosage guidelines. Higher doses can lead to side effects such as headaches, sleep disturbances, and mood changes. Toxic doses can cause diarrhea, blood loss for the intestinal tract, and more.
Androstenediol*,** Androstenedione*,**	Both are steroid molecules that the body can convert to testosterone and estrogen.	Supplementation does not significantly increase muscle size or otherwise improve athletic performance.	Probably not safe. Purity and potency varies. Increases cholesterol, raising the risk for heart disease. May masculinize women (increase facial hair) and shrink the testicles and increase breasts in men. Concerns exist about increasing cancers sensitive to reproductive hormones such as breast and prostate cancer.
Dehydroepiandrosterone (DHEA)**	The main use is for slowing some age changes, though evidence is scant. Also used to enhance sports performance. The body can change DHEA to androstenedione, a precursor to estrogen and testosterone.	The few studies have yielded conflicting results on muscle strength and athletic performance. May be helpful in older adults.	Appears safe at doses of less than 50 mg per day. Doses higher than 200 mg per day frequently cause side effects: acne, deeper voice, hair loss from scalp, insulin resistance, high blood pressure, and other symptoms.
Stimulants**	Examples include legal substances such as caffeine; banned supplements such as ephedra; prescription drugs such as methylphenidate (Ritalin) and amphetamine (Adderall); illegal drugs such as cocaine and methamphetamine.	While stimulants may increase subjective feelings of endurance and "energy," most of these substances have too many side effects to be considered effective.	Safety varies from relatively safe (caffeine) to extremely dangerous (cocaine and methamphetamine). Stimulation of the cardiovascular system and central nervous system produces increased heart rate and blood pressure, nervousness, tremors, restlessness, insomnia, decreased appetite, and weight loss. Seizures, heart attacks, strokes, and death are possible with the more dangerous stimulants.

*The Anabolic Steroid Control Act of 2004 reclassified androstenediol and androstenedione from dietary supplement (available over the counter) to anabolic steroid, which is a schedule III controlled substance. Schedule III means it has some potential for abuse but not as much as schedule I and II drugs. It can't be legally acquired without a prescription.

The National Collegiate Athletic Association (NCAA) bans androstenediol, androstenedione, and DHEA. You can visit http://www.ncaa.org/wps/wcm/connect/public/NCAA/Health+and+Safety/Drug+Testing/ Resources/NCAA+banned+drugs+list **to read a complete list of banned substances.

Name of supplement	What it is	Effectiveness	Safety
Erythropoietin (EPO)**	In the body, the kidney makes this hormone, which stimulates red blood cell production. It's given by injection to anemic people, usually those on dialysis for chronic kidney disease. Athletes have illegally injected themselves, a practice called "blood doping."	Does increase red blood cells, which carry oxygen from the lungs to cells.	Common side effects include fever, nausea, vomiting, rash, headache, cough, and pain in joints, muscles, and bones. Blood clots can lead to heart attacks and strokes.
Herbal supplements	Asian herbs such as ginseng that have long been used to enhance recovery from stress. Caffeine-containing plants (coffee, tea, yerba mate, kola nut, chocolate).	Research on ginseng and similar herbs in healthy, fit adults generally does not show significant performance benefits. Caffeine stimulates the respiratory, cardiovascular, and nervous systems. It can enhance some aspects of exercise performance but does not increase energy—something only macronutrients provide.	Ginseng is generally safe when taken within recommended dosage guidelines in healthy adults. Not recommended in pregnant women. Caffeine can contribute to insomnia, nervous tension, headaches, elevated blood pressure, and rapid heart rate.
*The Anabolic Steroid Control Act of 2004 reclassified androstenediol and androstenedione from dietary supplement (available over the counter) to anabolic steroid, which is a schedule III controlled substance. Schedule III means it has some potential for abuse but not as much as schedule I and II drugs. It can't be legally acquired without a prescription.			
The National Collegiate Athletic Association (NCAA) bans androstenediol, androstenedione, and DHEA. You can visit http://www.ncaa.org/wps/wcm/connect/public/NCAA/Health+and+Safety/Drug+Testing/Resources/NCAA+banned+drugs+list **to read a complete list of banned substances.			

Source: Natural Medicines Comprehensive Database. Stockton, CA: Therapeutic Research Faculty; 2013.

http://naturaldatabase.therapeuticresearch.com. Updated July 2, 2013. Accessed Updated July 2, 2013.

Avoiding Injuries Related to Heat and Cold

Our bodies have several mechanisms for maintaining a core temperature of about 98.6°F. When temperature rises, blood vessels to the skin dilate (become wider). Skin flushes and heat radiates away from the body. Sweat glands in the skin produce sweat, which, when it dries, removes heat. The kidneys conserve body water. Thirst drives us to replace lost liquids.

When temperatures fall, the blood vessels constrict (narrow), thus conserving core body heat. Tiny muscles make hair shafts stand more upright, which traps warmer air near the skin. If we're cold enough, skeletal muscles produce shivering, which generates heat. Movement generates even more heat. We cover up, drink warm liquids, and eat to replace lost calories. People with more body fat are better insulated.

There are limits to the body's ability to maintain a stable core temperature. Extremes of heat and cold stress the system and create illness, injury, and even death.

Climate change has led to hotter summers. Because exercise generates body heat, summertime activities present the risk of heat injury. Humidity compounds the problem because sweat evaporates less readily. Excess body fat further heightens the risk of overheating. Slight rises in body temperature are normal. **Hyperthermia** means above-normal body temperature. Dehydration often accompanies this condition. Two main types of heat-related illness are heat exhaustion and heat stroke.

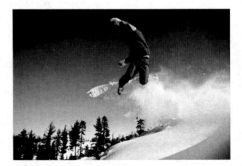

© Thinkstock

hyperthermia

Persistent elevation of body temperature above normal.

heat exhaustion

A heat-related condition marked by dizziness, weakness, nausea, and vomiting.

heat stroke

A life-threatening condition marked by elevated body temperature, flushed and dry skin, rapid pulse and respiratory rate, headache, muscle aches, and confusion or loss of consciousness.

hypothermia

Having an abnormally low body temperature.

frostbite

A condition that occurs when the tissue actually freezes, forming ice crystals that damage cells.

Heat exhaustion can produce dizziness, weakness, nausea, and vomiting. Rather than looking flushed, the skin may be pale, warm, and damp. The best strategy is to quit exercising, move to a cooler place, remove clothing, and drink fluids.

Confusion, inability to follow simple commands, and, eventually, loss of consciousness indicate the development of **heat stroke**. Other signs of this life-threatening condition are hot, flushed, dry skin and rapid breathing and heart rate. The body temperature rises to 104°F or higher. Seizures (convulsions) can occur.

Heat stroke requires rapid medical attention. After calling 911, you can help by moving the person to a cooler place, removing clothing, covering him or her with a sheet or other material soaked in cold water, and applying ice packs to armpits, groin, and neck. Because diminished consciousness raises the risk of choking, don't offer the person a beverage.

To reduce the risk of heat-related illness, schedule your outdoor exercise in the relative cool of morning and evening. Wear thin, loose, light-colored clothing. Gradually increase the pace of your activity. Drink plenty of water. Work out with a buddy so you can monitor each other's condition. If warning signs develop, take action.

Winter, depending on the location, can make possible activities like skiing, snowboarding, skating, and sledding. Damp and windy conditions speed the loss of precious body heat. Fingers, toes, noses, cheeks, and ears are most at risk for injury.

Unless the weather is extreme, winter shouldn't keep you from exercising outdoors. Instead, protect yourself by wearing adequate clothing—jacket, socks, reasonably thick athletic pants, hat, gloves, neck warmer, or scarf. Dress in layers. If clothes become damp with sweat, change into dry clothes as soon as you finish exercising.

Hypothermia is a condition of abnormally low body temperature. Symptoms and signs include chills, shivering, clumsiness (particularly in cold hands), confusion, slurred speech, and exhaustion. Left unchecked, it leads to coma and death. The best remedy is moving to a warm, dry place. Contrary to myths, drinking alcohol worsens the situation because it opens blood vessels in the skin, further dissipating precious body heat. Signs of severe hypothermia warrant a 911 call.

Frostbite occurs when the tissue actually freezes, forming ice crystals that damage cells. Signs that extremities have become cold-injured include pain, burning, tingling, numbness, and difficulty moving. Early on, frostbite resembles a second-degree burn, with redness, swelling, and blisters. The skin then becomes yellow or white and, eventually, turns black. If your hands get cold while you're outside, one remedy is to remove your gloves and place your hands in your armpits or over your abdomen until they warm up. If you suspect frostbite, get to shelter, avoid further exposure, and get immediate medical assistance. The rewarming process is tricky and best left to medical professionals.

Managing Athletic Injuries

Physical activity has many health benefits and, like anything else, some risks. Even with the use of proper equipment and technique, injuries happen. Most minor injuries heal quickly on their own, provided sufficient rest. Others require medical attention. When in doubt, call your health care practitioner.

Abrasions (scrapes), small **lacerations** (cuts), and punctures can be managed at home. Wash with mild soap and lots of running water. If you have "road rash," you may need to scrub a bit to remove asphalt and other grit that, left in the wound, could cause an infection or produce a long-term tattoo. If that hurts too much or seems to risk further injuring tissue, proceed to the nearest clinic. You don't need to apply rubbing alcohol, which isn't a great disinfectant and irritates tissue. Apply antibiotic ointment and cover with a clean bandage.

Bleeding, in limited quantities, helps flush microbes from the wound. The problem with puncture wounds is that there's little bleeding to remove microbes and it's harder to irrigate them with water. To stop bleeding, cover with a piece of gauze or clean cloth and apply steady pressure. If possible, elevate the wound above the heart. If 15 minutes of steady pressure doesn't stop the bleeding, seek medical assistance. For deep wounds with extensive bleeding, call 911.

If you're helping a bleeding buddy, wash your hands before and afterward or use a waterless hand sanitizer. If you have latex gloves (not something stocked in the average college dorm room), put them on. If someone else's blood contacts your own open wound, alert your health care provider right away.

Sutures (stitches) may be needed for a couple of reasons: the wound is deep, a laceration gapes open, or the wound's edges are ragged. Sutures can reduce scarring. For that reason, a doctor may elect to suture even small facial lacerations. If you have any doubt about whether a wound needs suturing, seek medical assistance.

Sprains occur when the ligaments holding a joint in place become stretched or torn. Wrists, ankles, thumbs, and knees are common sprain locations. Usually a fall or twisting motion forces the joint out of its normal alignment. **Strains** occur when a muscle or the tendon that attaches it to the bone becomes pulled or twisted. Both sprains and strains produce pain, swelling, and sometimes bruising. Symptoms can be mild or so severe as to interfere with normal movement. Severe sprains can be difficult to distinguish from a bone fracture.

Mild strains and sprains can often be managed by following a procedure known as RICE, which stands for rest, ice, compression, and elevation. The objective of this treatment is to reduce further swelling. Lie down, elevate the injured limb above your heart, and cover the injury with a cloth and, atop it, a cold pack. If you don't have a commercial cold pack, a plastic bag of ice or bag of frozen vegetables works fine. Do not apply ice directly to the skin. Remove after 10 minutes. Repeat the cold pack applications every 30 minutes. Sore muscles sometimes feel better after alternations of cold and hot packs.

Compression helps stabilize injured joints. Most drugstores and supermarkets carry elastic bandages and compression sleeves. The goal is not to cut off circulation. Make sure you can slide your index finger under the wrap. Over-the-counter medications include ibuprofen (Advil and Motrin) and naproxen (Aleve, Anaprox, Naprosyn), which reduce pain and inflammation, and acetaminophen (Tylenol), which reduces pain.

If symptoms of mild sprain or strain don't improve within 72 hours, make an appointment to see your doctor. Severe sprains, strains, and suspected bone fractures (exquisite pain over the bone, swelling, bruising, deformity, loss of function) all warrant medical attention. If the limb appears deformed or the bone is protruding from the skin, call 911. For suspected injuries to the neck or other parts of the spine, you should also call 911 and refrain from moving the injured person.

One injury that merits a physician evaluation is a head injury. A **concussion** is a mild traumatic brain injury caused by impact to the head. The word "mild" does not mean the condition should be taken lightly. Any head injury, even if you simply "got your bell rung," is a serious medical condition. You can develop a concussion from hitting your head against another object or from a whiplash movement, which causes your brain to bang against your skull.

Traumatic brain injury has gained some much-deserved attention of late. Even seemingly mild injuries, especially if they're recurrent, can lead to long-term neurologic problems. Combat soldiers and athletes engaging in contact sports are particularly vulnerable. Symptoms and signs range from subtle to dramatic. Red flags include brief loss of consciousness, dizziness, confusion, poor concentration and attention, memory loss, nausea, vomiting, headache, and trouble with balance and coordination. If even one of these signs or symptoms is present, the person should be referred to a physician immediately. Head-injured athletes should not return to the playing field or any other physical activity until completely cleared by a physician.

sprains

Painful stretching or tearing of the ligaments (the tough, fibrous bands that connect your bones and hold together joints).

strains

Injuries to a muscle or tendon connecting muscle to bone; also called pulled muscles.

concussion

An injury to the brain caused by blunt force trauma to the head. Also called closed-head injury or mild traumatic brain injury.

When to Seek Help for Injuries

For any serious injury, call 911:

- Any suspected concussion; head injury with loss of consciousness, nausea, vomiting, confusion, and double vision requires immediate attention

- Any suspicion of injury to the neck or the rest of the spine, in which case the injured person should not be moved until help arrives

- Eye injury

- Signs of heat exhaustion, heat stroke, hypothermia, or frostbite

- Injury to a limb produces significant pain, swelling, or bruising

- It hurts to bear weight on an injured leg

- Injury to a joint limits the usual range of motion

- In caring for an injured person, his or her blood contacts your own open wound

- Bleeding continues after 15 minutes of steady pressure

- A laceration is deep, gapes open, crosses a joint, or is on the face

- You are unable to remove debris from a wound

- You have diabetes and have a wound

- You sustain a break in the skin and are unsure whether your tetanus vaccination is up to date

KEY TAKEAWAYS

- Proper clothing can help you move comfortably and reduce the risk of becoming overheated or chilled. Depending on the sports you engage in, it's also important to invest in safety gear such as shin guards, helmets, and gloves.

- Basic measures to enhance your recovery from exercise include staying hydrated, consuming a healthy diet, cooling down afterward, and taking an occasional rest day.

- While sport supplements are popular, most have not been well studied. Some have only marginal benefits, some have none, and some can be dangerous. Before using supplements, check credible sources and discuss them with your doctor.

- Injuries can happen. Some respond to rest and basic remedies such as icing. If you have any doubt about the severity of your injury, contact a qualified medical practitioner.

DISCUSSION QUESTIONS

1. Imagine you have never gone snowboarding and intend to try it out over your winter break. What steps might you take to prevent injury?

2. A friend from the gym recommends a sports supplement he's been taking. He even offers to give you a free week's supply. What do you do?

3. It's summer. You head out for a run a bit later than planned. On the return trip, you start to feel light-headed and nauseated. What should you do?

4. While playing with friends, you jump up to grab a Frisbee. When you land, your ankle turns painfully. It hurts to bear weight on that foot. What should you do?

4. RECOMMENDED RESOURCES

4.1 Organizations and Websites

American College of Sports Medicine. http://www.acsm.org.

Centers for Disease Control and Prevention. http://www.cdc.gov/physicalactivity/everyone/guidelines/adults.html.

Exercise Is Medicine. http://exerciseismedicine.org.

US Department of Health and Human Services, Physical Activity Guidelines. http://www.health.gov/paguidelines.

ENDNOTES

1. Fussman C. Jack LaLanne: what I've learned. Originally published in *Esquire*. 2004 Aug. Available at: http://www.esquire.com/features/what-ive-learned/ESQ0804-AUG_WIL. Updated January 24, 2011. Accessed August 8, 2011.

2. Centers for Disease Control and Prevention. Summary health statistics for US adults: national health interview survey, 2009. National Center for Health Statistics. Available at: http://www.cdc.gov/nchs/fastats/exercise.htm. Updated February 21, 2012. Accessed July 28, 2011.

3. Centers for Disease Control and Prevention. Physical inactivity estimates, by county. Available at: http://www.cdc.gov/features/dsphysicalinactivity. Updated March 9, 2011. Accessed August 1, 2011.

4. Schoenborn CA, Barnes PM. Leisure-time physical activity among adults: United States, 1997–98. Advance Data: From Vital and Health Statistics; no. 325. Hyattsville, MD: National Center for Health Statistics; 2002. Available at: http://www.cdc.gov/nchs/data/ad/ad325.pdf. Accessed August 2, 2011.

5. Madsen K. Promoting the health of our youth: why physical activity policies are critical. *Arch Pediatr Adolesc Med*. 2011. doi:10.1001/archpediatrics.2011.1245.

6. The President's Council on Physical Fitness and Sports (PCPFS) Research Digest. Definitions: health, fitness, and physical activity. Department of Health and Human Services. Available at: http://www.fitness.gov/digest_mar2000.htm. Accessed July 28, 2011.

7. Hunter GR, Brock DW, Byrne NM, Chandler-Laney PC, Del Corral P, Gower BA. Exercise training prevents regain of visceral fat for 1 year following weight loss. *Obesity (Silver Spring)*. 2010 Apr;18(4):690–695. Available at: http://www.ncbi.nlm.nih.gov/pmc/articles/PMC2913900/?tool=pubmed. Accessed September 17, 2011.

8. Energy expenditure in different modes of exercise. *ACSM Current Comment*. American College of Sports Medicine. Available at: http://www.acsm.org/docs/current-comments/energyexpendindifferentexmodes.pdf. Accessed July 9, 2013.

9. Garber CE, Blissmer B, Deschenes MR, et al. Quantity and quality of exercise for developing and maintaining cardiorespiratory, musculoskeletal, and meromotor fitness in apparently healthy adults: guidance for prescribing exercise. *Med Sci Sports Exerc*. 2011;43(7):1334–1359. Available at: http://journals.lww.com/acsm-msse/Fulltext/2011/07000/Quantity_and_Quality_of_Exercise_for_Developing.26.aspx. Accessed November 5, 2011.

10. Herbert RD, de Noronha M, Kamper SJ. Stretching to prevent or reduce muscle soreness after exercise. *Cochrane Database Syst Rev*. 2011 Jul 6;(7):CD004577.

11. Sherman KJ, Cherkin DC, Wellman RD, et al. A randomized trial comparing yoga, stretching, and a self-care book for chronic low back pain [Epub ahead of print]. *Arch Intern Med*. 2011 Oct 24;171(22):2019–2026. doi:10.1001/archinternmed.2011.524.

12. da Costa BR, Vieira ER. Stretching to reduce work-related musculoskeletal disorders: a systematic review. *J Rehabil Med*. 2008 May;40(5):321–328.

13. Manson JE, Greenland P, LaCroix AZ, et al. Walking compared with vigorous exercise for the prevention of cardiovascular events in women. *N Engl J Med*. 2002 Sep 5;347(10):716–725. Available at: http://www.nejm.org/doi/full/10.1056/NEJMoa021067. Accessed August 1, 2011.

14. Centers for Disease Control and Prevention. Physical activity and the health of young people. Available at: http://www.cdc.gov/healthyyouth/physicalactivity/pdf/facts.pdf. Accessed August 1, 2011.

15. Mäkinen TE, Borodulin K, Tammelin TH, Rahkonen O, Laatikainen T, Prättälä R. The effects of adolescence sports and exercise on adulthood leisure-time physical activity in educational groups. *Int J Behav Nutr Phys Act*. 2010 Apr 12;7:27. Available at: http://www.ncbi.nlm.nih.gov/pmc/articles/PMC2873576/?tool=pubmed. Accessed August 1, 2011.

16. Cymet TC, Sinkov V. Does long-distance running cause osteoarthritis? *J Am Osteopath Assoc*. 2006;106(6):342–345.

17. Felson DT, Lawrence RC, Dieppe PA, et al. Osteoarthritis: new insights. Part 1: the disease and its risk factors. *Ann Intern Med*. 2000 Oct 17;133(8):635–646. Available at: http://www.annals.org/content/133/8/635.long. Accessed August 3, 2011.

18. Juster FT, Ono H, Stafford FP. Changing times of American youth: 1981–2003. Ann Arbor, MI: Institute for Social Research, University of Michigan; November 2004. Available at: http://ns.umich.edu/Releases/2004/Nov04/teen_time_report.pdf. Accessed July 28, 2011.

19. Media multi-tasking: changing the amount and nature of young people's media use [news release]. The Henry J. Kaiser Family Foundation. Available at: http://www.kff.org/entmedia/entmedia030905nr.cfm. Accessed July 27, 2011.

20. Danaei G, Ding EL, Mozaffarian D, et al. The preventable causes of death in the United States: comparative risk assessment of dietary, lifestyle, and metabolic risk factors. *PLoS Med*. 2009 Apr 28;6(4):e1000058. Available at: http://www.ncbi.nlm.nih.gov/pmc/articles/PMC2667673/?tool=pubmed. Accessed August 1, 2011.

21. Patel AV, Bernstein L, Deka A, et al. Leisure time spent sitting in relation to total mortality in a prospective cohort of US adults. *Am J Epidemiol*. 2010;172(4):419–429.

22. Booth FW, Chakravarthy MV, Gordon SE, Spangenburg EE. Waging war on physical inactivity: using modern molecular ammunition against an ancient enemy. *J Appl Physiol*. 2002 Jul;93(1):3–30. doi:10.1152/japplphysiol.00073.2002. Available at: http://jap.physiology.org/content/93/1/3.long. Accessed August 1, 2011.

23. Danaei G, Ding EL, Mozaffarian D, et el. The preventable causes of death in the United States: comparative risk assessment of dietary, lifestyle, and metabolic risk factors. *PLoS Med*. 2009 Apr 28;6(4):e1000058. Available at: http://www.ncbi.nlm.nih.gov/pmc/articles/PMC2667673/?tool=pubmed. Accessed August 1, 2011.

24. Anderson LH, Martinson BC, Crain AL, et al. Health care charges associated with physical inactivity, overweight, and obesity. *Prev Chronic Dis*. 2005 Oct;2(4):A09. Available at: http://www.ncbi.nlm.nih.gov/pmc/articles/PMC1435706/?tool=pubmed. Accessed August 1, 2011.

25. Walker DK, Dickinson JM, Timmerman KL, et al. Exercise, amino acids, and aging in the control of human muscle protein synthesis. *Med Sci Sports Exerc*. 2011 Dec;43(12):2249–2258.

26. Kelley GA, Kelley KS, Tran ZV. Aerobic exercise and lipids and lipoproteins in women: a meta-analysis of randomized controlled trials. *J Womens Health*. 2004 Dec;13(10):1148–1164. Available at: http://www.ncbi.nlm.nih.gov/pmc/articles/PMC2447858/?tool=pubmed. Accessed July 28, 2011.

27. Kelley GA, Kelley KS, Franklin B. Aerobic exercise and lipids and lipoproteins in patients with cardiovascular disease: a meta-analysis of randomized controlled trials. *J Cardiopulm Rehabil*. 2006 May–Jun;26(3):131–139. Available at: http://www.ncbi.nlm.nih.gov/pmc/articles/PMC2447859/?tool=pubmed. Accessed July 28, 2011.

28. Angevaren M, Aufdemkampe G, Verhaar HJ, Aleman A, Vanhees L. Physical activity and enhanced fitness to improve cognitive function in older people without known cognitive impairment. *Cochrane Database Syst Rev*. 2008 Jul 16;(3):CD005381.

29. Bekinschtein P, Oomen CA, Saksida LM, Bussey TJ. Effects of environmental enrichment and voluntary exercise on neurogenesis, learning and memory, and pattern separation: BDNF as a critical variable [Epub ahead of print 2011 Jul 7]? *Seminars in Cell & Developmental Biology*. 2011 Jul;22(5):536–542.

30. Foster PP, Rosenblatt KP, Kuljiš RO. Exercise-induced cognitive plasticity, implications for mild cognitive impairment and Alzheimer's disease. *Front Neurol*. 2011;2:28. Available at: http://www.ncbi.nlm.nih.gov/pmc/articles/PMC3092070/?tool=pubmed. Accessed July 30, 2011.

31. Martin SA, Pence BD, Woods JA. Exercise and respiratory tract viral infections. *Exerc Sport Sci Rev*. 2009 Oct;37(4):157–164. Available at: http://www.ncbi.nlm.nih.gov/pmc/articles/PMC2803113/?tool=pubmed. Accessed August 3, 2011.

32. Eliakim A, Nemet D. Exercise training, physical fitness and the growth hormone-insulin-like growth factor-1 axis and cytokine balance. *Med Sport Sci*. 2010;55:128–140.

33. Chien LY, Liou YM, Chang P. Low defaecation frequency in Taiwanese adolescents: association with dietary intake, physical activity and sedentary behaviour. *J Paediatr Child Health*. 2011 Jun;47(6):381–386. doi:10.1111/j.1440-1754.2010.01990.x.

34. Johannesson E, Simrén M, Strid H, Bajor A, Sadik R. Physical activity improves symptoms in irritable bowel syndrome: a randomized controlled trial. *Am J Gastroenterol*. 2011;106(5):915–922.

35. Pate RR, Pratt M, Blair SN, et al. Physical activity and public health. A recommendation from the Centers for Disease Control and Prevention and the American College of Sports Medicine. *J Am Med Assoc*. 1995;273:402–407.

36. Booth FW, Gordon SE, Carlson CJ, Hamilton MT. Waging war on modern chronic diseases: primary prevention through exercise biology. *J Appl Physiol*. 2000 Feb;88(2):774–787. Available at: http://jap.physiology.org/content/88/2/774.long. Accessed August 1, 2011.

37. Achour EC, Barthelemy JC, Lionard KC, et al. Level of physical activity at the age of 65 predicts successful aging seven years later: the PROOF study. *Rejuvenation Res*. 2011 Apr;14(2):215–221.

38. Schoenborn CA, Stommel M. Adherence to the 2008 adult physical activity guidelines and mortality risk. *Am J Prev Med*. 2011 May;40(5):514–521.

39. Hu FB, Willett WC, Li T, Stampfer MJ, Colditz GA, Manson JE. Adiposity as compared with physical activity in predicting mortality among women. *N Engl J Med*. 2004 Dec 23;351(26):2694–2703.

40. Melov S, Tarnopolsky MA, Beckman K, Felkey K, Hubbard A. Resistance exercise reverses aging in human skeletal muscle. *PLoS One*. 2007 May 23;2(5):e465. Available at: http://www.ncbi.nlm.nih.gov/pmc/articles/PMC1866181/?tool=pubmed. Accessed February 3, 2012.

41. Biddle SJ, Asare M. Physical activity and mental health in children and adolescents: a review of reviews [Epub ahead of print 2011 Aug 1]. *Br J Sports Med*. 2011 Sep;45:886–895. doi:10.1136/bjsports-2011-090185.

42. Brown J, Brown S. Exercise for dysmenorrhoea. *Cochrane Database Syst Rev*. 2010 Feb 17;(2):CD004142.

43. Daley A. Exercise and premenstrual symptomatology: a comprehensive review. *J Womens Health*. 2009 Jun;18(6):895–899.

44. Koivusilta LK, Nupponen H, Rimpelä AH. Adolescent physical activity predicts high education and socio-economic position in adulthood [Epub ahead of print 2011 Apr 7]. *Eur J Public Health*. 2011. doi:10.1093/eurpub/ckr037.

45. Saltin B, Blomqvist G, Mitchell JH, Johnson RL Jr, Wildenthal K, Chapman CB. Response to exercise after bed rest and after training. *Circulation*. 1968 Nov;38(5)(suppl):VII1–78.

46. McGuire DK, Levine BD, Williamson JW, et al. A 30-year follow-up of the Dallas Bedrest and Training Study: II. effect of age on cardiovascular adaptation to exercise training. *Circulation*. 2001 Sep 18;104(12):1358–1366. Available at: http://circ.ahajournals.org/content/104/12/1358.long. Accessed August 4, 2011.

47. McGavock JM, Hastings JL, Snell PG, et al. A forty-year follow-up of the Dallas Bed Rest and Training study: the effect of age on the cardiovascular response to exercise in men. *J Gerontol A Biol Sci Med Sci*. 2009 Feb;64(2):293–299. Available at: http://www.ncbi.nlm.nih.gov/pmc/articles/PMC2655009/?tool=pubmed. Accessed August 4, 2011.

48. Hall HL, Flynn MG, Carroll KK, Brolinson PG, Shapiro S, Bushman BA. Effects of intensified training and detraining on testicular function. *Clin J Sport Med*. 1999 Oct;9(4):203–208.

49. Jenkins DW, Cauthon DJ. Barefoot running claims and controversies: a review of the literature. *J Am Podiatr Med Assoc*. 2011 May–Jun;101(3):231–246.

50. De Pauw K, De Geus B, Roelands B, et al. Effect of five different recovery methods on repeated cycle performance. *Med Sci Sports Exerc*. 2011 May;43(5):890–897.

51. Lustig RH. Fructose: metabolic, hedonic, and societal parallels with ethanol. *J Am Diet Assoc*. 2010;110(9):1307–1321.

52. Johnson RJ, Murray R. Fructose, exercise, and health. *Curr Sports Med Rep*. 2010 Jul–Aug;9(4):253–258.

53. Casa DJ, Clarkson PM, Roberts WO. American College of Sports Medicine Roundtable on hydration and physical activity: consensus statements. *Curr Sports Med Rep*. 2005;4(3):115–127. Available at: http://www.acsm.org/search-results?q=sports%20hydration. Accessed November 16, 2011.

54. Menzies P, Menzies C, McIntyre L, Paterson P, Wilson J, Kemi OJ. Blood lactate clearance during active recovery after an intense running bout depends on the intensity of the active recovery. *J Sports Sci*. 2010;28(9):975–982.

CHAPTER 10
Body Weight

Americans are preoccupied with their appearance, especially with their size and shape. A survey of American college students found that nearly 22 percent of college students—almost 26 percent of women and 14 percent of men—felt distressed about the way they look.[1] Many of us worry about being overweight. More often than not, we are.

Currently, two-thirds of American adults are overweight or obese. In addition to the associated psychological anguish, excess body fat heightens the risk of a number of medical conditions. Health experts have proclaimed the worldwide boom in obesity a public health crisis. Some also predict that obesity rates among our children will halt the trend of steadily increasing longevity.

This chapter will discuss body composition, body image, overweight and obesity, and eating disorders. Because of the epidemic in overweight and obesity, much of the chapter will focus on underlying causes and tips for achieving and maintaining an optimal body weight. The emphasis is on building a positive body image and healthy attitude about food. The last section of the chapter reviews body image disturbances and eating disorders.

You are imperfect, permanently and inevitably flawed. And you are beautiful.

- *Amy Bloom, American writer*

1. BODY IMAGE AND BODY COMPOSITION

LEARNING OBJECTIVES

1. Define body image and explore cultural influences and impact on health.
2. Discover strategies for achieving a positive body image.
3. Define body composition.
4. Discuss methods of assessing body weight and body composition.
5. Explain positive and negative energy balance.

1.1 Body Image

Your **body image** is your mental image of your physical appearance. Family, peers, important institutions (school, religious organizations, etc.), and the greater cultural milieu shape your concept of a pleasing appearance. Your *perception* of the way people respond to you also shapes your body image.

body image

One's mental image of one's physical appearance.

Changing ideals of feminine beauty: From voluptuous to lean. Left: Marilyn Monroe, American actress from the 1950s. Right: Naomi Campbell, English fashion model.

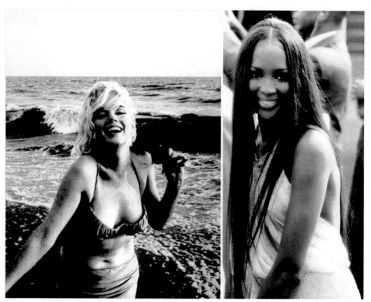

Source: Barris G. 1962. Available at: http://commons.wikimedia.org/wiki/File:Barris_Marilyn_Monroe.jpg (left); Biard G. Naomi Campbell at the Cannes film festival. 2008. Available at: http://commons.wikimedia.org/wiki/File:Naomi_Campbell_Cannes.jpg (right).

Because culture shapes body image, the assessment is subjective and subject to change. In earlier times, extra body fat was a sign of health and prosperity. You were scrawny because you fell ill, your crops failed, or you lacked skill with a bow and arrow. Now a thin, well-toned body may suggest sufficient wealth to hire a personal trainer and chef. In truth, maintaining a healthy body shouldn't require much money.

Around the world, cultures have long valued strong men and beautiful women. Symmetrical physical features, a marker of general health, represent an enduring criterion for physical attractiveness. Other standards shift with the times and cultural expectations.

The current ideal is for women to be thin, physically fit, and beautiful and for men to be ruggedly handsome, tall, and muscular. But people come in a variety of shapes, sizes, and hues. Furthermore, although female fashion models have grown thinner over recent decades—compare voluptuous Marilyn Monroe to lean Naomi Campbell and Adriana Lima—the average woman has grown fatter. Over time, the male ideal has become more muscular, even as fewer men engage in the daily physical labor that maintains muscle mass. Male models sport six packs; many men have love handles.

As a result, women and men are too often unhappy with their bodies. Collectively, Americans have lofty standards about physical attractiveness and miserable images of their own bodies. Two-thirds of adolescent girls are dissatisfied with their weight.[2] Over 90 percent of college women engage in "fat talk," making self-deprecating remarks like, "I'm so fat," "I need to lose weight," and "This ice cream is going straight to my hips."[3] Apparently, it's relatively uncommon for women to say anything positive about their own bodies.

Contentment with physical appearance varies by age, gender, ethnicity, and relative portion of body fat. White adolescent girls seem to excel at self-criticism. Many children start out feeling pleased about their looks. Satisfaction declines during adolescence—more so with gains in body fat. Boys and men can be just as dissatisfied as girls and women. The difference lies in the nature of the concern. Men want to be more muscular; women want to be thinner.

Of all the ethnic groups, black children and teens—especially boys—are the most satisfied with their bodies and therefore less likely to embark on weight-loss diets.[4] Among college women, white and Latina women desire thinner bodies than do black women.[5] Though there is little research on Asian American women, initial studies suggest that they are as vulnerable as white women to unhealthy weight-control measures.[6]

While girls may aspire to thinness, many boys and young men feel pressured by parents, peers, coaches, and the media to become both leaner and more muscular. In the past, if young men changed their dietary and physical activity habits, their goal was to gain muscle mass. With the uptick in overweight and obesity, boys and men may also be trying to lose body fat. Boys and men have become increasingly victim to unhealthy weight-control behaviors such as incorrect dieting, fasting, excessive exercise, and abusing muscle-enhancing substances, including anabolic steroids.[7]

Curiously, men don't have an accurate picture of themselves, often thinking that they are smaller than they actually are. Also, being muscular doesn't extinguish the drive for muscularity; both "undersized" and "buff" men want to be more muscular.[8]

Both men and women can harbor misperceptions about the norms for body size and shape. A study of college students found that the typical college woman wanted to be thinner and men wanted to be brawnier than the actual norms.[9] Put another way, women underestimated the leanness of other women, and men overestimated the muscularity of other men, as well as other men's ideals for muscularity.

In addition, men and women were often wrong about what the opposite sex wanted. Women mistakenly believed men preferred women who were thinner and less muscular than men's stated preferences. Likewise, men thought women wanted a more muscular guy than women actually preferred.

Such discrepancies between perception and reality can get us into trouble. We often fall short of our notions of the ideal body. We compare ourselves unfavorably to our peers. We imagine we're not attractive to potential partners. In a nutshell, we set ourselves up for unnecessary disappointment and distress.

For men and women, preoccupation with a negative body image adversely affects health. For one, it can cause psychological anguish, low self-esteem, and increased risk of depression.[10],[11] For another, it can sabotage healthy behaviors. Feeling ashamed of being seen in gym shorts or a bathing suit can become an excuse not to exercise. Negative thinking can devolve into despair and hopelessness: "I'm already fat. I might as well eat this pint of ice cream." Preoccupation with weight and food can lead to disordered eating and worsened health.

Indeed, body-size dissatisfaction and stigmatization (e.g., being teased or excluded due to overweight) *increase* the risk of gaining body fat.[12] Furthermore, exaggerated concerns about weight correlate with periodic overeating (binging), fasting, poor nutrition, and a number of unhealthy weight-loss behaviors, such as smoking, self-induced vomiting, and taking illicit amphetamines, laxatives, and diuretics. A 2012 study showed that half of adolescent girls and a quarter of adolescent boys had tried weight-loss diets in the previous year.[13] Ten years later, the prevalence remained unchanged.

Unfortunately, unhealthy attempts to avoid weight gain usually backfire. Adolescents who adopt unhealthy weight-control behaviors are two to three times more likely to *gain* weight.[14] Later in this chapter, we'll examine successful strategies for attaining a healthy body weight.

No matter what you look like and how you feel, it's important to accept and love yourself—as you are right now. If you don't, other people will have trouble doing so. Become aware of your body, your health, your actions, and your behaviors without judging yourself harshly. Life is too short to spend it in the abyss of self-reproach, shame, and guilt.

Your emotional response to your body depends in large part on your *self-concept*, your overall perception of yourself as a multidimensional person. Recall from Chapter 5 (Psychological Health) that self-awareness, self-respect, self-confidence, self-esteem, self-acceptance, and self-forgiveness combine to create your self-concept. Your body image is yet another component of self-concept. Your personality also tempers your feelings about your body.

Here are some examples. A woman may be 10 pounds above ideal body weight and feel either tremendous shame or generally feel good about her collective attributes: her ability to play lacrosse, solve algebraic equations, or sing in a band. A shorter-than-average guy may either feel self-conscious about his height or feel proud of his skill at dribbling a soccer ball, playing banjo, or telling jokes. The problem comes with focusing on what you perceive to be your flaws when, in fact, you have so many things going for you.

Particularly when you're young, it's easy to waste time worrying about your facial features and bodily proportions. However, you are so much more than the size and shape of any given body part. The older you get, the more such trivia fade when compared to the content of your heart and mind, the quality of your relationships, and the virtue of your actions. After all, Albert Einstein isn't remembered as a short guy with wild hair and a big nose. Former First Lady Eleanor Roosevelt, who did not fit conventions for female beauty, was a celebrated champion for civil rights, an author, a speaker, and a politician.

More important than your bodily proportions is the image you project. Someone could be as handsome as a Greek god or goddess, yet so unhappy, insecure, angry, or unkind as to drive people away. How many people do you find attractive mainly because they smile and express an interest in you? Most of us love babies, perhaps because they smile and don't go around saying, "Does this diaper make my backside look big?" The occasional self-deprecating remark can be disarming and even funny. But don't overdo it. Swinging your self-image into the positive zone will sway other people's opinion in that direction too.

Developing a Positive Body Image

Regardless of the messages you have received from family, peers, coaches, and the media, you deserve to develop a bright image of yourself. If you're reading this book, you're probably a college student, which means you must have a lot going for you. Here are some ideas for seeing yourself in rose-colored light.

- **Be happy with yourself now.** Don't wait until you morph into some idealized and perhaps unattainable size and shape. Self-love and compassion will actually make it easier to make lifestyle changes.

- **Accept reality.** Few people grow up to look like Beyoncé or Brad Pitt. But we are all, in our own ways, beautiful.

- **We are all works in progress.** Within limits, you can change for the better. From conception onward, you've been engaged in the process of transformation. The remodeling process continues daily. As we'll discuss later, optimal diet, physical activity, sound sleep, and the ability to cope effectively with stress will improve anyone's appearance.

- **What you do and think make you beautiful.** Take stock of all the great things you do and the people who care about you. Attractiveness springs from sources below the skin.

- **Remember that looks can be deceiving.** For instance, a thin person may not be as healthy as another person who weighs 10 to 20 pounds more. The skinny person might be ill, malnourished, and poorly muscled. Handsome doesn't mean happy.

- **Celebrate all the things your body can do.** It digests your food; gets you to class; comprehends a lecture; communicates with people; and senses textures, colors, sounds, tastes, and smells; thinks; talks; sings; dreams; and dances.

- **Surround yourself with people who accept you.** If you hang out with people who obsess about being fat, flabby, or puny, you may fall into the trap of putting yourself down too. Steer clear of those who criticize you. True friends should like you for who you are.

- **Wear clothes that flatter your figure and fit your contours.** You'll feel better about yourself if you do. Also, wearing clothes that fit right will also provide you cues about your current weight. People have gained weight without realizing it when routinely wearing loose clothing. Clothes that are too tight can irritate skin and mood and inhibit digestion and breathing.

- **Become aware of media messages.** Reject the ones that that don't fit your philosophy. Remember that all kinds of photography tricks—not to mention makeup, cosmetic surgery, and unhealthy eating behaviors—can make models and actors look better on camera than they do in real life.

- **Be kind to your body.** Pamper it. Give it enough rest. Massage it. Appreciate the feeling of warm water against your skin when you shower.

- **Think about other people.** If you're feeling self-absorbed, divert some of that energy into caring for someone else. Bring flowers to a friend. Offer encouragement. Tutor a peer. Volunteer at a soup kitchen. You'll feel better about yourself, and you'll learn that people will like you for your kind actions, not your looks.

Magazine Bans Adolescent, Malnourished Models

One problem with the fashion industry is that some of the models have scarcely entered puberty. Another is that some of the young women and men have used risky means to become thin and extremely muscular, respectively. Actors may undergo cosmetic surgery. In addition, photography software can mask flaws. As a result, the media portrays an unhealthy message about beauty.

In May 2012, *Vogue* magazine issued a statement that it would not work with models who are younger than 16 or who appear to have an eating disorder. Other media have begun to make use of more generously proportioned models and actors, and to otherwise introduce variety into our ideals of beauty.

Support media that portray the human body in a healthy fashion. Consider boycotting magazines, movies, and television shows that send the wrong message. For one, these media may create unhealthy working conditions for teens and young adults. For another, when we consumers internalize the message, we end up feeling dissatisfied with our bodies.

1.2   Body Composition

Body composition is a term used to describe how much of the body is fat and how much isn't. **Fat-free mass** includes muscle, bone, teeth, water, and organ tissues. Muscle and bone comprise the bulk of fat-free mass. Fat is stored primarily in **adipose tissue**. It's made of *adipocytes*, or fat cells.

There are two types of adipose tissue: **subcutaneous fat** (fat stored underneath the skin) and **visceral fat** (fat stored around the organs in the abdomen). **Abdominal fat**, also referred to as "belly" fat, includes visceral fat and the subcutaneous fat under the skin at the waist.

Fat has benefits. It forms the cell membranes (outer layer of cells) and is critical to the health of the brain, eyes, and other nerve tissue. Adipose tissue cushions your bones and organs, protecting them from injury. It insulates you from the cold. That's why thin people and old people (who lose subcutaneous fat) get cold more easily. Age-related loss of subcutaneous fat also increases the risk of bone fractures after a fall and makes faces look more hollowed and wrinkled.

Your amount of body fat depends on many factors: genetics, sex, age, activity level, diet, and metabolic rate. Genetics determine how many fat cells you have at birth and how they're distributed. Sex determines the relative amounts of male and female hormones. Throughout life, females have a greater proportion of fat relative to lean body mass.[15]

Disparities in body composition are much less apparent during childhood than during adolescence. During that time, girls develop breasts (which contain glandular tissue and fat) and more voluptuous hips; boys tend to lose fat and gain muscle and bone mass. From an evolutionary viewpoint, extra fat in women provides the energy necessary for pregnancy and breast-feeding. In that sense, the media message that thin is beautiful counters biology.

In modern society, most men and women gradually lose lean body mass starting in the third decade of life and accumulate body fat through the seventh decade. After age 70, many men and women begin to lose weight (both fat and lean body mass).

Distribution of fat also differs by sex. Men tend to carry extra fat in their abdomens; women pack fat on their thighs and hips. Hormones influence that distribution. Extra abdominal fat (visceral fat plus subcutaneous fat around the waistline) creates an apple shape. Extra subcutaneous fat around the thighs and hips creates a pear shape.

1.3   Assessing Body Weight and Body Composition

Everyone needs a certain amount of body fat. But how much is too much? The recommended body fat percentage ranges from 21 to 24 for fit women and from 14 to 17 for fit men.[16] A percentage higher than 30 in women and 25 in men indicates obesity. You have a number of ways of learning whether your weight and body composition are healthy.

A simple method is to step on a scale. However, you can't determine from body weight alone the relative proportions of fat and lean body mass. After measuring height, you can determine whether a person's weight falls within the range of normal for that height. Better still is a measurement called **body mass index** (BMI). BMI is weight in kilograms divided by height in meters squared, or BMI = weight in kilograms ÷ (height in meters)^2.

Many Americans don't work in the metric system. To convert pounds to kilograms, multiply weight in pounds by 2.2. To convert height in inches to meters, multiply the height by 0.0254. Here's another, shorter formula: BMI = weight (pounds) ÷ [height (inches)]^2 × 703. You can also use the BMI calculator on the Centers for Disease Control and Prevention's website: http://www.cdc.gov/healthyweight/assessing/bmi/adult_bmi/english_bmi_calculator/bmi_calculator.html.

Overweight and overfat are not the same thing. For that reason, BMI provides limited information. Here's an example. Looking at the graph in Figure 10.1, you'll see, for example, that a man who's 5 feet 11 inches tall and weighs 200 pounds falls into the overweight range. But you don't know how much of that extra weight comes from thick bones and muscles and how much comes from fat.

Despite its limitations, BMI nevertheless serves as a proxy for body fat. The measurement is simple and inexpensive, requiring only a measuring stick and a scale. For those reasons, you'll see it used by many authorities to determine whether or not people are overweight or underweight.

---

body composition

Describes the percentage of the body that is fat versus fat-free mass.

fat-free mass

Any tissues in the body that are not adipose tissue. It's mainly composed of bone and muscle.

adipose tissue

A body tissue that stores fat.

subcutaneous fat

Fat stored under the skin.

visceral fat

Fat stored around the internal organs.

FIGURE 10.1 Body Mass Index Chart

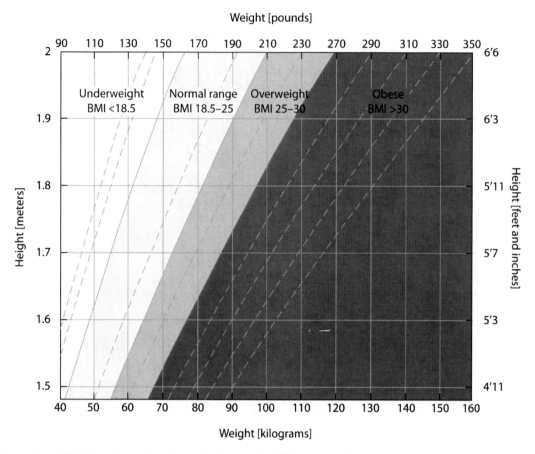

Source: InvictaHOG. 2006. Available at: http://commons.wikimedia.org/wiki/File:Body_mass_index_chart.svg.

This image shows a man with central obesity. The excess of visceral fat creates an apple shape. Until they reach menopause, women tend to deposit more fat around their hips and thighs than in their abdomens, creating a more pear-shaped appearance. Another influence on body fat percentages is age, especially for women. At menopause, female sex hormones (estrogen and progesterone) fall, and fat becomes more likely to be stored in the abdomen. In other words, overweight older women become less pear shaped and more apple shaped. In men, testosterone declines somewhat with age, which shifts body composition (from less fat-free mass to more fat mass).

Measuring a person's **waist circumference** would give you an idea of how much fat is packed around the middle. To learn yours, wrap a tape measure around your waist at the level of your navel. Higher waist circumference (waist size greater than 35 inches for women or 40 inches for men) indicates a heightened risk of heart disease and diabetes. However, this measurement doesn't differentiate fat versus lean tissue in the abdomen.

A better indicator is the **waist-to-hip ratio**. To calculate your ratio, wrap a tape measure around your waist, then around your hips at the widest part of your buttocks. Divide the measurement of your waist by the measurement of your hips. (You can also find a waist-to-hip calculator here: http://www.healthcalculators.org/calculators/waist_hip.asp.)

For men, a normal waist-to-hip ratio is 1.0 or less. For women, the ratio should be under 0.8. Higher numbers indicate a great amount of visceral fat, which indicates risk for conditions such as cardiovascular disease and diabetes. Larger waist circumference and waist-to-hip ratios *correlate* with body fat but don't actually measure it.

Skin fold measurements provide an estimate of subcutaneous fat. After the skin is pinched to trap two layers of skin and underlying adipose tissue, calipers measure the thickness. The data from those sites are then entered into mathematical formulas to calculate the percentage of body fat. While not very accurate, skin fold measurements can help monitor changes in body fat over time.

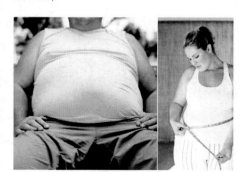

© *Thinkstock*

Hydrostatic testing, also called hydrodensitometry or underwater weighing, involves a person being in a tank of water. The amount of water you displace provides an estimate of body composition. Following the same principle, a computerized device called the BOD POD calculates a person's body composition based on air displacement. After a subject enters the egg-shaped machine, air displacement is used to estimate body fat percentage.

Bioelectrical impedance analysis passes a harmless electrical current through your body. Because fat offers more resistance to an electrical current than water-filled lean tissues, body composition can be estimated. Your level of hydration influences the results.

FIGURE 10.2
Skin Fold Measurement

Skin fold calipers estimate the amount of adipose tissue under the skin.

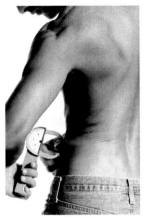

© Thinkstock

FIGURE 10.3   The Limits of Waist Circumference as a Predictor of Abdominal Fat

A higher waist circumference correlates with greater abdominal fat, which is a combination of the subcutaneous and visceral fat around the middle. But the correlation is far from perfect. See the scans of men with the same waist circumference. The scan captures a cross section of the body from belly button (top) to back. The darkest areas are muscle. You can also see the intestinal track and a vertebra. The light areas are fat (adipose tissue). Subcutaneous fat lies between the skin and the abdominal and back muscles. Visceral fat surrounds the organs. Notice that the first section has the least fat and the last has the most (as measured in liters). Presumably the men in the first few images exercised to stay lean. The last men were thin because of either dietary restrictions or illness.

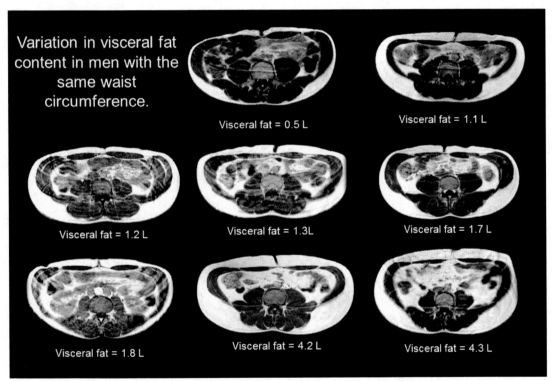

Source: ImagingFat. 2012. Available at: http://commons.wikimedia.org/wiki/

File:Variation_in_visceral_fat_in_men_with_the_same_waist_circumference.jpg.

Dual energy X-ray absorptiometry (DEXA), a test often used to measure bone density, can also assess the amount of body fat and muscle. The test entails lying on an X-ray table for a few minutes. It's relatively expensive but accurate. Other scanning procedures include magnetic resonance imaging (MRI) and computed tomography (CT).

1.4   Energy Balance

Energy balance is the ratio of energy intake (calories consumed) to energy expenditure (calories your body burns). What you eat and drink determine your energy intake. Energy expenditure is determined by your metabolic rate.

energy balance

Amount of calories your body burns versus the amount consumed.

Metabolic rate is the speed at which your body consumes calories. Metabolism refers to the chemical reactions occurring in your body. You break down food into small chemicals. Cells burn some of those chemicals. What's left over is stored. From these building blocks, your body makes proteins, fats, carbohydrates, bone, hormones, new cells, and more. Muscles enable you to chew, swallow, breathe, pump blood, talk, and move your body. The energy to do so is released from glucose and other energy molecules. It costs energy to break down molecules and to make new ones.

Basal metabolic rate (BMR) is the minimum level of energy to sustain vital processes such as breathing and circulating blood. When you digest food or move your body, your metabolic rate rises and you burn more calories. (Digesting food also leads to an input of calories.)

Lean body mass (especially muscle) demands more energy, thereby increasing BMR. The greater your muscle mass, the more calories you burn at rest. You also develop those muscles through regular physical activity, which adds to your total energy expenditure. In comparison, fat is not as metabolically active. If you compare two people who both weigh 160 pounds—one a weight lifter and the other a sedentary librarian, the weight lifter will burn more calories at rest.

FIGURE 10.4 Caloric Balance

If the calories consumed match your metabolic demands, you stay at the same weight. Energy in = energy out.

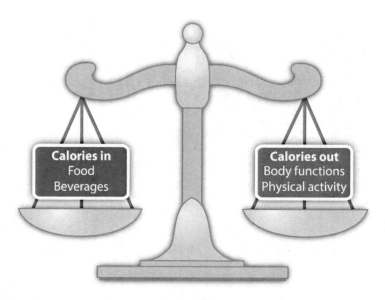

Source: Adapted from Centers for Disease Control and Prevention. Balancing calories. 2011. Available at: http://www.cdc.gov/healthyweight/calories/index.html.

If you're a woman 19 to 30 years old, your daily caloric needs are as follows: sedentary, 2,000; moderately active, 2,000–2,200; active, 2,400. A man in the same age bracket requires 2,400 calories a day if sedentary; 2,600–2,800 calories if moderately active; and 2,000–2,600 if active. For more information about calorie requirements based on age, sex, and activity level, go to this page at the National Heart Lung and Blood Institute: http://www.nhlbi.nih.gov/health/public/heart/obesity/wecan/healthy-weight-basics/balance.htm.

You may be wondering why men have slightly higher energy requirements than women. That's because male hormones create thicker bones and muscles. Under the influence of female hormones, women have relatively more fat around hips and in the breasts. Muscles, as you already know, burn more calories than fat.

Eating fewer calories than your body burns puts you into *negative energy balance*. Eventually, negative energy balance leads to weight loss. Put mathematically: Energy in < energy out = weight loss. *Positive energy balance* arises when you ingest more calories than your body burns. Because extra calories are stored as fat, positive energy balance leads to weight gain. Phrased as a mathematical equation: Energy in > energy out = weight gain. In America, sedentary lifestyles and easy access to high-calorie food has tipped many people into chronic positive energy balance.

KEY TAKEAWAYS

- Americans are preoccupied with physical appearance. Sadly, many young people are dissatisfied with their appearance. Dissatisfaction can lead to negative body image.
- Our culture prizes youth and beauty. A common cultural criterion for beauty is having a lean body.
- Regardless of size, shape, and age, everyone deserves to have a positive body image.
- Body composition describes the proportion of fat and lean tissue (also called fat-free mass). Muscle and bone form the majority of fat-free mass. A number of factors influence a person's body composition.
- A variety of measurements are used to determine body weight and body composition.
- When calories consumed from food match the body's energy expenditure, energy balance is achieved. Positive energy balance (more calories consumed than burned) leads to weight gain. Negative energy balance (more calories burned than consumed) leads to weight loss.

DISCUSSION QUESTIONS

1. Where do you get your ideas about personal beauty? What or who has influenced you the most?
2. Name one person who fails to meet the cultural norms of beautiful or handsome, but whom you nonetheless find appealing. What qualities make you find him or her attractive?
3. Describe in one to three sentences your body image. Now create two columns. On the left side, note attributes you wish you could change. On the right side, list your winning attributes.
4. In this exercise, you're going to write 10 positive personal statements. The first step is to identify negative thoughts about your body. Write them down. Now replace them with positive statements. That's not the same as writing the opposite. For instance, "I have thunder thighs," could become "My strong legs will take me farther each day." Post these 10 statements where you will see them every day.
5. BMI gives an indication of whether a person's body weight is normal for his or her height. Does it provide information about body composition? Explain your answer.

2. OVERWEIGHT AND OBESITY

LEARNING OBJECTIVES

1. Define overweight and obesity.
2. Discuss the prevalence of overweight and obesity globally and nationally.
3. Explore causes and environmental shifts thought to contribute to rising rates of obesity.
4. Describe the health consequences of overweight and obesity.
5. Identify strategies to prevent and treat overweight and obesity.

Overweight (BMI of 25 to 29.9) and **obesity** (BMI of 30 and up) have become a worldwide epidemic. The World Health Organization estimates that some 1.5 billion adults are overweight and 500 billion are obese.[17] Most live in the developed world. In high- and middle-income countries, more than half of adults carry excessive body fat.

In a study of trends of obesity in several developed countries, the United States had, hands down, the highest prevalence of obesity.[18] According to the Centers for Disease Control and Prevention (CDC), more than two-thirds of American adults weigh too much for their height, about a third are overweight but not obese, and over a third are obese.[19] Over the past three decades, the proportion of obese adults doubled from 15 percent to nearly 36 percent, and the proportion of obese young adults went from 8 percent to 24 percent. Obesity rates are highest among non-Hispanic blacks.

Overweight in childhood used to be uncommon. Not any longer. Over the past couple of decades, the number of overweight kids has tripled.[20] Over 30 percent of children and adolescents are overweight or obese.[21] Childhood overweight is significant because it often persists into adulthood.[22] A survey of college students found that 21 percent were overweight and 11 percent were obese.[23]

According to the CDC, obesity has topped 20 percent in all 50 states. In 12 states (Alabama, Arkansas, Kentucky, Louisiana, Michigan, Mississippi, Missouri, Oklahoma, South Carolina, Tennessee, Texas, and West Virginia), more than 30 percent of residents are obese.[24]

overweight

Having a BMI of 25 to 29.9.

obesity

Having a BMI of 30 and higher.

FIGURE 10.5 Prevalence of Self-Reported Obesity among US Adults, 2011

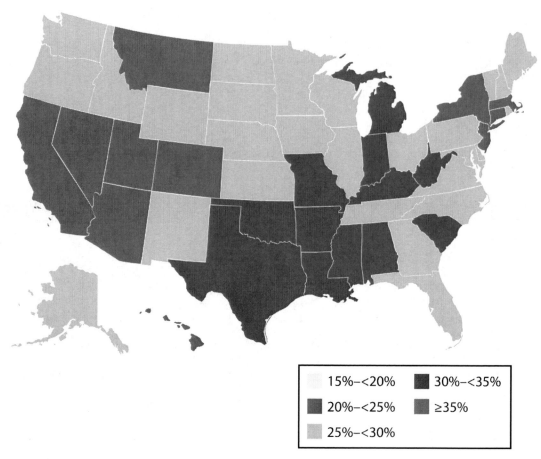

15%–<20%		30%–<35%
20%–<25%		≥35%
25%–<30%		

Source: Adapted from Centers for Disease Control. Adult obesity facts. 2012. Available at: http://www.cdc.gov/obesity/data/adult.html.

Most Americans gain weight steadily and inexorably—at the rate of just under a pound a year. Despite our best intentions, the pound added over the winter holidays never comes off. Seemingly small dietary change like washing down lunch with a soda instead of water and choosing the side of chips rather than the apple also contribute to a gradual accrual. This animated map from the CDC shows how obesity rates have increased from 1990 to 2010 in the United States: http://www.cdc.gov/obesity/data/adult.html#History.

2.1 What Causes Overweight and Obesity?

The simple answer is getting stuck in positive energy balance—that is, habitual intake of calories in excess of calories burned. Overeating and physical inactivity are the main culprits but other factors influence appetite, hunger, distribution of fat, and metabolic rate. One thing is clear: obesity is a medical condition, not a character flaw.

While inactivity is an important contributor, the main driver behind global obesity is consumption of excessive calories.[25] Between 1971 and 2004, calorie consumption among American adults increased 22 percent in women (from 1,542 to 1,886 calories a day) and 10 percent in men (from 2,450 to 2,693 calories a day).[26] Most of those extra calories came from carbohydrates, specifically starches, refined grains, sugar-sweetened beverages, other sugary snacks, and commercially prepared food (particularly fast food).

At first blush, the solution seems obvious: eat less and exercise more. Why can't we just do it? For one, access to food has increased. In the developing world, we have long ceased to rely on hunting and foraging for food. Relatively few of us grow our food. Developments in agriculture and government subsidies of some foods have led to the mass production of readily available, affordable, convenient, high-calorie food. In most cities and towns, you can hardly walk a block without passing a restaurant, market, or street vendor. Public buildings house cafés or, at least, vending machines. You can find snacks at gas stations, airports, sports arenas, theaters, and train and bus stations. The type of food so widely available is alien to the food our ancestors ate. Most of these energy-dense, palatable snacks come packaged from factories.

The food variety has also escalated. Restaurant menus fill several pages. Cafeteria lines stretch for yards. Not long ago, breakfast options were limited: eggs and bacon or oatmeal. Now breakfast foods fill an entire supermarket aisle. Making decisions can become exhausting. It's tempting to think, *Why not try a little of everything?*

Plates have gotten larger, as have the food portions covering them. At some restaurants, if you order steak, you get not a three-ounce serving (the size of a deck of cards), but a hunk bigger than your face. You're served not a roll, but an entire breadbasket. Convenience stores sell sodas in packs. Packaged foods come in "family-sized" boxes.

We dine out more often. Women, the traditional guardians of the kitchen, are often too busy with work to cook. Restaurateurs entice us to return with those high-fat, high-carbohydrate foods we're genetically groomed to prefer. Foods are fried or drenched in oil and butter. Restaurants also lure us with all-you-can eat buffets and inexpensive and swiftly delivered items. If you (and your kids) are strapped for cash and time, fast food becomes pretty appealing.

The media eggs us on, barraging us with advertisements for food, mainly processed, packaged food that's high in sugar and fat. When was the last time you saw an ad for celery sticks? Just seeing an ad for a juicy morsel can trigger an anticipatory rise in hormones and enzymes that send you running for the pantry. Basically, we are surrounded. We have literally become kids in the candy store.

Willpower is a finite resource. You may restrain yourself from eating the platter of donuts someone left in the dorm's common area the first two times you pass by. On the third, you may suddenly find yourself licking sugary glaze from your fingers.

There's even a genetic reason junk foods are hard to resist. Our species evolved in an environment of physical activity and occasional food scarcity. Our senses are primed to react enthusiastically to high-calorie foods. Also, in nature, sweet foods are usually nontoxic. No wonder sodas and other sugary beverages have nudged aside water as a rehydration fluid.

As compared to our ancestors, we don't even have to climb a tree to snag a sweet, juicy fruit. We're not sprinting across the savannah, hunting gazelles. Most of us don't push plows, harvest crops, milk cows, or tend goats. Motorized vehicles transport us. Thanks to drive-through restaurants, we don't even need to climb out of the car to eat. Or we can just stay home and open a cupboard.

As from excessive caloric consumption and inactivity, other factors do increase the risk of obesity.

Family History

If one parent is obese, the child's risk is two-and-a-half to four times greater. If both parents are obese, the risk is 10-fold.[27] But families share more than genes. Parents and other caregivers control what food comes into the home. In addition to food choices and availability, they influence attitudes about food and when, where, and how rapidly food is eaten. Some families eat to fill time. Some parents reward their children with food, punish them by withholding food, or insist the kids "clean their plates." All these behaviors can create unhealthy habits and attitudes.

The fact remains that inheritable factors shape body size and body composition. Studies in twins and adopted children indicate that genetics influences BMI. For instance, BMI of adopted children correlates more strongly with biological than adoptive parents.[28]

Aside from a near universal preference for energy-dense foods, some people have inherited genes that elevate the odds of overweight and obesity when food is abundant. Some people have what are called "thrifty metabolisms." They make efficient use of every calorie that comes their way, allowing them to survive lean times. Overabundance of energy-dense foods can lead to obesity. A case in point is the Pima Indians, native to the American Southwest, who thrived for millennia on their traditional diet, only to be stricken with obesity and diabetes with the transition to a modern lifestyle. In addition to affecting metabolism, genes can influence appetite and fat distribution. Many obesity genes have yet to be discovered.

The genetic makeup of populations shifts at a glacial pace. Therefore, genetics can't be blamed for the dramatic escalation in global obesity. However, genetic predisposition can explain who becomes obese in the face of societal changes (sedentary lifestyles and overnutrition).[29]

Early Childhood Influences

In addition to genetics, early life experiences cause *epigenetic changes*, modifications in the way genes are expressed. The genes have not altered, but their end products have. Epigenetic changes pass to the next generation.

For instance, babies born to mothers who were undernourished or overnourished during pregnancy are at risk for overweight. So are infants born to mothers who have diabetes. Often these infants are initially underweight but endowed with epigenetic modifications for thrifty metabolisms. In the face of abundant food, they can grow into overweight children and adults.

Prenatal and early childhood stressors can lead to an overactive stress response later in life. As will soon be discussed, stress can lead to overeating and visceral fat deposition. One profound early childhood influence is the maternal-child bond. A poor-quality bond is associated with overweight and obesity in adolescence.[30]

The type of food eaten in early childhood matters too. Foods a mother favors during pregnancy can bias an infant's palate. Compared to formula-fed babies, breast-fed babies have a reduced risk of obesity. Also, food preferences can be set early. Toddlers enjoy trying lots of different foods. They become pickier in preschool. That's why introducing healthy foods early—before their tastes narrow—is important.

 Video Clip 10.1

Genetic Predisposition Is Not Destiny
This video (fast forward to 3:11) provides evidence that genes indicate predisposition but don't dictate your fate. It features a scientific experiment with mice that carry the agouti gene. Most mice with this gene are yellow and obese. However, when a mother is fed a diet rich in supplements containing methyl groups (e.g., some B vitamins), epigenetic changes occur. Specifically, the methyl groups silence the agouti gene, resulting in normal weight, dark-coated offspring. Take-home message: no matter your genetic heritage, you can take steps to reduce your chances for becoming overweight.

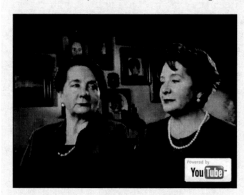

View the video online at: http://www.youtube.com/v/Xjq5eEslJhw

Physical Activity Levels

Physical activity levels affect body weight and body composition. People who are more physically active have more lean body mass and less fat than sedentary people—even if they're genetically predisposed to being overweight. Studies of identical twins show that genetic predisposition toward overweight is mainly apparent among people who don't vigorously exercise.[31] In other words, physical activity reduces the influence of genetic tendencies to develop high BMI and abdominal obesity. Furthermore, research suggests that exercise might most benefit people at greatest genetic risk for obesity.[32]

Sleep Deprivation

Sleep deprivation is a newly recognized risk factor for increased body fat. Over the past century, nightly sleep durations have declined an hour and a half. Meanwhile, obesity rates have risen. Sleep deprivation leads to changes in nervous system function, hormone release, and inflammatory chemicals that increase hunger, decrease satiety, and favor visceral fat deposition. People also are less likely to exercise when they feel tired.

Studies have linked chronic sleep deprivation, night-shift work, jet lag, and nocturnal behaviors (eating late, going to bed late, arising late) with weight gain.[33] A study of children aged three to seven found that the kids who didn't sleep enough were at significantly increased risk of becoming overweight.[34] In addition to short sleep cycles (6 hours and under), sleeping significantly more than 8 hours a night favors weight gain in adults. Research is under way to determine whether bumping volunteers' nightly sleep from under 6 hours to 7.5 hours will help them lose weight.[35]

Stress

There are several reasons that psychological stress can promote weight gain.[36] The majority of stressed people (women in particular) go for high-calorie "comfort" foods.[37] Complicated mechanisms link increased activation of the stress response to overeating and overweight. The stress hormone cortisol increases appetite, with a preference for sugary, fatty foods—just the kind of food you'd want after fleeing a tiger. This hormone also promotes deposition of visceral fat. Stress induces shifts in other hormones that can also increase food intake.

Lastly, stress influences the pleasure-reward system in the brain. Acute stress releases natural opioids such as endorphins, which relieve pain and make us feel good—in the short term. Chronic stress is not pleasurable. Eating good food is. It also releases endorphins, which make us feel better. When something is rewarding, we like to repeat it. Some researchers believe that repeated pleasure-reward system activation by episodes of stress and/or hedonic (for pleasure) eating lead to nervous system alterations that promote compulsive overeating and food addictions.[38]

Emotional Eating and Psychological Disorders

Many people eat in an attempt to cope with negative emotions such as anger, fear, and anxiety.[39] Eating disorders such as binge eating raise the risk of overweight and obesity. For complex reasons, depression, bipolar disorder, psychosis (e.g., schizophrenia), and some anxiety disorders are linked to a higher risk of overweight and obesity.[40],[41] Associated changes in body chemistry affect appetite. Having these conditions is stressful and may disrupt sleep. People may attempt to cope by smoking and drinking alcohol. Some medications used to treat the conditions promote weight gain. Finally, social stigmas against obesity can lead to depression and anxiety.

Racial and Socioeconomic Disparities

Overweight and obesity, as well as obesity-related diseases, are more common among minorities.[42] The prevalence of obesity is 36 percent for blacks, nearly 29 percent for Hispanics, almost 25 percent for non-Hispanic whites, and 7 percent for Asian Americans.[43] Compared to whites, obesity is also more prevalent among American Indians, Alaska Natives, Native Hawaiians, and Pacific Islanders.

Both genetics[44],[45] and multiple socioeconomic factors influence weight among different racial and ethnic groups. For instance, the idealized female size is larger for black women than for white women. Some traditional ethnic foods are higher in fat. Minorities more often face economic challenges and live in low-income, stressful neighborhoods. In the developed world, the highest obesity rates occur in the poorest, least educated populations.[46] Not surprisingly, the poorest states in the nation—Louisiana, Mississippi, and West Virginia—report the highest obesity rates.

Compared to poorer people, affluent people are more likely to be better educated about healthy food choices and more physically active. Prosperous neighborhoods have safer streets for walking, skating, and cycling and are more likely to have public parks, recreation centers, health clinics, and high-quality grocery stores.[47]

Lack of access to healthy food and fitness facilities, as often occurs in low-income neighborhoods, is associated with more obesity.[48] The correlation seems paradoxical. You might think that food insecurity would lead to weight loss. However, the food that's available and cheap is often high in refined grains, fats, and added sugars, but lacking in important nutrients. The result is a person on a processed-food diet can end up fat and malnourished.

Sometimes moving up is enough to improve weight and health. One study showed that black women and children who moved from high-poverty public housing to lower-poverty housing had subsequent declines in the rates of obesity and improvements in their diabetes.[49] The researchers didn't encourage the participants to eat better, exercise more, or make any other lifestyle change. The women and children simply moved to healthier neighborhoods.

Social Networks

Our relationships powerfully influence our behaviors. *Social contagion theory* postulates that conditions such as obesity spread within social networks (families, friends, workplaces, etc.).[50],[51] Social groups establish body weight norms, such that being overweight becomes ordinary and acceptable. Furthermore, individuals may adopt the eating and exercise habits of influential peers and family members.[52] A counter theory is that overweight people may hang out together because leaner peers have marginalized them.[53] Nevertheless, a useful tool is harnessing the power of social networks to improve diet and physical activity to promote weight loss.

Technological Innovations

Machines reduce energy expenditure. They transport us, manufacture our food, heat and cool our homes, and wash our clothes and dishes. Electronic devices make our work easier and entertain us. They can also lull us into a sedentary lifestyle. We spend hours in front of monitors of one sort or another, often grazing on food as we gaze.

People who watch more television are more likely to gain weight[54] because they're sitting instead of moving, many of the ads recommend high-calorie foods and beverages, and they often mindlessly snack in front of the television.

Environmental Chemicals

A modern complication is the development of myriad synthetic chemicals called *endocrine disruptors*, which interfere with hormone function. The list includes chemicals contained in plastics (bisphenol A and phthalates), flame retardants, cleaning products, personal care products, pesticides, and more. These chemicals have been linked to cancer, diabetes, infertility, and—yes, obesity.[55]

 Video Clip 10.2

A Historical Perspective on the American Diet
Stephan Guyenet, PhD, explains how changes in the American diet have resulted in an increase in caloric intake. You can learn more about the causes of obesity on Dr. Guyenet's blog, WholeHealthSource.com.

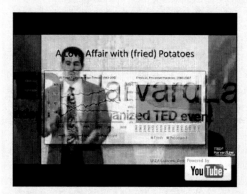

View the video online at: http://www.youtube.com/v/HC20OoIgG_Y
Source: TEDx, independently organized TED events.

Foods That Make Us Fat

A landmark 2011 study by Harvard University researchers examined the effect of changes in diet and lifestyle on weight gain.[56] The following foods were most strongly associated with weight gain (numbers in parentheses are pounds gained every four years): potato chips (1.69 extra pounds), potatoes (1.28 average, 3.35 for french fries), sugar-sweetened beverages (1.00), unprocessed and processed red meats (about 0.94), and refined grains, sweets, and desserts (all three about 0.4). Basically, starchy, sweet, and fatty foods add pounds. From a weight standpoint, white bread is just as bad as dessert. Furthermore, preliminary research indicates that refined carbohydrates can be downright addicting.[57]

Many health experts blame our burgeoning waistlines on our increased consumption of sweetened beverages:[58] sodas, juices, iced tea, "energy" drinks, coffee drinks containing added sugar and fat, and sports beverages. Most are sweetened with sucrose (table sugar) or high-fructose corn syrup. For complex reasons, high-fructose corn syrup appears to be more effective than other sugars at promoting fat deposition[59] and less effective at triggering satiety or decreasing appetite.[60]

Sweet drinks represent a major source of added (and readily absorbable) sugars, have scant nutritional value, do little to satisfy appetite, and add calories to our diets. The average 12-ounce can of carbonated soft drink contains 140 to 150 calories (and about 10 teaspoons of sugar). An 8-ounce cup of juice is often over 100 calories. A typical 12-ounce sports beverage is 75 calories. One study found that women who increased their sugar-sweetened beverage intake from one or fewer per week to one or more a day gained, on average, 10.3 pounds in four years—about 2.5 pounds a year.[61]

Unfortunately, these beverages represent a significant and increasing proportion of our daily intake. In fact, they're the single largest source of added dietary sugar. Between 1965 and 2002, calories from beverages increased by nearly 50 percent (an extra 222 calories a day).[62] Between 1977 and 2001, energy intake from sweetened beverages rose 135 percent,[63] and obesity rates doubled.[64] Subsequent studies show that the trend continues.[65] Consumption is highest among young adults, particularly minorities.

Lessons from the Bottomless Soup Bowl

We need to consume food to grow from infancy to full-fledged adulthood. Thereafter we need to replace the energy supplies that power cellular processes. When you pause to think about it, the process seems nothing short of miraculous. You chew and swallow a carrot and—presto—some of those orange pigments end up in the back of your eye, allowing you to see shades of gray under low illumination. The fat in the salmon you ate for lunch becomes incorporated into brain cells.

You don't think, "I'm feeling a little low on carotenes or essential fatty acids or amino acids." You simply hunger for the foods that might replace those nutrients. You're not eating out of concern for individual cells and their chemical processes. Most of us—registered dietitians excepted—don't select food based on nutritional content and the required ounces per serving.

When asked why they eat, many of my students respond that they eat when they're hungry. Period. Yet Americans often eat when we're not hungry. A multitude of other cues encourage putting food into our mouths: aromas, tastes, sights, social situations, advertisements, tradition, the way our clothes fit, and the time of day (if the clock says noon, it's time to eat lunch).

Sight, it turns out, is a powerful cue. You eyeball how much you think you should put on your plate and eat till it's done. Many of us were raised to "clean our plates." We graduated from childhood well suited for polishing off supersized servings.

Brian Wansink, PhD, director of the Cornell University Food and Brand Lab and author of *Mindless Eating: Why We Eat More Than We Think*, has executed a number of clever experiments illustrating our weird relationship with food. In one, he and his colleagues served free five-day-old popcorn to people attending a 1 p.m. movie. Most had recently eaten lunch. They randomly received medium, large, and supersized buckets of the stale popcorn. While watching the show, they palmed popcorn to their mouth. Afterward, all agreed the popcorn tasted no better than Styrofoam peanuts. Most believed they recognized fullness and therefore stopped eating. In reality, they ate much more (an average of 173 calories or 21 handfuls more) if given the biggest bucket. Furthermore, the participants underestimated both the volume consumed and the caloric content.

In another of Wansink's experiments, volunteers ate tomato soup. What they didn't realize was that half of the soup bowls were essentially bottomless. Tubing ran from a nearby pot into a hole at the bottom of the bowl. After 20 minutes, the researchers stopped the meal. People with normal bowls ate about 9 out of the 18-ounce servings. People with bottomless bowls consumed an average of 15 ounces; some consumed more than 32 ounces (a quart)! Everyone underestimated the number of calories consumed. Obese people, it turns out, underestimate food consumption to a greater degree than lean people.

Other experiments by Wansink demonstrate people eat more from larger packages, and they eat more if they anticipate the food will be great—if the menu is written in French rather than English, if they think the Two Buck Chuck in their wine glasses came from California versus North Dakota, if the Super Bowl is on, and if their clothes are loose.

Assess Yourself: Do You Eat When You're Not Hungry?

In order to get a handle on your eating triggers, answer the following questions.

	Never	Rarely	Sometimes	Often	Always
I eat when the clock says it's time to eat.					
I eat when I have something to celebrate.					
I eat when I'm angry, sad, or stressed.					
I snack while studying.					
I eat when I see or smell my favorite foods.					
I eat when I see advertisements for savory foods on television.					
I snack while watching television or movies.					
I eat when other people are eating.					
I eat until my plate is empty.					

Tally how many answers you have in the "often" or "always" column. What matters most is whether you do these behaviors when you're not actually hungry. If you checked yes to two or more of these things, you may be succumbing to mindless overeating. If you answered yes to the second or third questions, you may be an emotional eater. Becoming aware of your eating triggers can help you better manage your weight.

2.2 Consequences of Obesity

The World Health Organization calls overweight and obesity "a rapidly growing threat to the health of populations in an increasing number of countries."[66] Obesity is the fifth leading preventable cause of premature death—behind tobacco, high blood pressure, high blood sugar, and physical inactivity. Even in the developing world, obesity has begun to displace infectious diseases and undernutrition as major reasons for poor health.

Overweight and obesity contribute to a number of chronic, noncommunicable diseases: specifically heart disease, high blood pressure, stroke, diabetes, and some cancers. These diseases are the major killers in America. Furthermore, excessive body weight stresses the joints, increasing low back pain and osteoarthritis (joint inflammation caused by wear and tear). All these conditions can lead to decreased quality of life and physical disability.

Obesity shortens lifespan, more so for obese young adults than obese elders. In one study, severe obesity in adults aged 20 to 30 years reduced life expectancy up to 13 years of life for white men and 8 years for white women; 20 years for black men and 5 years for black women.[67] Due to overweight and obesity, children now have chronic illnesses normally occurring only in adults. Experts predict that, unless we take steps to prevent overweight, the current generation of young people will be the first to live a shorter time than their parents.

What's Wrong with Belly Fat?

Until recently, scientists regarded fat as a passive storage depot for excess calories. It turns out that adipose tissue—particularly visceral fat—has a number of biological activities. For instance, it makes hormones and releases inflammatory chemicals. For instance, adipose tissue processes and makes sex hormones, including estrogen. That's why overweight men develop breast tissue.

Adipose tissue makes *leptin*, a hormone that decreases appetite. Restriction of caloric intake and weight loss decrease leptin. The brain's response is to increase appetite and inhibit energy expenditures. Upon discovering leptin, scientists thought it would make a great obesity treatment. But that prediction didn't prove true. Regulating appetite is much more complex.

Adipose tissue, especially visceral fat, releases inflammatory chemicals and a number of proteins. As fat storage rises, levels of hormones produced or influenced by adipocytes shift. The net result an increased risk for high blood pressure, atherosclerosis (narrowing and hardening of the arteries due to fatty deposits), type 2 diabetes (a condition of high blood sugar due to decreased cellular response to the hormone insulin), metabolic syndrome (a clustering of risk factors for cardiovascular disease and diabetes), and colon cancer.[68] In women, visceral fat has been linked to breast cancer and gallstones.

The combination of excess weight on the joints and increased inflammation can lead to arthritis.

In addition to physical ailments, obesity has psychological, social, and economic consequences. Societal biases lead to social, academic, and workplace discrimination—even in health care settings.[69]

The economic consequences are multiple. Employer prejudice can hinder employment. Illnesses related to overweight and obesity increase absenteeism. Chronic illnesses are expensive to treat. Compared to their normal-weight peers, obese people spend about 30 percent more on health care.[70] Obesity-related disabilities erode quality of life and can lead to early retirement.

Stereotypes abound. Fat people are assumed to be jolly, lazy, stupid, unsexy, and unsuccessful. The media perpetuates these typecasts. Another misconception is that overweight arises simply from lacking the self-discipline and willpower to push away from the dinner table.

Societal attitudes also erode self-esteem, warp body image, generate psychological distress, and raise the risk of depression and anxiety.[71] Overweight children and teens face teasing, bullying, and other means of psychological torment from their peers. Such maltreatment stimulates binge eating[72] and reduces participation in physical activities,[73] creating a vicious cycle. Sadder still, it elevates the risk of attempted suicide.[74]

Such attitudes spawn shame and guilt among overweight people, which can thwart weight-loss strategies. For instance, overweight and obese people may be too embarrassed to exercise in public. Shame also hinders medical treatment. Worse, prejudice against obese patients exists among may exist among health care staff. Specifically, health care providers may spend less time on the health education of their heavier patients and be less likely to perform certain screening tests.[75] Sensing discrimination, patients may then postpone or avoid follow-up appointments.

TABLE 10.1   Medical Conditions Associated with Overweight and Obesity[76]

Metabolic syndrome (a combination of conditions that increase the risk for cardiovascular disease and diabetes)
High blood pressure
Atherosclerosis (a condition in which fatty deposits narrow and harden the arteries)
Heart disease
Blood clots in the deep veins
Type 2 diabetes (a condition in which poor response to the hormone insulin elevates blood sugar)
Arthritis (osteoarthritis and gout)
Cancer (cancer of the colon, breast, prostate, uterus, esophagus, kidney, and pancreas)[77]
Erectile dysfunction
Impaired fertility and complications during pregnancy
Nonalcoholic fatty liver disease (accumulation of fat in the liver not caused by alcoholism)
Obstructive sleep apnea (breathing stops multiple times during the night due to obstruction of the upper airway)
Stroke
Gallbladder disease
Gastroesophageal reflux disease (backwash of stomach contents into the esophagus)
Psychological distress and depression
Alzheimer's disease (a type of dementia)
Possibly asthma in children
Reduced quality of life
Premature death

Source: Kumanyika SK, Obarzanek E, Stettler N, et al. American Heart Association Statement. Population-based prevention of obesity. Circulation. 2008;118(4):428–464. Available at: http://circ.ahajournals.org/content/118/4/428.long#T1. Accessed July 20, 2012.

2.3   Preventing Overweight and Obesity

Obesity is a serious but largely preventable disease. It's particularly important to work toward preventing overweight and obesity in childhood. That means that efforts to improve diet and activity need to target pregnant women and children.

Though everyone should take personal responsibility for health, obesity is more than an individual problem; it's a global population problem. In addition to helping individuals eat better and exercise more, society should also work toward improving home, school, and work environments to promote good nutrition and physical activity. Regardless of body weight or age, we should all adopt healthy behaviors to improve quality of life and reduce disease risks. That said, efforts to improve lifestyles among individuals at school, at work, and in the greater community can work to reduce weight problems, are cost effective, and can even save money.[78]

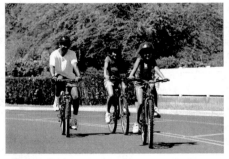
© Thinkstock

The first task is to increase availability of healthy foods to all people and limit access to obesity-promoting food. So what foods should people eat? From the previous discussion, it's clear about the importance of consuming more fruits, vegetables, grains, and nuts and restricting high-fat, sugary, starchy foods.[79] Low-fat and nonfat yogurt may be beneficial because it favorably alters intestinal bacteria.

Low-income neighborhoods need to have grocery stores that stock healthy foods. Increased access to supermarkets leads to consumption of more fruits and vegetables and a reduced risk of obesity.[80] Shifts in government subsidies away from obesity-promoting foods and toward fruits and vegetables would help make healthy foods affordable. Education about selecting and preparing healthy foods is also important. Initiatives to create organic farms in low-income neighborhoods can also increase access to fresh produce. When neighbors cooperate in growing foods, they develop a strong sense of community and a sense of pride, self-sufficiency, and ownership that encourages healthy eating.

At the same time, junk foods need to become less affordable and less available. In 2012, the federal government made changes in government-subsidized school meals to add more fruits and vegetables to kids' diets and to reduce fat and salt.[81] All milk must be low fat, and whole grains rather than refined grains must be used. Age-appropriate limits on caloric content per meal were also set. Unfortunately, the food industry lobbied to block a reduction in fat-promoting starchy foods such as potatoes. Because it contains tomato paste, pizza counts as a vegetable serving.

School-based interventions to include more fruits and vegetables in meals and increase physical activity have reduced overweight and obesity.[82] On the other hand, efforts to educate children and teens about healthy food and physical activity have met with little success.[83] Education alone doesn't change obesity-inducing environments.

As a way of improving school environments, some states have enacted laws curbing sales of sweetened drinks and other junk foods from vending machines. One report showed that, five years after California took steps to reduce junk food in schools, students did indeed consume less fat and sugar than kids who lived in schools without such laws.[84] A 2012 study showed positive changes following state bans on junk food in schools.[85] Specifically, the researchers calculated BMI on students in 40 states in fifth grade and again in eighth grade. Students in states with strong laws gained less weight and were less likely to become or remain overweight or obese with age.

The food industry could help by reducing the fat, sugar, and salt content of foods and by making healthy foods affordable. The industry should make more responsible marketing decisions. However, most industries are not very good at policing themselves.

For that reason, some experts favor regulating the marketing of junk food. According to the Yale Rudd Center for Food Policy and Obesity, the food industry invests more than $1.6 billion each year marketing food—the vast majority of it is promoting obesity—to kids.[86] Each child sees an average of 13 food commercials each day, 5,900 a year. Kids also see ads at school and on public transportation, mobile phones, and the Internet. Children then beg their parents to buy these unhealthy foods.

Another strategy is to increase taxes on unhealthy foods, to place nutrition labels on the front of packages to catch consumers' attention and to prominently display nutritional information at fast-food restaurants. For instance, you may be less likely to eat Chicken McNuggets if you knew 10 of them packed 510 calories. On the other hand, you would choose them if you were broke and hungry and those fried chicken morsels seemed to be the best option.

We all need to do a better job of working physical activity into our days. To prevent weight gain, 60 minutes a day of moderate-intensity exercise is recommended. In addition to individuals making moving a priority, cities may need to make infrastructure improvements that promote physical activity. Better city planning could reduce the suburban sprawl linked to weight gain. Better public transportation encourages people to leave their cars at home.

To encourage physical activity, cities can establish bicycle lanes, create sidewalks that safely buffer pedestrians from motor vehicles, and build pedestrian and cyclist bridges over or under busy intersections. Some cities have adopted bike-sharing programs, which allow people to check out bicycles to travel to their destinations. Placing new recreation centers near schools makes it easier for kids and their parents to exercise.

Municipalities can work toward increasing urban green spaces. That means building more parks, playgrounds, and community gardens, especially in lower-income neighborhoods. Children and teens living in greener neighborhoods are less likely to gain excessive body weight with age.[87]

Workplaces can support healthy food choices, regular physical activity, and healthy changes in weight. Employers that model such behaviors can inspire employees to follow suit. Schools and day care centers can ensure that ample physical activity is woven into every school day.

Parents and teachers can encourage kids to play outside. Studies in children show that children allowed to play outdoors increase their physical activity and reduce their risk of being overweight by 27 to 41 percent.[88] The same likely holds true for adults. That means we all need safe neighborhood places to recreate outdoors.

Food Patterns That Prevent Overweight and Obesity

While foods like potatoes and white bread tend to promote weight gain, others tend to curb it. People who consume more fruits and vegetables have a lower risk of weight gain.[89]

A study that tracked the influence of dietary choices on weight changes over time found that people who included more whole grains, vegetables, and fruits in their diets tended to lose weight.[90] That may be because these foods took the place of items such as potato chips.

Adding nonfat or low-fat yogurt to the diet is associated with weight loss. Yogurt may be beneficial because it favorably alters intestinal bacteria. Fascinating lab research suggests the gut microbes affect weight.[91],[92]

Eating nuts in moderation—since they're high in both calories and nutrients—is associated with healthy weight.[93] Studies have also linked regular consumption of dark chocolate, which is high in health-promoting chemicals called polyphenols, with a lower BMI.[94] A small square of dark chocolate can also produce a sense of satisfaction at the end of a meal. Keep in mind that, due to saturated fats and added sugars, a chocolate bar can pack up to 200 calories. So either limit your daily chocolate consumption to one ounce or add cocoa powder (which contains the polyphenols but little fat) to nonfat milk or yogurt.

2.4   Benefits of Losing Weight

For people who are overweight or obese, losing weight has many benefits, even when BMI doesn't drop within the range of normal. Here's why:

- Weight loss prevents and helps manage cardiovascular disease and diabetes.
- Dropping 10 pounds of excess body fat can lower blood pressure, cholesterol, and triglycerides (blood fat).
- Weight loss can resolve obstructive sleep apnea, promoting more restful sleep.
- Joints hurt less, and physical activity becomes easier.
- Body-wide inflammation declines.
- Weight loss can also relieve embarrassing problems such as urinary incontinence (leakage) in overweight women. In obese men, weight loss can make it easier to urinate.
- Slimming down can improve sex life. Men and women may feel better about their bodies. Sexual desire rises. For obese men, weight loss can improve erectile function.[95]
- Successful weight loss enhances overall well-being and boosts self-confidence, self-esteem, and self-efficacy.

2.5   Strategies for Successful Weight Loss

Although not always easy, losing extra pounds is entirely possible. To do it, you have to shift into a negative energy balance. A pound of body fat is just over 3,500 calories. If, for example, you wanted to lose a pound in one week, you would need to run a 3,500-calorie deficit from dietary restriction or increased physical activity. (Note: This 3,500-calorie formula, which was derived from short-term studies of men on very restricted diets, provides a very rough estimate of weight loss.[96] ,[97] It doesn't account for individual variations in metabolism and body composition and doesn't apply to long-term lifestyle modifications.) Most experts believe that the best weight-loss plans combine reduced-calorie diets and exercise. They also recommend people lose no more than two pounds a week.[98]

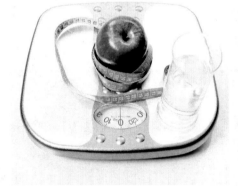

© Thinkstock

Eating less and exercising more sounds deceptively simple. Increasing physical activity, once we overcome the inertia of the couch, is fairly straightforward. Choosing a weight-loss diet is not. Every day, there's a new book or blog hawking the latest diet. Unfortunately, the word "diet" connotes deprivation. Deprivation promotes cravings. If you stop eating your favorite foods, you'll spend most of the day thinking about them and finding ways to cheat. You make many food decisions over the course of the day and possess limited willpower. Eventually, we tend to wear out and give in. The best diet doesn't feel like a "diet." It's tasty, satisfying, healthy, and sustainable.

As a case in point, a 2011 study found that a reduced-calorie diet that allowed a daily sweet (a chocolate or nonchocolate snack) led to reductions in weight, fat mass, and waist and hip circumference.[99]

Studies show that a variety of weight-loss diets work regardless of the portion of protein, carbohydrate, and fat. As long as a diet puts you into negative energy balance, you will lose weight. Some diets help by limiting food variety, which reduces frequent food decisions and temptations. Severely restricted food options are boring, are challenging to maintain, and may compromise health and well-being.

Steer clear of extreme measures for rapid weight loss. These include starvation diets, unbalanced diets (eating only meat or only grapefruit), liquid meals, self-induced vomiting, laxatives, and diuretics. For one, these measures can harm your health.

Two, rapid weight loss is, for most people, neither sustainable nor enjoyable. Some studies, however, do show that initial rapid weight loss works for some people.[100] However, study volunteers embark on more intensive weight-loss regimes under professional supervision.

One problem with very low-calorie diets is that your body responds by slowing metabolism. You also tend to move less, which is another means of reducing your energy expenditure.[101] That's how humans survive lean times.

In addition, as pounds are shed, hormones regulating appetite shift. For example, ghrelin (which stimulates hunger) rises and leptin (which signals satiety) falls. A 2011 yearlong study found that these counterproductive alterations persist.[102] In other words, perseverance is required.

Compared to extreme diets, modest changes in caloric intake have three advantages. One, your psychological outlook is also more positive when dietary changes feel enjoyable rather than punitive. Two, you're less likely to cheat and more likely to persist. Three, small fluctuations in calories won't send your body into metabolic slowdown.

For instance, if you cut 100 to 200 calories from your diet each day, you won't feel hungrier and your metabolism won't switch into starvation mode. As long as you don't make up the calories in some other way, you'll steadily lose weight. In fact, a habitual deficit of 100 to 200 calories a day will lead to a weight loss of 10 to 20 pounds a year.

You don't even have to give up your favorite, high-calorie foods. You simply need to consume less of them. Most sweetened drinks are about 100 calories per eight-ounce cup. A simple solution is to substitute water or diet soda for sugar-sweetened soda. You could eat a half cup of vanilla ice cream (145 calories) topped with fresh berries rather than a full cup serving. Drink nonfat (86 calories per cup) rather than full-fat milk (150 calories per cup). Take the bread off a sandwich. Try one cookie instead of two. Eat the hamburger topped with lots of lettuce and tomato, rather than cheese and bacon. When ordering pizzas, hold the pepperoni and request half as much cheese. These compromises can work because you diminish calories but not pleasure.

Bottom line about diet: rather than going on a "diet," make modest changes to your food patterns.

The Skinny on Weight-Loss Diets

An ongoing discussion is whether and how the proportion of macronutrients—carbohydrate, protein, and fat—affects weight gain. Your body stores extra calories—regardless of whether they're from carbohydrate, protein, or fat—as fat. If you reduce daily caloric intake, you will lose weight. You can eliminate junk food and lose no weight if you make up the calories with other foods (e.g., steak). Comparisons of several popular diets show they can all be successful.[103]

A current popular belief is that high-protein, low-carbohydrate diets help people lose weight. Three things are true: One, we need adequate amounts of dietary protein to maintain lean body mass. Two, dietary protein and fat provide a sense of satiety. Three, compared to carbohydrates and fat, the digestion, absorption, and metabolism of protein consumes more energy. Again, you only lose body fat if your total caloric intake declines below calories burned.

Some experts worry about the health consequences of consuming lots of animal protein and fat. Short-term consequences of such weight-loss diets include bad breath, headache, and constipation. Potential long-term consequences include heart disease, cancer, and some colon conditions. For more information about popular weight-loss diets, consult the reviews of each on WebMD at http://www.webmd.com/diet/evaluate-latest-diets.

Here are some other tips for successful weight loss. Note that if you are pregnant, breast-feeding an infant, or have a chronic medical condition, discuss your weight-loss plans with your physician. Parents of overweight children should work with their pediatrician to learn safe ways to manage weight.

- **Tell yourself that you can change your behaviors.** After all, you abandoned all kinds of routines to attend college. College is an excellent time to reinvent yourself.

- **Set specific, attainable goals.** Having a long-term goal is good, but it also helps to have mini goals for each week or month. Write your intentions and post them where you can see them. For example, you might write, "I want to fit into the jeans I wore when I started college." The most you should aim to lose in a week is one to two pounds. For some people, a more realistic, maintainable goal is a pound a month.

- **Formulate an eating plan.** Identify two or three modest changes you think you can make. For example, you may resolve to give up or reduce cheese, switch from sodas to water, and cover half your plate with vegetables.

- **Move your body.** Studies confirm that regular exercise—ideally 60 to 90 minutes a day—is essential to successful weight loss. Exercise can be broken into 10-minute increments. Benefits are multiple.

  Activity burns calories. Because muscle is more metabolically active than fat, gains in muscle mass increase your basal metabolic rate (the rate at which your body consumes energy at rest). Pleasurable exercise relieves stress and gives you something else to do aside from eating. Even without losing significant amounts of weight, exercise reduces the risk of diseases associated with overweight such as heart disease and diabetes.[104]

Instead of gathering with friends to eat, walk, dance, or play a sport together. (Note: Spot exercises such as sit-ups will tone your abdominal muscles but won't melt away visceral fat. Focus instead on aerobic and resistance training.)

■ **Eat when you're hungry.** There are two messages here: (1) Don't eat if you're not hungry—no matter whether the clock suggests it's mealtime, there's still food on your plate, your friends are eating, or emotions send you to the fridge; and (2) don't skip meals. People who skip meals with hopes of losing weight are typically so famished by the next meal that they overeat. A 2012 study found that teenage girls who ate fewer meals gained more body fat.[105] Between-meal snacking is fine if you're hungry and if you eat real food (as opposed to chips and ice cream).

■ **Eat real food.** The less processed your food, the better. Go for whole foods: vegetables, fruits, nuts, fish, lean meats, and eggs. Raw fruits and vegetables contain water, which take up room in your gut. Consume whole grains and nonfat dairy in moderation. The fiber in plants slows absorption of sugars and creates a sense of fullness because it's poorly absorbed from the intestines. Nonfat dairy such as plain yogurt provides calcium and hunger-curbing protein.

■ **Emphasize vegetables.** At mealtime, cover two-thirds of your plate with them. Start meals with leafy greens. Volume eaten is a key cue to satiety. That's why two-thirds of a cup of juicy grapes slakes hunger better than a quarter cup of raisins, even though both pack 100 calories. The goal is to make that volume both low in calories and high in nutrients. Vegetables fit the bill—as long as you avoid calorie-packed, creamy salad dressings and sauces. Try lightly dressing greens with olive oil and vinegar (or minus herbs).

■ **Make time for breakfast.** For many people, the morning meal is essential to satisfying hunger and maintaining energy. Some studies show that eating breakfast protects against being overweight.[106] The high protein content of eggs fends off hunger longer than a high-carbohydrate breakfast such as a bagel with jam.

■ **Drink water.** Green tea is another good choice, but curb your consumption to five cups a day. It contains less caffeine than coffee and health-promoting flavonoids, including catechins, which may stimulate the body to burn fat.[107] Limit or eliminate soda, juice, sports beverages, fatty and sugary coffee drinks, "energy" drinks, and other sweetened beverages. Many sodas now come in containers that far exceed eight ounces.

If you love soda, swap it for an artificially sweetened beverage. Then try to wean off sodas, as even when artificially sweetened they seem to increase the risk of excessive weight gain and other chronic conditions.[108] If you enjoy coffee drinks, choose black coffee (plus or minus a teaspoon or two of half and half or milk) or espresso drinks made with nonfat milk. Give up caffeinated drinks blended with syrup and cream. Instead of using sports beverages, drink water and follow an exercise session with a wholesome snack. Substitute that morning glass of orange juice (112 calories per 8-ounce cup) with an orange, which contains only 70 calories and is more filling than juice. Or steadily dilute the orange juice with water. You may eventually be able to switch to water with a squeeze of lemon juice.

Minimize alcohol intake. A 12-ounce can of beer contains about 150 calories. A glass of wine (3.5 ounces) is 85 calories. A shot (1.5 ounces) of the average hard liquor is 97 ounces.

■ **Shop the periphery of the supermarket,** which is where you'll find unprocessed food. Start in the produce section. Unless you're a vegetarian, head to the seafood and meat counters next. Select lean cuts and trim away visible fat before cooking. Avoid or restrict fried foods, bakery items, sugary yogurts, juice, soda, and anything else that is high in trans fats and simple carbohydrates.

■ **Keep healthy snacks on hand.** When you're shopping, pick out healthy snack foods such as carrots, celery, apples, nuts, hummus, and peanut butter. That way, when you're ravenous, you won't be tempted to cheat with potato chips and other fat-promoting snacks.

■ **Read nutritional labels.** You'll learn about ingredients and the caloric content. If a product announces it's low fat, check how many of the calories are from refined carbohydrates. A little butter or vegetable oil is better for you than sugar or high-fructose corn syrup. Also, people tend to eat more of a low-fat product, which may not be that much lower in calories than the regular-fat product. What counts is calories.

■ **Use low-fat cooking methods.** Depending on the food, you can bake, broil, roast, or cook with water or broth (poach, braise, steam, or stew). If you find steamed vegetables too bland, try sautéing onions in a little olive oil then adding other vegetables and broth to keep things moist. Keep in mind that your body needs some dietary fat and that fat satisfies hunger. Your body doesn't need fried foods.

- **Eat your food from a plate or bowl.** It's easier to lose track of how much you've devoured if you're reaching into a family-sized box or bag. Instead, arrange the whole meal on the plate so you can see it. We tend to estimate how much we're going to eat with our eyes and continue chewing until it's all gone.

- **Use smaller plates.** The goal is to put smaller portions onto your plate—about 10 to 20 percent less than usual. People routinely and unwittingly scoop heartier servings onto larger plates. A three-ounce serving of steak (the size of a deck of cards) looks much more substantial on a small plate. Serve desserts on saucer-sized plates. WebMD has a useful online tool to visualize appropriate portion sizes at http://www.webmd.com/diet/healthtool-portion-size-plate. You can download and print a pocket-sized guide.

- **Eat slowly and mindfully.** People who eat hastily tend to gain more weight than those who eat slowly.[109] One of your cues for satiety is how long you've been eating. You can wolf down a 270-calorie candy bar in less than a minute and still feel unsatisfied. Instead, engage all your senses. If you're eating an orange, pay close attention to the sights, smells, textures, and tastes as you peel the rind. Separate the sections, place them one at a time on your tongue, chew, and swallow. Compare that experience to eating an orange (or any other food) while reading, driving, or watching television.

  A leisurely pace also helps when dining with friends. Culture dictates that we remain at the table until everyone has finished. The longer you sit, the more you're tempted to eat. If you take your time, pausing between bites, you'll eat less.

- **Push away from the table sooner.** People from countries like Japan and France stop before they're full and leave food on their plates. In workman-like fashion, Americans tend to clean their plates. Those additional last bites don't taste better than the first. Don't wait until you feel full. You stop feeling hungry well before you appreciate a full belly. In fact, it can take up to 20 minutes for your stomach to appreciate that it's had enough.

- **Pack up leftovers.** When you're paying for a dinner out, you may find yourself thinking, "But I paid good money for this food." That doesn't mean you need to eat it all at one sitting. "Doggy bags" are always an option. Another dining-out tactic is to split an entrée with a friend. In American restaurants, a main course often contains enough food to feed at least two people.

- **Steer clear of fast-food restaurants.** Granted, quickly prepared meals aren't necessarily promoting obesity. But many of us can't resist the fried chicken, double-cheese hamburgers, fries, extra-large soda, and the white-bread sandwich with pastrami, cheese, and mayonnaise. A 20-year-long study found that young adults who ate more often in fast-food versus sit-down restaurants were more likely to gain weight, expand their girths, and increase levels of fat in the blood.[110] If you frequent fast-food places in the interest of convenience and economy, consider packing your lunch.

- **Get smart about cafeteria lines.** A variety of food offerings trigger an urge to sample everything. If you're eating on campus, you may have noticed this phenomenon. Particularly fiendish is the restaurant habit of putting desserts at the start of the line. Start with the salad bar. Next consider fruits, cooked vegetables, meat, and whole grains. Limit your selections to two or three things and put them all on one plate. Plan on filling half the plate with vegetables. If you're still hungry, you can always go back for more.

- **Store food out of sight.** People snack more when food is visible and within arm's length. Make tempting foods inconvenient. Following that general principle, you might want to stand farther from the table laden with pretzels and chips at parties.

- **Manage stress.** As noted earlier, chronic stress can increase hunger, cravings for junk foods, and deposition of abdominal fat. When researchers taught mindfulness-based stress reduction to overweight and obese people, the results were reductions in anxiety and the stress hormone cortisol and eating in response to external cues (rather than hunger). Among volunteers with a significant decrease in chronic stress, abdominal fat also declined.[111] Other methods for countering stress include exercising, practicing yoga and tai chi, meditating, connecting with friends, and journaling. See Chapter 3 for other ideas about staying calm.

- **Find healthy outlets for negative emotions.** Emotional eating, which tends to result in guilt and shame, typically comes on suddenly and has nothing to do with the emptiness of one's stomach. It's difficult to eat mindfully when you're upset. Eating won't solve your emotional challenges and might even aggravate them. Rather than smothering anxiety, anger, and sadness with a sundae, do something beneficial—jog, record your feelings in a journal, create art, listen to (or make) music, dance, talk to a friend.

- **Seek social support.** Enlist the backing of friends and family. Team up with others who are also trying to lose weight. The campus health clinic may offer group classes. Studies show that both in-person and remote (telephone, e-mails, texts) reinforcement from weight-loss coaches enhances weight loss.[112]

- **Harness the power of social networks.** Just as the widening waistlines of friends and family can sway you to join in, weight loss in friends and family seems to also be "contagious."[113] Hang out with lean, physically active people who eat wisely. Find a buddy who is also trying to exercise and cut out fatty, sugary food. In lieu of lounging on the couch, snacking, and watching televised football, suggest to your friends to go outside for a game of touch football. At parties, turn on the dance tunes and move.

- **Get enough sleep.** You already know that chronic sleep deprivation triggers the stress response and promotes weight gain. See Chapter 4 for tips on sleeping well.

- **Limit television viewing** and other passive forms of entertainment. One study found that doing just that reduced BMI in adolescents.[114]

- **Seek treatment for psychiatric conditions.** Depression, anxiety, and eating disorders will limit your success in managing weight.

- **Monitor your progress.** Record your weight at the same time and day each week. Create a graph or use smartphone and Internet apps. It's normal to move two steps forward and one step back. If you gain back some weight, don't despair and don't quit. Look for overall positive trends. Also, pay attention to other signs of forward progress: your clothes fitting more comfortably, better sleep, more energy, greater ease in climbing stairs and reaching your shoelaces, compliments from friends, a rosier self-image, and so on.

- **Celebrate progress.** Just don't make food rich in sugar and fat the reward. Go to a movie, concert, or a sporting or cultural event. Treat yourself to flowers, body lotion, or sports paraphernalia. If your jeans are now loose and you can afford a shopping spree, buy a new, slimmer pair.

- **Maintain your excellent habits during the holidays.** Celebration doesn't need to entail gorging. Many adults gain a little weight over the winter holidays and never lose it: a pound a year, 10 pounds a decade, and so on.

- **Be patient and persistent.** It took time to gain the weight and it will take time to lose it. Small, positive changes in diet and physical activity eventually pay off.

If repeated attempts to lose weight are unsuccessful or you have any concerns about your weight, meet with your physician.

Medical and Surgical Treatments

Health practitioners start by recommending dietary changes and physical activity. More comprehensive treatments include a combination of lifestyle interventions. As part of such programs, overweight and obese individuals may receive education about diet, food journals (to record food intake and associated behaviors), incentives to exercise, periodic weight checks, and professional and peer counseling.

A popular therapy is **cognitive behavioral therapy**, which can help people revamp self-defeating thoughts, set goals, identify support systems, break down barriers to success, motivate, strategize, alter behaviors associated with eating, and track progress. Studies show that comprehensive programs can lead to steady, sustained weight loss and also improve self-concept and create a sense of self-efficacy.[115]

Here's an example of a successful behavioral weight-loss intervention. For six months, 472 obese volunteers attempted to reduce dietary intakes by 500 calories a day, adopt a healthy diet (vegetables, fruits, legumes, grains, low-fat or nonfat dairy, nuts, and lean meats with restricted sweets and fats), and increase physical activity to 180 minutes a week. During that time, they participated in 22 groups sessions led by behavioral counselors. In addition to tracking changes in weight, researchers also measured sleep times, insomnia, screen time, depression, and stress symptoms at the study's start and end.[116] The average weight loss was 12.6 pounds. Better sleep and lower stress at entry predicted greater success in losing weight. Furthermore, weight loss reduced symptoms of stress and depression.

When behavioral changes aren't enough to achieve and sustain weight loss, psychotherapy, medications, and surgery are options.

Prescription weight-loss medications are sometimes used to manage obesity in concert with lifestyle changes. The goal is to either suppress appetite, hasten feelings of satiety, increase the rate at which food energy is burned, or interfere with absorption. Drugs such as phentermine suppress appetite. Orlistat (marketed as Alli and Xenical) interferes with the absorption of fat from food. Belviq (lorcaserin), a newly approved prescription medication, activates brain receptors for serotonin, a naturally occurring chemical that fosters feelings of contentment and satiety.

Most of these medications have side effects. For instance, stimulants such as phentermine not only suppress appetite but may also cause upset stomach, nervousness, insomnia, and increased heart rate and blood pressure. Cardiovascular stimulation makes the medication unsafe for people with heart disease. Orlistat can cause flatulence, urgent bowel movements, incontinence, and oily stools.

Weight-Loss Supplements

The media bombards us with advertisements for weight-loss supplements. Store shelves groan with the weight of these products. Online retailers hawk the stuff too. Do they work? Oftentimes not. Or the weight lost boomerangs home once you stop the product. Worse, some come with unpleasant or dangerous side effects.

Chinese ephedra (*Ephedra sinensis*) is a case in point. The plant contains ephedrine alkaloids, including pseudoephedrine, the chemical in the decongestant Sudafed. These chemicals, which have an effect similar to the body's epinephrine (adrenaline), open the airways for easier breathing. For centuries, Asian healers blended ephedra with other herbs to treat respiratory conditions such as asthma and bronchitis. People didn't take the plant singly or in large doses.

More recently, some American weight-loss and sport supplement companies started combining concentrated ephedrine alkaloids with caffeine and caffeine-containing herbs—a combination that can prove dangerous, especially for people at risk of cardiovascular disease. Adverse effects included insomnia, irritability, rapid heart rate, heart palpitations, increased blood pressure, as well as cases of heart attack, cardiac arrest with sudden death, stroke, and seizures.[117] In 2004, the Food and Drug Administration removed all ephedra-containing products from the market. In Asia, the herb continues to be safely used in respiratory formulas.

As mentioned earlier, green tea extracts have met with some success in stimulating weight loss. Other herbal supplements (hoodia, Garcinia, bitter orange) haven't yet been proven effective and safe. Conjugated linolenic acid (a concentrated form of a group of fatty acids in dairy and meat) may improve body composition in obese people but without significantly reducing weight.[118]

This image shows a gastric band around the stomach. Food enters at the top, via the esophagus. Because the pouch is small, people feel full quickly. The food then passes slowly through the bottleneck to the rest of the intestinal tract.

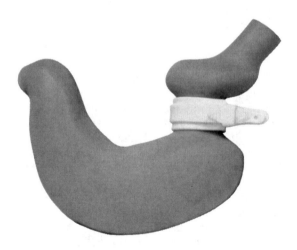

© Thinkstock

bariatric surgery

Weight-loss surgery.

Surgical treatments for weight loss, also called **bariatric surgery**, alter the digestive tract in such a way as to limit the amount of food that can be eaten and digested. It's generally reserved for people with a BMI over 40 or obese people with a lower BMI (35 to 4) who have developed significant health problems. In either case, lifestyle changes have not been able to achieve lasting weight loss.

Three main types of bariatric surgery are currently done. The least invasive is *gastric banding surgery*, which restricts the size of the stomach with an adjustable band. Food passes through the narrowing created by the band more slowly. *Gastric sleeve surgery*, also called *gastroplasty*, involves stapling the stomach to make it smaller. *Gastric bypass surgery* reduces the size of the stomach and then reattaches the small intestine to this pouch.

The benefits include significant weight loss and improvements in quality of life and in associated conditions such as diabetes, high blood pressure, obstructive sleep apnea, and arthritis. Risks include pain or infection at the surgical site, as well as nutritional deficiencies, heartburn, nausea, vomiting, diarrhea, and gallstones. Rare but serious complications include blood clots, ulcers, and leakage of stomach contents into the abdomen (after gastric bypass surgery).

KEY TAKEAWAYS

- Overweight and obesity have become a worldwide public health crisis.
- Compared to environmental changes, genetics play a relatively minor role in the rise in overweight and obesity. While some genes may predispose us to gaining fat, they only do so in the presence of excessive intake of high-calorie foods. The food industry—whose motivation is profit, not public health—has made fattening foods readily available.
- Two main factors lead to a positive energy balance: increased caloric intake and decreased physical activity. Factors such as poverty, lack of education, racial inequalities, psychological distress, and sleep deprivation also contribute to obesity.
- Overweight and obesity reduce longevity and raise the risk for a number of chronic conditions, including cardiovascular disease and diabetes. Obese individuals are also at risk for social stigmatization.
- Lifestyle modifications can prevent and treat overweight and obesity. The best strategies are to reduce caloric intake (without sacrificing optimal nutrition) and to increase physical activity.
- In the case of obesity that can't be controlled with lifestyle changes, doctors may prescribe medications or recommend bariatric surgery.

DISCUSSION QUESTIONS

1. In May 2012, Michael Bloomberg, Mayor of New York City, announced a ban on the sale of large-sized (greater than 16 ounces) sodas and other sugary drinks at movie theaters, restaurants, and street carts. The justification was that such a move might counter obesity. Read more about the subject at either the *New York Times* (http://www.nytimes.com/2012/05/31/nyregion/ bloomberg-plans-a-ban-on-large-sugared-drinks.html) or *MedPage Today* (http://www.medpagetoday.com/PrimaryCare/DietNutrition/33013?utm_content=&utm_medium= email&utm_campaign=DailyHeadlines&utm_source=WC&eun=g236011d0r&userid=236011 &email=lwhite27@mscd.edu&mu_id=5231323). In 100 to 250 words, write your well-reasoned opinion of the proposed ban.

2. How many calories do you need to maintain your current weight? Go to http://www.cancer.org/healthy/ toolsandcalculators/calculators/app/calorie-counter-calculator, fill out the form, and record your result.

3. Imagine that you want to lose weight or are helping a friend who wants to lose four pounds in a month. That's a pound a week for four weeks. Recall that a rough formula for short-term weight loss is 3,500 calories per pound of fat. To lose a pound a week means that the average daily calorie deficit is 500 (3,500 divided by 7).

    Your job is to design a daily plan of action for both changing diet and activity levels. Write down a Sunday-through-Saturday schedule. For each day, note the following: (1) The type of physical activity, duration performed, and anticipated calories expended; and (2) the food normally eaten that you plan to give up and how many calories that change represents.

    Note: To find out how many calories various activities expend, go to this US Department of Agriculture's website: http://www.choosemyplate.gov/physical-activity/calories-burn.html. To determine caloric content of foods, try http://www.thecaloriecounter.com/Search.aspx or the Food-o-Meter at WebMD (http://www.webmd.com/diet/healthtool-food-calorie-counter). Alternatively, you can also find smartphone apps to track calories and physical activity. For additional ideas about creating a food and fitness plan, go to the WebMD Food & Fitness Planner at http://www.webmd.com/diet/ food-fitness-planner/default.htm.

3. BODY IMAGE DISTURBANCES AND EATING DISORDERS

LEARNING OBJECTIVES

1. Examine the more common body image disturbances.
2. Identify key signs and risk factors for eating disorders.
3. Discuss the health consequences of eating disorders.
4. Recognize the need for timely professional treatment of eating disorders.

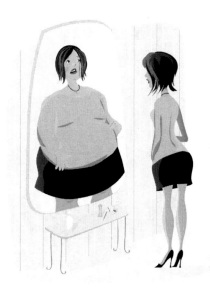

© Thinkstock

body dysmorphic disorder

A disorder characterized by distressing or impairing preoccupation with a slight or imagined defect in physical appearance.

muscle dysmorphia

An abnormal preoccupation with muscularity that causes compulsive exercising and other means to build muscle; also called muscle dysmorphic disorder or "bigorexia."

Body image can become warped. People with a *negative body image* have distorted perception of physical appearance, especially the size and shape of their bodies. They feel ashamed and anxious about their bodies and imagine that other people see them through a dark lens.

The severity of body image disturbances varies. Some people are simply overly preoccupied with and critical of their bodies. They constantly compare themselves—usually unfavorably—to others. Extreme dissatisfaction characterizes a condition called **body dysmorphic disorder**. In this condition, people obsess over minor and imagined flaws. They may spend much of the day worrying about the straightness of their teeth, the size of their noses, or the clarity of their skin. They may spend hours fixing their hair. They convince themselves they're unattractive, perhaps downright ugly. Many seek cosmetic treatments from doctors. The condition, which usually starts during adolescence, is debilitating and distressing. It erodes self-esteem and can lead to anger, aggression, depression, and even suicide.[119]

The perceptions in body image disturbances may have little basis in reality. In fact, they can be completely delusional. In a moment, we'll discuss the body image distortion that can occur with anorexia nervosa, wherein a skeletally thin person believes she or he is fat.

Another example is **muscle dysmorphia**, also called muscle dysmorphic disorder or "bigorexia." In this mental disorder, people—usually young men—become obsessed with muscularity to the extent that it impairs psychological and social function. Body image is so disturbed that a body builder would look in the mirror and see a 90-pound weakling. The incidence has been steadily rising, a fact experts blame on societal pressure for men to be "ripped."[120] Athletes can be particularly vulnerable.

The preoccupation with muscularity leads to compulsive exercising, particularly resistance training. It can also lead to the adoption of strict or extreme diets (e.g., very high in protein and very low in fat and carbohydrates), abuse of anabolic steroids, excessive intake of sports supplements, and rigid rituals about diet and exercise.

Notice that body dysmorphic disorder and muscle dysmorphia both contain the suffix "dys," which means bad, and root word "morph," which means form or shape. In both conditions, the person has delusional beliefs that he or she is malformed. Both cause significant distress and impairment. Both are variants of obsessive-compulsive disorder (see Chapter 5 for a definition). Both are treated with psychotherapy and medications.[121]

The difference is the nature of the preoccupation. In body dysmorphic disorder, the dissatisfaction could be about any physical feature. In muscle dysmorphia, the perceived flaw is being inadequately lean and muscular.

Assess Yourself: Do You Use Unhealthy Weight-Loss Measures?

It's not uncommon for people to go to extreme lengths to manage their weight. These methods aren't sustainable, can damage health, and usually backfire. In yo-yo like fashion, any weight loss is typically soon regained. One study found that frequent incorrect dieting paradoxically increased susceptibility to weight gain.[122]

Another example is the misguided use of cigarette smoking to lose weight. Short-term effects of smoking are increased energy expenditure and decreased appetite.[123] (Sense of smell influences taste; smoking impairs olfaction, which can reduce appetite.) However, chronic, heavy smokers tend to weigh more than nonsmokers (and have more abdominal fat).

A study of college students found taking up smoking correlated with declining physical activity and spending more time eating in front of the television and dining at restaurants that served high-calorie food—all of them behaviors that promote weight gain.[124] Smokers are also more likely to drink alcohol, which can be chock-full of calories. Most importantly, tobacco is an addicting substance and the single most preventable cause of premature death.

Check off any methods you've tried. If you're still doing them and can't give them up, contact your doctor.

_____severely restricting caloric intake (starvation diet)

_____skipping meals

_____fasting (skipping two or more meals for reasons other than religious tradition)

_____smoking cigarettes

_____using food substitutes such as special drinks and powders mixed with water

_____taking nonprescription "diet pills"

_____taking laxatives or diuretics

_____making yourself vomit after a meal

3.1 Eating Disorders

Eating disorders include a range of psychological disorders characterized by abnormal eating behaviors. Though each is different, they share some common characteristics:

- Disturbed body image.
- Abnormal diets. Depending on the disorder, people either eat extremely small amounts of food or vastly overeat.
- Preoccupation with food, with a focus on resisting it. The fixation can become obsessive.
- A sense of shame or lack of control about eating.
- Secrecy about eating behaviors. Reluctance to eat around others.
- Distress and anxiety about body weight and eating.
- Use of unhealthy or extreme means of controlling weight.

For all the eating disorders, the American Psychiatric Association's *Diagnostic and Statistical Manual of Mental Disorders* establishes the criteria for diagnosis. An important point here is that the conditions are psychological in nature (rather than character flaws) and need to be treated as such.

Clearly, eating disorders are about much more than food. Several factors increase the risk.[125]

- **Family history.** These conditions can run in families. Research indicates that genetics play a role.
- **Developmental stage.** With the onset of puberty, bodies change, self-consciousness increases, peer acceptance matters even more, and media messages gain credence. Both boys and girls may gain weight in advance of the growth spurt. The development of breasts and hips can distress some girls, particularly those involved in activities where thinness matters (e.g., gymnastics, ballet, running).
- **Preexisting psychological issues.** These include low self-esteem, loneliness, a sense of lack of control, anger, anxiety, and depression. Psychological trauma, particularly sexual abuse, can trigger an eating disorder.
- **Interpersonal problems.** Examples include difficult relationships with family members and peers. Teasing about body weight can trigger disordered eating.
- **Cultural ideals.** Societal pressures to conform to lofty standards of beauty, especially thinness, can warp body image.

Eating disorders are most common among adolescent girls. However, boys are not immune. Because these conditions are less common in males, eating disorders are less often recognized and treated in boys and men. Alarmingly, these conditions have become more common during childhood.[126] At some point during their lives, 2.7 percent of adolescents—twice as many girls as boys—have had an eating disorder.[127]

While eating disorders often become apparent during adolescence, the behaviors can persist into adulthood. In one study, between 50 and 60.7 percent of girls and young women and 22 to 28 percent of boys and young men engaged in unhealthy weight-control behaviors, which is a key sign of an eating disorder. Extreme weight-control measures actually increased from 8.4 percent in early adolescence to just over 20 percent in young adulthood. Binge eating also increased with time.[128]

Eating disorders are all too common among college students. A recent survey found that 13.5 percent of college women and 3.6 percent of college men had an eating disorder.[129] Many had persistent symptoms at the two-year follow-up. Unfortunately, only 20 percent of these students had received mental health treatment during the previous year. Such treatment is important for recovery. All eating disorders increase the risk of death, none more so than anorexia nervosa.

People with eating disorders often can't heal themselves. In fact, they often deny or hide their illness and avoid professional help. Treatment depends on the severity of the condition. Comprehensive treatment includes psychotherapy (individual, group, and family therapy), nutrition counseling, medications (usually antidepressants), and medical monitoring. Milder cases are managed on an outpatient basis, meaning people continue to live at home and make periodic clinic visits. For severe cases, hospitalization or a stay in a residential treatment center may be necessary.

Assess Yourself: Do You Have an Eating Disorder?

Two simple screening tools are often used to examine people for eating disorders: the ESP (**e**ating disorder **s**creen for **p**rimary care) and the SCOFF[130] (which stands for key signs noted below) questionnaires. For both questionnaires, zero to one abnormal answers indicate a lack of an eating disorder; two or more abnormal responses suggest an eating disorder. In one study, the ESP was a slightly better tool.[131]

ESP

(A "no" response to the first question is considered abnormal. For all other questions, a "yes" response is a worrisome sign.)

- Are you satisfied with your eating patterns?
- Do you ever eat in secret?
- Does your weight affect the way you feel about yourself?
- Have any members of your family suffered with an eating disorder?
- Do you currently suffer with or have you ever suffered in the past with an eating disorder?

SCOFF

(A "no" response to any answers is considered abnormal.)

- Do you make yourself **S**ick because you feel uncomfortably full?
- Do you worry you have lost **C**ontrol over how much you eat?
- Have you recently lost more than **One** stone (14 pounds) in a three-month period?
- Do you believe yourself to be **F**at when others say you are thin?
- Would you say that **F**ood dominates your life?

Note: If you have any concerns about your eating habits or your weight, make an appointment with your doctor.

Video Clip 10.3

The Face of Anorexia Nervosa
This CBS news segment portrays model Isabelle Caro, who became a "poster child" for a campaign against anorexia nervosa.

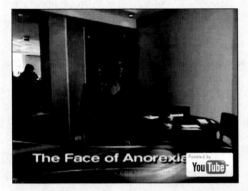

View the video online at: http://www.youtube.com/v/VS2mfWDryPE

Anorexia nervosa is a life-threatening condition in which people starve themselves and use other extreme measures to lose weight. A person may begin by restricting calories to lose an appropriate amount of weight, then finding she is unable to stop. Other means of achieving thinness include compulsive exercising, self-induced vomiting, taking diet pills, and abusing laxatives and diuretics.

"Anorexia," which means "without appetite," is a misnomer. People with anorexia nervosa are, in fact, hungry, but they deny themselves food out of an intense fear of gaining weight. Although people with anorexia nervosa look emaciated, their body image distortion leads them to believe they are fat.

Eating, food, and weight control become obsessions for people with anorexia. They may cook for other people but refuse to eat the food. They often have strict rituals, such as eating sparingly of low-calorie foods then exercising for hours. Perfectionism, self-criticism, insecurity, and an eagerness to please others are common traits. Eventually, however, they may withdraw from friends and family. Over a lifetime, nearly 1 percent of women and 0.3 percent of men develop anorexia nervosa.[132] The peak onset is during the latter part of adolescence.

Anorexia nervosa takes a serious toll on the body. People feel tired, lethargic, and light-headed. Starvation lowers metabolism and leads to malnutrition. The following signs and symptoms can develop:

- fatigue and lethargy
- cold, dry, and sometimes yellowish skin that's covered with fine hair (*lanugo*)
- brittle and sparse scalp hair
- severe constipation
- thinning of bones (with a risk of osteoporosis and bone fractures)
- depletion of fat stores and loss of muscle mass
- absent menstrual cycles and infertility
- depression
- neurologic damage, including brain damage
- slow heart rate and low blood pressure
- organ failure
- cardiac arrest
- death

Of all the psychiatric disorders, anorexia nervosa has the highest death rate. Although estimates vary, a recent analysis determined overall mortality (death) at about 4 percent.[133] Each year, 5 out of 1,000 people with anorexia nervosa die; 1 in 5 deaths are suicides.[134]

Several factors inherent to the condition can create barriers to treatment: denial of the condition, low motivation to change behaviors, the strong drive to thinness, and a high resistance to achieving and maintaining a normal body weight. Nevertheless, with professional treatment, people with anorexia nervosa can and do recover. The goals are to correct malnutrition, restore health and normal weight, resolve the underlying psychological issues, and restructure thoughts and behaviors to prevent relapse.

anorexia nervosa

An eating disorder characterized by self-starvation, emaciation, and severe body image disturbance.

bulimia nervosa

An eating disorder characterized by recurrent episodes of binge eating followed by purging and other means of compensating for food intake.

binge eating

Consuming large quantities of food within a relatively short period of time.

purging

Using laxatives and enemas or inducing oneself to vomit to rid the body of food. Diuretics may also be abused in a misguided attempt to compensate for eating.

Bulimia nervosa can also threaten lives. Frequent binging and purging characterize this condition. **Binge eating** involves consuming huge quantities of food in a discrete period of time (usually within two hours). **Purging** refers to compensating for eating by self-induced vomiting or abusing laxative or diuretics. People with bulimia nervosa may also follow binging with fasting, exercising, and taking diuretics. Binging and purging can occur from once a week to several times in a day.

In *purging disorder*, binging is infrequent but purging occurs more than once a week. In other words, people are trying to rid themselves of normal amounts of food. As with anorexia nervosa, binging and purging often begin in adolescence and more commonly afflicts girls than boys. About 1 percent of teenage girls have bulimia nervosa, and 2 to 3 percent have purging disorder.[135] Unlike those who have anorexia nervosa, people who have bulimia nervosa and purging disorder are of normal weight or somewhat overweight. A deep-seated fear of overweight is common theme for all three conditions.

Bulimia nervosa causes numerous health problems. Purging causes most of them. Vomiting and using laxatives and diuretics promote dehydration, loss of acid-base balance in the body, and derangement of electrolytes (minerals such as sodium, chloride, potassium, and calcium). Not only do these changes make you feel ill, but they can also lead to muscle cramps, bone loss, and, worse, heart rhythm disturbances and death. The other conditions are caused by chronic exposure to the acidic stomach contents. These health problems include

- dehydration
- electrolyte and acid-base imbalances
- muscle cramps
- tooth decay and erosion of tooth enamel
- thinning bones (osteoporosis)
- chronic sore throat
- inflammation and tears in the esophagus
- tender, swollen salivary glands
- heart attack due to electrolyte imbalance

binge eating disorder

A condition in which frequent binge eating is not followed by compensatory measure such as purging, fasting, and exercising.

In **binge eating disorder**, binging is frequent, but compensatory purging, fasting, and exercising are rare or absent. Food is consumed rapidly and secretively in the absence of hunger and in the presence of a full belly. The lack of control against the compulsion to binge causes distress, self-disgust, guilt, shame, and depression.[136]

Although obesity isn't a requirement for diagnosis, most people who come to medical attention are overweight or obese. However, not all obese people have a binge eating disorder. Binge eating disorder affects 2 to 5 percent of the general population and an estimated 30 percent of obese people seeking weight-control treatment.[137]

The majority of people with eating disorders don't fulfill the criteria for any one disorder. These cases are given the diagnosis *eating disorder not otherwise specified*.[138] People fall into this diagnostic category when their symptoms are borderline or when they have a blend of signs and symptoms of a couple eating disorders.

When a Friend Has an Eating Disorder

We all want to help our friends. But we also respect their privacy and treasure their trust in us. What do you do when you suspect a friend, family member, or roommate has an eating disorder? The same thing you would do if they had any other serious mental disorder: encourage them to get professional help.

You now know the signs of eating disorders. But how do you detect them in someone else, especially in someone who hides and denies their condition? The following changes are red flags:

- a radical change in diet or adoption of an extremely restricted diet
- lots of talk about being "fat"; complaining of fat on belly, hips, and thighs when none exists
- excessive exercising
- wearing baggy clothes to hide dramatic weight changes
- preparing meals for other people, then declining to eat it
- disappearing into the bathroom after meals
- hoarding and hiding food for later binging in secret
- erosion of tooth enamel
- social withdrawal

If you suspect someone you know has an eating disorder, find time to speak to the person privately. Start with positive statements about the person's accomplishments. Tell him or her what you've observed. Express your concern. Listen without judgment. Stay calm if he or she angrily denies a problem. Say you've heard treatment can help but don't insist. You're not a doctor and not responsible for your friend's eating behavior. If you are worried about your friend's mental and physical health, contact someone at the college health clinic or counseling center. When someone's life depends on adequate treatment, it's time to sidestep confidentiality.

KEY TAKEAWAYS

- With severe body image disturbances, people are chronically dissatisfied and preoccupied with their appearance. They may become delusional—that is, falsely believing they're fat or inadequately muscled.
- Two examples of body image disturbances are body dysmorphic disorder and muscle dysmorphia.
- Eating disorders are psychological conditions characterized by severe body image disturbance, abnormal eating patterns, and unhealthy weight-management behaviors. They adversely affect mental, emotional, physical, and social health. If left untreated, these conditions can cause premature death. Anorexia nervosa is particularly deadly.
- Eating disorders more commonly affect women. However, lack of recognition has caused underdiagnosis among men.
- Denial, shame, and low motivation to change create barriers to seeking treatment for body image disturbances and eating disorders. However, treatment can be effective and saves lives.

DISCUSSION QUESTIONS

1. What factors raise the risk for body image disturbances and eating disorders? Include in your discussion the influence of family, friends, coaches, the media, and individual factors.
2. Science Daily has a website on eating disorders research. Go to http://www.sciencedaily.com/news/ health_medicine/eating_disorders/. Select a study, read about it, and summarize the key points in your own words.

4. RECOMMENDED RESOURCES

4.1 Websites

Centers for Disease Control and Prevention: Overweight and Obesity. http://www.cdc.gov/obesity.

National Association of Anorexia Nervosa and Associated Disorders. http://www.anad.org.

National Eating Disorders Association. http://www.nationaleatingdisorders.org.

National Institutes of Mental Health, Eating Disorders. http://www.nimh.nih.gov/health/publications/eating-disorders/index.shtml.

Obesity Society. http://www.obesity.org.

Weight Control Information Network. http://win.niddk.nih.gov.

Yale Rudd Center for Food Policy and Obesity. http://www.yaleruddcenter.org.

WebMD. http://www.webmd.com/diet/default.htm.

World Health Organization: Obesity. http://www.who.int/topics/obesity/en.

4.2 Books

American Heart Association. *American Heart Association No-Fad Diet: A Personal Plan for Healthy Weight Loss*. 2nd ed. New York, NY: Clarkson Potter; 2011.

Wansink B. *Mindless Eating: Why We Eat More Than We Think*. New York, NY: Bantam; 2006.

Rolls V. *Volumetrics Weight-Control Plan: Feel Full on Fewer Calories*. New York, NY: William Morrow; 2000.

4.3 Smartphone and Tablet Apps

Lose It. Helps you track weight loss, daily food intake, and physical activity. https://itunes.apple.com/us/app/lose-it!/id297368629?mt=8.

MyNetDiary Calorie Counter. You can use it to record meals, exercise, weight, and other functions. http://www.mynetdiary.com.

Other free apps. http://www.shape.com/weight-loss/weight-loss-strategies/best-free-apps-help-you-lose-weight.

ENDNOTES

1. American College Health Association–National College Health Assessment. Spring 2011 reference group executive summary. Available at: http://www.achancha.org/docs/ACHA-NCHA-II_ReferenceGroup_ExecutiveSummary_Spring2011.pdf. Accessed August 9, 2012.

2. Moore DC. Body image and eating behavior in adolescents. *J Am Coll Nutr*. 1993 Oct;12(5):505–510.

3. Salk RH, Engeln-Maddox R. If you're fat, then I'm humongous!: frequency, content, and impact of fat talk among college women. *Psychol Women Q*. 2011;35:18–28.

4. Mikolajczyk RT, Iannotti RJ, Farhat TM, Thomas V. Ethnic differences in perceptions of body satisfaction and body appearance among US schoolchildren: a cross-sectional study. *BMC Public Health*. 2012 Jun 12;12(1):425.

5. Gordon KH, Castro Y, Sitnikov L, Holm-Denoma JM. Cultural body shape ideals and eating disorder symptoms among white, Latina, and black college women. *Cultur Divers Ethnic Minor Psychol*. 2010 Apr;16(2):135–143.

6. Nouri M, Hill LG, Orrell-Valente JK. Media exposure, internalization of the thin ideal, and body dissatisfaction: comparing Asian American and European American college females. *Body Image*. 2011 Sep;8(4):366–372.

7. Cafri G, Thompson JK, Ricciardelli L, McCabe M, Smolak L, Yesalis C. Pursuit of the muscular ideal: physical and psychological consequences and putative risk factors. *Clin Psychol Rev*. 2005;25:215–239.

8. McCreary DR, Karvinen K, Davis C. The relationship between the drive for muscularity and anthropometric measures of muscularity and adiposity. *Body Image*. 2006 Jun;3(2):145–152.

9. Grossbard JR, Neighbors C, Larimer ME. Perceived norms for thinness and muscularity among college students: what do men and women really want? *Eat Behav*. 2011 Aug;12(3):192–199.

10. Friedman KE, Reichmann SK, Costanzo PR, Musante GJ. Body image partially mediates the relationship between obesity and psychological distress. *Obes Res*. 2002;10(1):33–41.

11. McCreary D, Sasse DK. An exploration of the drive for muscularity in adolescent boys and girls. *J Am Coll Health*. 2000;48(6):297–304.

12. Haines J, Neumark-Sztainer D, Wall M, Story M. Personal, behavioral, and environmental risk and protective factors for adolescent overweight. *Obesity (Silver Spring)*. 2007 Nov;15(11):2748–2760.

13. Neumark-Sztainer D, Wall M, Larson NI, Eisenberg ME, Loth K. Dieting and disordered Eating Behaviors from adolescence to young adulthood: findings from a 10-year longitudinal study. *Journal of the American Dietetic Association*. 2011 Jul;111(7):1004–1011. Available at: http://www.ncbi.nlm.nih.gov/pmc/articles/PMC3140795/?tool=pubmed. Accessed July 23, 2012.

14. Neumark-Sztainer D, Wall M, Guo J, Story M, Haines J, Eisenberg M. Obesity, disordered eating, and eating disorders in a longitudinal study of adolescents: how do dieters fare 5 years later? *Journal of the American Dietetic Association*. 2006 Apr;106(4):559–568.

15. Kirchengast S. Gender differences in body composition from childhood to old age: an evolutionary point of view. *J Life Sci*. 2010;2(1):1–10. Available at: http://www.krepublishers.com/02-Journals/JLS/JLS-02-0-000-10-Web/JLS-02-1-000-10-Abst-PDF/JLS-02-1-01-10-052-Kirchengast-S/JLS-02-1-1-10-052-Kirchengast-S-Tt.pdf. Accessed July 30, 2012.

16. What are the guidelines for percentage body fat loss? Ask an ACE expert. American Council on Exercise. December 2, 2009. Available at: http://www.acefitness.org/acefit/expert-insight-article/3/112/what-are-the-guidelines-for-percentage-of. Accessed March 11, 2013.

17. World Health Organization (WHO). Obesity and overweight. Fact sheet No. 311. February 2011. Available at: http://www.who.int/mediacentre/factsheets/fs311/en. Accessed June 15, 2012.

18. Bleich SN, Cutler D, Murray C, Adams A. Why is the developed world obese? *Annu Rev Publ Health*. 2008;29:273–295.

19. Adult obesity facts. Overweight and obesity. Centers for Disease Control and Prevention. Available at: http://www.cdc.gov/obesity/data/adult.html. Accessed July 22, 2012.

20. Harris KM, Perreira KM, Lee D. Obesity in the transition to adulthood: predictions across race/ethnicity, immigrant generation, and sex. *Arch Pediatr Adolesc Med*. 2009;163:1022–1028.

21. Ogden CL, Lamb MM, Carroll MD, Flegal KM. Obesity and socioeconomic status in children and adolescents: United States, 2005–2008. NCHS data brief, no. 51. Hyattsville, MD: National Center for Health Statistics; 2010:1–8.

22. The NS, Suchindran C, North KE, Popkin BM, Gordon-Larsen P. Association of adolescent obesity with risk of severe obesity in adulthood. *JAMA*. 2010;304(18):2042–2047.

23. American College Health Association–National College Health Assessment. Spring 2011 reference group executive summary. Available at: http://www.achancha.org/docs/ACHA-NCHA-II_ReferenceGroup_ExecutiveSummary_Spring2011.pdf. Accessed August 9, 2012.

24. Centers for Disease Control and Prevention. National obesity trends. Data from the National Health and Nutrition Examination Survey (NHANES). Available at: http://www.cdc.gov/obesity/data/trends.html. Accessed August 2, 2011.

25. Bleich S, Cutler D, Murray C, Adams A. Why is the developed world obese? *Annu Rev Publ Health*. 2008;29:273–295.

26. National Health and Nutrition Examination Survey (NHANES) as reported in: Roger VL, Go AS, Lloyd-Jones DM, et al. American Heart Association Statistics Committee and Stroke Statistics Subcommittee. Executive summary: heart disease and stroke statistics—2012 update: a report from the American Heart Association. *Circulation*. 2012 Jan 3;125(1):188–197.

27. Reilly JJ, Armstrong J, Dorosty AR, et al.; Avon Longitudinal Study of Parents and Children Study Team. Early life risk factors for obesity in childhood: cohort study. *BMJ*. 2005 Jun 11;330(7504):1357.

28. Stunkard AJ, Sørensen TI, Hanis C, et al. An adoption study of human obesity. *N Engl J Med*. 1986 Jan 23;314(4):193–198.

29. Choquet H, Meyre D. Molecular basis of obesity: current status and future prospects. *Curr Genomics*. 2011;12(3):154–168.

30. Anderson SE, Gooze RA, Lemeshow S, Whitaker RC. Quality of early maternal-child relationship and risk of adolescent obesity. *Pediatrics*. 2011 Dec 26. doi:10.1542/peds.2011-0972.

31. McCaffery JM, Papandonatos GD, Bond DS, Lyons MJ, Wing RR. Gene X environment interaction of vigorous exercise and body mass index among male Vietnam-era twins. *Am J Clin Nutr*. 2009 Apr;89(4):1011–1018.

32. Mustelin L, Silventoinen K, Pietiläinen K, Rissanen A, Kaprio J. Physical activity reduces the influence of genetic effects on BMI and waist circumference: a study in young adult twins. *Int J Obes (London)*. 2009 Jan;33(1):29–36.

33. Garaulet M, Ordovás JM, Madrid JA. The chronobiology, etiology and pathophysiology of obesity. *Int J Obes (London)*. 2010 Dec;34(12):1667–1683.

34. Carter PJ, Taylor BJ, Williams SM, Taylor RM. Longitudinal analysis of sleep in relation to BMI and body fat in children: the FLAME study. *BMJ*. 2011;342:d2712. doi:10.1136/bmj.d2712.

35. Cizza G, Marincola P, Mattingly M, et al. Treatment of obesity with extension of sleep duration: a randomized, prospective, controlled trial. *Clin Trials*. 2010 Jun;7(3):274–285.

36. Wardle J, Chida Y, Gibson EL, Whitaker KL, Steptoe A. Stress and adiposity: a meta-analysis of longitudinal studies. *Obesity (Silver Spring)*. 2011 Apr;19(4):771–778.

37. Epel E, Lapidus R, McEwen B, Brownell K. Stress may add bite to appetite in women: a laboratory study of stress-induced cortisol and eating behavior. *Psychoneuroendocrinology*. 2001 Jan;26(1):37–49.

38. Adam TC, Epel ES. Stress, eating, and the reward system. *Physiol Behav*. 2007;91(4):449–458.

39. Macht M, Simons G. Emotions and eating in everyday life. *Appetite*. 2000 Aug;35(1):65–71.

40. Strine TW, Mokdad AH, Dube SR, et al. The association of depression and anxiety with obesity and unhealthy behaviors among community-dwelling US adults. *Gen Hosp Psychiatry*. 2008 Mar–Apr;30(2):127–137.

41. Grossniklaus DA, Dunbar SB, Tohill BC, et al. Psychological factors are important correlates of dietary pattern in overweight adults. *J Cardiovasc Nurs*. 2010 Nov–Dec;25(6):450–460.

42. Zhang H, Rodriguez-Monguio R. Racial disparities in the risk of developing obesity-related diseases: a cross-sectional study. *Ethn Dis*. 2012 Summer;22(3):308–316.

43. Kirby JB, Liang L, Chen HJ, Wang Y. Race, place, and obesity: the complex relationships among community racial/ethnic composition, individual race/ethnicity, and obesity in the United States. *Am J Public Health*. 2012 Aug;102(8):1572–1578.

44. Klimentidis YC, Miller GF, Shriver MD. The relationship between European genetic admixture and body composition among Hispanics and Native Americans. *Am J Hum Biol*. 2009 May–Jun;21(3):377–382.

45. Cheng CY, Reich D, Coresh J, et al. Admixture mapping of obesity-related traits in African Americans: the Atherosclerosis Risk in Communities (ARIC) Study. *Obesity (Silver Spring)*. 2010 Mar;18(3):563–572.

46. Drewnowski A, Specter SE. Poverty and obesity: the role of energy density and energy costs. *Am J Clin Nutr*. 2004 Jan;79(1):6–16.

47. Morland K, Diez Roux AV, Wing S. Supermarkets, other food stores, and obesity: the atherosclerosis risk in communities study. *Am J Prev Med*. 2006 Apr;30(4):333–339.

48. Black JL, Macinko J, Dixon LB, Fryer GE Jr. Neighborhoods and obesity in New York City. *Health Place*. 2010 May;16(3):489–499.

49. Ludwig J, Sanbonmatsu L, Gennetian L, et al. Neighborhoods, obesity, and diabetes—a randomized social experiment. *N Engl J Med*. 2011;365:1509–1519.

50. Christakis NA, Fowler JH. The spread of obesity in a large social network over 32 years. *N Engl J Med*. 2007;357:370–379.

51. Hill AL, Rand DG, Nowak MA, Christakis NA. Infectious disease modeling of social contagion in networks. *PLoS Comput Biol*. 2010 Nov 4;6(11):e1000968.

52. Shoham DA, Tong L, Lamberson PJ, et al. An actor-based model of social network influence on adolescent body size, screen time, and playing sports. *PLoS One*. 2012;7(6):e39795.

53. de la Haye K, Robins G, Mohr P, Wilson C. Homophily and contagion as explanations for weight similarities among adolescent friends. *J Adolesc Health*. 2011 Oct;49(4):421–427.

54. Reilly JJ, Armstrong J, Dorosty AR, et al.; Avon Longitudinal Study of Parents and Children Study Team. Early life risk factors for obesity in childhood: cohort study. *BMJ*. 2005 Jun 11;330(7504):1357.

55. De Coster S, van Larebeke N. Endocrine-disrupting chemicals: associated disorders and mechanisms of action. *J Environ Public Health*. 2012;2012:713696. Available at: http://www.ncbi.nlm.nih.gov/pmc/articles/PMC3443608. Accessed December 2, 2012.

56. Mozaffarian D, Hao T, Rimm EB, Willett WC, Hu FB. Changes in diet and lifestyle and long-term weight gain in women and men. *N Engl J Med*. 2011;364:2392–2404.

57. Lennerz BS, Alsop DC, Holsen LM, Stern E, et al. Effects of dietary glycemic index on brain regions related to reward and craving in men. *Am J Clin Nutr*. Jun 26, 2013. In press.

58. Malik VS, Schulze MB, Hu FB. Intake of sugar-sweetened beverages and weight gain: a systematic review. *Am J Clin Nutr*. 2006 Aug;84(2):274–288.

59. Jurgens H, Haass W, Castaneda TR, et al. Consuming fructose-sweetened beverages increases body adiposity in mice. *Obes Res*. 2005;13:1146.

60. Havel PJ. Dietary fructose: implications for dysregulation of energy homeostasis and lipid/carbohydrate metabolism. *Nutr Rev*. 2005;63:133–157.

61. Schulze MB, Manson JE, Ludwig DS, et al. Sugar-sweetened beverages, weight gain, and incidence of type 2 diabetes in young and middle-aged women. *JAMA*. 2004 Aug 25;292(8):927–934.

62. Duffey KJ, Popkin BM. Shifts in patterns and consumption of beverages between 1965 and 2002. *Obesity (Silver Spring)*. 2007;15:2739–2747.

63. Nielsen SJ, Popkin BM. Changes in beverage intake between 1977 and 2001. *Am J Prev Med*. 2004;27:205–210.

64. Flegal KM, Campbell SM, Johnson CL. Prevalence and trends in obesity among US adults, 1999–2000. *JAMA*. 2002;288:1723–1727.

65. Bleich SN, Want YC, Want Y, Gortmaker SL. Increasing consumption of sugar-sweetened beverages among US adults: 1988–1994 to 1999–2004. *Am J Clin Nutr*. 2009;89(1):372–381. Available at: http://www.ajcn.org/content/89/1/372.long. Accessed August 6, 2012.

66. World Health Organization. Obesity: preventing and managing the global epidemic. WHO Technical Report Series 894. 2000. Available at: http://www.who.int/nutrition/publications/obesity/WHO_TRS_894/en. Accessed July 20, 2012.

67. Fontaine KR, Redden DT, Wang C, Westfall AO, Allison DB. Years of life lost due to obesity. *JAMA*. 2003 Jan 8;289(2):187–193.

68. Kershaaw EE, Flier JS. Adipose tissue as an endocrine organ. *J Clin Endocrinol Metab*. 2004;89(6):2548–2556. doi:10.1210/jc.2004-0395. Available at: http://jcem.endojournals.org/content/89/6/2548.full.pdf+html. Accessed July 22, 2012.

69. Puhl RM, Andreyeva T, Brownell KD. Perceptions of weight discrimination: prevalence and comparison to race and gender discrimination in America. *Int J Obes*. 2008;32:992–1000.

70. Withrow D, Alter DA. The economic burden of obesity worldwide: a systematic review of the direct costs of obesity. *Obesity Reviews*. 2011;12(2):131–141.

71. Friedman KE, Reichmann SK, Costanzo PR, Zelli A, Ashmore JA, Musante GJ. Weight stigmatization and ideological beliefs: relation to psychological functioning in obese adults. *Obes Res*. 2005;13:907–916.

72. Neumark-Sztainer D, Falkner N, Story M, Perry C, Hannan PJ, Mulert S. Weight-teasing among adolescents: correlations with weight status and disordered Eating Behaviors. *Int J Obes Relat Metab Disord*. 2002;26:123–131. Available at: http://www.nature.com/ijo/journal/v26/n1/full/0801853a.html. Retrieved June 8, 2011.

73. Storch EA, Milsom VA, DeBraganza N, Lewin AB, Geffken GR, Silverstein JH. Peer victimization, psychosocial adjustment, and physical activity in overweight and at-risk-for-overweight youth. *J Pediatr Psychol*. 2007;32:80–89.

74. Falkner NH, Neumark-Sztainer D, Story M, Jeffery RW, Beuhring T, Resnick MD. Social, educational, and psychological correlates of weight status in adolescents. *Obes Res*. 2001 Jan;9(1):32–42.

75. Hemminki K, Li X, Sundquist J, Sundquist K. Obesity and familial obesity and risk of cancer. *Eur J Cancer Prev*. 2011 May 20 [Epub ahead of print]. Abstract available at: http://www.ncbi.nlm.nih.gov/pubmed/21606843. Accessed June 8, 2011.

76. American Heart Association statement. Population-based prevention of obesity. *Circulation*. 2008;118(4):428–464. Available at: http://circ.ahajournals.org/content/118/4/428.long#T1. Accessed August 15, 2012.

77. Demark-Wahnefried W, Platz EA, Ligibel JA, et al. The role of obesity in cancer survival and recurrence. *Cancer Epidemiol Biomarkers Prev*. 2012 Jun 13 [Epub ahead of print]. doi:10.1158/1055-9965.EPI-12-0485.

78. Lehnert T, Donntag D, Konnopka A, Riedel-Heller S, Konig HH. The long-term cost-effectiveness of obesity prevention interventions: systematic literature review. *Obesity Reviews*. 2012;13(6):537–553.

79. Mozaffarian D, Hao T, Rimm EB, Willett WC, Hu FB. Changes in diet and lifestyle and long-term weight gain in women and men. *N Engl J Med*. 2011;364:2392–2404.

80. Morland K, Diez Roux AV, Wing S. Supermarkets, other food stores, and obesity: the atherosclerosis risk in communities study. *Am J Prev Med*. 2006 Apr;30(4):333–339. Abstract available at: http://www.ncbi.nlm.nih.gov/pubmed/16530621.

81. Nixon R. New rules for school meals aim at reducing obesity. *New York Times*. January 12, 2012. Available at: http://www.nytimes.com/2012/01/26/us/politics/new-school-lunch-rules-aimed-at-reducing-obesity.html. Accessed August 13, 2012.

82. Shamah Levy T, Morales Ruán C, Amaya Castellanos C, et al. Effectiveness of a diet and physical activity promotion strategy on the prevention of obesity in Mexican school children. *BMC Public Health*. 2012 Mar 1;12:152.

83. Flynn MA, McNeil DA, Maloff B, et al. Reducing obesity and related chronic disease risk in children and youth: a synthesis of evidence with "best practice" recommendations. *Obesity Reviews*. 2006;7(suppl 1):7–66.

84. O'Connor A. Bans on school junk food pay off in California. *New York Times*. May 12, 2012. Available at: http://well.blogs.nytimes.com/2012/05/08/bans-on-school-junk-food-pay-off-in-california. Accessed August 13, 2012.

85. Taber DR, Chriqui JF, Perna FM, Powell LM, Chaloupka FJ. Weight status among adolescents in states that govern competitive food nutrition content. *Pediatrics*. 2012. doi 10.1542/peds.2011-3353.

86. Yale Rudd Center for Food Policy. Food marketing to youth. Available at: http://www.yaleruddcenter.org/what_we_do.aspx?id=4. Accessed August 13, 2012.

87. Bell JF, Wilson JS, Liu GC. Neighborhood greenness and 2-year changes in body mass index of children and youth. *Am J Prev Med*. 2008 Dec;35(6):547–553. Available at: http://www.ncbi.nlm.nih.gov/pmc/articles/PMC2649717/?tool=pubmed. Accessed June 8, 2011.

88. Cleland V, Crawford D, Baur LA, Hume C, Timperio A, Salmon J. A prospective examination of children's time spent outdoors, objectively measured physical activity and overweight. *Int J Obes*. 2008 Nov;32(11):1685–1693.

89. Buijsse B, Feskens EJ, Schulze MB, et al. Fruit and vegetable intakes and subsequent changes in body weight in European populations: results from the project on Diet, Obesity, and Genes (DiOGenes). *Am J Clin Nutr*. 2009 Jul;90(1):202–209.

90. Mozaffarian D, Hao T, Rimm EB, Willett WC, Hu FB. Changes in diet and lifestyle and long-term weight gain in women and men. *N Engl J Med*. 2011;364:2392–2404.

91. Tilg H. Obesity, metabolic syndrome, and microbiota: multiple interactions. *J Clin Gastroenterol*. 2010 Sep;44 Suppl 1:S16–8.

92. DiBaise JK, Zhang H, Crowell MD, Krajmalnik-Brown R, Decker GA, Rittmann BE. Gut microbiota and its possible relationship with obesity. *Mayo Clin Proc*. 2008;83(4):460–469. doi:10.4065/83.4.460. Available at: http://www.mayoclinicproceedings.com/content/83/4/460.long. Accessed June 25, 2011.

93. Bes-Rastrollo M, Wedick NM, Martinez-Gonzalez MA, Li TY, Sampson L, Hu FB. Prospective study of nut consumption, long-term weight change, and obesity risk in women. *Am J Clin Nutr*. 2009 Jun;89(6):1913–1919.

94. Golomb BA, Koperski S, White HL. Association between more frequent chocolate consumption and lower body mass index. *Arch Intern Med*. 2012 Mar 26;172(6):519–521.

95. Khoo J, Piantadosi C, Duncan R, et al. Comparing effects of a low-energy diet and a high-protein low-fat diet on sexual and endothelial function, urinary tract symptoms, and inflammation in obese diabetic men. *J Sex Med*. 2011. doi:10.1111/j.1743-6109.2011.02417.x.

96. Casazza K, Fontaine KR, Astrup A, et al. Myths, presumptions, and facts about obesity. *N Engl J Med*. 2013 Jan 31;368(5):446–454. doi:10.1056/NEJMsa1208051.

97. Hall KD. What is the required energy deficit per unit weight loss? *Int J Obes (London)*. 2008 Mar;32(3):573–576. doi:10.1038/sj.ijo.0803720.

98. What are the guidelines for percentage body fat loss? Ask an ACE expert. American Council on Exercise. December 2, 2009. Available at: http://www.acefitness.org/acefit/expert-insight-article/3/112/what-are-the-guidelines-for-percentage-of. Accessed March 11, 2013.

99. Piehowski KE, Preston AG, Miller DL, Nickols-Richardson SM. A reduced-calorie dietary pattern including a daily sweet snack promotes body weight reduction and body composition improvements in premenopausal women who are overweight and obese: a pilot study. *Journal of the American Dietetic Association*. 2011 Aug;111(8):1198–1203.

100. Nackers LM, Ross KM, Perri MG. The association between rate of initial weight loss and long-term success in obesity treatment: does slow and steady win the race? *Int J Behav Med*. 2010 Sep;17(3):161–167. doi:10.1007/s12529-010-9092-y.

101. Rosenbaum M, Kissileff HR, Mayer LE, Hirsch J, Leibel RL. Energy intake in weight-reduced humans. *Brain Research*. 2010 Sep 2;1350:95–102. Available at: http://www.ncbi.nlm.nih.gov/pmc/articles/PMC2926239/?tool=pubmed. Accessed January 7, 2012.

102. Sumithran P, Prendergast LA, Delbridge E, et al. Long-term persistence of hormonal adaptations to weight loss. *N Engl J Med*. 2011. 365;1597–1604.

103. Dansinger ML, Gleason JA, Griffith JL, Selker HP, Schaefer EJ. Comparison of the Atkins, Ornish, Weight Watchers, and Zone diets for weight loss and heart disease risk reduction: a randomized trial. *JAMA*. 2005 Jan 5;293(1):43–53.

104. McInnis KJ. Exercise and obesity. *Coronary Artery Disease*. 2000 Mar;11(2):111–116.

105. Ritchie LD. Less frequent eating predicts greater BMI and waist circumference in female adolescents. *Am J Clin Nutr*. 2012 Feb;95(2):290–296.

106. Haines J, Neumark-Sztainer D, Wall M, Story M. Personal, behavioral, and environmental risk and protective factors for adolescent overweight. *Obesity (Silver Spring)*. 2007 Nov;15(11):2748–2760.

107. Phung OJ, Baker WL, Matthews LJ, et al. Effect of green tea catechins with or without caffeine on anthropometric measures: a systemic review and meta-analysis. *Am J Clin Nutr*. 2010;91:73–81.

108. Swithers S. Artificial sweeteners produce the counterintuitive effect of inducing metabolic derangements. *Trends Endocrinol Metab*. July 2013. In press. Available at: http://download.cell.com/images/edimages/Trends/EndoMetabolism/tem_888.pdf. Accessed July 16, 2013.

109. Leong SL, Madden C, Gray A, Waters D, Horwath C. Faster self-reported speed of eating is related to higher body mass index in a national survey of middle-aged women. *Journal of the American Dietetic Association*. 2011;111(8):1192–1197.

110. Duffey KJ, Gordon-Larsen P, Steffen LM, Jacobs DR Jr., Popkin BM. Regular consumption from fast food establishments relative to other restaurants is differentially associated with metabolic outcomes in young adults. *J Nutr*. 2009 Nov;139(11):2113–2118.

111. Daubenmier J, Kristeller J, Hecht FM, et al. Mindfulness intervention for stress eating to reduce cortisol and abdominal fat among overweight and obese women: an exploratory randomized controlled study. *J Obes*. 2011;2011:651936.

112. Appel LJ, Clark JM, Yeh H-C, et al. Comparative effectiveness of weight-loss interventions in clinical practice. *N Engl J Med*. 2011;365;21:1959–1968.

113. Woodard GA, Encarnacion B, Peraza J, Hernandez-Boussard T, Morton J. Halo effect for bariatric surgery: collateral weight loss in patients' family members. *Arch Surg*. 2011 Oct;146(10):1185–1190.

114. French SA, Mitchell NR, Hannan PJ. Decrease in television viewing predicts lower body mass index at 1-year follow-up in adolescents, but not adults. *J Nutr Educ Behav*. 2012 May 14 [Epub ahead of print].

115. Lloyd-Richardson EE, Jelalian E, Sato AF, et al. Two-year follow-up of an adolescent behavioral weight control intervention. *Pediatrics*. 2012;130(2):e281–e288. doi:10.1542/peds.2011-3283.

116. Elder CR, Gullion CM, Funk KL, Debar LL, Lindberg NM, Stevens VJ. Impact of sleep, screen time, depression and stress on weight change in the intensive weight loss phase of the LIFE study. *Int J Obes (London)*. 2012 Jan;36(1):86–92. doi:10.1038/ijo.2011.60.

117. Haller CA, Benowitz NL. Adverse cardiovascular and central nervous system events associated with dietary supplements containing ephedra alkaloids. *N Engl J Med*. 2000;343:1833–1838.

118. Riserus U, Smedman A, Basu S, Vessby B. Metabolic effects of conjugated linoleic acid in humans: the Swedish experience. *Am J Clin Nutr*. 2004;79(suppl 6):1146S–8S.

119. Phillips KA, Rogers J. Cognitive-behavioral therapy for youth with body dysmorphic disorder: current status and future directions. *Child Adolesc Psychiatr Clin N Am*. 2011 Apr;20(2):287–304.

120. Leone JE, Sedory EJ, Gray KA. Recognition and treatment of muscle dysmorphia and related body image disorders. *J Athl Train*. 2005 Oct–Dec;40(4):352–359. Available at: http://www.ncbi.nlm.nih.gov/pubmed/16404458. Accessed August 17, 2012.

121. Ipser JC, Sander C, Stein DJ. Pharmacotherapy and psychotherapy for body dysmorphic disorder. *Cochrane Database Syst Rev*. 2009 Jan 21;(1):CD005332.

122. Pietiläinen KH, Saarni SE, Kaprio J, Rissanen A. Does dieting make you fat? A twin study. *Int J Obes (London)*. 2012 Mar;36(3):456–464. doi:10.1038/ijo.2011.160.

123. Chiolero A, Faeh D, Paccaud F, Cornuz J. Consequences of smoking for body weight, body fat distribution, and insulin resistance. *Am J Clin Nutr*. 2008:87(4):801–909. Available at: http://ajcn.nutrition.org/content/87/4/801.full. Accessed March 11, 2013.

124. Carroll SL, Lee RE, Kaur H, Harris KJ, Strother ML, Huang TT. Smoking, weight loss intention and obesity-promoting behaviors in college students. *J Am Coll Nutr*. 2006 Aug;25(4):348–353.

125. Portela de Santana ML, da Costa Ribeiro Junior H, Mora Giral M, Raich RM. Epidemiology and risk factors of eating disorder in adolescence: a review. *Nutr Hosp*. 2012 Apr;27(2):391–401.

126. Nicholls DE, Lynn R, Viner RM. Childhood eating disorders: British national surveillance study. *Br J Psychiatry*. 2011 Apr;198(4):295–301.

127. Merikangas KR, He JP, Burstein M, et al. Lifetime prevalence of mental disorders in US adolescents: results from the National Comorbidity Survey Replication—Adolescent Supplement (NCS-A). *J Am Acad Child Adolesc Psychiatry*. 2010 Oct;49(10):980–989.

128. Neumark-Sztainer D, Wall M, Larson NI, Eisenberg ME, Loth K. Dieting and disordered eating behaviors from adolescence to young adulthood: findings from a 10-year longitudinal study. *Journal of the American Dietetic Association*. 2011 Jul;111(7):1004–1011. doi:10.1016/j.jada.2011.04.012.

129. Eisenberg D, Nicklett EJ, Roeder K, Kirz NE. Eating disorder symptoms among college students: prevalence, persistence, correlates, and treatment-seeking. *J Am Coll Health*. 2011;59(8):700–707.

130. Morgan JF, Reid F, Lacey JH. The SCOFF questionnaire: assessment of a new screening tool for eating disorders. *BMJ*. 1999 Dec 4;319(7223):1467–1468.

131. Cotton MA, Ball C, Robinson P. Four simple questions can help screen for eating disorders. *J Gen Intern Med*. 2003;18(1):53–56. Available at: http://www.pubmedcentral.nih.gov/articlerender.fcgi?artid=1494802. Accessed August 17, 2012.

132. Hudson JI, Hiripi E, Pope HG Jr, Kessler RC. The prevalence and correlates of eating disorders in the National Comorbidity Survey Replication. *Biol Psychiatry*. 2007 Feb 1;61(3):348–358.

133. Crow SJ, Peterson CB, Swanson SA, et al. Increased mortality in bulimia nervosa and other eating disorders. *Am J Psychiatry*. 2009;166(12):1342–1346.

134. Arcelus J, Mitchell AJ, Wales J, Nielsen S. Mortality rates in patients with anorexia nervosa and other eating disorders. A meta-analysis of 36 studies. *Arch Gen Psychiatry*. 2011 Jul;68(7):724–731.

135. Field AI, Sonneville KR, Micali N, et al. Prospective association of common eating disorders and adverse outcomes. *Pediatrics*. 2012;13(2):e289–3295. doi:10.1542/peds.2011-3633.

136. American Psychiatric Association. *Diagnostic and Statistical Manual of Mental Disorders*. 4th ed. Washington, DC: American Psychiatric Association; 1994.

137. de Zwaan M. Binge eating disorder and obesity. *Int J Obes*. 2001;25(suppl 1):S51–S55.

138. Fairburn CG, Cooper Z. Eating disorders, DSM-5 and clinical reality. *Br J Psychiatry*. 2011;198(1):8–10.

CHAPTER 11
Substance Use Disorders and Addictive Behaviors

Humans have long used substances that alter consciousness. Since ancient times, they employed psychoactive plants such as psilocybin mushrooms and peyote in ceremonies. Opium poppies relieved pain. Coca leaves and similar plants suppressed appetite in the face of food scarcity and helped sustain hard physical labor. Whether by accident or design, humans fermented plants, yielding mead from honey and water; whiskey from a number of grains; wine from grapes; sake from rice; and vodka from grains, potatoes, and other crops.

This chapter will explore the attraction of mind-altering substances and behaviors, the effects of such substances on the brain, the risk factors for dependency and abuse, the consequences of addictive behaviors, strategies for steering clear of abuse, and resources for kicking unhealthy habits.

I thought I'd wake up on my first day here full of health, wisdom, and academic vigor, but instead I just get the usual: shame, self-loathing and nausea, and a vague feeling that waking up needn't always be like this.

- David Nicholls, Starter for Ten

Talented English singer and songwriter Amy Winehouse died of alcohol poisoning in 2011.

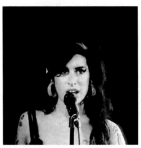

Source: Hommel F. Available at: http://commons.wikimedia.org/wiki/File:AmyWinehouseBerlin2007.jpg.

1. DEFINING SUBSTANCE USE DISORDERS

LEARNING OBJECTIVES

1. Understand the meaning of key terms, such as psychoactive, illicit, abuse, addiction, dependency, and tolerance.
2. Provide statistics that indicate the scope of substance use.
3. Explain why people use substances.
4. Identify risk and protective factors for substance use disorders.
5. Explain how addictive substances change the brain.

The use of alcohol, caffeine, and drugs is widespread in the United States. Part of our culture is inclined toward quick fixes. Most diseases are treated with medications. Have a headache? Take an aspirin. For a variety of reasons, many people also reach for **psychoactive substances**—those that affect the brain to alter mood and mental state. Some are natural and some are synthetically derived. Some are physician prescribed. Many are not, including alcohol, tobacco, caffeine, and illicit drugs. All have pharmacological (drug) effects.

A **drug** is any chemical that alters bodily processes. Some people use the word *medication* to refer to prescription or over-the-counter drugs intended to treat illnesses and the word *drug* to indicate a substance likely to cause harm, abuse, and dependence. In this chapter, the word *substance* will broadly refer to any psychoactive compound with the potential for abuse or addiction.

An **illicit drug** is illegal to produce or possess. Examples of illicit drugs include marijuana (excluding medical marijuana in states that have legalized it), hashish, heroin, cocaine (including crack), hallucinogens such as LSD and PCP, inhalants, and any psychoactive drug used for nonmedical purposes. Examples of legally produced medications that are used for nonmedical reasons include

psychoactive substances

Drugs and other substances containing chemicals that affect the brain to alter mood and mental state.

illicit drug

A drug that is illegal to produce or possess.

narcotic pain relievers and stimulants intended for people with attention deficit hyperactivity disorder (ADHD) or obesity.

Acute use of a psychoactive substance produces physical, mental, and emotional changes generally referred to as **intoxication**. With repeated use, biological adaptations lead to **tolerance**, which means the person requires a higher dose to get the same effects. While the person doesn't feel "high" with lower amounts, the substance may nonetheless harm the body.

Repeated use can also escalate into illnesses generally referred to as *substance use disorders*. The fourth edition of the American Psychiatric Association's (APA) *Diagnostic and Statistical Manual of Mental Disorders (DSM-4)* lumped these disorders into two main categories: substance abuse and substance dependence.[1] The two can occur independently or together. Nevertheless, it's worth examining abuse and dependence separately.

Substance **abuse** has four primary characteristics:

- failure to fulfill obligations at home, work, and school due to recurrent use
- continued use despite harmful effects on health and interpersonal relationships
- use in situations that could result in bodily harm to self and others (e.g., driving a car)
- legal problems

According to the APA, substance **dependence** requires the occurrence of three or more of the following criteria within a 12-month period:

- spending a great deal of time seeking, using, and recovering from the substance
- taking the substance in larger amounts or for longer periods of time than intended
- requiring higher doses to achieve the desired effects (tolerance)
- experiencing considerable discomfort when the substance is discontinued
- continuing use despite recognition of physical and psychological harm
- withdrawing from engagement in professional, social, or recreational activities due to substance use
- failing to cut back or quit without *relapsing* (returning to substance use), despite a desire to do so

While the DSM-4 avoided the word "addiction," the fifth edition (DSM-5), published in 2013, combines substance abuse and substance dependence into a single category called *addictions and related disorders*.[2] Each substance disorder is discussed separately (e.g., alcohol-use disorder). In addition to addictive substances, the DSM-5 covers addictive disorders marked by compulsive behaviors associated with gambling, eating, exercising, and sex. These behavioral addictions lack some of the characteristics of dependence.

Experts often use the words "substance dependence" and "addiction" interchangeably. The National Institute on Drug Abuse (NIDA) defines **addiction** as a chronic, relapsing brain disease characterized by compulsive use of a substance in spite of harmful consequences.[3] Note that the definition uses the words "brain disease." That's because all addicting drugs change the brain's structure and function—often for a long time. Addiction is not a moral failing—something you can quickly recover from simply by willing it so. Later, this chapter will discuss how substances change the brain in more detail.

Addiction has both psychological and physiological (pertaining to functioning of the body) components. With *psychological dependence*, the user believes that he or she needs the substance to function normally. If you've ever had trouble sleeping without a favorite blanket or stuffed animal, you understand that psychological dependence can feel very real. Separation from the object triggers emotional distress (irritability, anxiety, cravings) and a fierce motivation to get the thing back.

With repeated use, substances can lead to **physical dependence**, which changes in the brain. The end result is that, when the substance is removed, the unpleasant symptoms of **withdrawal** occur. The exact withdrawal symptoms vary with the substance. However, for all substances, seeking the pleasure associated with intoxication takes a back seat to avoiding withdrawal symptoms. People go from wanting the drug to feel better to needing the drug to feel normal. Withdrawal symptoms make it difficult to quit and easy to relapse. Cravings for the substance may continue long after quitting.

Addiction and physical dependence are not identical. For instance, someone with chronic pain could become dependent upon physician-prescribed morphine. Stopping the drug leads to withdrawal symptoms. However, if this patient doesn't compulsively use the drug, he or she is not an addict.[4]

With addiction, the combination of physical and psychological dependence leads to a preoccupation with acquiring and compulsively using the substance, regardless of the harm. Clearly, the surest way to avoid problems is to shun substances altogether. However, not everyone who tries a psychoactive substance becomes an addict. Later, we'll discuss how factors associated with the user, the substance, and the way the substance enters the body influence addiction.

---

intoxication

Changes to mental, emotional, and physical functioning that occur in response to acute administration of a psychoactive substance. In the absence of tissue damage, these effects resolve with time.

tolerance

A state in which higher doses of substances are needed to achieve the same effect.

abuse

Recurrent use of a substance despite interference with role obligations, adverse health, and social and legal consequences.

dependence

A substance use disorder marked by the inability to function normally without the substance and withdrawal symptoms upon discontinuing the substance.

addiction

A chronic, relapsing brain disease characterized by compulsive use of a substance, despite harmful consequences; often used synonymously with dependence, though the latter has a narrower meaning.

withdrawal

The development of unpleasant symptoms when the substance is removed.

The Scope of Substance Use Disorders

Substance dependence and abuse are common worldwide and nationally.

- In the United States, nearly 15 percent of adults have a substance abuse disorder during their lifetimes.[5] In 2010 alone, 22.1 million Americans 12 and up (8.7 percent of the population) had a dependence or abuse problem with alcohol and/or illicit drugs.[6] Of the illicit drugs, dependence and abuse was most common with marijuana, followed by narcotic pain relievers and cocaine.

- Every year, the abuse of illicit drugs and alcohol kills more than 100,000 Americans. Tobacco claims another 440,000 lives.[7]

- Substance use and abuse often takes root during adolescence. A national 2012 survey of adolescents found that by age 18, 78 percent had consumed alcohol, 47 percent drank regularly, and 15 percent already met criteria for abuse.[8] Nearly 43 percent used illicit drugs and just over 16 percent abused drugs. On the bright side, between 2000 and 2011, tobacco use among high schoolers fell from 34 to 23 percent and from 15 to 7 percent in middle schoolers.[9]

- Abuse of prescription drugs is, according to the Centers for Disease Control and Prevention (CDC), "the fastest growing drug problem in the United States."[10] *Nonmedical use of prescription drugs* is the practice of taking a medication, whether or not it was prescribed for you, for reasons other than its intended use. Examples include narcotic pain relievers (also called opioid analgesics), stimulants, and sedatives. Users often combine the drugs with alcohol and marijuana. Teens who misuse these medications have a much higher risk of abuse and dependence.[11]

1.1   Why People Use Substances

Our brains are wired in such a way that we're drawn to pleasurable activities. To explain this link, we need to get into a bit of brain anatomy and physiology. When something pleasurable happens, a network of brain cells popularly referred to as the **reward pathway** become activated. (Some authorities call it the "pleasure pathway" or the "pleasure-reward pathway.") As a result, a neurotransmitter (nerve chemical) called **dopamine** rises. The message is: "That felt good. Repeat that." You become motivated to obtain another pulse of dopamine.

A number of behaviors important to our survival increase dopamine: intimate touch, sex, or eating good food. Unless you engage in those behaviors excessively, your health and well-being rises. You get a burst of dopamine when you bite into a juicy peach, find a convenient parking place on your campus, finally grasp a scientific concept, do well on an exam, hug a friend, fly down a hill on a mountain bike, and swoop the hills and valleys of a roller coaster ride.

Clearly, the situation and your sense of control will affect your brain's response. If the parking space is in a nearly empty parking lot, you won't feel much pleasure. The same is true if your brakes give out on the mountain bike or the roller coaster ride goes on for two hours rather than the expected two minutes. And as we'll discuss later, some life-affirming activities such as eating and having sex can get out of control.

Anticipation alone can activate the reward pathway. Let's say a loved one is flying into town. Your dopamine may rise as you drive to the airport to meet him or her. If you're looking forward to a cold beer at the end of the day, your dopamine rises as you unlock the door and head to the refrigerator.

Perhaps because we're programmed for pleasure, humans generally seek to feel better. We start self-soothing in the womb. Fetuses sometimes emerge with small blisters from sucking on their hands and forearms. Infants also calm themselves by sucking. One of parents' jobs is to teach their children to help themselves feel better. When babies cry, parents rock, swaddle, and sing to them. They help their children recognize what's the matter, which helps identify the solution. If you're hungry, eat. If you're tired, take a nap. If you're restless, move your body. If you feel lonely, seek out a friend. If you're sad or angry, learn to talk about it. If you're feeling bored, change your scenery.

In addition to modifying behavior, we also take advantage of medicinal plants and synthetic drugs to feel better. We use ginger ale for upset stomachs, aspirin (derived from a plant) for headaches, coffee to enhance alertness, and, yes, alcohol to relax. Indeed, we are inclined to deliberately alter consciousness.

So why do humans turn to substances that may harm them? Some people either haven't learned or have limited access to healthy means of feeling better. Or the usual remedies don't work. Or their lives are generally hard and unrewarding. Media images signal that users are cool. Peer pressure and the desire to gain social acceptance can compel young people to try substances to gain social acceptance. Scientists speculate that, for some people, problems with the dopamine system may drive substance use and other risky behaviors.

Most people don't begin with the intention of becoming addicts. They tell themselves they could quit anytime. And they believe it—until they find out how wrong they are.

reward pathway

A region of the brain activated during pleasurable activities; also called the "pleasure pathway" or the "pleasure-reward pathway."

dopamine

The key neurotransmitter (nerve chemical) associated with the reward pathway in the brain.

1.2 Risk Factors for Substance Use Disorders

So why is it that one person can drink socially and another becomes an alcoholic? Why does one person experiment briefly with cocaine and another ends up an addict? It depends on genetics, environment, and personal characteristics. No one risk factor can increase vulnerability or doom a person to abuse and addiction.

1. **Genetics.** Family history of alcoholism and substance abuse. Substance disorders tend to cluster in families due to a combination of shared genes and shared environments. Studies in twins and adopted children demonstrate that genetics confer vulnerability.[12] If substance abuse runs in your family, you may be at risk, but you are not destined to addiction.

2. **Environmental factors.**

   - **Ready availability of the substances.**

   - **Substance use by influential peers and family members.**

   - **Stress.** Stress increases the risk of using substances, becoming dependent upon them, and relapsing after quitting. There seem to be critical periods for programming a predisposition to substance use. Specifically, prenatal (before the birth) and early childhood adversity can render people particularly vulnerable to substance abuse.[13] Children who experience trauma—loss of a parent, physical or sexual abuse, witnessing violence—are more at risk for starting substances early and developing dependencies.[14] Growing up in a chaotic, dysfunctional family also increases risk.

     However, significant stress later in life continues to serve as a risk factor. Poverty, unsafe neighborhoods, and low social standing count as serious stressors. Selling drugs can also seem a justifiable job in the face of poverty. Other life stressors include dysfunctional marriage, divorce, and job loss. If life seems otherwise unrewarding, substance use can seem a reasonable escape. Furthermore, people who haven't learned positive coping skills often find substances a quick, albeit fleeting, remedy. Unfortunately, substance abuse is, itself, a stressor.

3. **Personal characteristics.** Stressful environments and personal characteristics interact. More resilient personality types won't be as adversely affected by trauma. And stress can underlie some of the characteristics listed.

   - **Early initiation of substance use.** Adolescence represents a susceptible period for substance disorders. Most substance dependence and abuse begins during late adolescence and early adulthood. Onset later in life is rare.[15] Younger users develop abuse and dependence problems more swiftly and are more likely to continue to use substances.

   - **Male sex.** Compared to women, men are twice as likely to experience alcohol and substance use disorders.[16] Men are more inclined to use substances for thrills and social status. Women use substances to improve mood and confidence. Because of biological differences, women may be more vulnerable to intoxication and dependence once they begin using substances.

   - **Race and ethnicity.** Substance dependence and abuse is lowest among Asians, Native Hawaiians, and other Pacific Islanders and highest for American Indians and Alaskan Natives. While genetic variations are a possible influence, social factors such as cultural values, poverty, and discrimination play a greater role.

   - **Education level.** People with lower levels of education are more likely to smoke and less likely to quit.[17] They're also at higher risk for using illicit drugs. Conversely, illicit drug use reduces educational attainment.

   - **Psychological characteristics.** Negative traits include anxiety, anger, guilt, and sad mood. Having an untreated psychological illness—depression, anxiety, bipolar disorder, schizophrenia, or posttraumatic stress disorder (PTSD)—fuels substance use. In addition to possible biological influences, people may use substances to relieve psychological issues.[18] Unfortunately, substance use only worsens these conditions.

     Poor self-image, low self-esteem, and lack of self-control—all of which may reflect unhappy childhoods—also foster substance use. Risk takers are more likely to become involved with potentially addictive behaviors.

   - **Poor academic performance.** Apathy about school, skipping class, and low grades correlate with substance use. These factors, in turn, predict low educational attainment, which is another risk factor for substance use disorders.

- **Fighting and delinquent behavior.** Youths who get into fights, belong to gangs, commit assault, carry guns, steal, sell drugs, and so on are more likely to develop drug and alcohol problems.

- **Sleep deprivation.** A study for the CDC found that teens who routinely sleep less than eight hours a night are more likely to smoke, drink, take drugs, and engage in other unhealthy behaviors.[19]

The Perils of Early Substance Use

During adolescence, brain areas that govern learning, memory, judgment, and other so-called executive function skills haven't finished developing. That means two things: (1) Teens may not make the wisest decisions about using substances, and (2) substances can have toxic effects on young brains, arresting development and worse. A third problem occurs no matter what age substance abuse and dependence begins: undesirable brain changes that can take a very long time to revert to normal.

Adolescents who start using substances face a quicker time to addiction, a greater chance of long-term use, and lower likelihood of quitting. Early initiation of less risky substances can progress to dangerous drug use. Alcohol and tobacco are usually the first psychoactive drugs used by young people. Long-term problems with alcohol and drugs are a common consequence.[20],[21] The most widely used illicit drug among teens is marijuana.

1.3 Protective Factors against Substance Misuse

Many things that protect us from substance use disorders are the opposite of the risk factors. Researchers have found the following items to be particularly helpful:

- Coming from a family and greater community that discouraged substance use.
- Perceiving that substances are potentially harmful.
- Feeling disapproval of peers who use substances.
- Attending religious services. However, a spiritual community doesn't necessarily involve religion. It might entail belonging to an environmental organization, practicing yoga with others, or any other activity that enhances spiritual growth.
- Growing up in a supportive, peaceful, and reasonably prosperous environment. When parents and their kids communicate easily and openly, kids are less likely to use or abuse substances. For adolescents, parental involvement (e.g., limiting nights out with friends, checking on homework completion, showing up for school events, expecting kids to do chores, and praising them for a job well done) reduces substance use and abuse.
- Feeling engaged with academics, athletics, work, community service, and other worthy pursuits. These activities provide a sense of meaning and purpose.
- Possessing good mental and emotional health. Relevant elements of psychological health include the following:
  - positive self-image and healthy self-esteem
  - self-assertiveness and independent thinking skills
  - self-control
  - overall positive mood and optimistic attitude about the future
  - a sense of meaning and purpose
  - resilience and the ability to cope with stress in healthy ways

What about substance abuse awareness education? Some studies do suggest they work. Campaigns to increase public awareness of the dangers of smoking, as well as laws that restrict smoking in public places, have led to a decline in tobacco use. Interventions to prevent alcohol abuse on campuses also work.[22] Simply providing scary facts about substance abuse isn't enough. It's not easy to say no to people you like and admire. Individual and group training provide students with skills to resist or reduce use of substances.[23] Such skill-based interventions improve self-esteem, teach self-assertiveness, and enhance decision-making ability.

Video Link 11.1

Anyone Can Become Addicted to Drugs

The National Institute on Drug Abuse explains why no one is immune to drug addiction and briefly reviews risks factors for heightened vulnerability. Click on the video called "Anyone Can Become Addicted to Drugs."

http://www.drugabuse.gov/related-topics/addiction-science

Assess Yourself: Are You Vulnerable to Substance Use Disorders?

While many young adults experiment with drugs, most eventually quit as they assume responsibilities with work and family. However, some people are more vulnerable than others to developing substance use problems. Take the following assessment to determine if you might be one of them.

- Do your close friends use substances?
    ___Yes ___No
- Is it easy for you to acquire substances?
    ___Yes ___No
- Do your biological parents or siblings have substance use problems?
    ___Yes ___No
- Did you experience early childhood adversity (economic hardship; parental neglect; or physical, psychological, or sexual abuse)?
    ___Yes ___No
- Do you have untreated depression, anxiety, bipolar disorder, or PTSD?
    ___Yes ___No
- Do you have trouble controlling your impulses?
    ___Yes ___No
- Do you easily become emotionally upset or angry?
    ___Yes ___No
- Do you feel lonely?
    ___Yes ___No
- If you're already using a substance, did you begin before age 17?
    ___Yes ___No
- Do you feel stressed out most days?
    ___Yes ___No

The more affirmative answers you have, the greater your risk. If you answered yes to the first two questions, you're more likely to try substances but not necessarily at risk for dependence. The rest of the questions address biological and psychological characteristics associated with vulnerability to substance abuse and dependence. If you already use substances and answered yes to more than three questions, proceed to the self-assessment for drug and alcohol dependence. If you answered yes to several questions and do not use substances, congratulate yourself and continue to maintain abstinence.

1.4 Consequences of Substance Use and Abuse

Intoxication can impair judgment, trigger impulsive behavior, slow reflexes, and diminish coordination. Those effects lead to the following problems:

- **Poor academic performance.** Intoxicating substances aren't compatible with studying. By definition, substance dependence and abuse are enormously time consuming. School and other important pursuits become secondary to financing, acquiring, and using the substance.

- **Social and interpersonal problems.** People with substance use problems may neglect friends and family and become secretive. Some substances alter personality in ways that interfere with healthy relationships.

- **Unintentional injuries.** Central nervous system depressants such as Valium-like drugs, alcohol, and opiates/narcotics impair mental and physical function. Marijuana and hallucinogens alter mental function and sensory perception. The most dangerous activity is driving a motorized vehicle while intoxicated.

- **Intentional injuries.** Addicts may go to great lengths for the next fix. Depending on the substance, users may become violent or vulnerable to victimization (e.g., physical and sexual assault and robbery). Crack cocaine, amphetamines, and alcohol are notorious for triggering violent behavior. Drug rings that trade in illegal substances come at the cost of much violence. Substance use also greatly heightens the risk of suicide.

- **Unsafe sexual behaviors.** Some substances increase sexual desire, release inhibitions, and cloud judgment, elevating the risk of risky sexual behaviors. Intoxication raises the risk of rape. Addicts may trade sex for money or drugs. For all these reasons, the risk of unintended pregnancy and sexually transmitted infections rises.

- **Compromised health and reduced longevity.** Undesirable side effects of the substance used can produce both acute toxicity and, with long-term use, chronic disease. Addicts may also neglect to eat well, which can lead to malnutrition. The risk of intentional suicide and overdose rises.

     A recent study found a fivefold increased risk of death from continued use of "hard drugs" (cocaine, opioids, amphetamines) into middle age relative to peers who had quit substances after early adulthood.[24] Most of the users were not addicts but recreational "dabblers."

- **Transmission of blood-borne infections with injected drugs.** Drugs such as heroin, amphetamines, and cocaine can be injected with needles. To save money, some drug users share needles, a risky practice that can result in spreading bacteria and viruses. Bacteria transmitted via needles can infect the heart, lungs, and other organs. Deadly viruses such as human immunodeficiency virus (HIV) and hepatitis viruses can lead to chronic illness and premature death. Viruses may survive attempts to sterilize needles with boiling water and bleach.

- **Financial ruin.** Substance use problems raise the risk of disability, absenteeism, unemployment, and repeated hospitalizations, creating an enormous economic burden. Furthermore, poorer people appear to be more vulnerable to substance abuse. People with chronic substance dependencies can become homeless.

- **Legal consequences.** People may commit crimes to get the funds to pay for substances. Furthermore, possessing, using, and selling illicit drugs can lead to arrest and incarceration. The "War on Drugs," championed by the US government starting in 1972, hasn't done much to curtail drug use but has put a lot of people behind bars. Unfortunately, blacks are far more likely than whites to be sent to prison on drug-related charges—at great cost to them and their communities.[25]

How Substances Affect the Brain

As we explore the different substances, we'll discuss particular effects of each. For some substances, every organ in the body is affected. For others, the effects are relatively limited. All substances cause *epigenetic* changes, alterations in the way genes are expressed.[26] The end result is impairments in neurologic function. While other brain areas can be affected, one that's most critical to the addiction process is the **reward pathway.**

     Recall from Chapter 5 that *neurons* (nerve cells) communicate using electrical and chemical signals. The chemicals (*neurotransmitters*) are released into the synapse (the tiny gap separating neurons), allowing the electrical message from neurons to get transmitted to the next neuron. Neurotransmitters attach to *receptors* (structures on cell surfaces designed to bind to particular molecules) thereby initiating changes within the cell.

     The amount of neurotransmitter in the synapse (space between neurons or nerve cells) depends on how much the first (transmitting) neuron released, the number of receptors for that neurotransmitter on the second (receiving) neuron and how quickly the neurotransmitter is cleared from the synapse. Neurotransmitters are either broken down by enzymes or taken up by the first neuron for repackaging.

     In the brain's reward pathway, the dominant neurotransmitter is *dopamine*. Whereas normal rewards stimulate a blip of dopamine, most substances associated with abuse and dependence release a tsunami. The premier dopamine booster is cocaine. It blocks the reuptake of dopamine, resulting in higher levels in the synapse. Repeated exposure to high levels of dopamine causes the second neuron to pull back its receptors. The process is akin to clapping your hands over your ears if someone keeps shouting at you.

     While this receptor "downregulation" is a key mechanism by which **tolerance** develops, there are exceptions. For instance, increased efficiency of liver enzyme systems results in tolerance to alcohol.

     While all substances raise dopamine (albeit sometimes indirectly) in the reward pathway, they can also affect other neurotransmitters. For instance, stimulants increase norepinephrine, which is chemically similar to epinephrine (adrenaline). Narcotics increase natural opioids such as endorphin, which have an analgesic (pain-relieving) effect. Nicotine, the addicting substance in tobacco, binds to receptors for acetylcholine, a prominent neurotransmitter in the autonomic (involuntary) nervous system and in brain centers involved in with maintaining alertness. Alcohol and other central nervous system depressants augment the effects of gamma-aminobutyric acid (GABA), which has a relaxing effect.

FIGURE 11.1 Dopamine Pathways in the Brain

In the reward pathway, dopamine is made in a brain region called the ventral tegmental area (VTA) and released in the nucleus accumbens. A branch to the frontal cortex (a higher brain region) creates a sense of reward and reinforces the behavior. Other dopamine pathways influence movement.

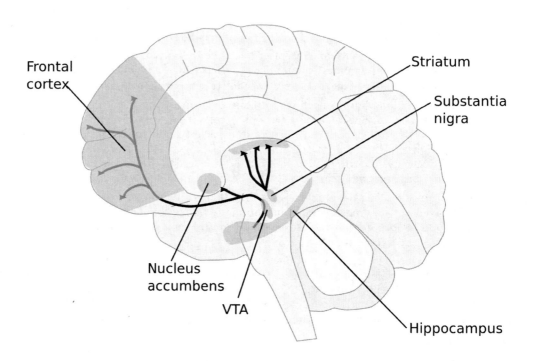

Source: Quasihuman. Available at: http://commons.wikimedia.org/wiki/File:Dopamine_pathways.svg, adapted from the National Institute on Drug Abuse.

Once the nervous system adapts, it doesn't function well in the absence of the substance. Withdrawal symptoms occur. Also, naturally pleasurable events no longer seem, well, pleasurable. A kiss from a loved one isn't enough to get a feel-good rise in dopamine. Unfortunately, addictive substances change the brain in ways that endure a long time after the drug is stopped. Quitting, however, is possible.

  Video Link 11.2

Why Are Drugs So Hard to Quit?

This National Institute on Drug Abuse video explains why brain changes associated with addiction makes it hard (but not impossible) to quit. Click on the video called "Why Are Drugs So Hard to Quit?"

http://www.drugabuse.gov/related-topics/addiction-science

How Substances Affect the Body

A number of factors influence a substance's acute effect and how fast addiction develops. The two main variables are the drug itself and the individual characteristics of the person taking the drug.

Human factors:

- **Body mass.** The same dose will have a bigger drug effect on a person who weighs 100 pounds than 180 pounds. Body composition also figures in. Many substances dissolve in water. For two people of the same weight, the one with more lean body mass (which contains water) will feel the impact of the drug less than the individual with relatively greater fat mass.

- **Ingestion of food.** If an individual has just eaten, an ingested substance will take longer to absorb into the blood. Specific foods have effects that can raise or lower blood levels of some drugs. For instance, grapefruit juice inhibits enzymes that break down certain drugs in the gut, thereby increasing blood levels.

- **Metabolic processes.** A number of biochemical processes remove drugs from the body. Your most important detoxification organs are the liver and kidneys. Poor function of either will increase the time a drug lingers in the body. Also, even when detoxification organs function normally, the speed of metabolism of particular chemicals varies from person to person.

- **Mental and emotional state.** Expectations are key. If you think a drug (or any other intervention) will have a particular effect, it likely will. Positive expectations produce the *placebo effect*. In this case, a pill without the active chemical causes effects normally associated with the drug.

- **Genetics.** As mentioned, genetics contribute to vulnerability to addiction. It can also affect the rate at which you detoxify and eliminate substances.

- **Repetition.** Addiction usually requires the user try the substance several times. If the user found the first experience to be particularly profound and pleasurable, he or she may keep taking the substance to try recapturing that initiation—though the first time is often the best.

Drug factors:

The type of substance, the dose taken, and the way the substance enters the body all influence the effect on the individual. The more intensely pleasurable and rewarding the substance, the greater the speed of addiction.

- **The nature of the substance itself.** Different substances have different effects on bodily function. Alcohol and sedatives depress the central nervous system. Stimulants activate the nervous system. Some drugs act more quickly and are more addicting, no matter how they're taken.

- **Dose.** The more of the substance taken in a period of time, the greater the level of intoxication. Taking the same dose in a relatively short period also increases the high.

- **Route of administration.** The way in which a drug enters the body influences the rapidity and intensity of the high. At some point, psychoactive substances enter the bloodstream and cross into the brain. Those that quickly and intensely affect the nervous system are typically more swiftly addictive.

  - **Oral administration.** Ingesting by mouth is the slowest route. If you swallow a substance, it may first have to be digested. Food in the stomach slows the process. Purified, small molecules are absorbed from the intestinal tract into the bloodstream.

  - **Intranasal administration.** Drugs that are "snorted" pass easily from the linings of the nose into the underlying blood vessels.

  - **Inhalation.** Drug inhaled deep into lungs move quickly into the blood.

  - **Injection.** Drugs can be injected into the muscle (intramuscular), under the skin (subcutaneous), or directly into a vein (intravenous). Intravenous (IV) administration acts more quickly than intramuscular and subcutaneous injections. The intense and nearly immediate effects cause IV drug use to be extremely addicting and dangerous.

  - **Transdermal absorption.** Some drugs can be absorbed across the skin. Few drugs of abuse are delivered that way. However, nicotine skin patches can ease withdrawal symptoms in people quitting tobacco.

  - **Rectal suppositories and colonic enemas.** Rectal suppositories, though not a typical way of taking illicit drugs, involve mixing drugs with waxy substances that dissolve inside the body, allowing the drug to be absorbed across the mucous membranes of the rectum. Enemas entail introducing liquids into the colon via the anus. There have been reports of people trying coffee and also alcohol enemas. Dangers include damage to the anus and colon, disturbances in electrolytes (blood minerals), and unpredictably high blood levels of the drug.

- **Interactions with other substances.** Illicit, prescription, and over-the-counter drugs and the chemicals in dietary supplements can interact. Two chemicals with similar actions—for instance, a sedative drug and alcohol—can produce an additive effect.

Assess Yourself: Drug and Alcohol Dependence

The transition from using a substance for recreational and social reasons to developing abuse and dependence problems is slippery. Sometimes friends and family recognize the problem before the user. If you have any doubts about your own relationship with substances, speak to your doctor about whether it's time for treatment.

In the meantime, do your best to respond honestly to the following statements.

- I spend a good chunk of my waking hours planning how to get, acquire, and use a substance.
  ___Yes ___No
- I spend a significant proportion of any given month recovering from the use of this substance.
  ___Yes ___No
- Since I began using this substance, I now need more of it to get the desired effects.
  ___Yes ___No
- I've failed in my attempts to reduce or stop my use of this substance.
  ___Yes ___No
- I keep using the substance even though it's caused problems with my physical and mental health.
  ___Yes ___No
- Using this substance has caused me to miss out on important activities.
  ___Yes ___No
- I continue to use the substance despite resultant problems with work, school, athletics, or other important activities.
  ___Yes ___No
- Use of this substance has caused problems with my relationships with family and friends.
  ___Yes ___No
- I've put myself or others at risk while under the influence of this substance.
  ___Yes ___No
- Use of this substance has caused me to get into trouble with the law.
  ___Yes ___No

Adapted from questions used in the 2010 National Survey on Drug Use and Health from the Substance Abuse and Mental Health Services Administration. Available at: http://www.samhsa.gov/data/NSDUH/2k10NSDUH/2k10Results.htm#3.1.6

1.5 Treatment of Substance Use Disorders

Because the brain changes caused by addiction can endure a long time, proper treatment is important. However, few people receive the treatment they need. In 2010, of the 23.1 million Americans in need of specialty treatment for an illicit drug or alcohol use problem, only about 1 percent received it.[27] Ninety-five percent didn't believe they needed treatment. Of the minority who recognized they needed treatment, more than 3 percent didn't make an effort to get it, and 1.7 percent tried but couldn't get treatment—mainly because they lacked health insurance coverage and couldn't afford the cost. People also worried about the impact of treatment on their jobs and their reputations.

However, treatment is often essential to recovery and, in some cases, to avert life-threatening withdrawal reactions. People may need to detoxify ("detox") in a hospital's rehabilitation unit. Medications can make withdrawal safer and easier and reduce cravings.

Long-term services involve psychotherapy to help people identify triggers, change self-defeating thoughts, modify behaviors, learn to manage cravings, and help rectify underlying social and psychological problems that paved the way to addiction. Therapists can also teach life skills to help recovering addicts cope in the outside world: find work, manage money, communicate effectively, and generally reintegrate themselves into society. A stay in a halfway house can provide an intermediate training ground between release from a treatment center and independent living.

Most colleges provide counseling, prevention, and treatment services. If you think you're at risk, the first place to start is the campus health center. Most cities have private and public rehabilitation centers. The United States Substance Abuse and Mental Health Services Administration website has a behavioral health treatment facility locator (http://findtreatment.samhsa.gov/TreatmentLocator/faces/geographicSearch.jspx). Also, national recovery programs (e.g., Alcoholics Anonymous) usually have local chapters. Programs are also available to support and educate family and friends of addicts.

General Strategies for Breaking Addictive Behaviors

Much of the work of breaking addiction is internal. The first step is recognizing you have a problem. The second is believing the substance problem poses serious risks for you and others. The third is deciding you're ready to change. The fourth is actually doing something about the problem.

Be prepared for competing desires. If you see or are reminded of the substance, you may feel torn and think, "It would feel great to have some." "If I do, I won't finish studying." "I could get up early and study." "No, I'll feel guilty and hung over." "My friends are doing it. They seem OK…" The tug-of-war is exhausting. You only have so much energy to resist these urges. If you have become dependent or addicted to a substance, your resolve can be on especially thin ice. So you need tools.

- **Acknowledge and accept the problem.** Write it down. Record everything you don't like about your relationship with alcohol, tobacco, or drugs.

- **Establish underlying causes.** What initially made you start to smoke, drink, or take drugs? Are those motivators still important to you? How else can you satisfy them? Do you need the help of mental health expert to overcome feelings of low self-esteem, depression, or anxiety? Can you find healthier ways to release negative emotions?

- **Remove temptations.** Until you have fully recovered (a process that can take a long time), rid your life, as much as possible, of the substance. Toss the tobacco and drugs or pour the alcohol down the drain.

- **Identify patterns.** For example, you may have developed strong associations between breakfast and coffee, studying and cigarettes, football games and beer, celebrations of any sort and alcohol, and listening to music and marijuana.

- **When possible, break those associations.** You may have to change friends or stop frequenting bars. You can't, of course, avoid any reminders of the substance. In that case, you need other tools to resist the urge to cave in.

- **Find substitutions.** Sip a nonalcoholic substance at parties. Suck on a licorice stick (the actual root if you can find it in health food stores) or crunch a celery stick or chew gum when you feel like bringing a cigarette to your lips.

- **Create distractions.** The anxiety and restlessness associated with craving don't last forever. Have a ready list of things you can do until they pass. Examples include journaling, praying, and exercising. You can also try watching a short video or doing a hobby (especially those that use your hands or require concentration—knitting, drawing, sculpting, playing music). Creative pursuits can also release the negative feelings that drive the addiction.

- **Quiet your mind.** That's asking a lot. The cravings, restlessness, and anxiety of withdrawal can rock tranquility. Yet deliberately calming and focusing works. Studies show that slow, deep breathing and mindfulness meditation helps people break through addictions, resist cravings, and prevent relapse.[28] ,[29] Try going outside and staring at the ever-changing sky or a growing plant.

- **Think positively.** Unhelpful thoughts go something like this: "I feel awful. I want X. X would make me feel better." Are those assessments actually true? How else could you feel better, stronger, more in control? Try thinking, "I can learn to feel good without X. I know I can do this. I am sticking to my plan to quit. I will feel better tomorrow if I do."

- **Seek social support.** Tell your friends and family about your desire to give up a substance. Once you come out, you may feel even more committed to success. Find someone you can call and talk to when needed. Team up with someone who's also trying to quit.

- **Track your behavior.** Make a list of the times you feel a craving, what that urge felt like physically and emotionally, what the situation was, whether you used the substance, and what the consequences were of doing so. Be honest. It's sometimes hard to see a record, but you may also learn what's getting in your way. Better yet, you may see evidence of improvement.

- **Accept occasional setbacks.** Many people have to quit substances more than once before they're completely clean. Don't give up. Analyze what happened. What triggered the relapse? What did you do? How might you respond differently the next time?

- **Become more health conscious.** Regardless of which substance you're quitting, you're doing yourself a favor. Your health will improve soon. Move your whole life into a healthier zone. Think of it this way: You're giving up something harmful and adopting life-affirming habits. Exercising can help relieve the tension and anxiety that accompanies cravings. It's also a good distraction. Improving your diet will also heighten well-being.

- **Notice good things about not using.** Once withdrawal symptoms subside, you may sleep better, wake up more refreshed, think more clearly, get along better with people, feel more cheerful and motivated, and enjoy everyday pleasures again (the smell of food, the sight of flowers or fall foliage). It might be easier to study or exercise. You may get along better with people. Maybe your clothes, hair, and room smell better. Maybe you look healthier.

- **Celebrate progress—without getting high.** Make a list of things that please you. Take up a new hobby. Visit a museum or a farmers' market. Catch a film. Go for a bike ride. Buy a magazine or a novel.

- **Don't hesitate to get professional help.** Medications, counseling, and professional support groups can improve the odds of success.

DISCUSSION QUESTIONS

1. This section discussed reasons people use and abuse substances. In your own words, discuss three factors that you think are most important in determining whether or not a person develops a problem with substances. Use a combination of facts and personal observations. For facts, cite your resource. Resources might include this text, other books, and credible Internet sites.
2. Explain the biological adaptations that lead to tolerance.
3. What is the difference between substance abuse and substance dependence?
4. Why is early initiation of substance use particularly dangerous?

2. TOBACCO

LEARNING OBJECTIVES

1. Examine the toll tobacco use takes on society.
2. Examine the chemicals in tobacco.
3. Define environmental tobacco smoke.
4. Detail the health effects of tobacco products.
5. Review specific treatments for nicotine withdrawal.

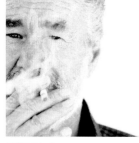

© Thinkstock

While a few substances discussed in this chapter have both potential health benefits and adverse consequences, smoking cigarettes will gain you nothing. On the contrary, tobacco use diminishes health and abbreviates life. It's the *leading* preventable cause of death. The only possible merit of tobacco is its sacred use in Native American ceremonies.

Here are some statistics about tobacco:

- Worldwide, tobacco use kills 6 million people a year, and experts predict the annual death toll will reach 8 million by 2030.[30] In the United States, tobacco use causes 1 in 5 deaths, or about 467,000 deaths a year.[31]
- An estimated 69.6 million—more than 27 percent—Americans 12 and older use some kind of tobacco product.[32]
- Cigarette smoking rates have fallen, but not far enough. Between 2005 and 2010, the percentage of American smokers fell from nearly 21 percent to 19.3 percent—a decline of three million.[33]
- Surveys show that 18.6 percent of college students smoke at least one cigarette month (nearly a third of whom smoke every day), and 9.2 percent smoked tobacco from a water pipe (hookah).[34] The good news is that college students and college graduates smoke less than people who don't attend college.
- Men smoke cigarettes and use other tobacco products more than women. Among ethnic groups, Asian Americans are the least likely to smoke and Native Americans the most likely. Poverty correlates with more smoking, despite the expense of tobacco products. Higher education seems to protect against smoking.
- While cigarette use declined dramatically between 2000 and 2011, use of loose tobacco (used for pipe smoking or roll-your-own cigarettes) and cigars rose 123 percent.[35] Economics drive that

shift. Differential taxes make large cigars and pipe tobacco less expensive than cigarettes and small cigars.

- According to the CDC, smoking costs us about $96 billion a year in medical costs and $97 billion in lost productivity from premature death.[36] More is lost when workers call in sick because of smoking-related maladies. Nevertheless, the tobacco industry continues to generate multibillion-dollar sales. If you're wondering how it remains fashionable and profitable to promote poison, check out this link on Tobacco.org: http://www.tobacco.org/resources/history/strategieslb.html.

2.1 What's in Tobacco?

Tobacco products are made from dried leaves of the tobacco plant. It contains more than 7,000 chemicals.[37] In addition, ingredients may be added to enhance flavor or reduce the irritation of the smoke.

Nicotine is the addictive substance. Within seconds of drawing in a lungful of tobacco smoke, this chemical reaches the brain, where it briefly enhances attention and concentration and immediately stops cravings. The instant gratification makes nicotine the most addictive drug.

Over 40 chemicals in tobacco smoke are *carcinogens*, or cancer-causing substances. Tobacco smoke also contains carbon monoxide, which binds more tenaciously to hemoglobin (an oxygen-carrying molecule in red blood cells) than oxygen. The end result is it lowers the oxygen-carrying capacity of blood. Poisonous substances include arsenic, cadmium, acetone (which is in nail polish remover), butane (lighter fluid), ammonia, toluene (an industrial solvent), and hydrogen cyanide.

The particles in tobacco smoke condense into a sticky, toxic substance called *tar*. It's the brown stuff on the end of a cigarette filter. It stains fingers and blackens the lungs.

nicotine

The chemical in tobacco that leads to dependence.

 Video Clip 11.1

How Nicotine Affects the Body
This video explains the effects of nicotine and withdrawal from nicotine.

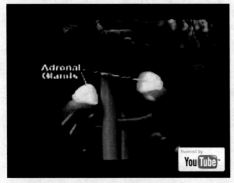

View the video online at: http://www.youtube.com/v/HlclKekEldg

2.2 Environmental Tobacco Smoke

Smoke released by burning tobacco is called **environmental tobacco smoke (ETS)**. The smoke inhaled and exhaled by the smoker is called **mainstream smoke**. **Sidestream smoke**, which is the majority of environmental smoke, comes from the burning end. Because sidestream smoke is unfiltered, it contains a higher content of nicotine, tar, carbon monoxide, and other noxious substances. Smokers and innocent bystanders inhale this polluted air. **Passive smoking** refers to the inhalation of ETS without actually putting a burning tobacco product to your lips.

ETS is also referred to as *second-hand smoke*. However, ETS also creates *third-hand smoke*, the residual chemicals that settle on indoor surfaces as well as clothes and hair.[38] Nonsmoking adults, infants, and children pick up these toxins from furniture, drapes, bedding, walls, and carpets. Airing out the room doesn't eliminate this residue. In fact, it can build up over time.

Among people who don't smoke, about 40 percent have blood levels of a chemical (cotinine) that indicates they've been subjected to other people's smoke. Worse, the exposure is highest (54 percent) among children 3 to 11 years old. Tobacco smoke undermines everyone's health—smokers and nonsmokers. Exact health hazards are detailed in the next section. Suffice it to say, ETS contributes to about 49,000 deaths in the United States each year.[39]

environmental tobacco smoke (ETS)

Smoke from a burning tobacco product that enters the environment; also called second-hand smoke.

passive smoking

Inhaling environmental tobacco smoke, whether you want to or not.

2.3   Tobacco Products

Tobacco comes in several forms.

- **Cigarettes.** These are the most common form of tobacco product. Most commercial brands have filters that reduce some of the dangerous substances inhaled. However, the better the filter, the deeper smokers "drag" on the cigarette, delivering more noxious substances into the lungs. That's why low-tar and low-nicotine cigarettes are no healthier than other products.

- **Clove cigarettes** (also called kreteks). These contain ground cloves, a spice that has the numbing chemical eugenol. While the smoke may feel less irritating, the fact that it is often inhaled more deeply can make it more hazardous to your health. The same is true of *menthol* cigarettes. *Bidis* are hand-rolled, often flavored cigarettes that come from Southeast Asia and India. They contain three to five times as much nicotine as regular cigarettes.[40]

- **Pipe tobacco and cigars.** Food and Drug Administration (FDA) regulations about flavoring, labeling, and marketing don't apply to these products. When burned, they release the same toxic chemicals as in cigarette smoke. Unlike cigarettes, the mainstream smoke isn't filtered. In some cultures, *hookahs* (water pipes) are used. While the water-cooled smoke feels less harsh, it is no less harmful.

- **Smokeless tobacco.** These products include chewing tobacco and snuff. The leaves of chewing tobacco are often treated with molasses and flavorings. A small amount is usually placed between the teeth and lower lip. The increase in saliva causes users to spit frequently. Snuff, which is more finely ground, can be placed between teeth and gums and sniffed up the nose. While these substances don't entail inhaling noxious substances into your lungs, they cause nicotine dependence, gingivitis (gum inflammation), and changes in the mucous membranes of the mouth called *leukoplakia*, which can lead to cancer.

- **Dissolvable tobacco.** Tobacco companies such as R. J. Reynolds have come out with finely ground flavored tobacco in the form of pellets, strips applied to the tongue, and toothpicks that allow nicotine to dissolve in the mouth. People who aren't already smokers can become hooked on these products, which deliver more nicotine than cigarettes. Critics accuse tobacco companies of using these products to boost flagging cigarette sales and to keep people addicted.

2.4   Health Consequences of Tobacco

Unless you work with toxic chemicals, tobacco smoke is probably the most significant air pollutant to which you're exposed. There is no safe level of tobacco. It causes oxidative damage to tissues all over the body.

- **Decreased longevity.** Compared to nonsmokers, smokers lose about 13 to 14 years of potential life.[41]

    Smokers are more likely to be sedentary, binge drink, and use illicit drugs—all habits that reduce quantity and quality of life. Even if other health habits are excellent, tobacco use causes several chronic, life-shortening diseases.

    - **Atherosclerosis.** This disease is marked by the deposition of fat and other substances within the arteries.

    - **Heart disease and stroke.** Most smokers die from cardiovascular diseases (diseases of the arteries and heart). Compared to nonsmokers, smokers are two to four times more likely to develop heart disease and about twice as likely to have a stroke.[42]

    - **Cancer.** It probably seems obvious that tobacco might cause cancer in tissues that directly contact smoke or chewed leaves, such as the mouth, throat, larynx (voice box), esophagus, and lungs. Because many carcinogenic (cancer-causing) substances easily move into the blood, cells everywhere are exposed. Bladder, cervical, pancreatic, and stomach cancer are more common in smokers.

    - **Chronic obstructive pulmonary (lung) disease (COPD).** COPD encompasses two main conditions: chronic bronchitis and emphysema. *Bronchitis* means inflammation of the bronchi (the tubular structures that deliver air to the bottom of the lungs). Whereas infections cause most cases of acute bronchitis, the main cause of chronic (persistent) bronchitis is tobacco smoke. The airways narrow and produce excessive mucus. Habitual smokers have their most productive coughs in the morning. That's because, during the night, the cilia lining the airways recovered from their tobacco smoke-induced daytime paralysis and nudged the heavy carpet of mucus upward.

Smoking also causes *emphysema*, a permanent destruction of the walls of the alveoli (the delicate air sacs where gas exchange occurs between the lungs and the bloodstream). People with COPD are more vulnerable to acute respiratory infections. Despite campaigns to discourage smoking, COPD recently became the number three cause of death in America, bumping stroke down to number four.[43]

- **Erectile dysfunction.** All parts of your body need a healthy blood flow—including the reproductive organs. As noted, smoking is a huge risk factor for arterial diseases such as atherosclerosis, and arterial disease is a common cause of erectile dysfunction.
- **Ulcers.** Smokers have a higher risk of peptic ulcers (painful erosions into the lining of the stomach and/or first part of the small intestine).
- **Miscellaneous chronic conditions.** These include gum disease, cataracts, and osteoporosis (with a resultant increased risk of bone fractures). Skin also ages prematurely.

Tobacco carries unique problems for pregnant women and children. Women who smoke have reduced fertility. Smoking during pregnancy is the primary preventable cause of illness and death among pregnant women and infants. It raises the risk of miscarriage, detachment of the placenta from the uterus, premature delivery, low-birth-weight babies, birth anomalies, and sudden infant death syndrome.[44] ,[45]

Infants born to smoking mothers may be born with reduced lung function and have lower levels of HDL cholesterol, a blood lipid that protects against heart disease.[46] They're more likely to develop colic,[47] anxiety, depression, and behavior problems. Despite these risks, 10 to 12 percent of pregnant American women smoke.[48]

Kids who breathe environmental tobacco smoke are at increased risk of asthma, hay fever, respiratory infections, middle ear infections, anxiety, and attention deficit hyperactivity disorder (ADHD).[49] Not surprisingly, they miss more school than kids not subjected to tobacco smoke. Worse, like the smokers they live with, they're more at risk for cancer.

FIGURE 11.2 How Tobacco Affects the Body

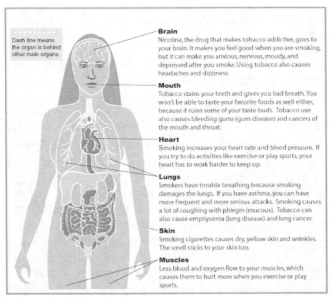

Source: Office on Women's Health in the Office of the Assistant Secretary for Health. How tobacco affects your body. Available at:

http://commons.wikimedia.org/wiki/File:Tobacco_diagram.png.

2.5 Quitting Tobacco

Nicotine addiction is tough to kick. However, the returns, including more years of life, are priceless. Some benefits are immediate. For instance, you smell better to others and your sense of smell returns. Food tastes better. Irritated respiratory linings busily repair themselves. The body recovers from tobacco-induced inflammation and free-radical damage. Within three years, an ex-smoker's risk of cardiovascular calamity drops to that of a nonsmoker and the risk of dying after a heart attack drops about 50 percent.[50] ,[51]

A lot of people, especially young people, talk about quitting in the future. They say things like, "I only smoke socially. I don't really have a problem. I could quit anytime. And I will, as soon as…" Don't fall into this trap. If you smoke, stop now. A number of treatments can help. Here are some options.

- **Nicotine replacement.** While the goal is to overcome nicotine cravings, sometimes it's easier to gradually taper off. To that end, nicotine replacement can be used. That way, the person can at least eliminate exposure to harmful chemicals in tobacco. A number of nicotine products are available.

  While nicotine gums and patches may help people in research studies quit, recent surveys show they don't seem to make much difference in real-world settings.[52] Nevertheless, many experts believe that nicotine replacement products—used as recommended—help people manage their cravings.

  Electronic cigarettes (E-cigarettes) are devices resembling cigarettes or pipes that deliver nicotine but do not burn tobacco. When the user inhales through the mouthpiece, a heating element warms a cartridge containing nicotine, allowing it to be aerosolized. Concerns about these products are that manufacturers can sell products that deliver concentrations of nicotine higher than the amount contained in cigarettes (about one to two milligrams).[53] Ten milligrams is enough to kill a child. Some refills may contain enough nicotine to kill an adult.

- **Other prescription medications.** Bupropion (Wellbutrin, Zyban, and other trade names) contains no nicotine. It does, however, boost brain levels of dopamine and improves cravings and withdrawal symptoms such as anxiety and depressed mood. Because it partially blocks the effects of nicotine, it renders smoking less rewarding. Studies show that this medication can double the rate at which people quit tobacco.[54]

  Varenicline (Chantix) influences the binding of nicotine to nervous system receptors. Studies show that it reduces cravings, withdrawal symptoms, and satisfaction from smoking.[55] It can triple success rates in quitting.[56] The main side effect is nausea, which usually subsides with time.

- **Cognitive behavioral therapy.** Such treatment helps people learn to avoid triggers, diminish cravings, and manage other withdrawal symptoms.

- **Social support.** Many states have quitlines you can phone. The National Cancer Institute also maintains a smoking quitline at 1-877-44U-QUIT (1-877-448-7848), as well as a live online chat (https://livehelp.cancer.gov/app/chat/chat_launch). You can also call the national 800-QUIT-NOW. More resources are available at http://smokefree.gov. Another option is to contact your campus health center about support groups.

- **Dietary improvements.** If you feel the urge to smoke, gnaw on a carrot, celery stick, or apple. These foods are not just good for you but low in calories, which can decrease the likelihood of gaining weight as you recover from tobacco. In a recent 14-month study, people who ate four or more servings of fruits and vegetables a day were about three times more likely to stay away from tobacco.[57]

- **Breathing techniques and meditation.** In one study, yogic breathing techniques not only enhanced immune function but also helped people quit tobacco.[58] A recent study found that mindfulness meditation reduced cravings when volunteers were presented with visual triggers and also reduced brain activity in regions associated with cravings.[59]

- **Acupuncture.** A number of studies have shown that acupuncture, including ear acupuncture, improves success in quitting smoking.[60] Acupuncturists can also place tiny seeds on particular points in the outer ear that recovering smokers can press when withdrawal symptoms surface.

KEY TAKEAWAYS

- Smoking is the leading cause of preventable death.
- While the rates of cigarette smoking have declined in this country, use of loose tobacco (for pipe smoking or roll-your-own cigarettes) and cigars and other tobacco substances is on the rise.
- A number of factors increase the likelihood of tobacco use.
- Nicotine is the addicting substance in tobacco. Tobacco also contains numerous carcinogens and other poisons.
- The consequences of smoking to health are enormous.
- Benefits of quitting start immediately.
- Multiple treatment options can help people kick the habit.

3. ALCOHOL

LEARNING OBJECTIVES

1. Define blood alcohol concentration, "one drink," and binge drinking.
2. Explain how the body metabolizes alcohol.
3. Review factors that influence intoxication.
4. Discuss short- and long-term effects of alcohol.
5. Strategize ways to promote responsible drinking.
6. Review treatment options for alcohol use disorders.

Alcohol is America's number one substance of choice. Use is rampant on college campuses. Full-time college students drink more than part-time students and peers who don't go to college. Two-thirds of college students report at least some use during any given month. Most drink between one and nine days out of the month.[61] Because the legal age is 21, many college students drink illegally. According to the World Health Organization (WHO), 90 million people worldwide suffer from a disorder related to alcohol or drug use.[62]

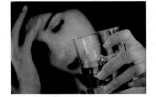

© *Thinkstock*

What exactly is alcohol? The short answer is yeast excrement. When yeast ferment sugars, they produce alcohol as a waste product. Alcohol, more correctly called ethyl alcohol or ethanol, is most commonly consumed as beer, wine, and hard liquor. It's quickly absorbed from the stomach and small intestine into the bloodstream, which delivers it to every cell in the body. **Blood alcohol content (BAC)**, the amount of alcohol in 100 milliliters of blood, rises rapidly. Within minutes, alcohol reaches your brain.

The liver does the lion's share of ridding the body of alcohol. Enzymes convert ethanol to acetaldehyde (a toxic chemical that causes many of the unpleasant side effects of alcohol consumption), which is eventually converted to acetic acid. Cells in the body either burn acetic acid for energy or store as fat. The kidneys, sweat glands, and lungs can also excrete a small amount of ethanol—hence the smell of alcohol on the breath. (A Breathalyzer estimates BAC based on the ethanol in exhaled air.)

The liver metabolizes (breaks down) alcohol at a slow, steady rate. The rate varies among individuals, with an average being about one standard drink an hour. Alcohol consumption can quickly outpace metabolism. The more you drink, the more intoxicated you feel.

blood alcohol content (BAC)

The amount of alcohol measured in grams in 100 milliliters of blood. For example, 0.08 grams (80 milligrams) in 100 milliliters is 0.08 percent, or a BAC of 0.08. Most people's function is impaired at that level, which is why 0.08 is the legal limit for drivers.

How Much Is One Drink?

Alcoholic beverages come in different sizes and vary in their ethanol concentration. One standard drink contains 14 grams, or 0.6 fluid ounces, of ethanol. Serving sizes, however, may be larger or smaller.

One drink = 1.5-ounce shot of 80-proof spirits* = 5 ounces of wine = 8 to 9 ounces of malt liquor = 12 ounces of beer

*Note: The *proof value* is two times the percentage of ethanol. In other words, 80-proof spirits contain 40 percent ethanol by volume.

Adapted from the National Institute on Alcohol Abuse and Alcoholism. Available at: http://pubs.niaaa.nih.gov/publications/Practitioner/YouthGuide/YouthGuidePocket.pdf **and** http://rethinkingdrinking.niaaa.nih.gov/WhatCountsDrink/WhatsAStandardDrink.asp.

How much alcohol is too much? For some people—children, pregnant women, nursing women, people on certain medications or who have certain diseases, and anyone who will soon operate a motor vehicle—any amount is unsafe. The limit for light to moderate drinking is up to two drinks per day for men and up to one drink per day for women. Heavy drinking is more than that.

A particularly dangerous pattern is **binge drinking**, the consumption of alcohol resulting in a blood alcohol concentration (BAC) of 0.08 percent or higher. That threshold is usually reached at four or more alcoholic drinks within two hours for women and five or more drinks within two hours for men. It's a deadly habit—one that's become more common in the United States.

Binge drinking is most prevalent among young adults. Over 80 percent of binge drinkers are men. (In general, far more men—nearly 20 percent—abuse alcohol than women—7.5 percent.) Unfortunately, over 44 percent of full-time college students binge drink—more so than part-time students and peers who don't attend college.[63] When students were asked how many drinks they had the last time they "partied," nearly 25 percent of women and nearly 40 percent of men admitted to having five or more drinks.[64] On the other hand, almost a quarter of college students say they don't drink.

The question is why do Americans—especially young Americans—drink so much? Alcohol is a pervasive part of our culture. It's readily available and, compared to most substances of abuse, inexpensive. Say the word "celebration" or "party" and what comes to mind? If we believed advertisements, we'd assume it was impossible to have fun without it. Stereotypic gender roles also factor in. Part of the myth of masculinity is that real men drink. Women are less likely to rely on alcohol and have "drinking buddies" than men.[65]

3.1 Effects of Alcohol

- Low concentrations (BAC of 0.03 to 0.059) can make people a bit stimulated, relaxed, and talkative. Concentration is slightly impaired.

- Moderate concentrations (BAC of 0.06 to 0.09) cause people to lose their normal inhibitions and act more extroverted. Reasoning, judgment, and sensory perception (especially for hearing and vision) falter.

- High concentrations (BAC 0.1 to 0.19) cause mood swings. People may cry, lash out in anger, and become aggressive. Speech slurs. Coordination and reflexes are impaired. Walking a straight line becomes impossible. Sexual desire and function drops. Men may have erectile dysfunction.

- Higher levels become even more toxic. The central nervous system is severely depressed. People have memory blackouts, loss of consciousness, and severe motor impairment. Eventually breathing and heart rate become abnormally slow. Coma occurs at a BAC of 0.35. The risk of death rises steeply.

Factors Affecting Intoxication

A number of factors affect an individual's reaction to alcohol. They include the following:

- **Age.** With advancing age, body composition typically shifts to a greater proportion of fat relative to lean tissue. Lean body mass contains water. The result is that older people have less body water for alcohol to dissolve into, which makes them more sensitive to alcohol.

- **Sex.** Women become intoxicated more easily than men and can therefore develop problems at lower drinking levels. Compared to men, they tend to be smaller and have less lean body mass, which means alcohol is distributed into a smaller volume of water. Hormonal differences between women and men may also contribute. Women are also more vulnerable to the health consequences of regular alcohol use.

- **Body size.** If you take two people of similar body composition (i.e., the same ratio of fat to lean mass), the larger person will become intoxicated less easily than the small one.

- **Speed of consumption.** Gulping an alcoholic beverage will lead to more rapid intoxication than sipping.

- **The relative emptiness of the stomach.** The presence of food in the stomach will slow the absorption of alcohol.

- **Carbonation.** It speeds alcohol absorption. That's why champagne can make you feel intoxicated faster than wine.

- **Speed of metabolism.** Enzymes in the liver break down most of the alcohol a person consumes. Some alcohol is excreted unprocessed by the kidneys, sweat glands, and lungs. (That's why you can smell alcohol on the breath.) Individuals vary in the efficiency at which they eliminate alcohol.

- **Sleep deprivation.** It amplifies the effects of alcohol.

- **Drugs.** Prescription medications (e.g., sedatives such as Valium, Ativan, and Xanax; opiate drugs such as Vicodin) and over-the-counter drugs (e.g., antihistamines) that depress the central nervous system will have an additive effect with alcohol. The same is true of illicit sedative drugs. Combining alcohol with some medications can lead to adverse effects such as nausea and vomiting.

- **Genetics.** People with family members who have alcohol problems may find they don't handle alcohol very well. Some ethnic groups, mainly those of Asian ancestry, don't tolerate alcohol. That's mainly because genetic differences affect the liver's processing of ethanol, causing acetaldehyde to rise rapidly. Acetaldehyde is toxic. Rapid rises can lead to flushing, feeling hot, faster pulse and breath rate, headache, upset stomach, and hives.

Keeping Afloat When Alcohol Abounds

Maybe you never drink. Or maybe you can't resist the ready availability on college campuses. If you're going to drink, be smart about it. Here are some tips.

- Put food into your stomach first. That will slow the absorption of alcohol.

- Pace yourself. Sip, don't gulp. Don't consume more than one drink in an hour.

- If you're at a party, hold a glass containing a nonalcoholic beverage. If your hands are empty, someone may thrust a drink into them. You can also alternate an alcoholic drink with a nonalcoholic drink. Doing so will prevent dehydration.

- Avoid punch bowls and "Jell-O shots." It's far too easy to underestimate how much alcohol you've consumed. You may not realize you've had too much until you're drunk. Also, you have no way of knowing whether someone spiked the concoction with drugs.

- Practice control. While one drink may relax you and lift your spirits, more will not make you feel (or look) better.

- Don't mix. Alcohol and sedatives create a double-whammy depressant effect. Stimulants, including caffeine, won't make you less drunk. They can make you feel more alert, which can disguise your level of intoxication. Compared to people who only drink alcohol, those who combine caffeine and alcohol are more likely to drive—a risky maneuver.

- Designate a driver who abstains from alcohol and other skill-impairing substances. Alcohol impairs your judgment about many things, including your ability to drive.

- Listen to your conscience. If a small, internal voice says, "I really shouldn't be doing X," don't do X. Wait until you're sober, then decide if you really want to become intimate with someone, climb the fence to swim in a private pool, or have your current beloved's name tattooed across your back.

- Look out for your friends. Never leave someone who passed out to "sleep it off." He or she might never wake up. If a friend loses consciousness and can't be awakened, take him or her to the emergency room.

FIGURE 11.3 How Alcohol Affects the Body

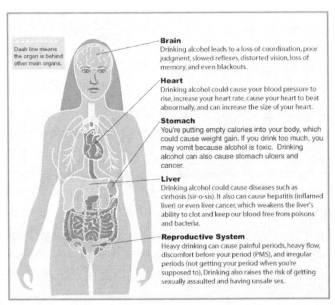

Source: Office on Women's Health in the Office of the Assistant Secretary for Health. How alcohol affects your body. Available at:

http://commons.wikimedia.org/wiki/File:Alcohol_diagram.png.

Consequences of Excessive Alcohol Consumption

In 2010, almost 18 million Americans 12 and up—7 percent of the population—abused or were dependent on alcohol.[66] Many more make the occasional mistake of drinking too much. The results are not pretty. Binge drinking can be deadly.

Problems associated with acute intoxication:

The problems listed are caused by both ethanol and the toxic metabolite acetaldehyde.

- **Depression of the central nervous system (brain and spinal cord).** Inhibition of nerve impulses results in slurred speech, delayed reflexes, incoordination, dizziness, poor judgment, and loss of normal inhibitions. People under the influence often say and do things they later regret.

- **Intensified emotions.** Some people become more jovial, some become sad and weepy, some become angry and aggressive. Often the emotions are inappropriate for the situation.

- **Unintentional injuries (e.g., falls, drowning, motor vehicle accidents).** Each month, 23 percent of college students drink and drive and a shocking 3 percent binge drink before climbing behind the wheel.

- **Intentional injuries.** Alcohol contributes to upward of 37 percent of violent crimes.[67] Alcohol increases the likelihood of being a perpetrator or a victim of physical and sexual assault and homicide. Drinking also raises the risk of suicide.

- **Nausea, vomiting, and headache.**

- **Poor sleep.** Alcohol may make it easier to fall asleep but disrupts normal sleep stages and can interrupt sleep later in the night.

- **Hangover.** Once the alcohol wears off, unpleasant symptoms such as headache, nausea, diarrhea, fatigue, mental fog, and shakiness occur.

- **Sexual dysfunction.** Drunk men may experience erectile dysfunction (impotence). Long-term alcohol abuse can eventually damage arteries to the penis, producing enduring dysfunction.

- **Sexually transmitted diseases and unintended pregnancy.** Alcohol and other central nervous system depressants release normal inhibitions and hinder judgment, leading to unsafe sex. Sexual assault is also a factor. (Having sex with a person who is drunk or unconscious, and who therefore can't consent, is considered sexual assault.)

- **Alcohol poisoning and death.** Drinking large amounts of alcohol in a short period of time swiftly raises the BAC into the toxic range. Ethanol is a central nervous system depressant. Higher doses cause loss of consciousness. People may pass out and suffocate on their own vomit and die. Very high doses can also directly cause respiratory failure.

Problems associated with chronic heavy use:

- **Poor performance at work, school, athletics, and other activities.** Alcohol abuse and dependence costs people their careers.

- **Interpersonal problems.** Alcohol-use disorders wreak havoc on social relationships. Partners and children of alcoholics often suffer enormously.

- **Weight gain due to the extra calories in alcoholic beverages.** Ethanol supplies 7 calories per gram—about 100 calories in a seven-gram serving. Because alcoholic beverages also contain carbohydrates, the actual calorie count is usually higher. For instance, a serving of beer contains about 150 calories. Sweetened cocktails contain more.

- **Immune impairment.** Chronic, excessive alcohol ingestion suppresses several aspects of immune function.

- **Fetal alcohol spectrum disorders.** Alcohol is particularly toxic to developing brains. Drinking during pregnancy causes birth defects resulting in physical, mental, and behavioral impairments. Of the collected disorders, the worst is fetal alcohol syndrome. Characteristics include low birth weight, small head circumference, facial abnormalities, and mental deficiencies that result in learning and behavioral problems. While this syndrome is more likely with higher levels of consumption, there is no safe threshold for alcohol during pregnancy. Doctors advise that women abstain from alcohol for the duration of the pregnancy.

- **Cardiovascular diseases: high blood pressure, irregular heart rhythm, damage to heart muscle (cardiomyopathy), and stroke.** While some studies have suggested that mild to moderate drinking may benefit cardiovascular health, scientists have lately questioned that belief.[68] Red wine contains flavonoids and other antioxidants that benefit the cardiovascular system. But so do red grapes and grape juice.

- **Liver diseases: alcoholic fatty liver disease, hepatitis (liver inflammation), cirrhosis (scarring and loss of function), and liver failure.**

- **Stomach inflammation (gastritis) and ulcers.**
- **Pancreatitis.** This condition involves pain and inflammation of the pancreas, the organ that makes two hormones that regulate blood sugar (insulin and glucagon) and digestive enzymes.
- **Aggravation of diabetes due to the sugars in alcoholic beverages.**
- **Neurologic damage, including nerves outside and within the central nervous system (brain and spinal cord).** Infants of mothers who drink can be born with nerve damage. Underage drinking appears to impede brain development. Teen drinkers score lower on some memory and learning tests. Alcoholics also have shrinkage of the cerebellum (the area that controls muscle coordination), limbic system (important for memory and emotions), and cerebral cortex (the outer part of the brain that controls higher functions such as thinking, planning, and civilized behavior). Certain B vitamin deficiencies common in alcoholics can lead to dementia (persistent loss of mental abilities).
- **Cancer.** Acetaldehyde, the toxic metabolic byproduct of alcohol, is a carcinogen (promotes cancer). Drinkers face an increased risk of cancer of the breast, liver, mouth, throat, colon, and rectum.[69]

FIGURE 11.4 The Face of Fetal Alcohol Syndrome

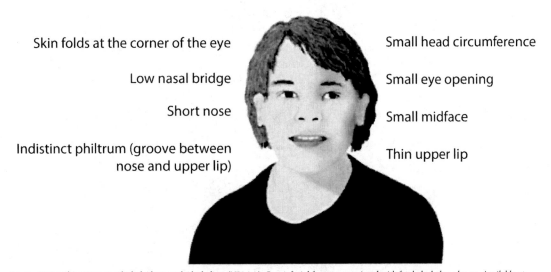

Facial Features of FAS

Skin folds at the corner of the eye

Low nasal bridge

Short nose

Indistinct philtrum (groove between nose and upper lip)

Small head circumference

Small eye opening

Small midface

Thin upper lip

Source: National Institute on Alcohol Abuse and Alcoholism (NIAAA). Craniofacial features associated with fetal alcohol syndrome. Available at: http://commons.wikimedia.org/wiki/File:FASkid.gif.

Withdrawal Symptoms

Alcoholism, the most serious alcohol use disorder, is marked by tolerance, cravings, loss of control over drinking, and physical dependence. The cardinal sign of dependence is withdrawal symptoms.

Alcohol is so socially accepted in our culture that it may surprise you that withdrawing from it can be life threatening. The severity of symptoms depends on how much and how long the person has been drinking, as well as his or her overall state of health. Symptoms and signs range from tremors ("the shakes") to a rebound hyperactivity of the central nervous system. The acute withdrawal period begins 6 to 12 hours after the last drink and continues for 5 to 7 days.[70] During that time, medical supervision is important.

The first symptoms are tremors, flushing, rapid heart rate, sweating, loss of appetite, agitation, restlessness, insomnia, brisker reflexes, increased respiratory rate, and elevated heart rate and blood pressure. A small amount of alcohol relieves the symptoms but doesn't address the underlying problem (i.e., dependence). Symptoms then progress to delirium tremens, a state that includes more exaggerated central nervous system excitation along with delirium (confusion, disorientation, and hallucinations). Seizures can ensue. Dehydration and other imbalances can lead to heart failure and death. Some alcoholics continue to experience milder withdrawal symptoms such as anxiety, depression, insomnia, and hand tremors for a year.

Assess Yourself: Do You Have a Problem with Alcohol?

The following questions can help you identify problem drinking. The more items you respond to affirmatively, the more likely it is that you have an *alcohol-use disorder*. Affirmative responses to items 11 to 16 indicate physical dependence (a condition often referred to as *alcoholism*). Contact the college health center or your family doctor if you think you have a problem with alcohol.

1. Do you ever consume more than three drinks (if you're a woman) or four drinks (if you're a man) within a few hours?
2. How often do you drink heavily? ____Once a month. ____Once a week. ____More than once a week.
3. If you're a woman, do you consume more than 7 drinks in a week? If you're a man, do you consume more than 14 drinks in a week?
4. Have you had a memory blackout while intoxicated?
5. Have you gotten into fights while intoxicated?
6. Have you lost consciousness (unintentionally passed out) while intoxicated?
7. Have you had unplanned or unprotected sexual intercourse while drinking?
8. Has drinking caused you to miss classes or fail to turn in assignments on time? Have your grades dropped since you started drinking?
9. Have you put yourself or others at risk while intoxicated? (For example, have you driven a car while intoxicated?)
10. Have you gotten into legal problems because of your drinking?
11. Have you noticed that you can drink more without feeling the effects of alcohol?
12. Have you continued to drink even though it made you feel sad, anxious, or aggressive?
13. Is it difficult to stop at one drink?
14. Have you tried more than once to cut down or quit drinking but found you couldn't?
15. If you don't drink, do you feel restless, irritable, nauseated, sweaty, or shaky? Do you have trouble sleeping? Do you feel your heart racing? Have you ever had a seizure or sensed things that weren't there?
16. Have friends or family members let you know they view your drinking as a problem?

Tools for Cutting Back

As with most substance abuse problems, you may need professional help to get alcohol out of your life. There are some steps you can work on yourself.

1. Evaluate the impact of alcohol on your life. Write down things you like in one column and things you hate in the other.
2. Identify patterns. The NIAA's Rethinking Drinking website has a drinking analyzer card that you can print and carry with you. It helps enhance your awareness of situations that make you feel like downing a drink and what happens when you do. Go to http://rethinkingdrinking.niaaa.nih.gov/ToolsResources/DrinkingTrackerCards.asp.
3. Track your alcohol intake. The same website has a card you can print and carry with you. A written record can help you cut back, stop rationalizing, and recognize progress. An inability to stick to your goals signals the need for professional help.
4. Use the other strategies laid out in "General Strategies for Breaking Addictive Behaviors."

How to Talk to a Friend about Alcohol Abuse

Confronting our friends about difficulties can be challenging. Nevertheless, your friend's behavior not only harms him or her but creates stress and anxiety for you. A few basic principles can help you navigate a conversation.

1. Express your concern in an empathetic way. "I've noticed that you seem to be drinking more."
2. Refrain from judgment.
3. Listen to your friend's response.
4. Consider offering to go with him or her to the college health center (or whatever local treatment center is available). You can also call the National Drug and Alcohol Treatment Referral Routing Service at 1-800-662-HELP.

5. Try not to take a negative response (angry denial, clamming up) personally.

6. Close by saying you believe in your friend. Point out his or her strengths. If your friend agrees to the need for treatment, support him or her in that decision.

3.2   Treatment of Alcohol Use Disorders

Some reactions associated with withdrawal from alcohol can be life-threatening. For that reason, people with severe alcoholism require professional treatment. About 90 percent of colleges provide counseling and treatment services.[71]

Disulfiram (Antabuse) inhibits the liver enzyme that changes acetaldehyde to acetic acid. Rising levels of acetaldehyde produce unpleasant symptoms such as flushing and nausea—symptoms that can discourage people from drinking. Cognitive behavioral therapy and support groups can help people learn to handle urges to drink.

Many people find organizations such as Alcoholic Anonymous (AA) invaluable for recovery. AA follows a 12-step program. Key steps include (1) acceptance of the problem ("I'm an alcoholic."); (2) belief in a higher power that can help the person overcome the substance use problem; (3) abstinence; (4) frequent meetings; and (5) assignment to a support person who can be called at any time to talk a person through cravings. Some organizations omit the religious component.

Organizations such as Al-Anon help families and friends of alcoholics. One skill is identifying ways that might have enabled substance abuse. For instance, they may make excuses for the person. "He had a rough life or a rough day at work." Or they may cover for the person. "He can't come to work because he has the flu." They may even supply the substances. Instead, friends, family, teachers, and employers need to hold the alcoholic responsible—without withdrawing compassion.

3.3   Reducing College Student Drinking

Efforts to reduce alcohol consumption on campuses can work. Some methods attempt to heighten awareness about alcohol misuse, help people examine their personal beliefs about alcohol, review drinking history, identify patterns of alcohol use, and self-monitor alcohol intake. Studies show that they reduce drinking and the negative consequences of alcohol misuse such as ill health, academic decline, fights, and property damage. Researchers note that interventions need to target at-risk groups such as Greeks (fraternities and sororities) and athletes.[72]

Peer counseling can support students who want to cut back and students who wish to abstain. Unfortunately, people who don't drink often feel like odd ducks swimming in the campus punch bowl. College administrators also can help by providing substance-free housing, which does cut down on binge drinking.[73] They can take steps to make alcohol less readily available on campus. Bars can stop the practice of making cheap alcohol available to students.

KEY TAKEAWAYS

- Alcohol is a central nervous system depressant.
- Surveys show two-thirds of college students drink. Binge drinking is a problem in teens and young adults.
- Factors such as age, sex, body size, and genetics affect an individual's reaction to alcohol.
- Negative consequences of acute intoxication include injuries, unsafe sex, nausea and vomiting, and death.
- Chronic heavy use of alcohol impairs performance at work and school, leads to interpersonal problems, and damages many organ systems.

4. OPIOIDS, DEPRESSANTS, AND STIMULANTS

LEARNING OBJECTIVES

1. Discuss the effects opioids, depressants, and stimulants have on the body.
2. Provide examples of each class of drug.
3. Discuss dangers of misuse, abuse, and dependence.

4.1 Opioids

The word *opioid* means "opium-like," referring to the fact that these substances are derived from the opium poppy. The plant's Latin name, *Papaver somniferum*, essentially means sleep-inducing poppy. In the *Wizard of Oz*, Dorothy and friends lie down in a poppy field and fall deeply asleep. In truth, the flower's scent has no psychoactive effect.

Cultivation of the opium poppy began with the Sumerians in 3400 BC.[74] Opium, which is basically sap collected from the flower's seedpods, acts as a highly effective analgesic (pain killer), cough suppressant, and antidiarrheal agent. Derivations of opium include morphine; heroin; semisynthetic drugs such as oxycodone and hydrocodone; and completely synthetic drugs fentanyl, meperidine, methadone, propoxyphene, and tramadol.

By definition, **opioids** activate the opiate receptors in the body. Most of these receptors are in the central nervous system and gastrointestinal tract. In the brain, opioids act to reduce pain and dull the senses.

You may have heard the words "opiate," "opioid," and "narcotic" used interchangeably to refer to this class of drugs. "Narcotic" is an imprecise term. For a time, scientists called naturally derived drugs like opium and morphine "opiates" and the synthetic drugs "opioids." Now doctors refer to natural, semisynthetic, and synthetic narcotics as opioids.

A bit of backstory explains all. The first thing scientists understood was the similar chemical structure of opium-derived substances, which they categorized as opiates. During the 1970s, while searching for the means by which opioids produced their effects, scientists discovered that these drugs bind to specific receptors, which they named "opiate receptors."

Why would the brain have receptors for opium-based drugs? It turns out that the body manufactures similar compounds, which they called *endogenous* (originating from within) *opioids*. Still later, scientists identified three different classes of these endogenous opioids: endorphins, enkephalins, and dynorphins. During the stress response, the body makes and releases these chemicals, which explains why you might not at first feel the pain of injuries incurred in the line of battle or on the playing field. These chemicals also contribute to the famed "runner's high."

opioids

Natural and synthetic substances that bind to the body's opiate receptors to relieve pain. Other effects include euphoria, drowsiness, and constipation. Also called narcotics.

Doctors prescribe opioid drugs to treat pain and diarrhea. Effects include euphoria, drowsiness, dizziness, sedation, decreased respiratory rate, confusion, nausea, vomiting, and constipation. Higher doses can cause unconsciousness, coma, respiratory arrest, and death. Repeated use leads to tolerance and dependence—even when used as prescribed for longer periods of time.

Opium, which is no longer used in modern medicine, can be refined to create morphine, which is still prescribed for severe pain. Heroin, which is processed from morphine, has no legitimate medical use. It's sold illegally as either a black, gummy substance or white or brownish powder. Street names include "H," "smack," and "junk." According to the 2011 National Survey on Drug Use and Health, 620,000 Americans aged 12 and older used heroin at least once in the previous year and 369,000 were dependent on the drug.[75] Heroin is usually snorted, injected, or smoked.

Of the opioids used in medicine, doctors most often prescribe semisynthetic or synthetic opioid analgesics (pain relievers). Some of the drugs are combined with acetaminophen (Tylenol), a nonsteroidal (non-narcotic) analgesic. Short-term use to manage pain is relatively benign. Long-term use to manage chronic pain results in dependence. At some point in their lives, nearly 32 million Americans take prescription opiates.

Recent years have seen an epidemic of nonmedical use and addiction for opioids such as oxycodone (OxyContin, Roxicodon), oxycodone plus acetaminophen (Percocet, Roxicet, Tylox), and hydrocodone plus acetaminophen (Vicodin, Lorcet). Opioid-use disorders jumped nearly 240 percent during the decade between 1991 and 2001.[76] In 2010, upward of 12 percent of people 18 to 25 years old (the age group most likely to abuse these drugs) took opioids for nonmedical reasons.[77] The CDC blames the upswing in misuse of prescription opioid analgesics for an increase in deaths from prescription drug overdoses. In the past decade, fatal overdoses have more than tripled and now exceed the deaths from heroin and cocaine combined.[78],[79]

Medical support is often needed to navigate withdrawal, manage cravings, and otherwise support recovery. Doctors may prescribe methadone, a synthetic opioid, to people recovering from heroin and other opioids. It reduces withdrawal symptoms without creating the high.

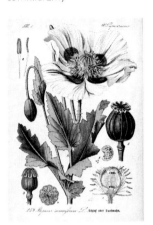

FIGURE 11.5
Opium Poppy (*Papaver somniferum*)

Source:

http://commons.wikimedia.org/wiki/ File:Illustration_Papaver_somniferum0.j

   Video Clip 11.2

Heroin Addicts Speak
This National Geographic segment portrays the daily grind of heroin addicts.

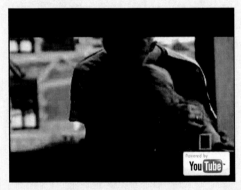

View the video online at: http://www.youtube.com/v/kOPOK24g9Cc

4.2   Central Nervous System Depressants

The central nervous system (CNS) includes the brain and spinal cord. The brain controls the state of alertness; creates thoughts and emotions; and governs heart rate, respiratory rate, and most other bodily functions. **Central nervous system (CNS) depressants** slow nervous system activity by increasing the activity of an inhibitory neurotransmitter called gamma-aminobutyric acid (GABA).

Thoughts dull, alertness wanes, anxiety diminishes, inhibitions fade, reflexes slow, coordination falters, and respiratory rate slows. Because these drugs induce *sedation* (a calm, relaxed, drowsy state), they're often referred to as *sedatives*. At high doses, CNS depressants induce coma, respiratory arrest, and death.

Alcohol is the most commonly used CNS depressant. Doctors prescribe sedative drugs to people with insomnia, sleep disorders such as sleepwalking, anxiety disorders (particularly acute stress reactions), and seizure disorders. They're also used to relax people before surgical procedures. Combining alcohol with sedating drugs creates a dangerous double whammy.

central nervous system (CNS) depressants

Substances that depress (slow) central nervous system activity, resulting in decreased anxiety, drowsiness, decreased coordination, and slowed breathing; also called sedatives, tranquilizers, and "downers."

These substances should not be taken before doing any activity that requires mental focus and physical coordination. Examples include swimming, riding a bike or motorcycle, driving a car or boat, or piloting a plane.

Once people become dependent upon CNS depressants, withdrawal symptoms can range from insomnia and anxiety to seizures and delirium. Medical supervision is important for safe, successful withdrawal. Cognitive behavioral therapy also helps.

There are three main classes of sedative drugs:

1. **Barbiturates** were once used to relieve anxiety, induce sleep, and control seizures (convulsions). Examples include phenobarbital and seconal. Street names include "barbs," "yellow jackets," "red birds," and "reds." They're addictive and carry a significant risk of overdose, particularly when combined with other central nervous system depressants such as alcohol. Actress Marilyn Monroe is said to have died of an overdose of barbiturates. Withdrawal signs and symptoms are similar to those with chronic, heavy alcohol use. Because these drugs can be life threatening, doctors rarely prescribe them and, when they do, recommend close medical supervision.

2. **Benzodiazepines** are a newer, relatively safer category of depressant. Examples include diazepam (Valium), alprazolam (Xanax), and lorazepam (Ativan). Doctors may prescribe them to treat insomnia, anxiety, stress reactions, panic attacks, and seizures. People can become dependent upon them. Cessation of the drug can cause the original symptoms (insomnia, anxiety) to rebound.

3. **Hypnotics** are sleep-inducing medicines. In the past, doctors prescribed barbiturates and, later, benzodiazepines for insomnia and other sleep problems. Imidazopyridine medications are a newer, safer class of hypnotics. Examples include zolpidem (Ambien), zaleplon (Sonata), and eszopiclone (Lunesta). Though they have less potential for abuse and addiction, people can become dependent upon them to sleep. Discontinuation may lead to a rebound in insomnia, as well as fatigue, irritability, anxiety, and other symptoms.

4.3 Central Nervous System Stimulants

central nervous system (CNS) stimulants

Substances that stimulate central nervous system activity; effects include enhanced alertness, nervousness, insomnia, increased motor activity (movement), and elevated heart rate and respiratory rate.

Central nervous system (CNS) stimulants increase activity in the brain. They directly increase neurotransmitters such as norepinephrine (which is similar in structure to epinephrine, also called adrenaline). Stimulants all enhance the sympathetic ("fight or flight") nervous system, the same system activated during stress. As such, they all elevate heart rate, blood pressure, and respiratory rate. CNS effects include enhanced alertness, decreased appetite, and interference with sleep. Higher doses cause nervousness, insomnia, and headache. Stronger drugs dilate the pupils of the eyes and cause muscle twitches and tremors. The intensity of the effects depends on the drug taken and the dose. Of the drugs listed next, caffeine is the most benign.

Caffeine

Caffeine is the most widely used psychoactive substance. Many Americans are dependent on it. The effects of mild to moderate doses are enhanced mood, alertness, wakefulness, and attention. Reaction times are swifter. Athletic performance may improve. People who don't usually consume caffeine may get relief of migraine headaches.

Caffeine interacts with the sympathetic nervous system. High doses produce restlessness, nervousness, anxiety, rapid heart rate, increased blood pressure, muscle twitches, hand tremors, upset stomach, and frequent urination. Insomnia may occur when consuming even low doses later in the day.

Caffeine blocks the binding of adenosine to brain receptors. (Adenosine levels rise during the course of cellular activity and makes us sleepy.) As with most substances, tolerance develops with caffeine. However, most people are fairly steady and consistent in their consumption of caffeinated beverages.

Withdrawal symptoms do, however, occur soon after cessation of caffeine. In fact, the morning mental fog is a withdrawal symptom—one quickly remedied by a cup of coffee or tea. (People who don't use caffeine and who get enough sleep awaken clear-headed.) Other withdrawal symptoms include impaired concentration, fatigue, muscle tension, headache, and, less often, nausea and vomiting.

The good news is that caffeine doesn't influence dopamine levels in brain areas that govern addiction and abuse. As a result, caffeine doesn't cause the serious behavioral problems associated with other substances. In fact, beverages made from caffeine-containing plants (coffee, green and black tea, guarana, and yerba mate) have health benefits. The same goes for cocoa and chocolate, which are made from cacao. In addition to caffeine, these plants contain antioxidants and other beneficial chemicals.

For instance, coffee and tea drinkers enjoy a reduced risk of type 2 diabetes[80] and some cancers and protection against some brain disorders.[81],[82] The same benefits apply to tea, especially green tea.[83] So if you're going to consume caffeine, get it from tea and coffee. Skip the sugar. If you like to add dairy, go with lower-fat options.

Steer clear of sugary cola-based sodas (Coke, Pepsi) and "energy" drinks to which synthetic caffeine has been added (Monster, Red Bull, Rockstar). Sodas contribute mightily to unhealthy weight gain, diabetes, and cardiovascular disease. In addition, the so-called energy drinks (which only provide energy in the form of sugar) can cause serious health risks. The Substance Abuse and Mental Health Services Administration recently reported a surge in emergency room (ER) visits by people who had consumed too much of these drinks or had combined them with alcohol or drugs.[84]

Unfortunately, 50 percent of children, teens, and young adults consume energy drinks. Of the 13,114 ER visits in 2009, the vast majority were young men, ages 8 to 34.

Keep in mind that caffeine lingers in the body. It takes three to seven hours to eliminate half of the caffeine circulating in your blood—double that time in women who are pregnant or on oral hormonal contraceptives. If you want to sleep, avoid late afternoon and evening consumption. Because caffeine affects the developing fetus, pregnant women should avoid it altogether.

Cocaine

Cocaine is derived from the leaves of the coca plant, which grow in the Andes in South America. Native people chew the leaves to provide physical stamina, increase alertness, and relieve hunger. The leaves also have ceremonial reasons. The stimulating effects are subtle. (Note that chocolate and cocoa come from a different plant with a somewhat similar name: cacao. While pleasurable and possibly habit-forming, these foods are not addictive substances.)

Pure cocaine, on the other hand, is far from subtle. The powdered hydrochloride salt ("coke") is snorted (taken intranasally) or dissolved in water for intravenous injection. Doctors once used it to as a local anesthetic (numbing medicine) and to stop bleeding (as in severe nose bleed). Before cocaine use became prohibited, Coca-Cola contained some cocaine. Dr. Sigmund Freud, the founder of psychoanalysis, thought that cocaine's ability to induce euphoria made it a good treatment for depression. In fact, he used it himself. However, cocaine's addictive nature and the fact that a common withdrawal symptom is low mood rendered it inappropriate as a psychiatric drug.

Effects of cocaine include euphoria, increased energy and alertness, and numbness. As mentioned earlier, cocaine directly raises dopamine in the reward pathway by interfering with its reuptake (a process that clears the neurotransmitter from the synapse).

Historically, the powdered form of cocaine was snorted (inhaled into the nose). Not all users become addicted. Repeated use does, however, lead to tolerance and physical dependence. In the 1970s, crack, the freebase form of cocaine, was developed. The rocklike pieces can be smoked, leading to rapid brain delivery and a short, intense high. Cheaper than the powder form, crack ravaged impoverished inner-city neighborhoods during the mid-1980s. Like crack, intravenous cocaine reaches the brain quickly and is more addicting and dangerous than intranasal use.

A hazardous but common habit is combining alcohol and cocaine, which raises toxicity due to the creation of a substance called cocaethylene, which is more toxic than cocaine. Furthermore, the stimulating effect of cocaine allows people to continue drinking longer, thus allowing for greater damage. ER reports confirm that alcohol and cocaine vastly increase problems such as stroke, heart damage, heart arrhythmias, heat attack, and sudden death.[85] Stroke and heart attack can occur with the first use of cocaine (plus or minus alcohol).

FIGURE 11.6 Coca Leaf

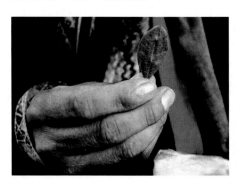

Source: Marcello Casal Jr./ABr, Agência Brasil. Available at: http://commons.wikimedia.org/wiki/File:Folha_de_coca.jpg.

FIGURE 11.7 III Effects of Crack Cocaine

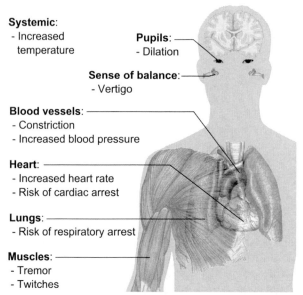

Systemic:
- Increased temperature

Pupils:
- Dilation

Sense of balance:
- Vertigo

Blood vessels:
- Constriction
- Increased blood pressure

Heart:
- Increased heart rate
- Risk of cardiac arrest

Lungs:
- Risk of respiratory arrest

Muscles:
- Tremor
- Twitches

Source: Häggström M. Available at: http://commons.wikimedia.org/wiki/File:Physiological_effects_of_Crack_cocaine.png.

Because of appetite suppression, chronic use can lead to malnutrition. Snorting cocaine repeatedly can lead to loss of a sense of smell, hoarseness, persistent runny nose, nosebleeds, and ulceration (destruction) of tissue in the nose. Ingested cocaine can reduce blood flow in the intestinal tract to such an extent that gangrene develops. Intravenous use raises the risk of serious infection diseases such as HIV and hepatitis.

Crack cocaine damages the lungs. Intravenous cocaine and crack can lead to paranoia and aggression. Use during pregnancy causes serious problems, including premature labor, low birth weights, and smaller heads in infants. The 1980s saw a rash of "crack babies," who started out life going through drug withdrawal.

Another problem is that cocaine (as well as many other drugs) may be adulterated ("cut" or "laced") to enhance profits. Adulterants include methamphetamine, caffeine, lidocaine (an anesthetic), and various sugars.

Withdrawal symptoms occur soon after a cocaine binge ends. They include sleepiness, irritability, difficulty feeling pleasure, and anxiety. Heavy users may become severely agitated and paranoid.

Methamphetamine

Methamphetamine ("meth") has a similar chemical structure as amphetamine. Doctors can prescribe both, though amphetamine is much more common, for instance in attention deficit hyperactivity disorder and narcolepsy (a disorder in which people have sleep attacks). Both drugs increase the neurotransmitters dopamine and norepinephrine.

Compared to amphetamine, meth has much greater abuse and dependence potential. It's the most powerful and toxic stimulant. Addiction occurs quickly.

Most of this drug is illegally imported or made in domestic labs. Street names are speed, crank, crystal, glass, and ice. The ability to make the meth in home-based laboratories, cheaply and from readily available chemicals, has led to rampant addictions and related violence. In the mid-1990s, many crack smokers switched to crystalline methamphetamine ("crystal meth"), which is cheaper, more potent, and creates a much longer high. While crack was an inner-city scourge, the advent of do-it-yourself meth labs blighted whole regions of rural America.[86]

Meth is a white powder that dissolves readily into water. It can be swallowed, snorted, injected, and smoked. Solutions can be swallowed or injected into the vein. The powder can be snorted. Dealers often cut it with other substances to increase profits.

Like cocaine, the effect is euphoria and stimulation of the cardiovascular, respiratory, and central nervous systems. At low doses, users feel alert, energetic, and confident. At higher doses, toxic effects set in.

Meth is particularly toxic to the brain. Scans of users' brains show damage to areas related to memory and emotion. People can become paranoid, aggressive, and violent. Mood disturbance, anxiety, and confusion occur. Cardiovascular consequences include elevated blood pressure, arrhythmias, heart attack, and stroke. Use during pregnancy can lead to premature labor and babies born small for their age and with neurologic damage.

Heavy meth users go days without sleep. Malnutrition, severe weight loss, and tooth damage ("meth mouth") are common. A sensation of insects crawling on or under the skin can cause meth users to pick or scratch. The resultant sores can become infected. Prolonged, heavy use can also lead to psychosis—intense paranoia, hallucinations (hearing, seeing, and feeling things that aren't there), and delusions (false beliefs).

When heavy meth use is stopped, the user "crashes." Symptoms include agitation, depression, lethargy, and catch-up sleep. Because depression can continue for days, the risk of suicide is high.

On a brighter note, surveys show that methamphetamine use among high-school seniors has dropped from 4.7 percent in 1999 to 1.2 percent in 2009. Use among Americans over age 12 has also declined to 314,000 users in 2008.[87]

 Video Clip 11.3

Faces of Meth
This series of before-and-after mug shots of methamphetamine users speaks volumes about the toll the drug takes.

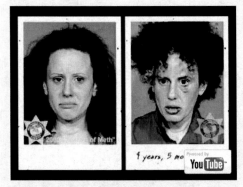

View the video online at: http://www.youtube.com/v/bVEulrvBwsA

Video Clip 11.4

World's Most Dangerous Drug
This National Geographic segment discusses the dangers of methamphetamine.

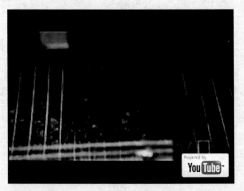

View the video online at: http://www.youtube.com/v/at3Sg6qvgTE

Nonmedical Use of Prescription Stimulants

An increasingly common practice is the illicit use of stimulant medications such as Ritalin, Dexedrine, and Adderall intended to treat attention deficit hyperactivity disorder (ADHD). To a lesser extent, prescription diet pills are also taken, as well as nonstimulant drugs used to treat ADHD.

A large survey published in 2007 found that 2 percent of adults 18 to 49 engaged in nonmedical use of stimulant ADHD medications within a year.[88] The prevalence was highest—4.3 percent—among those 18 to 25. While about a quarter of nonmedical users did so for recreational reasons, the main motivation was for performance enhancement. Some people aren't simply swallowing the pills but instead snorting crushed pills or dissolving them into water for injection. Such methods produce an intense, quick rise in dopamine that heightens the risk of dependence.

Regardless of whether or not you have ADHD, stimulants increase attention and focus—as long as they're taken within a normal dosage range. These so-called study drugs do not make you smarter. The question is, if a student is desperate for an academic edge or needs to stay awake to finish writing a paper, why not pop someone else's pills? Here are five reasons not to take the risk.

1. Doing so is illegal. Selling or sharing prescription drugs is a criminal offense. Legal consequences vary from state to state and can include fines and imprisonment.

2. Taking drugs to gain an advantage is unethical. For the person who actually has ADHD, these medications level the playing field.

3. The person who actually has ADHD should be taking the medication rather than diverting them to illicit use.

4. It's not safe. Even taken as prescribed, the medications have side effects. Long-term use poses a particular risk to people vulnerable to cardiovascular disease (many of whom are unaware of that vulnerability). Ramping up the dosage or opening the capsule and snorting the medication escalates the risk of toxicity and dependence. Combining stimulants with other drugs and alcohol further ratchets up the risks.

5. People can become psychologically dependent in the absence of physical dependence. More specifically, students without ADHD may start to believe that they can't perform well academically unless they take the medications.

 Video Clip 11.5

Addiction to Prescription Stimulants
The news segment portrays young people addiction to ADHD medication.

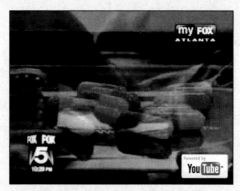

View the video online at: http://www.youtube.com/v/E0ihO1KFxkQ

KEY TAKEAWAYS

- Opioids bind to opiate receptors in the nervous system and other tissues. Endogenous opioids such as endorphins rise during strenuous exercise, stress, and pain to decrease pain and create a sense of well-being. Drugs derived from the opium poppy create more powerful effects. The most dangerous opioid drug is heroin. However, an epidemic misuse and abuse of prescription opioids has had serious adverse consequences.

- CNS depressants include alcohol and drugs such as barbiturates, benzodiazepines, and imidazopyridines (Ambien and others). They slow activity in the brain. Depending on the dose, effects range from relaxation to coma and death.

- CNS stimulants span the spectrum from relatively benign (caffeine) to perilous (crack cocaine and methamphetamine). Misuse of prescription stimulants has become common in teens and young adults.

5. MARIJUANA, HALLUCINOGENS, CLUB DRUGS, AND INHALANTS

LEARNING OBJECTIVES

1. Discuss the effects, potential adverse consequences, and potential medical uses of substances derived from cannabis.
2. Review the main effects of hallucinogens and provide examples of hallucinogenic substances.
3. Discuss the risks of "club drugs" and inhalants.

5.1 Marijuana (Cannabis)

FIGURE 11.8 Marijuana (Cannabis)

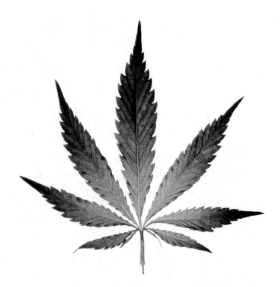

© *Thinkstock*

Marijuana is the most commonly used illicit drug in the world. Of the three million Americans who begin using illicit drugs each year, the majority (almost 62 percent) start with marijuana.[89] Nearly 41 percent of Americans 12 and up try it at least once.[90] In any given month, about 19 percent of college students use marijuana.[91] In 2010, nearly 16 percent of marijuana users—about 4.6 million people—used it almost every day. About the same number had abuse or dependence problems.[92]

Two main plant species are used: *Cannabis sativa* and *Cannabis indica*. They differ in appearance and in their chemical composition. Subspecies are cultivated to manipulate the chemical profile. "Cannabis," the plant's genus name, refers broadly to the plant and substances derived from it. The word "marijuana," a Spanish derivation, describes varieties bred for recreational and medicinal uses. The word can also more narrowly refer to the dried flowers and leaves.

Cannabis is chemically complex, including more than 100 cannabinoids. **Cannabinoids** bind to cannabinoid receptors in the *endocannabinoid system*. Endocannabinoids (cannabinoids our bodies make) also bind to these receptors.[93] There are at least two types of receptors—one that exists mainly on nervous system cells, including the brain, and another found on immune system cells. Depending on the amount and kind of receptor activation, effects can include euphoria, muscle relaxation, anxiety, dry mouth, hunger, and a decrease in pain and inflammation.

Two main cannabinoids in marijuana have been the subject of much research: tetrahydrocannabinol (THC) and cannabidiol (CBD). THC is responsible for the plant's psychoactive effects. CBD is not intoxicating and has been linked with a host of beneficial actions.

The flowers and leaves of cannabis plants yield resinous products. The term "marijuana" often refers to dried flowers ("buds"), which are usually smoked or consumed in cooked foods. The leaves, though less potent, are also used. *Kief* is a more potent product containing only the resinous trichomes (hairs on the flowers). To make *hashish*, the trichomes are pressed into a paste or more solid block. "Hash oil" refers to extractions of THC into oil.

Acute effects of recreational use of marijuana can include an enhanced sense of well-being, relaxation, sedation, poor concentration, impaired learning and memory, reddened eyes, dry mouth, and increased appetite. Instead of relaxation, some people experience anxiety and paranoia. These symptoms dissipate, although cognitive (thinking) impairments may persist a full day later.[94] Because reaction times may also be diminished, people should not drive while under the influence of cannabis products.

As with other substances, the initiation of marijuana at a younger age (which has become quite common) is associated with more health problems. Chief among them is **dependence**, which occurs in about 10 percent of regular users, more with early initiation.[95] Withdrawal symptoms include cravings, headaches, mood changes, and sleep disturbances. Other adverse effects also become more likely when regular use starts early.

Chronic use has been linked to **cognitive (mental) impairments**. One large study examined the effect of regular use of cannabis before age 18 on IQ (intelligence quotient).[96] The researchers tested the volunteers' IQs between ages 7 and 13 and then again at age 38. Nonusers exhibited a slight rise in IQ. Heavy users during adolescence exhibited a significant dip in IQ by age 38, as well as poorer scores on other tests of mental function such as memory, attention, and processing speed. Alarmingly, mental impairment persisted after abstinence. Another study showed memory impairment—even after 28 days of abstinence.[97] Adult-onset use, however, doesn't appear to reduce IQ. Bottom line: early marijuana use may be toxic for the developing brain.

Given these findings, perhaps it's not surprising that teens and college-aged young adults who regularly use marijuana are at risk for **reduced educational attainment**.[98] In addition to direct brain toxicity, marijuana reduces motivation.

Like tobacco smoke, marijuana smoke contains a range of harmful chemicals. However, the inhalation pattern (deep inhalation and breath holding) from marijuana smoking results in comparatively greater exposure to these chemicals.[99] Habitual pot smokers are at risk for acute and chronic **bronchitis** (airway inflammation). Morning cough to clear excess respiratory mucus is common. Lung **cancer** may also be a risk. A recent study associated marijuana use with a doubling in the risk of testicular cancer, the most common cancer in young men 15 to 45.[100]

Frequent marijuana use during adolescence correlates with an increase in **anxiety** later in life.[101] However, it's possible that some people began using marijuana in an attempt to remedy preexisting anxiety.

Regular use of marijuana during adolescence and young adulthood seems to elevate the risk for using other illicit and licit (e.g., tobacco and alcohol) substances.[102] However, many marijuana users do not progress to "harder" drugs.

The Medical Marijuana Debate

For thousands of years, marijuana has been used for medicinal purposes. Records indicate use of the plant in ancient China, Egypt, India, Persia, Rome, and Greece. European physicians once prescribed it. From 1850 to 1942, marijuana was listed in the United States Pharmacopoeia, the official listing of medicines.[103] Starting in the 1970s, research indicated that marijuana could be used to manage glaucoma, a condition in which elevated pressure within the eye leads to vision loss. Since then, it's been

cannabinoids

Compounds present in cannabis that bind to receptors (cannabinoid receptors) to provide a variety of effects; endocannabinoids refer to similar compounds made by the body.

used to increase appetite and curb weight loss associated with conditions such as AIDS and cancer and to help manage muscle spasms in conditions such as multiple sclerosis.

As mentioned earlier, cannabidiol (CBD) produces a number of benefits without intoxication or other serious side effects. Effects include anti-inflammatory, antioxidant, antinausea, antianxiety, and nerve protection. It also appears to have anticancer effects.[104] Exploratory research suggests CBD may have applications in managing schizophrenia,[105] anxiety, nausea and vomiting,[106] multiple sclerosis,[107] inflammatory bowel disease,[108] insomnia, arthritis, and some types of dementia.[109],[110] Scientists have recently bred strains of cannabis plants that are low in THC but higher in CBD, thereby creating a nonpsychoactive product.[111] THC does, however, hold therapeutic benefits for some conditions.

In fact, in 1985, the Food and Drug Administration (FDA) approved dronabinol (another name for THC, which is sold under the trade name Marinol).[112] It was first used to treat nausea and vomiting resulting from cancer treatment and, later, to increase appetite and counter weight loss. In the mid-1980s, the FDA also approved a synthetic derivative of dronabinol called Cesamet. The drug disappeared from the American market but continues to be used in Canada and some European countries. Sativex, an extract containing both THC and CBD, is also available in Canada and some European countries.

In 1998, states began to legalize crude forms of marijuana (rather than purified chemicals or synthetic drugs) for medical use. Marijuana leaves and flowers are smoked (the traditional method); vaporized (a method that heats the plant at a lower temperature than the burning point so that smoke is not inhaled); or extracted into cooked food ("edibles"), honey or oil, or alcohol (a tincture).

To date, 16 states—Alaska, Arizona, California, Colorado, Connecticut, Delaware, Hawaii, Maine, Michigan, Montana, Nevada, New Jersey, New Mexico, Oregon, Rhode Island, Vermont—plus the District of Columbia have legalized medical use of marijuana. Some states require patients to carry special ID cards; some allow patients to cultivate their own plants. All states limit the amount of plant a patient can possess. However, medical marijuana possession remains illegal under federal law—a paradox that has created a legal quagmire.

What Is Hemp?

The word *hemp* refers to cannabis plants that are cultivated for nondrug purposes. Hemp products are not psychoactive. Fiber from cannabis stalks is used to make clothes, rope, and paper. Seeds are used as food and to generate hemp seed oil. The seeds and oil contain both omega-3 and omega-6 fatty acids, which have health benefits. The seeds are rich in protein and fiber and also contain vitamins A, C, D, E, and some B vitamins.[113]

Video Link 11.3

Medical Marijuana: Benefits and Limitations

This PBS report interviews patients and doctors about the potential benefits, controversies, and legal complications associated with medical marijuana.

http://video.pbs.org/video/2103797319

5.2 Hallucinogens

Hallucinogens alter sensory perceptions and consciousness. The effects range from mild sensory distortions to outright hallucinations. Paranoia and delusions can also occur. Some plants are naturally hallucinogenic. Examples include **psilocybin** mushrooms ("magic mushrooms") and **peyote** (a kind of cactus that contains the chemical *mescaline*). Native peoples used such plants for medicine and rituals. Synthetic hallucinogens include **LSD** (lysergic acid) and **PCP** (phencyclidine).

LSD ("acid," "yellow sunshine," and others) is extremely potent. In addition to visual hallucinations and delusions, effects include pupil dilation, increased heart rate and blood pressure, elevated temperature, insomnia, mood changes, and appetite lost. The changes can induce fear and panic. Effects (the "trip") can last 12 hours.[114] LSD is sold as a liquid, tablet, and "blotter" (absorbed onto paper).

PCP (angel dust) was developed for use as an intravenous anesthetic in the 1950s but never approved for humans due to adverse effects.[115] It's sold in powder, tablet, and capsule form. It distorts visual and auditory perceptions and causes *dissociation* (a feeling of detachment from self and

hallucinogens

Substances that alter sensory perception and consciousness.

surrounding environment). Some of the effects mimic schizophrenia, with hallucinations, delusions, paranoia, and disorganized thinking. High doses can cause seizures. Response to the drug can be unpredictable. People suffering from schizophrenia-like symptoms have committed suicide, destroyed property, and harmed others.

5.3 Club Drugs

"Club drugs" refer to drugs taken by young adults at parties, clubs, and concerts. In addition to LSD, the NIDA includes GHB (gamma-hydroxybutyrate), flunitrazepam (Rohypnol), ketamine, and MDMA (methylenedioxymethamphetamine, Ecstasy). Effects vary.

Ketamine, a drug once used to induce general anesthesia, causes hallucinations, amnesia, and dissociation. **GHB** is now rarely used in medicine. Overdose of this central nervous system depressant leads to death and unconsciousness. **Rohypnol** is an extremely potent benozdiazepine (a type of sedative) capable of producing amnesia for events while under the influence. Street names include "roofies," "forget-me pill," and "roche." Because of Rohypnol's ability to "knock people out," the drug has earned the name "date rape drug." GHB and ketamine can also be slipped into drinks to facilitate sexual assault, physical assault, robbery, and other crimes.[116] The addition of alcohol augments the sedating effects and toxicity.

MDMA is a synthetic drug taken as a pill. Note that the long name—methylenedioxymethamphetamine—contains "methamphetamine." Not surprisingly, MDMA acts as a stimulant. It also increases emotional warmth and empathy (earning names like "hug drug" and "lover's speed"), boosts self-confidence, and enhances sensory perception. Adverse effects include elevated heart rate and blood pressure, nausea, vomiting, chills, sweating, dehydration (and disturbances in blood electrolytes, or salts, if users overcompensate by drinking a lot of water), rapid eye movement, and teeth clenching. It can also produce hyperthermia (abnormally high body temperature). Deaths have occurred.

While toxicity is significant, the general public hasn't yet appreciated how damaging this drug can be. Within the body, MDMA causes oxidative stress, which generates free radicals.[117] DNA and cellular structures called mitochondria, which generate energy for cells, can be damaged. The brain, heart, liver, kidneys, and other organs can be injured. Production of reproductive and other hormones is impaired. Combining MDMA with alcohol or caffeine escalates toxicity.

Regular users have abnormalities on brain scans (including loss of gray matter), depletion of the neurotransmitter serotonin (which, along with other functions, regulates mood), depression, and impairments of memory and thinking.[118] ,[119] ,[120] Prolonged abstinence may restore serotonin levels.

5.4 Inhalants

Chemicals that readily move into a gaseous state can be inhaled through the nose ("sniffing") or mouth ("huffing"). Those that have mind-altering effects include gasoline, paint thinner, cigarette lighter fluid, nail polish remover, spray paints, nitrous oxide, amyl nitrate, and the fluorinated hydrocarbons in aerosolized products such as hairspray and whipped cream.

Most of the chemicals inhaled depress the CNS to cause sedation, euphoria, lack of coordination, and incoherent speech. Some inhaled chemicals trigger hallucinations and delusions. Other potential adverse effects include damage to the nervous systems, kidneys, liver, and bone marrow. Blood cells can also be unfavorably altered or destroyed. Sudden death is the worse consequence. Use is most common in teenagers.

KEY TAKEAWAYS

- Marijuana, hashish, and kief all come from the cannabis plant. Cannabis contains compounds called cannabinoids, which bind to special receptors—receptors originally designed to receive the body's own endocannabinoids. THC is the cannabinoid responsible for the plant's "high." Regular, heavy marijuana users can develop dependence, as well as lung damage, memory impairment, and mood disturbances. The cannabis plant and medications derived from it have applications in managing certain disease conditions.

- Hallucinogenic substances include LSD, peyote, psilocybin, and PCP. They alter sensory perceptions, thinking, and mood. MDMA (Ecstasy) also has both hallucinogenic and stimulant effects.

- Club drugs (MDMA, Rohypnol, BHB, ketamine, PCP) and inhalants can have dangerous side effects.

DISCUSSION QUESTIONS

1. What is your opinion about medical marijuana? Should people with legitimate complaints be able to grow, possess, and use limited amounts? Where do you stand on the legalization of marijuana for recreational use? Should government regulate it in the same way it does tobacco and alcohol? Do you think that marijuana is more or less harmful than alcohol and tobacco?

2. Which of the hallucinogenic substances can trigger extreme agitation and violent behavior?

3. In your experience, how common is "club drug" use at your college? Do you know anyone who has had a bad experience? What happened?

---

6. BEHAVIORAL ADDICTIONS

LEARNING OBJECTIVES

1. Differentiate between habit and addiction.
2. Identify characteristics of addictive behaviors.
3. Provide examples of common behavioral addictions.

All of us have habits. Many of them keep us happy, healthy, and successful. Going to bed and rising at more or less the same time helps us feel rested. Regular meals give us the energy to work and play. Daily physical activity and getting together with friends promote health and longevity. We have study habits and work habits.

But some of those very same activities required for well-being and survival can get out of control. People can compulsively and excessively eat, exercise, and work. What's the line between normal habits and addictions?

As with drug and alcohol abuse and dependence, similar red flags show the behavior has become pathologic.

1. The person becomes preoccupied with the activity, spending much of his or her waking hours thinking about it.

2. The person engages compulsively in the activity—to the exclusion of other previously pleasurable or important pursuits.

3. Time spent doing the activity escalates to the point the person loses control and can no longer quit.

4. An inability to do the activity generates distress.

5. Harmful consequences surface. Other responsibilities and interests suffer. Mental preoccupation and compulsive engagement of the activity interfere with social relationships, school, work, hobbies, sleep, and eating. Some activities can lead to financial ruin.

Brain regions affected on scans overlap those associated with drug addictions (dopamine availability in the reward pathway) and poor impulse control. As with drug addiction, people with behavioral addictions may have a genetic predisposition. Early childhood factors may play a role. Failure to learn how to regulate emotions, delay gratification, and effectively manage stress can all factor in. The behavior begins as a way to relieve stress and generally feel better.

Behavioral addictions can involve gambling, shopping, playing video games, watching television, cleaning, working, exercising, having sex, and eating. Compulsive gambling has moved beyond the horse ring and casino. You can now easily burn time and money gambling on your computer. Shopaholics buy things they don't even need and bury themselves in debt. Compulsive exercisers often also have body image disturbances such as muscle dysmorphia (bigorexia) or anorexia nervosa. Compulsive eaters can develop obesity. Workaholics become nearly unable to relax and do things unrelated to work. Some people become preoccupied with sex, spending much of their time trying to find a partner. Others become adrenaline junkies and can't seem to feel good unless they're parachuting, bungee jumping, white-water kayaking, or rappelling down a cliff.

A relative newcomer is techno addiction, which includes compulsive use of the Internet and smartphones. People with this problem compulsively text, e-mail, Google, Tweet, and access social media sites and/or sexual websites. In addition to the classic signs of addiction, particular problems can occur. Repetitive use injuries can affect the hands, wrists, and spine. Several people have died in China and Korea after days of nonstop online video playing.[121] If you suspect you might be such a person, give yourself breaks. Tell yourself those things can wait. Go out with friends or go outside—without your phone. You might check out a new book called *iDisorder* by California psychologist Larry Rosen, PhD.

Treatment of behavioral addictions is similar to that for drug and alcohol addiction: 12-step programs, cognitive behavioral therapy, and other types of individual and group therapy. The goal is to restrict time spent doing the activity, manage the cravings and moodiness associated with discontinuing the activity, and increase time doing other, healthier activities. If you think you have a problem, contact your college health center or family doctor for a referral.

6.1   Conclusion: Promoting a Healthy Campus Environment

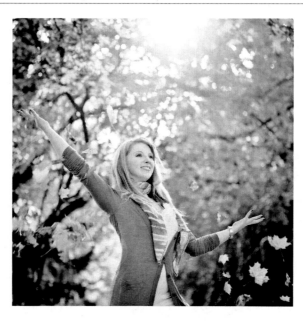

© Thinkstock

Abuse and addiction of substances degrades communities, including college campuses. Perhaps you're weary of sidestepping puddles of puke on your way to the shower. Maybe you've seen substance use hurt you or your friends.

Know that you have the power to effect change. You may find peers and college administrators happy to support your goals. Here are some tips to help you:

- Remember that moderation and abstention are normal. Don't be shy about politely saying, "No, thanks."
- Support friends who don't drink or want to cut back or quit.
- Find a peer group that shares your values.
- Find a living situation where you feel safe. If you're uncomfortable with the substance use patterns in your dorm, contact the housing office. Many colleges have the option of substance-free living quarters. While, in reality, they aren't completely substance-free, far fewer students binge drink and take drugs than in traditional dorms.[122]
- Keep in mind that, from a legal standpoint, all dormitories should be substance free. Public indoor spaces should be smoke-free. Students under age 21 aren't supposed to drink. And illicit drugs are, by definition, illegal. Colleges could enforce those rules. But often they don't.
- Decline to support the multibillion-dollar tobacco industry, an industry that markets to children, teens, and people in the developing world who can ill afford the health consequences.
- Lobby against alcohol-related sponsorship of events.
- Advocate for activities that don't involve substance use. Invite people to your living space to play charades or board games. Take a dance class in a drug- and alcohol-free zone.

This table summarizes the addictive substances discussed in this chapter. Toxic effects refer to adverse events occurring at higher doses.

Table 11.1 summarizes the addictive substances discussed in this chapter. Toxic effects refer to adverse events occurring at higher doses.

TABLE 11.1 Summary of Addictive Substances

Substance	Examples	Acute effects	Potential adverse effects with abuse and dependence
Alcohol		Sedation, poor coordination, longer reaction times, impaired judgment, mood changes (reduced anxiety, anger, and aggression), sleepiness. Toxic effects: nausea, vomiting, blackouts, respiratory depression, death.	Accidents (including car crashes), social and academic problems, liver damage, brain damage, nerve damage, high blood pressure, stomach ulcers, malnutrition, bone loss, fetal alcohol syndrome.
Tobacco		First-time use: coughing, dizziness, nausea. With habitual use: subtle relaxation and reduction in anxiety, anger, and stress.	Cardiovascular disease, respiratory infections, asthma, chronic lung disease, cancer, premature birth, low-birth-weight infants.
Cannabis	■ marijuana (dried leaves and flowers) ■ hashish ■ kief	Sense of well-being, relaxation, sedation, poor concentration, impaired learning and memory, reddened eyes, dry mouth, airway irritation, increased appetite, decreased pain. Occasionally paranoia (esp. of products high in the psychoactive chemical THC).	Cognitive (mental) impairment, esp. for memory; chronic bronchitis; dependence; precancerous lung changes, with possible risk for cancer.
Opioids	■ opium ■ morphine ■ codeine ■ heroin ■ semisynthetic (oxycodone, hydrocodone) ■ synthetic (methadone, mepridine, fentanyl)	Pain relief, sedation, nausea, constipation, cough suppression, respiratory depression. Magnitude of symptoms depends on the type of opioid drug and the route of administration.	Fatal overdose.
CNS depressants	■ barbiturates ■ benzodiazepines ■ nonbenzodiazepine hypnotics	Sedation, decreased anxiety, incoordination, diminished reflexes, slowed respiratory rate, drowsiness.	Overdose can lead to respiratory failure and death.
CNS stimulants	■ caffeine ■ cocaine ■ methamphetamine ■ amphetamine ■ dextroamphetamine ■ methylphenidate	Increased alertness and wakefulness, euphoria, elevations in heart rate and blood pressure, decreased appetite, insomnia. Toxic effects (excluding caffeine): hallucinations, dangerously elevated body temperature.	Agitation, aggression, psychosis, paranoia, heart arrhythmias, heart attack, stroke, seizures, damage to the nose (cocaine), damaged teeth (meth), low-birth-weight infants.

Substance	Examples	Acute effects	Potential adverse effects with abuse and dependence
"Club" drugs	■ Methylenedioxymethamphetamine (MDMA, Ecstasy) ■ gamma-hydroxybutyrate (GHB) ■ flunitrazepam (Rohypnol) ■ ketamine ■ phencyclidine (PCP)	In addition to stimulant effects, a sense of heightened compassion and empathy, impulsiveness, anxiety, hallucinations, teeth clenching, insomnia, dehydration, and heat stroke. For GHB, flunitrazepam, and ketamine: sedation, amnesia, loss of consciousness, distorted perceptions (ketamine online). For PCP: Feelings of detachment and disconnection from reality. Toxic effects: agitation, aggression, seizures, respiratory depression.	Repeated MDMA use can lead to brain damage with emotional problems, memory deficits, and depression. Flunitrazepam use can lead to life-threatening withdrawal reactions. PCP use can lead to cognitive impairment.
Hallucinogens	■ LSD ■ psilocybin ■ peyote	Auditory and visual hallucinations, mood changes, shifts in perception and thinking. Heart rate and blood pressure may rise. Nausea, vomiting, anxiety, and sense of unease.	Usually not addicting.
Inhalants	■ solvents ■ aerosols ■ nitrites ■ anesthetic gasses	Depending on the chemical inhaled, sedation, elation, stimulation, slurred speech, incoordination, loss of consciousness, or death.	Damage to the brain, liver, kidney, and bone marrow.

KEY TAKEAWAYS

- The characteristics of behavioral addictions are the same as for any addiction. Compared to normal habits, addictions are associated with mental preoccupation, compulsive engagement, escalations in time spent doing the activity, and negative consequences.

- As with drug addictions, overcoming behavioral addictions can require professional treatment.

DISCUSSION QUESTION

1. Do you know anyone with a behavioral addiction? (That someone could be you.) Describe the behaviors that indicated something was wrong. What were the negative consequences? Did this person receive treatment? Was the treatment successful?

7. RECOMMENDED RESOURCES

7.1 Organizations and Websites

American Council for Drug Education. http://www.acde.org.

Americans for Nonsmokers' Rights—provides information about colleges and universities with smoke-free policies. http://www.no-smoke.org/goingsmokefree.php?id=447.

Office of National Drug Control Policy. http://www.whitehouse.gov/ondcp.

National Center on Addiction and Substance Abuse at Columbia University. http://www.casacolumbia.org/templates/Home.aspx?articleid=287&zoneid=32.

National Clearinghouse for Alcoholism and Drug Dependence. http://www.ncadd.org.

National Institute on Alcohol Abuse and Alcoholism. http://www.niaaa.nih.gov.

National Institute on Drug Abuse. http://www.drugabuse.gov.

Substance Abuse and Mental Health Services Administration. http://www.samhsa.gov.

ENDNOTES

1. DSM-IV substance abuse criteria. Available at: http://www.sis.indiana.edu/DSM-IV-Criteria.aspx. Accessed September 24, 2012.

2. Substance-related and addictive disorders. *Diagnostic and Statistic Manual of Mental Disorders* (DSM-5). American Psychiatric Association. Available at: http://www.dsm5.org/Documents/Substance%20Use%20Disorder%20Fact%20Sheet.pdf. Accessed May 30, 2013.

3. What is drug addiction? Drug Abuse and Addiction. National Institute on Drug Abuse. Available at: http://www.drugabuse.gov/publications/science-addiction/drug-abuse-addiction. Accessed September 24, 2012.

4. The science of drug abuse and addiction. National Institute on Drug Abuse. Available at: http://www.drugabuse.gov/publications/media-guide/science-drug-abuse-addiction. Accessed September 26, 2012.

5. Kessler RC, Berglund P, Demler O, Jin R, Merikangas KR, Walters EE. Lifetime prevalence and age-of-onset distributions of DSM-IV disorders in the National Comorbidity Survey Replication. *Arch Gen Psychiatry*. 2005;62:593–602.

6. Results from the 2010 National Survey on Drug Use and Health: summary of national findings. US Department of Health and Human Services. Substance Abuse and Mental Health Services Administration. Center for Behavioral Health Statistics and Quality. Available at: http://www.samhsa.gov/data/NSDUH/2k10Results.htm#2.13. Accessed September 9, 2012.

7. Why study drug abuse and addiction? The Science of Drug Abuse and Addiction. National Institute on Drug Abuse. Available at: http://www.drugabuse.gov/publications/media-guide/science-drug-abuse-addiction. Accessed September 24, 2012.

8. Swendsen J, Burstein M, Case B, Conway KP, Dierker L, He J, Merikangas KR. Use and abuse of alcohol and illicit drugs in US adolescents: results of the national comorbidity survey-adolescent supplement. *Arch Gen Psychiatry*. 2012 Apr;69(4):390–398.

9. Arrazola RA, Dube SR, Engstrom M. Current tobacco use among middle and high school students—United States, 2011. *MMWR Morb Mortal Wkly Rep*. 2012;61:581–585.

10. Paulozzi L, Baldwin G, Franklin G, et al. CDC grand rounds: prescription drug overdoses—a U.S. epidemic. *MMWR Morb Mortal Wkly Rep*. 2012 Jan 13; 61(1):10–13. Available at: http://www.cdc.gov/mmwr/preview/mmwrhtml/mm6101a3.htm. Accessed September 29, 2012.

11. McCabe SE, West BT, Morales M, Cranford JA, Boyd CJ. Does early onset of non-medical use of prescription drugs predict subsequent prescription drug abuse and dependence? Results from a national study. *Addiction*. 2007;102(12):1920–1930.

12. Kendler KS, Prescott CA, Myers J, Neale MC. The structure of genetic and environmental risk factors for common psychiatric and substance use disorders in men and women. *Arch Gen Psychiatry*. 2003 Sep;60(9):929–937.

13. Frye CA, Paris JJ, Osborne DM, Campbell JC, Kippin TE. Prenatal stress alters progestogens to mediate susceptibility to sex-typical, stress-sensitive disorders, such as drug abuse: a review. *Front Psychiatry*. 2011;2:52. Published online 2011 October 17. doi:10.3389/fpsyt.2011.00052.

14. Whitesell NR, Beals J, Mitchell CM, Manson SM, Turner RJ; the AI-SUPERPFP TEAM. Childhood exposure to adversity and risk of substance-use disorder in two American Indian populations: the meditational role of early substance-use initiation. *J Stud Alcohol Drugs*. 2009 November;70(6):971–981.

15. Compton WM, Thomas YF, Stinson FS, et al. Prevalence, correlates, disability, and co-morbidity of DSM-IV drug abuse and dependence in the United States: results from the National Epidemiologic Survey on Alcohol and Related Conditions. *Arch Gen Psychiatry*. 2007;64:566–576.

16. Merikangas KR, McClair VL. Epidemiology of substance use disorders. *Hum Genet*. 2012;131:779–789.

17. Kandel DB, Griesler PC, Schaffran C. Educational attainment and smoking among women: risk factors and consequences for offspring. *Drug Alcohol Depend*. 2009 Oct 1;104(Suppl 1):S24–S33.

18. Kashdan TB, Vetter CJ, Collins RL. Substance use in young adults: associations with personality and gender. *Addict Behavs*. 2005;30:259–269.

19. Eaton DK, Lowry R, Croft JB, Presley-Cantrell L, Perry GS. Relationships between hours of sleep and health-risk behaviors in US adolescent students. *Prev Med*. 2011 Oct;53(4–5):271–273. doi:10.1016/j.ymed.2011.06.020.

20. Dawson DA, Goldstein RB, Chou SP, Ruan WJ, Grant BF. Age at first drink and the first incidence of adult-onset DSM-IV alcohol use disorders. *Alcohol Clin Exp Res*. 2008 Dec;32(12):2149–2160.

21. Grant BF, Dawson DA. Age of onset of drug use and its association with DSM-IV drug abuse and dependence: results from the National Longitudinal Alcohol Epidemiologic Survey. *J Subst Abuse*. 1998;10:163–173.

22. Carey KB, Scott-Sheldon LA, Carey MP, DeMartini KS. Individual-level interventions to reduce college student drinking: a meta-analytic review. *Addict Behavs*. 2007 Nov;32(11):2469–2494. Available at: http://www.ncbi.nlm.nih.gov/pmc/articles/PMC2144910/?tool=pubmed. Accessed August 16, 2011.

23. Faggiano F, Vigna-Taglianti FD, Versino E, Zambon A, Borraccino A, Lemma P. School-based prevention for illicit drugs use: a systematic review. *Prev Med*. 2008 May;46(5):385–396.

24. Kertesz SG, Khodneva Y, Richman J, et al. Trajectories of drug use and mortality outcomes among adults followed over 18 years. *J Gen Intern Med*. 2012 Jul;27(7):808–816.

25. Rice JD, Wakeman SE, Dickman SL. Medicine and epidemic of incarceration in the United States. *N Engl J Med*. 2011;364(22):2081–2082.

26. Kuhar M. *The Addicted Brain: Why We Abuse Drugs, Alcohol, and Nicotine*. Saddle River, NY: FT Press/Pearson; 2012.

27. Results from the 2010 National Survey on Drug Use and Health: summary of national findings. US Department of Health and Human Services. Substance Abuse and Mental Health Services Administration. Center for Behavioral Health Statistics and Quality. Available at: http://www.samhsa.gov/data/NSDUH/2k10Results.htm#2.13. Accessed September 9, 2012.

28. Skanavi S, Laqueille X, Aubin HJ. Mindfulness based interventions for addictive disorders: a review. *Encephale*. 2011 Oct;37(5):379–387. doi:10.1016/j.encep.2010.08.010.

29. Witkiewitz K, Bowen S, Douglas H, Hsu SH. Mindfulness-based relapse prevention for substance craving. *Addict Behavs*. 2012 Apr 6 [Epub ahead of print].

30. World Health Organization. *WHO Report on the Global Tobacco Epidemic, 2011*. Geneva, Switzerland: World Health Organization. Available at: http://www.who.int/tobacco/global_report/2011/en/index.html. Executive summary available at: http://whqlibdoc.who.int/hq/2011/WHO_NMH_TFI_11.3_eng.pdf. Accessed September 6, 2012.

31. Danaei G, Ding EL, Mozaffarian D, Taylor B, Rehm J, Murray CJ, Ezzati M. The preventable causes of death in the United States: comparative risk assessment of dietary, lifestyle, and metabolic risk factors. *PLoS Med*. 2009;6(4):e1000058. Available at: http://www.ncbi.nlm.nih.gov/pmc/articles/PMC2667673/?tool=pubmed. Accessed August 1, 2011.

32. Results from the 2010 National Survey on Drug Use and Health: summary of national findings. US Department of Health and Human Services. Substance Abuse and Mental Health Services Administration. Center for Behavioral Health Statistics and Quality. Available at: http://www.samhsa.gov/data/NSDUH/2k10Results.htm#2.13. Accessed September 9, 2012.

33. September 2011 vital signs issue: adult smoking in the US. CEC Vital Signs. Centers for Disease Control and Prevention. Available at: http://www.cdc.gov/vitalsigns/AdultSmoking/index.html. Accessed September 7, 2011.

34. Spring 2011 reference group executive summary. National College Health Assessment. American College Health Association. Available at: http://www.achancha.org/docs/ACHA-NCHA-II_ReferenceGroup_ExecutiveSummary_Spring2011.pdf. Accessed September 7, 2012.

35. Tynan MA, McAfee T, Promoff G, Pechacek T. Consumption of cigarettes and combustible tobacco: United States, 2000–2011. *MMWR Morb Mortal Wkly Rep*. 2012;61(30):565–569.

36. Smoking & tobacco use. Fast Facts. Centers for Disease Control and Prevention. Available at: http://www.cdc.gov/tobacco/data_statistics/fact_sheets/fast_facts. Accessed November 7, 2012.

37. What's in tobacco? Cigarette Smoking. American Cancer Society. Available at: http://www.cancer.org/Cancer/CancerCauses/TobaccoCancer/CigaretteSmoking/cigarette-smoking-tobacco. Accessed September 30, 2012.

38. Dale L. What is thirdhand smoke, and why is it a concern? Mayo Clinic. Available at: http://www.mayoclinic.com/health/third-hand-smoke/AN01985. Accessed September 30, 2012.

39. Centers for Disease Control and Prevention. Smoking-attributable mortality, years of potential life lost, and productivity losses—United States, 2000–2004. *MMWR Morb Mortal Wkly Rep*. 2008;57(45):1226–1228.

40. Delnevo CD, Pevzner ES, Hrywna M, Lewis MJ. Bidi cigarette use among young adults in 15 States. *Prev Med*. 2004;39:207–211.

41. Centers for Disease Control and Prevention. Annual smoking-attributable mortality, years of potential life lost, and productivity losses—United States, 1997–2001. *MMWR Morb Mortal Wkly Rep*. 2005;54(25):625–628. Available at: http://www.cdc.gov/rnmwr/preview/mmwrhtml/rnm5425a1.htm.

42. Smoking and tobacco use: heart disease and stroke. Centers for Disease Control and Prevention. Available at: http://www.cdc.gov/tobacco/basic_information/health_effects/heart_disease/index.htm. Accessed July 11, 2012.

43. *Chronic Obstructive Pulmonary Disease among Adults Aged 18 and over in the United States, 1998–2009*. Centers for Disease Control and Prevention; 2011. National Center for Health Statistics Data Brief, no. 63. Available at: http://www.cdc.gov/nchs/data/databriefs/db63.htm. Accessed July 1, 2011.

44. Centers for Disease Control and Prevention. Cigarette smoking among adults—United States, 2006. *MMWR Morb Mortal Wkly Rep*. 2007;56(44):1157–1161. Available at: http://www.cdc.gov/mmwr/preview/mmwrhtml/mm5644a2.htm.

45. Rogers JM. Tobacco and pregnancy: overview of exposures and effects. *Birth Defects Res C Embryo Today*. 2008;84:1–15.

46. Ayer JG, Belousova E, Harmer JA, et al. Maternal cigarette smoking is associated with reduced high-density lipoprotein cholesterol in healthy 8-year-old children. *Eur Heart J*. 2011. doi:10.1093/eurheartj/ehr174.

47. Milidou I, Henriksen TB, Jensen MS, Olsen J, Søndergaard C. Nicotine replacement therapy during pregnancy and infantile colic in the offspring. *Pediatrics*. 2012 Feb 20. doi:10.1542/peds.2011-2281.

48. Martin JA, Hamilton BE, Sutton PD, et al. Births: final data for 2005. *Natl Vital Stat Rep*. 2007;56:1–103.

49. Bandiera FC, Richardson AK, Lee DJ, He JP, Merikangas KR. Mental health risks: secondhand smoke exposure and mental health among children and adolescents. *Arch Pediatr Adolesc Med*. 2011;165(4):332–338.

50. Critchley JA, Capewell S. Mortality risk reduction associated with smoking cessation in patients with coronary heart disease: a systematic review. *JAMA*. 2003 Jul 2;290(1):86–97.

51. Gerber Y, Rosen LJ, Goldbourt U, Benyamini Y, Drory Y; Israel Study Group on First Acute Myocardial Infarction. Smoking status and long-term survival after first acute myocardial infarction a population-based cohort study. *J Am Coll Cardiol.* 2009 Dec 15;54(25):2382–2387.

52. Alpert HR, Connolly GN, Biener L. A prospective cohort study challenging the effectiveness of population-based medical intervention for smoking cessation. *Tob Control.* 2012. doi:10.1136/tobaccocontrol-2011-050129. Available at: http://hcc.musc.edu/research/programs/prevention/February%202012%20Journal%20Club%20Article.pdf. Accessed September 30, 2012.

53. Cobb NK, Abrams DB. E-cigarette or drug-deliver device? Regulating novel nicotine products. *N Engl J Med.* 2011;365(3):193–195.

54. Mooney ME, Sofuoglu M. Bupropion for the treatment of nicotine withdrawal and craving. *Expert Rev Neurother.* 2006 Jul;6(7):965–981.

55. Garrison GD, Dugan SE. Varenicline: a first-line treatment option for smoking cessation. *Clin Ther.* 2009 Mar;31(3):463–491.

56. Cahill K, Stead LF, Lancaster T. Nicotine receptor partial agonists for smoking cessation. *Cochrane Database Syst Rev.* 2007 Jan 24;(1):CD006103.

57. Haibach JP, Homish GC, Giovino GA. A longitudinal evaluation of fruit and vegetable consumption and cigarette smoking. *Nicotine Tob Res.* 2012 May. doi:10.1093/ntr/nts130.

58. Kochupillai V, Kumar P, Singh D, et al. Effect of rhythmic breathing (Sudarshan Kriya and Pranayam) on immune functions and tobacco addiction. *Ann NY Acad Sci.* 2005 Nov;1056:242–252.

59. Westbrook C, Creswell JD, Tabibnia G, et al. Mindful attention reduces neural and self-reported cue-induced craving in smokers. *Soc Cogn Affect Neurosci.* 2013 Jan;8(1):73–84. doi:10.1093/scan/nsr076.

60. Cheng HM, Chung YC, Chen HH, Chang YH, Yeh ML. Systematic review and meta-analysis of the effects of acupoint stimulation on smoking cessation. *Am J Chin Med.* 2012;40(3):429–442.

61. Spring 2011 reference group executive summary. National College Health Assessment. American College Health Association. Available at: http://www.achancha.org/docs/ACHA-NCHA-II_ReferenceGroup_ExecutiveSummary_Spring2011.pdf. Accessed September 7, 2012.

62. Investing in mental health. World Health Organization. 2003. Available at: http://www.who.int/mental_health/en/investing_in_mnh_final.pdf. Accessed May 7, 2012.

63. Results from the 2010 National Survey on Drug Use and Health: summary of national findings. US Department of Health and Human Services. Substance Abuse and Mental Health Services Administration. Center for Behavioral Health Statistics and Quality. Available at: http://www.samhsa.gov/data/NSDUH/2k10NSDUH/2k10Results.htm#2.13. Accessed September 9, 2012.

64. Spring 2011 reference group executive summary. National College Health Assessment. American College Health Association. Available at: http://www.achancha.org/docs/ACHA-NCHA-II_ReferenceGroup_ExecutiveSummary_Spring2011.pdf. Accessed September 7, 2012.

65. Borsari B, Carey KB. How the quality of peer relationships influences college alcohol use. *Drug Alcohol Rev.* 2006 Jul;25(4):361–370. Available at: http://www.ncbi.nlm.nih.gov/pmc/articles/PMC2635065/?tool=pubmed. Accessed August 16, 2011.

66. Results from the 2010 National Survey on Drug Use and Health: summary of national findings. US Department of Health and Human Services. Substance Abuse and Mental Health Services Administration. Center for Behavioral Health Statistics and Quality. Available at: http://www.samhsa.gov/data/NSDUH/2k10Results.htm#2.13. Accessed September 9, 2012.

67. Alcohol and crime: Data from 2002 to 2008. Bureau of Justice Statistics. Available at: http://bjs.ojp.usdoj.gov/content/acf/ac_conclusion.cfm. Accessed September 19, 2012.

68. Hansel B, Kontush A, Bruckert E. Is a cardioprotective action of alcohol a myth? *Curr Opin Cardiol.* 2012 Sep;27(5):550–555.

69. Alcohol alert. No. 72. National Institute on Alcohol Abuse and Alcoholism. National Institutes of Health. July 2007. Available at: http://pubs.niaaa.nih.gov/publications/AA72/AA72.htm. Accessed October 1, 2012.

70. Substance abuse: CNS depressants-alcohol. Nurses Learning Network. Available at: http://www.nurseslearning.com/courses/corexcel/cxnrp-1600/Chap3/course/chap1/P10.html. Accessed September 29, 2012.

71. Wechsler H, Seibring M, Liu IC, Ahl M. Colleges respond to student binge drinking: reducing student demand or limiting access. *J Am Coll Health.* 2004 Jan–Feb;52(4):159–168.

72. Carey KB, Scott-Sheldon LAJ, Carey MP, DeMartini KS. Individual-level interventions to reduce college student drinking: a meta-analytic review. *Addict Behav.* 2007;32(11):2469–2494.

73. Wechsler H, Lee JE, Nelson TF, Lee H. Drinking levels, alcohol problems and secondhand effects in substance-free college residences: results of a national study. *J Stud Alcohol.* 2001 Jan;62(1):23–31.

74. Kim-Katz SY, Anderson IB. Prescription opiate/opioid drug abuse: a new epidemic. Pulmonary, Critical Care, Sleep Upate. 2011 Jan 11. Vol 25, Lesson 1.

75. Results from the 2011 National Survey on Drug Use and Health: summary of national findings. US Department of Health and Human Services. Substance Abuse and Mental Health Services Administration. Center for Behavioral Health Statistics and Quality. Available at: http://www.samhsa.gov/data/NSDUH/2k11Results/NSDUHresults2011.htm#8.4. Accessed September 29, 2012.

76. McCabe SE, Cranford JA, West BT. Trends in prescription drug abuse and dependence, co-occurrence with other substance use disorders, and treatment utilization: results from two national surveys. *Addict Behav.* 2008;33(10):1297–1305.

77. Results from the 2010 National Survey on Drug Use and Health: summary of national findings. US Department of Health and Human Services. Substance Abuse and Mental Health Services Administration. Center for Behavioral Health Statistics and Quality. Available at: http://www.samhsa.gov/data/NSDUH/2k10NSDUH/2k10Results.htm#2.13. Accessed September 9, 2012.

78. Substance Abuse and Mental Health Services Administration. Nonmedical users of pain relievers: characteristics of recent initiates. *The NSDUH Report.* Office of Applied Studies. 2006. Available at: http://www.oas.samhsa.gov/2k6/pain/pain.pdf. Accessed June 29, 2012.

79. Paulozzi L, Baldwin G, Franklin G, et al. CDC grand rounds: prescription drug overdoses—a U.S. epidemic. *MMWR Morb Mortal Wkly Rep.* 2012 Jan 13;61(1):10–13. Available at: http://www.cdc.gov/mmwr/preview/mmwrhtml/mm6101a3.htm. Accessed September 29, 2012.

80. Muley A, Muley P, Shah M. Coffee to reduce risk of type 2 diabetes? A systematic review. *Curr Diabetes Rev.* 2012 May;8(3):162–168.

81. Palacios N, Gao X, McCullough ML, et al. Caffeine and risk of Parkinson's disease in a large cohort of men and women. *Mov Disord.* 2012 Sep 1;27(10):1276–1282. doi:10.1002/mds.25076.

82. Butt MS, Sultan MT. Coffee and its consumption: benefits and risks. *Crit Rev Food Sci Nutr.* 2011 Apr;51(4):363–373.

83. Chacko SM, Thambi PT, Kuttan R, Nishigaki I. Beneficial effects of green tea: a literature review. *Chin Med.* 2010 Apr 6;5:13.

84. Harrison L. Surge reported in energy drink emergency department visits. *Medscape J Med.* 2011 Nov 28. Available at: http://www.medscape.com/viewarticle/754146?src=ptalk. Accessed September 19, 2012.

85. Farooq MU, Bhatt A, Patel M. Neurotoxic and cardiotoxic effects of cocaine and ethanol. *J Med Toxicol.* 2009 Sep;5(3):134–138.

86. Gfroerer JC, Larson SL, Colliver JD. Drug use patterns and trends in rural communities. *J Rural Health.* 2007 Fall;23 Suppl:10–15.

87. DrugFacts: methamphetamine. National Institute on Drug Abuse. Available at: http://www.drugabuse.gov/publications/drugfacts/methamphetamine. Accessed September 27, 2012.

88. Novak SP, Kroutil LA, Williams RL, Brunt DL. The nonmedical use of prescription ADHD medications: results from a national Internet panel. *Subst Abuse Treat Prev Policy.* 2007 Oct 31;2:32.

89. Results from the 2010 National Survey on Drug Use and Health: summary of national findings. US Department of Health and Human Services. Substance Abuse and Mental Health Services Administration. Center for Behavioral Health Statistics and Quality. Available at: http://www.samhsa.gov/data/NSDUH/2k10Results.htm#2.13. Accessed September 9, 2012.

90. Schulden JD, Thomas YF, Compton WM. Substance abuse in the United States: findings from recent epidemiologic studies. *Curr Psychiatry Rep.* 2009 Oct;11(5):353–359.

91. Spring 2011 reference group executive summary. National College Health Assessment. American College Health Association. Available at: http://www.achancha.org/docs/ACHA-NCHA-II_ReferenceGroup_ExecutiveSummary_Spring2011.pdf. Accessed September 7, 2012.

92. Results from the 2010 National Survey on Drug Use and Health: summary of national findings. US Department of Health and Human Services. Substance Abuse and Mental Health Services Administration. Center for Behavioral Health Statistics and Quality. Available at: http://www.samhsa.gov/data/NSDUH/2k10NSDUH/2k10Results.htm#2.13. Accessed September 9, 2012.

93. De Petrocellis L, Grazia Cascio M, Di Marzo V. The endocannabinoid system: a general view and latest additions. *Br J Pharmacol.* 2004 Mar;141(5):765–774. doi:10.1038/sj.bjp.0705666. Available at: http://www.ncbi.nlm.nih.gov/pmc/articles/PMC1574255. Accessed September 17, 2012.

94. Kuhar M. *The Addicted Brain: Why We Abuse Drugs, Alcohol, and Nicotine.* Saddle River, NY: FT Press/Pearson; 2012.

95. Kalant H. Adverse effects of cannabis on health: an update of the literature since 1996. *Prog Neuropsychopharmacol Biol Psychiatry.* 2004 Aug;28(5):849–863. doi:10.1016/j.pnpbp.2004.05.027.

96. Meier MH, Caspi A, Ambler A, et al. Persistent cannabis users show neuropsychological decline from childhood to midlife. *Proc Natl Acad Sci USA.* 2012 Aug 27. [Published online before print.] doi:10.1073/pnas.120682010.

97. Pope HG Jr, Gruber AJ, Hudson JI, et al. Early-onset cannabis use and cognitive deficits: what is the nature of the association? *Drug Alcohol Depend.* 2003 Apr 1;69(3):303–310.

98. Horwood LJ, Fergusson DM, Hayatbakhsh MR, et al. Cannabis use and educational achievement: findings from three Australasian cohort studies. *Drug Alcohol Depend.* 2010 Aug 1;110(3):247–253.

99. Taylor DR, Hall W; Thoracic Society of Australia and New Zealand. Respiratory health effects of cannabis: position statement of the Thoracic Society of Australia and New Zealand. *Intern Med J.* 2003 Jul;33(7):310–313.

100. Lacson JC, Carroll JD, Tuazon E, Castelao EJ, Bernstein L, Cortessis VK. Population-based case-control study of recreational drug use and testis cancer risk confirms an association between marijuana use and nonseminoma risk. *Cancer.* 2012. doi:10.1002/cncr.27554.

101. Degenhardt L, Coffey C, Romaniuk H, Swift W, Carlin JB, Hall WD, Patton GC. The persistence of the association between adolescent cannabis use and common mental disorders into young adulthood. *Addiction.* 2012 Jul 6. doi:10.1111/j.1360-0443.2012.04015.x [Epub ahead of print].

102. Swift W, Coffey C, Degenhardt L, Carlin JB, Romaniuk H, Patton GC. Cannabis and progression to other substance use in young adults: findings from a 13-year prospective population-based study. *J Epidemiol Community Health*. 2012 Jul;66(7):e26.

103. Brecher EM; the editors of *Consumer Reports Magazine*, 1972. The consumers union report on licit and illicit drugs. *Schaffer Library of Drug Policy*. Available at: http://www.druglibrary.org/schaffer/library/studies/cu/cu54.html. Accessed September 17, 2012.

104. Massi P, Solinas M, Cinquina V, Parolaro D. Cannabidiol as potential anticancer drug. *Br J Clin Pharmacol*. 2012 Apr 17. doi:10.1111/j.1365-2125.2012.04298.x [Epub ahead of print].

105. Zuardi AW, Crippa JA, Hallak JE, et al. A critical review of the antipsychotic effects of Cannabidiol: 30 years of a translational investigation. *Curr Pharm Des*. 2012 Jun 7 [Epub ahead of print].

106. Bergamaschi MM, Queiroz RH, Zuardi AW, Crippa JA. Safety and side effects of cannabidiol, a Cannabis sativa constituent. *Curr Drug Saf*. 2011 Sep 1;6(4):237–249.

107. Wade D. Evaluation of the safety and tolerability profile of Sativex: is it reassuring enough? *Expert Rev Neurother*. 2012 Apr;12(4 Suppl):9–14.

108. Esposito G, Filippis DD, Cirillo C, et al. Cannabidiol in inflammatory bowel diseases: a brief overview. *Phytother Res*. 2012 Jul 20. doi:10.1002/ptr.4781 [Epub ahead of print].

109. Zuardi AW. Cannabidiol: from an inactive cannabinoid to a drug with wide spectrum of action. *Rev Bras Psiquiatr*. 2008 Sep;30(3):271–280.

110. Scuderi C, Filippis DD, Iuvone T, Blasio A, Steardo A, Esposito G. Cannabidiol in medicine: a review of its therapeutic potential in CNS disorders. *Phytother Res*. 2009 May;23(5):597–602.

111. Mader LS. Is CBD the answer? Analyzing the role of cannabidiol in medical cannabis. *HerbalGram*. 2012 Aug–Oct;95:26–29.

112. Grotenhermen F. Cannabinoids and the endocannabinoid system. *Cannabinoids*. 2006;1(1):10–14. Available at: http://www.cannabis-med.org/data/pdf/en_2006_01_2.pdf. Accessed September 18, 2012.

113. Callaway JC. Hempseed as a nutritional resource: an overview. *Euphytica*. 2004;140(1–2): 65–72. doi:10.1007/s10681-004-4811-6.

114. Basic facts about drugs: PCP and LSD. American Council on Drug Addiction. Available at: http://www.acde.org/youth/Research.htm. Accessed September 28, 2012.

115. DrugFacts: hallucinogens—LSD, peyote, psilocybin, and PCP. National Institute on Drug Abuse. Available at: http://www.drugabuse.gov/publications/drugfacts/hallucinogens-lsd-peyote-psilocybin-pcp. Accessed September 28, 2012.

116. Date rape drugs fact sheet. US Department of Health and Human Services Office on Women's Health. WomensHealth.gov. Available at: http://www.womenshealth.gov/publications/our-publications/fact-sheet/date-rape-drugs.cfm. Accessed September 29, 2012.

117. Song BJ, Moon KH, Upreti VV, Eddington ND, Le IJ. Mechanisms of MDMA (Ecstasy)-induced oxidative stress, mitochondrial dysfunction, and organ damage. *Curr Pharm Biotechnol*. 2010 Aug 1;11(5):434–443.

118. Cowan RL, Roberts DM, Joers JM. Neuroimaging in human MDMA (Ecstasy) users: a cortical model. *Ann NY Acad Sci*. 2008 Oct;1139:291–298. doi:10.1196/annals.1432.007.

119. Rogers G, Elston J, Garside R, et al. The harmful health effects of recreational ecstasy: a systematic review of observational evidence. *Health Technol Assess*. 2009 Jan;13(6):iii–iv, ix–xii, 1–315.

120. McCardle K, Luebbers S, Carter JD, Croft RJ, Stough C. Chronic MDMA (ecstasy) use, cognition and mood. *Psychopharmacology* (Berl). 2004 May;173(3–4):434–439.

121. Flisher C. Getting plugged in: an overview of Internet addiction. *J Paediatr Child Health*. 2010;46(10):557–559. doi:10.1111/j.1440-1754.2010.01879.x.

122. Wechsler H, Lee JE, Nelson TF, Lee H. Drinking levels, alcohol problems and second-hand effects in substance-free college residences: results of a national study. *J Stud Alcohol*. 2001 Jan;62(1):23–31.

CHAPTER 12
Personal Safety

Accidents happen. Without meaning to, we can hurt ourselves and others. Humans can also deliberately harm one another. The yearly death total from both intended and unintended injuries tops 180,000, or about 1 death every 3 minutes.[1]

FIGURE 12.1 Injury Deaths Compared to Other Leading Causes of Death for Persons Ages 1–44, United States, 2007
Injury includes unintentional injuries and intentional injuries (e.g., homicides and suicides). Noncommunicable diseases include cardiovascular disease, cancer, stroke, and diabetes.

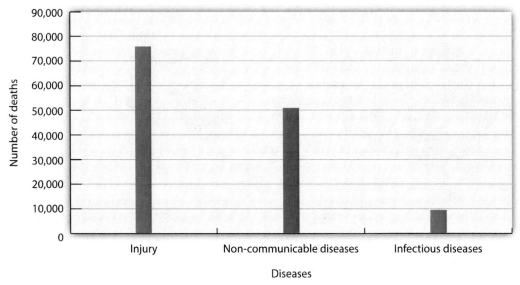

Source: Adapted from Centers for Disease Control and Prevention. Injury: the leading cause of death among persons 1–44. 2010. Data Source: National Vital Statistics System using CDC Wonder (http://wonder.cdc.gov). Available at: http://www.cdc.gov/injury/overview/leading_cod.html.

Teens and young adults are most at risks for dying of injuries. The top three causes of death for people ages 15 to 24 are accidents (unintentional injuries), suicides, and homicides.[2] As a nation, we don't compare well to other countries for injury-related deaths. Of 18 countries with detailed injury data, the United States is the fifth highest for fatal injuries in people ages 15 to 24. The only countries with higher death rates were Columbia, South Africa, Brazil, and Puerto Rico.[3]

The good news is you can both prevent and protect yourself from injuries. Of course, you can't prevent them all—short of confining yourself to a padded room, which would be bad for your health for other reasons. Part of the thrill of life is learning new skills and pushing the envelope for your personal best.

For instance, you could completely prevent cycling injury by never riding a bike. However, cycling has multiple personal and environmental health benefits. Just make sure to protect yourself by wearing a helmet and bike gloves and following the rules of the road. In other words, minimize your risks while engaging fully with life. To do so, recognize your limits, estimate reasonable risk, learn from inevitable mistakes, and take precautions to reduce potential harm to you and others.

This chapter will review the common causes and the possible solutions to both unintentional and intentional injuries. For information about preventing and managing athletic injuries and injuries related to temperature extremes, see Chapter 9 (Physical Fitness).

If we are to teach real peace in this world, and if we are to carry on a real war against war, we shall have to begin with the children.

- Mohandas "Mahatma" Gandhi

FIGURE 12.2 Five Leading Causes of Death, by Age Group
These pie charts demonstrate that the top killers of young Americans are unintentional injuries, homicides, and suicides. Notice the shift to chronic, noncommunicable diseases such as heart disease and cancer with advancing age.

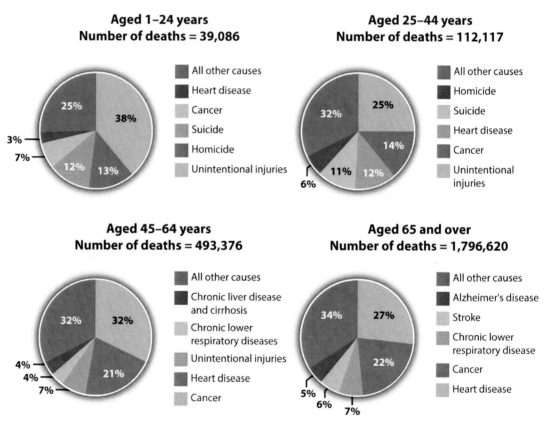

Source: Adapted from CDC/National Center for Health Statistics Death in the United States, 2010. National Vital Statistics System, Mortality, 2012. Data brief. Available at: http://www.cdc.gov/nchs/data/databriefs/db99.htm.

1. UNINTENTIONAL INJURIES

LEARNING OBJECTIVES

1. Distinguish between unintentional and intentional injuries.
2. Discuss statistics and risk factors for unintentional injuries.
3. Describe ways to prevent and protect against common injuries.

Unintentional injuries are unplanned occurrences that led to bodily harm. Experts prefer this term to *accidents*, which suggests a chance and unavoidable mishap. In reality, we often play a role in injuries, even when we didn't intend them to happen. **Intentional injuries**, on the other hand, are incidents that occurred with a goal of inflicting harm. We'll discuss these deliberate injuries later.

Each year, over 118,000 people die from unintentional injuries.[4] In 2010, accidents were the fifth most common cause of death for age groups combined. Motor vehicle accidents cause the most fatal accidents (34,485), followed by unintentional poisonings (31,758) and falls (24,792).

Young Americans take the brunt of the death toll. In people under age 45, unintentional injuries are the leading cause of death. In the 15- to 24-year-old age group, unintentional injuries account for nearly half of deaths. Most die in motor vehicle accidents. Other common causes are unintentional poisonings, drowning, and firearm accidents. As we'll discuss, young males are at particular risk for both unintentional and intentional injuries.

So why do so many young people become injured, sometimes fatally? A number of factors contribute.

- Compared to the older adults, young people tend to be more physically active. And while elders can and should exercise, they typically avoid high-risk sports. Visit any skate park in the national and check out the demographics. If you spot people with crow's feet, they're probably making videos of their kids.

- Independence from parents and other authority figures rises during adolescence. That's how it should be. On the other hand, older, wiser adults aren't on hand to point out possible perils.

- A sense of invulnerability and overconfidence in abilities promotes risk taking.

- Young people have a different assessment of potential harm. That's not an entirely irrational judgment. Put snowboarding pro Lindsey Jacobellis (born 1985) and a 60-year-old woman in the half pipe and it doesn't take a PhD to figure out who would more likely get hurt.

- Young people are relatively inexperienced. Expertise comes with repetition. The hazards are higher for a 16-year-old driver navigating the highway for the first time than for a 30-year-old taking the usual commute to work. Also, older adults have learned from their mistakes, including the injuries they've survived.

- Experimentation with alcohol and illicit drugs is common. Most of these substances impair judgment, reaction times, and physical function. Worse, high doses can be fatal.

- Peer pressure, which has a stronger hold on the young, can spur risky activities.

- The highest brain region doesn't finish maturing until your midtwenties. This area, the prefrontal cortex, reins in impulses, plans, reasons, and judges. It's what prevents you from piling into a car packed with drunken teenagers and speeding off.

Why Are Young Men Particularly Accident Prone?

The elderly are most at risk for fatal unintentional injuries, especially from falls. But if you exclude people above age 85, adolescent and young adult males are the most injury prone. In fact, throughout the life span, boys and men suffer more unintentional injuries. But why?

Compared to women, men are more likely to engage in risky behaviors such as binge drinking, drunken driving, driving without a seat belt, and aggressive driving. They're three times more likely than women to die in a car crash. They're also more likely to engage in extreme sports. And they more often perform manual labor that has a high potential for injury.[5] In 2008, 5,310 men and 580 women were hurt on the job.[6] While no women died, 37 men died due to occupational injuries.

What drives the gender differences in risk taking and injury? Culturally defined gender roles and biological differences both contribute. Our culture expects boys and men to behave in a more rough and tumble fashion. Yet some behavior differences seem to appear at an early age.

unintentional injuries

Injuries that occur without the intent of harm; also called accidents.

intentional injuries

Injuries arising from a goal to inflict personal harm.

Risk-taking fits stereotypes of masculinity. Guys are supposed to be bold, unafraid, and able to "hold their liquor." We expect men to do the heavy lifting and, thanks to biological differences in muscle mass, they can.

Furthermore, studies show that men and women assess risk differently. More specifically, women are more likely to perceive negative consequences and a relative lack of enjoyment from physically risky activities.[7]

In addition, adult role models too often instill a "boys don't cry" ethic. Such attitudes can hinder timely treatment when young men become injured working or recreating.

Unfortunately, the belief that it's somehow shameful to seek help can also prevent men from talking to their doctors about psychological pain. Untreated depression, combined with the fact that men more often own firearms, contributes to their higher suicide rate. Lastly, greater possession of firearms and other weapons also fuels a higher homicide rates among men—both as perpetrators and as victims.

1.1 Risks of the Road

Though many of us have a cavalier attitude about cars, driving is probably the most hazardous thing you do regularly. Occupants of trucks and cars, motorcyclists, scooter riders, bicyclists, and pedestrians—basically anyone traveling—bear certain risks and responsibilities. The greatest danger comes from being struck by a car or truck.

Motor Vehicle Accidents

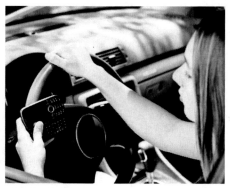

© Thinkstock

Of the approximately 34,500 deaths from motor vehicle crashes in 2009, 22 percent were in people 15 to 24 years old.[8] Excluding other types of unintentional injuries, car crashes are the leading cause of death in teens and young adults. Young males die at double the rate of females. Driver inexperience and alcohol underlie many accidents.

Driving while under the influence of alcohol or drugs is called **impaired driving**. In recent years, fewer people drink and drive. Nevertheless, almost a million high school students got behind the wheel after drinking.[9] The practice is common among college students too. Compared to older people, younger people more often drink with the goal of intoxication. In 2007, alcohol was behind fatal car crashes in 23 percent of teen drivers and 41 percent of young adults 20 to 24.[10] The CDC notes that alcohol-impaired driving causes a death every 48 minutes.[11]

Distracted driving has increasingly become a safety hazard. Driving requires multitasking. You're using your hands, feet, eyes, and ears. Your brain directs the show and processes sensory information related to the task. One second of inattention can be disastrous. Within that time frame, your car can swerve into another lane or collide with nearby objects.

Driver distraction includes taking your eyes of the road or your hands off the wheel or diverting your mental focus to anything other than the task at hand. In 2009, distracted driving killed nearly 5,550 people (an average of 15 people a day) and injured another 448,000.[12] Common distractions include talking to passengers, fiddling with the car sound system, reading maps, eating, drinking, grooming, and, especially, using cell phones.

About 20 percent of the distracted-driving fatal crashes involved **cell phone use**. In a 2011 survey of US drivers 18 to 65 years of age, more than two-thirds reported that they talked on their cell phones and a third had sent a text or e-mail message while driving during the previous 30 days.[13] Use is particularly high in teens and young adults. In a 2012 survey, more than half of high school seniors—people who haven't had a driving permit for very long—admitted to texting or e-mailing while driving.[14] Texting is particularly perilous. Between 2001 and 2007, the dramatic increase in texting contributed to an additional 16,000 road fatalities.[15]

A study of college students illustrates why people continue to drive and phone. Students filled out a survey in which they predicted their performance in a driving simulator with or without a simultaneous cell phone conversation. Then they got in the simulator. As expected, they didn't function as well while talking on the phone. Ironically, students who thought they were good at compensating for distractions and who overestimated their performance in a driving simulator often used their cell phones in the car. They also had "poorer real-world driving records" than infrequent cell phone users.[16]

Currently, 10 states and the District of Columbia ban handheld cell phone use while driving.[17] (However, hands-free devices may not make phone conversations any less dangerous.[18]) More states prohibit use for drivers under age 18. Thirty-nine states and the District of Columbia ban texting and driving. It's not yet clear how effective those bans have been on public safety, in part due to less than complete compliance with the laws. Breaking the law, even if no accidents occurred, can result in fines, criminal charges, jail or prison time, points on one's driving record, and suspension or revocation of one's driver license.

 Video Clip 12.1

Texting and Driving: A Lethal Combo
AT&T has started an It Can Wait campaign against driving and texting.

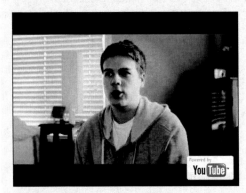

View the video online at: http://www.youtube.com/v/mjc_0JBlRgE

Another important cause of driver inattention is **drowsiness**. Drowsy drivers contribute to about 1,550 fatal and 40,000 nonfatal car crashes. Sleep deprivation, the main cause of daytime sleepiness, erodes mental and physical skills needed to drive safely. In fact, a sleep-deprived driver can drive as badly as a drunk driver. Plus, drowsy drivers can fall asleep at the wheel—in spite of their best attempts to remain awake.

Sedative medications (including antihistamines in many cold and allergy preparations) and alcohol also cause drowsiness. Furthermore, these substances interact with sleep deprivation. In other words, being tired increases the sedating effect of a single drink. Now consider that college is a time when many students drink and fail to get enough sleep.

Aggressive driving has become a serious problem. An aggressive driver puts people at risk by tailgating, speeding, repeatedly changing lanes, cutting off other motorists and cyclists, running red lights and stop signs, and making illegal turns. Such behavior can escalate into **road rage** on behalf of the aggressor and those transgressed against. People honk, shout, and gesture angrily. In extreme cases, enraged drivers have caused accidents and used firearms.

Each of us can take steps to reduce highway aggression. For many people, frustration mounts when traffic is sluggish. For some, irritation flares into fury. See the next section for tips on minimizing aggravation.

Environmental hazards account for a relatively small proportion of motor vehicle crashes. Nevertheless, it's important to respect and prepare for hazards posed by snow, rain, ice, wind, fog, glare, road construction, and anything else that limits visibility and tire traction on the road. Check weather reports when going on a trip. Drive cautiously to account for road conditions.

Preventing Motor Vehicle Accidents

Changes to highway infrastructure have led to a decline in car crashes. They include road improvements, wider median dividers, guardrails, and signs that break away to reduce crash impact. Legislation promoting highway safety includes mandatory seat belt laws, airbag installation in newer cars and trucks, programs wherein teen drivers gradually gain privileges (graduated driver license), and limitations on the number of passengers in cars driven by young drivers.

States have child safety seat laws, though exact regulations vary from state to state. In general, children should sit in the back seat. Infants less than 20 pounds should be in a rear-facing infant seat. Toddlers and preschoolers 20 to 40 pounds should be in a forward-facing car seat. Kids under age six or seven can sit in special booster seats.

Here are things you can do to maximize motor vehicle safety:

- Prepare. Before you turn on the engine, adjust your seat and mirrors, fasten your seat belt, check your map, and set up your audio system. Resist the temptation to change the music once you're rolling.
- Make sure your car is in good working order. Ensure that headlights, taillights, turn indicators, and wiper blades work. Check tires for wear and pressure. Use snow tires or all-weather tires if you travel in snowy areas. Refill washer fluid as necessary.

- Obey speed limits—no matter how late you are for an appointment. If you get a speeding ticket, you'll be further behind, including financially. If, in your haste, you cause an accident, the impact could last a lifetime.

- Allow ample time to reach your destination. Doing so reduces the temptation to speed and the aggravation of slow traffic and insufficient parking spots.

- Allow enough distance between you and the car ahead. Try the three-second rule. Select a fixed object ahead of the car in front. As soon as that car passes the landmark, start counting "one-one thousand, two-one thousand, three-one thousand." If you get to the object before the third second, you're too close. Drop back. If someone is tailgating you, pull into the slow lane or get off the road to let him or her pass.

- Follow the rules of the road. Halt at stop signs and red lights. A yellow light means slow, not go faster.

- Share the road. Yield to pedestrians. Give cyclists a wide berth.

- Use all your senses—except taste. Save the snacks for later. Keep your eyes on the road. Leave out the earbuds. You need to be able to hear squealing brakes, honking, sirens, and shouts.

- Put your cell phone safely out of reach. Those alerts for e-mail, texts, and phone calls can be hard to resist. But they really can wait. If you need to use your phone, pull over or ask a passenger to make or receive the call for you.

- If another driver behaves badly, don't retaliate. It's not worth it. Keep yourself safe by getting out of an aggressive driver's way. Note the license plate number and, after you pull off the road, call the police.

- Don't drink and drive. You may think alcohol hasn't impaired your skills. But that's because alcohol hinders your judgment. Take a cab or catch a ride with a sober driver.

- Decline rides with a driver who has been drinking. That's hard to do, but the difficulty pales compared to recovering physically and emotionally from an accident.

- When traveling with pets or small children, make sure they're secure before you switch on the ignition. It's hard to drive with a cat, dog, or child leaping around the car. Nor is it safe for them. If you're a passenger, holding a child in your lap is a terrible idea. In the event of a crash, your body weight will add to the forward velocity of the child.

- Adjust your driving for weather conditions. If fog, snow, or rain obscures your view, drive slowly and cautiously. If you can't see, pull over. Remember it takes longer to stop on wet and icy roads.

- If you're having trouble keeping your eyes open, pull over, let a passenger drive, or take a nap. If you can't do any of those, drink a caffeinated beverage. Just know it can take 30 minutes for the caffeine to take full effect.

Assess Yourself: Are You a Safe Driver?

Answer the following questions as honestly as possible. The more spaces you check, the greater your risk. You're at particularly high risk if you habitually use your cell phone or drive aggressively, while intoxicated, or when drowsy. It only takes one misstep to cause a fatal accident.

- Driver inexperience
  - ____ I am under age 24.
  - ____ I have only been driving for a year or less.
- General safety precautions
  - ____ I rarely wear a seat belt.
  - ____ The car I usually drive does not have air bags.
- Driver inattention
  - ____ I talk on the phone or to passengers when I drive.
  - ____ I read texts or e-mails while driving.
  - ____ I send texts while driving.
  - ____ I habitually drive when tired.
- Reckless driving
  - ____ I often exceed the speed limit.
  - ____ I cut in and out of lanes.
  - ____ I rarely signal my turns.
  - ____ I drive under the influence of alcohol, marijuana, or sedative drugs.
- Aggressive driving

_____ I'm easily angered while driving.

_____ I often honk, shout, curse, and make rude gestures.

_____ If the person ahead of me drives too slowly, I tailgate.

_____ When someone cuts me off or otherwise drives rudely, I want to retaliate.

Motorcycle Safety

In 2010, 4,500 motorcyclists died.[19] These deaths composed 14 percent of all road traffic deaths. That figure sounds low—until you consider that motorcyclists covered less than 1 percent of miles traveled in a motorized vehicle.

Helmets save lives and billions of dollars. In the event of a crash, they lower the risk of death by 37 percent and the risk of head injury by nearly 70 percent.[20] Yet only 20 states require that all motorcyclists wear helmets. Twenty-seven states have "partial helmet laws," which require riders and their passengers to wear helmets only if under a certain age or if riding with a learner's permit. Given the risks, there's no good reason *not* to protect the heads of anyone traveling on a motorcycle. You can hear and see fine while wearing them. Concerns about personal freedom and helmet hair seem trivial against the greater backdrop of brain injury and death.

Scooter Safety

Motorized scooters have become popular of late. They're lightweight, fuel efficient, and relatively easy to drive. Make sure you complete the required training before you ride one. While scooters may seem more toylike than motorcycles, you're just as vulnerable if a car or truck hits you.

Safety Tips for Motorcycles and Motorized Scooters

- Wear a helmet.
- Protect your eyes. Proper motorcycle helmets have visors to do just that. Otherwise, wear goggles. Heavier motorcycles should also have a windshield.
- Protect your skin with ample clothing. There's a reason motorcycle enthusiasts wear leather pants, jackets, and boots. Light colors and reflective fabric make you easier to see.
- Take particular care at intersections, which is where most crashes occur. Signal your turns.
- Use your horn to make drivers aware of your presence.
- Pay close attention to what drivers around you are doing.

Bicycle Safety

More Americans are taking up cycling as a way to improve fitness, have fun, and save money on gasoline and parking. When people commute by bike rather than motorized vehicle, they reduce the emission of climate-warming gases.

Unfortunately, relatively few cyclists wear bike helmets. Only 34 percent of college students regularly wear helmets[21]—perhaps due to a false belief that accidents don't happen on college campuses or that helmets look geeky. Helmet-free cyclists are three times more likely to die from a head injury than those who don helmets.[22]

In 2009, 51,000 bicyclists were injured and 630 died in traffic accidents.[23] Many more cyclists go to emergency rooms from some kind of bicycle-related injury. In 97 percent of the deaths, the cyclist wasn't wearing a helmet.[24] Wearing one lowers the risk of injury to the face by 65 percent and to the brain by 88 percent.

Tips for Making Your Bike Ride Safer

- Wear a helmet (and do fasten the strap under your chin) and cycling gloves. Heads and hands are difficult to put back together.
- Make sure your bike fits you. The seat should be just high enough that there's a slight bend at the knee when your leg is extended. Hand brakes should be within easy reach. (To avoid flipping over your bike, squeeze both hand brakes to stop.)
- Obey traffic signs and signals—even if you think you can make it safely across an intersection. When on the road, you're expected to follow the same laws as cars.
- Ride with not against traffic.
- Leave the sidewalk for pedestrians.

- Signal your turns.
- When passing parked cars, stay alert to drivers opening their doors or pulling away from the curb.
- Use lights at night. Mount a headlight and taillight on your bike. You might also want a light on your helmet, arm, or leg. A reflective jacket or vest makes you even more visible.
- Yield to pedestrians.
- Be courteous to drivers. You're in a more vulnerable position than they are.

 Video Clip 12.2

Fitting a Helmet
This National Highway Traffic Safety Association (NHTSA) video explains the importance of properly fitting bike helmets.

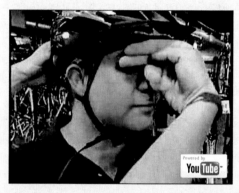

View the video online at: http://www.youtube.com/v/0yzSwxWlJTk

All-Terrain Vehicle (ATV) Safety

You don't normally see ATVs on city streets. Farmers, ranchers, and weekend enthusiasts drive them on dirt roads or in designated off-road regions. People can underestimate their risks because of their small size. The US Consumer Product Safety Commission estimates that 903 people died riding ATVs in 2006.[25] Seventy percent of fatalities occurred in children under age 16—who should not ride on adult ATVs. In 2009, emergency department staff treated 131,900 people with ATV injuries. These injuries stem from excessive speed, rollovers, and collisions.

If you're going to ride an ATV, take a safety training course; stay sober; and wear a helmet, boots, and gloves. Most ATVs aren't designed for passengers. Stay in areas designated for ATV use. Operating them off-road degrades the environment.

Pedestrian Safety

According to the National Highway Traffic Safety Association (NHTSA), traffic accidents killed nearly 4,400 pedestrians and injured another 69,000 in 2008.[26] On average, one pedestrian is injured every eight minutes and one is killed every two hours. About 70 percent of those killed were male. Kids under age five are another at-risk group.

To stay safe when walking, cross in crosswalks at intersections. Obey the signals. Look both ways before you step off the curve. Watch for cars coming around corners. Refrain from darting across streets between intersections. Wear light colors or reflective clothing or carry a flashlight if walking or jogging at night. If there's no sidewalk, walk facing traffic.

Some of your safety depends on infrastructure. Ideally, there's a buffer between the sidewalk and the road. Favor well-lit routes at night. Nearby buildings with windows facing the street (and occupants who might witness an accident or violent act) also increase your safety.

1.2 Home Safety

The expression "safe as houses" can provide a false sense of security about one's home. Injuries within the home are second only to motor vehicle accidents. Examples of accidents within the home include unintentional poisonings, falls, fires, choking, suffocation, and drowning. The age groups at highest risk for most of these calamities are small children and seniors.

Unintentional Poisoning

Poisonings follow motor vehicle accidents as a common cause of fatal unintentional injury. According to the CDC, 87 Americans die a day from unintentional poisoning and nearly 2,300 go to emergency departments for treatment.[27]

Poisons can be ingested, inhaled, injected, and even absorbed through the skin. The highest-risk age group for fatal poisonings are adults ages 45 to 49, mainly because of abuse of prescription medications. Men die at double the rate of women. The race at highest risk for fatal overdose is American Indians and Alaskan Natives.[28]

The very old and the very young are vulnerable to accidental poisoning. Seniors have reduced function of liver and kidney (the organs that break down medications), which increases their risk for toxicity from prescription medications. Because they explore the world with all their senses (including taste), small children are at risk for unintentional poisoning. Caregivers need to supervise small children at all times and keep medications, dietary supplements, personal care products, cleaning products, pesticides, gasoline, paint thinner, antifreeze, poisonous houseplants, and other toxins out of reach. Medications and toxic chemicals should have childproof caps.

Parents also need to double check the proper dosages for prescription and over-the-counter medications intended for children. Adults and children alike are at risk for unintentional overdose from acetaminophen (Tylenol and other brands). Because this medication reduces pain and fever, it's a frequent ingredient in over-the-counter cough, cold, flu, and sinus remedies. Also acetaminophen may be an ingredient in prescription painkillers such as Vicodin (hydrocodone and acetaminophen). Overdose leads to liver damage. In fact, acetaminophen is the most common cause of acute liver failure.[29]

Experts blame opioid pain relievers for the fivefold increase in drug overdose deaths in the United States since 1990.[30] This medication class is derived from the opium poppy and includes codeine, hydrocodone, oxycodone, and morphine. People overdose on their own prescription medications or misuse and abuse medications not intended for them. The illicit drug heroin is also responsible for fatal overdoses.

Sedative drugs (barbiturates, benzodiazepines such as Valium) and alcohol depress the central nervous system. People may lose consciousness and choke on their own vomit. Toxic overdoses also stop the brain's respiratory centers. Teens and young adults are notoriously at risk for alcohol toxicity. Overdose of stimulants such as amphetamines (including those used to treat ADHD), methamphetamine, and cocaine also kill.

If you suspect you or are someone else has ingested a poison, call the American Association of Poison Control Centers at 1-800-222-1222. The person answering can help you identify whether the substance was indeed poisonous and how to proceed. Unless an expert tells you to do so, do not automatically induce vomiting as some substances cause further harm when regurgitated. If someone clearly shows signs of toxicity (including loss of consciousness), take him or her to emergency treatment or call 911. Do not assume someone is simply "sleeping it off."

In terms of inhaled toxins, a common household hazard is *carbon monoxide*, an odorless, colorless gas released during combustion of fossil fuel. Hundreds of Americans die from inhalation each year. The gas is present in automobile exhaust, cigarette smoke, wood smoke, and smoke from charcoal grills.

Properly functioning heating systems, water heaters, gas driers, and gas stoves and ovens emit little carbon monoxide. Have yours—as well as fireplace chimneys—regularly inspected. Dwellings should have carbon monoxide alarms. Never idle a motor vehicle in a garage, even if the door is open. If you experience symptoms of carbon monoxide poisoning (headache, fatigue, shortness of breath, nausea, dizziness) open doors and windows, turn off appliances, and hurry outside. Have someone else take you to the emergency room.[31]

Falls

Each year, about 24,792 Americans die from falls.[32] The death rate is especially high in the very young and the very old. For most age groups, falls most often occur at home. The exceptions are teens and young adults, who spend more time outside the home.

For infants and children, adult vigilance is key to prevention. Caregivers should put infants to sleep in cribs with the slides pulled up. Block stairs with gates. Upstairs windows should be closed or open in such a way that the child could not squeeze through and topple out. Playgrounds are another place where kids need constant supervision.

Frail seniors also need to take precautions by removing scatter rugs and other hazard for tripping and installing handrails in stairways and bathrooms. Falls are especially problematic because, as bone strength declines with age, the risk of serious fractures rises.

People of all ages can take precautions. Here are some examples:

■ Place rubberized mats in the bathtub and liners under rugs.

- Pay attention when using stairs, particularly wet, slick, and icy steps outside the home.
- Watch out for pets, which cause a surprising number of falls by getting underfoot.
- Wear sensible shoes. Tie your shoelaces. Shoes with high platforms and heels can make for unsteady walking. Flip flops can also be hazardous, depending on the conditions.
- Use steady stepstools or ladders when reaching for high objects. If possible, do risky things like cleaning gutters and stringing holiday lights on the roof with a buddy.
- If you drink alcohol or take sedative medications (including antihistamines), be aware that your balance and coordination will be compromised.

Fires

Fires are the number three cause of fatal home injuries.[33] Most people die from inhalation of smoke and toxic gases rather than from burns. Risks for fires in homes stem from cooking, smoking tobacco, and natural gas explosions. Smokers are at particular risk if intoxicated, due to the risk of falling asleep while smoking. Other at-risk groups are children, seniors, and people living in substandard housing.

You can reduce your risk of fire injury. Here's how:

- Avoid intoxication with sedating substances. Alcohol contributes to about 40 percent of residential fires.
- Stay alert while smoking. Never smoke in bed. Better yet, quit.
- Make sure cigarettes, candles, incense, wood fires, and other burning things are properly extinguished.
- Maintain a safe distance between lamps and draperies.
- Clean the lint trap before you start the clothes drier.
- When cooking, make sure cooktops are properly vented. Keep fabric (dish cloths, pot holders, sleeves) away from burners.
- If you live in an old building, don't overload electrical circuits.
- Know the nearest exit in your building and other evacuation procedures.
- If you hear a fire alarm, take it seriously. Get out immediately. Don't delay to gather precious belongings.
- If you're caught inside a burning building, shout "Fire." If the door handle isn't hot, exit the building and then call 911. If a door handle is hot or smoke is coming under the door, don't open it. Put damp towels or other material at the bottom of the door to prevent smoke from entering the room. Call 911. Signal out the window (with a flashlight or colored piece of cloth). Stay low (below the smoke) until your rescuers arrive.
- If your clothes catch fire, stop, drop to the ground, and roll. Do not run.
- For more information, go to the Federal Emergency Management Agency (FEMA) website at ready.gov/fires.

 Audio Link 12.1

A Time to Act

The National Center for Injury Prevention and Control created this podcast to help keep you safe in the event of a fire.

http://www2c.cdc.gov/podcasts/player.asp?f=47788

Water Safety

Each day about 10 people drown.[34] Twenty percent of drowning victims are children under the age of 14. Small children are particularly at risk, mainly because they can't swim. Infants and toddlers can drown in small amounts of water—in bathtubs, toilets, puddles, and buckets. Other home-related risks include private swimming pools and hot tubs. Bodies of water outside the home add to the hazards. Even able-bodied adults have drowned in creeks after slipping and knocking themselves unconscious.

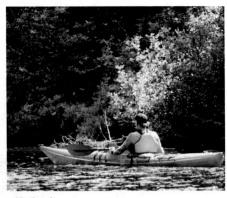
© Thinkstock

Anyone taking care of children needs to supervise them around water, even if they're wearing life jackets or other flotation devices. Barriers around pools and ponds offer some protection.

Do the following to keep yourself safe in the water:

- Take swimming lessons before you take the plunge.
- Never swim alone, immediately after eating, or while intoxicated.
- Wear a personal flotation device (life vest) when kayaking, rafting, boating, and water skiing.
- Don't operate watercraft while intoxicated.
- Be particularly cautious in cold water. You can become hypothermic and have difficulty swimming back to shore.
- Limit hot tub soaking to 15 minutes. The heat amplifies the effects of alcohol and sedative drugs. If you pass out in the hot tub, you could drown.
- Take a CPR (cardiopulmonary resuscitation) class so you know what to do if you encounter someone in the midst of drowning.

Suffocation and Choking

Infants and small children are at particular risk. Each year, nearly 1,000 children **suffocate** (die from an inability to breathe).[35] Newborn babies don't have the strength to raise their heads and turn over if bedding obstructs their mouth and nose. The American Academy of Pediatrics now recommends that infants under six months of age be put to bed lying on their backs on firm surfaces. Kids should also be closely watched so they don't encounter plastic bags or become trapped in refrigerators (or other unventilated spaces).

suffocation

Death from an inability to breathe or oxygen deprivation.

Choking is an inability to breathe because the throat or trachea (windpipe) is blocked. A common scenario is chunks of food (or other foreign objects) get stuck in the throat or "go down the wrong way," meaning into the trachea rather than the esophagus (tube connecting mouth and stomach). Air exchange with the lungs abruptly stops.

choking

An inability to breathe because the throat or trachea (windpipe) is blocked.

Again, children under age four are the high-risk group. They don't have all their teeth and lack complete muscle coordination for thoroughly chewing and swallowing. For that reason and others, infants should not be fed solid food (and then, only selected, pureed foods) until six months of age. Don't give small children foods that could stick in their throats. Examples include hot dogs, popcorn, nuts, peanuts, hard candy, chewing gum, raw carrots, whole grapes, and peanut butter. Small toys, which little children tend to put in their mouths, are another hazard.

Elderly people have weakened swallow, cough, and gag reflexes, which put them at risk for choking too. But people of all ages can choke when eating too quickly and trying simultaneously to swallow, talk, and breathe. Intoxication increases the risk of choking and of passing out and suffocating on one's own vomit.

Video Clip 12.3

How to Help a Choking Victim
As explained in this ABC *Good Morning, America* segment, if someone is choking, you can help by delivering five back blows and then five abdominal thrusts.

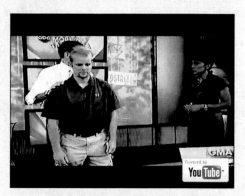

View the video online at: http://www.youtube.com/v/O9pgQ5bs2K4

Firearm Safety

In an analysis of firearm fatality in 23 high-income countries, 80 percent of all deaths occurred in the United States, and the vast majority of deaths were women and children. Unintentional firearm deaths alone were more than five times higher in developed countries.[36] Two-thirds of these accidents occur in the home.

The main reason for the staggering rate of firearm death and injury is accessibility. The United States is the most armed country in the world. Some 270 million Americans own guns.[37] A third of families with children have firearms in the home.[38] Whereas unintentional shootings account for 3 percent of firearm deaths overall, the statistic reaches 20 percent in children under age 14. Even a small child can figure out how to fire a gun. Compared to other developed countries, American children 5 to 14 years old are 11 times more likely to be accidentally shot to death.[39] The next section of this chapter will discuss their contribution to the death toll from homicides and suicides.

If you're around firearms, follow recommended safety tips:

- Don't operate a firearm without proper training.
- Keep the safety on, except when firing the weapon.
- Store firearms unloaded and in a locked cabinet. Make sure keys to the storage area are well hidden.
- If you pick up a gun, assume it's loaded.
- Never point a gun (even if you think it's unloaded) at another living creature, unless your intent is to wound or kill.
- Wear colorful clothing (red hat and vests) when outdoors during hunting season. Tie colorful material (e.g., red bandana, orange ribbons) to dogs and horses.

1.3 Wilderness Safety

While being out in nature has a number of health benefits, it's not without risks. You can become lost, injured, or engulfed in bad weather.

Here are a few tips for staying safe in the great outdoors:

- Learn orienteering skills, including using a map and a compass.
- Never hike, climb, ski, raft, canoe, kayak, or otherwise travel alone.
- Tell friends your itinerary.
- Stay on designated trails. You'll be easier to find and reduce your impact on fragile ecosystems.
- Bring more water, food, and clothing than you think you need. In many wilderness areas, weather can change quickly.
- If you get lost or if bad weather interferes with navigation, stay put.

- Learn the best ways to respond if you should encounter potentially dangerous wildlife such as mountain lions (cougars), bears, moose, and venomous snakes.
- Take a wilderness safety class. For more information, check out the Center for Wilderness Safety website, http://www.wildsafe.org.

 Video Clip 12.4

Aron Ralston Discusses His Near-Death Wilderness Experience

In 2003, Aron Ralston set out on a canyoneering adventure southeastern Utah. He traveled alone and without informing anyone of his itinerary. While he was at the bottom of a slot canyon, a boulder fell, crushing his arm. After five and a half days (with little food and water), he amputated his own arm and escaped. In this video, he discusses the meaning of this experience.

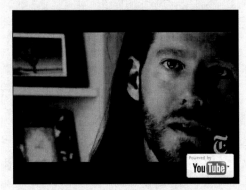

View the video online at: http://www.youtube.com/v/h91lptsl5CM

1.4 Workplace Injuries

This type of injury varies by occupation. Miners and computer programmers occupy entirely different environments. Nevertheless, most workers are vulnerable to two particular types of injury: repetitive strain injuries and back injuries.

Repetitive strain injuries arise when the same movement is repeated over and over. Damage occurs to soft tissues such as tendons, muscles, and nerves. Pain and impaired function result. The exact injury depends on the repeated action. For example, golfers, tennis players, and baseball pitchers tend to injure elbows and shoulders.

People who work at computer keyboards are vulnerable to **carpal tunnel syndrome**. Frequent use of a keypad on a phone or other device can also cause problems. The carpal tunnel is the narrow passageway at the base of the hand that's packed with bones, blood vessels, ligaments, tendons, and nerves. Repetitive motion inflames the tendons, which leads to compression of the median nerve. That nerve controls the fingers, except for the pinkie finger. Symptoms include pain, tingling, weakness, and numbness of the hand and wrist.

Anti-inflammatory medications, exercises, and wearing splints (to keep the wrist straight) can relieve carpal tunnel syndrome. Sometimes surgery is needed to relieve the pressure. Prevention is best. Position your keyboard and mouse at or below elbow height. If you work on a laptop, consider investing in an external keyboard. Place the monitor at a position that allows you to keep your head and neck in a neutral position. Take breaks to stretch your fingers and wrists, as well as your back, neck, and shoulders.

Back injuries are a common ailment in the United States. The usual cause of acute back injury is heavy lifting. If you need to lift something, put your feet hip distance apart and bend your knees and hips, keeping your back straight and your core muscles firm. If the object feels too heavy or too unwieldy, quit and ask for help.

repetitive strain injury

Pain and impaired function due to prolonged repetition of a movement.

Video Clip 12.5

Carpal Tunnel Syndrome
This video explains the causes and symptoms of carpal tunnel syndrome.

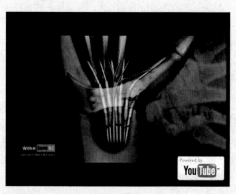

View the video online at: http://www.youtube.com/v/J11ElfiHMYw

Quick Wrist Relief from the Keyboard

After an hour of pecking on your keyboard and keypad, sit up straight or stand. Hold your right arm straight ahead of you at a 90-degree angle to your body. Rotate your elbow upward and extend your fingers toward the ground (thumb pointing to your side). Using the fingers on your left hand, pull your pinkie finger slowly toward your torso. Move sequentially, finger by finger, toward your thumb. Repeat on the other side.

Now hold your right arm straight ahead, palm up, as though you're stopping traffic. Curl your pinkie toward your palm, then the ringer, middle finger, index finger, and thumb. Now flex your wrist slowly, so that your knuckles angle toward the floor. Hold and feel the stretch. Release. Wave your hand. Repeat on the other side.

KEY TAKEAWAYS

- Unintentional injuries are the number one cause of death in people younger than 45. Young men are more likely to die from unintentional injuries than women.
- Motor vehicle accidents represent the most common cause of death due to unintentional injury. Other common fatalities stem from unintentional poisonings, drowning, and firearm accidents.
- The main causes of motor vehicle accidents are driver inattention (cell phone use); alcohol; drugs; drowsiness; and aggressive, reckless driving.
- Everyone can take steps to prevent and protect themselves from unintentional injuries.

DISCUSSION QUESTIONS

1. Given your daily routine, which of the common unintentional injuries are you most at risk for? What puts you at risk for this type of injury? What could you do right now to prevent or protect yourself from an accident?

2. Imagine you're taking care of a five-year-old. This child wants to ride his or her new bicycle but balks at putting on the helmets and gloves. How might you handle the situation? Why should you also wear a helmet when riding with him or her?

3. Currently, 21 states ban concealed weapons on college campuses. Some states leave the decision up to individual colleges. (For a list, go to http://www.ncsl.org/issues-research/educ/guns-on-campus-overview.aspx.) Colorado, Mississippi, Oregon, Utah, and Wisconsin allow concealed weapons on campus. What is the policy on your campus for owning a firearm? If your college or university allows students to possess a firearm, how must they be stored? Are guns allowed in dormitories? Do you think students should be able to carry concealed guns on campus? Explain your opinion.

2. INTENTIONAL INJURIES

LEARNING OBJECTIVES

1. Explore the factors contributing to violence in this country.
2. Identify, define, and review key facts about the different types of intentional injuries.
3. Explore ways to prevent and protect yourself from violent crimes.
4. Identify resources for people who experience or witness violent acts.

As mentioned, intentional injuries are those performed with the goal of inflicting psychological or physical harm. The word "violence" is often used synonymously with intentional injury. The World Health Organization (WHO) defines **violence** as "the intentional use of physical force or power, threatened or actual, against oneself, another person, or against a group or community, that either results in or has a high likelihood of resulting in injury, death, psychological harm, maldevelopment, or deprivation."[40]

Notice the definition says that force doesn't necessarily have to be delivered. Threatening harm can cause significant psychological and physical suffering. Also the violence can be directed at oneself, as in self-mutilation and suicide. Violence can occur among friends, family members, coworkers, and strangers. A single person or a group can be responsible for the attack.

A 2012 Federal Bureau of Investigation report revealed that violent crime dropped 4 percent in 2011, the fifth straight year of decline.[41] Homicides, aggravated assault (attempting to cause or causing bodily harm with a weapon), rape (a type of sexual assault involving sexual intercourse), and robbery all went down. So did property crimes such as automobile theft and burglary. The trend ran counter to prediction that the economic recession would spur crime. A review of the risk factors for violence reveals the rationale for that bleak prediction.

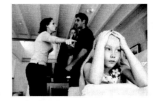

© *Thinkstock*

violence

The intentional use of actual or threatened physical force capable of resulting in physical injury, psychological harm, deprivation, or death.

2.1 Factors Contributing to Violence

Most violence is committed in association with another crime or in a moment of high emotion. Several factors increase the odds that individuals resort to violence.

- **Poor parenting.** Parents and other caregivers shape their children's empathy (the ability to understand another person's feelings). In the ideal, they help children develop empathy, compassion, respect, and self-control. They teach their children to temper strong emotions and solve conflicts with well-chosen words, not fists. They discipline with love and logic rather than punishing with blows, harsh words, and deprivation.

  Physical punishment of children has been linked to subsequent aggression and psychopathic and criminal behavior.[42] While many parents deem spanking an acceptable punishment, studies show that young children who are spanked have higher levels of aggression.[43] Kids who have witnessed family violence or have been hurt by a family member are more likely to become bullies and to use violence as a means of achieving personal ends.

- **Cultural beliefs.** Cultures around the world vary widely in their views about the acceptability of violence, including violence against women and minority groups. Even within the United States, rates of violence vary by region. Violent crimes tend to be higher in the South and West, perhaps, in part because of prevailing attitudes about the justification for such acts.

  Media violence is thought to desensitize people to violence. Children and teens who see more violence on television, the Internet, and in video games tend to behave more aggressively.[44],[45] It's not yet clear whether media exposure actually leads to violent crime.[46] The media also affects attitudes about gender-based violence, which is covered in a separate section. Critics point out that, while today's youth witness more media violence than previous generations, crime rates have steadily fallen.

- **Religious beliefs.** Strongly held religious beliefs can have expected and paradoxical effects on violent behavior. Most religions preach peace. But some religions also promote subjugation of women and intolerance of other religions and homosexuality. Violent acts, including wars, have ignited over religious hatred. Religious differences can also match with political differences to incite anger and civil unrest.

- **Availability of firearms.** As discussed in the section on unintentional injuries, firearms contribute hugely to injuries—both intended and unintended. (See the sidebar Section 2 for more details.)

- **Poverty and unemployment.** Low socioeconomic status is stressful. Unemployment creates a sense of hopelessness and desperation. Drug trafficking and other crimes can become tantalizing sources of income, an avenue that often spawns violence.

- **Inequality and discrimination.** Many countries exhibit a large divide between the rich and the poor. That phenomenon has become increasingly apparent in the United States. The inequality also extends to education, which further widens the rift. Discrimination based on social class, race, gender, sexual preference, and disability can breed resentment.

- **Gangs.** Poverty, unemployment, and neighborhood crime can herd people into gang associations. While gang membership may provide a sense of security, many gangs become involved with crime, which only degrades neighborhood safety.

- **Illicit drugs and alcohol.** These substances alter mental status, impairing judgment and reason. Furthermore, drug trafficking is a crime associated with violence.

- **Failure of criminal justice systems.** Jails and prisons are overcrowded and often lack the tools to rehabilitate criminals before release. Furthermore, some (usually poorer) neighborhoods are not as well policed as others.

- **Gender and race.** Men are more often perpetrators of violence. Women and children bear the brunt of domestic violence. When it comes to homicides and suicides, more men die than women. African American men under age 35 are the highest risk group.[47] For them, homicides are the leading cause of death.

- **Personal characteristics.** Poor anger management and impulsivity can cause people to act rashly in the heat of the moment.

FIGURE 12.3 Rate of Civilian Firearms Ownership by Country

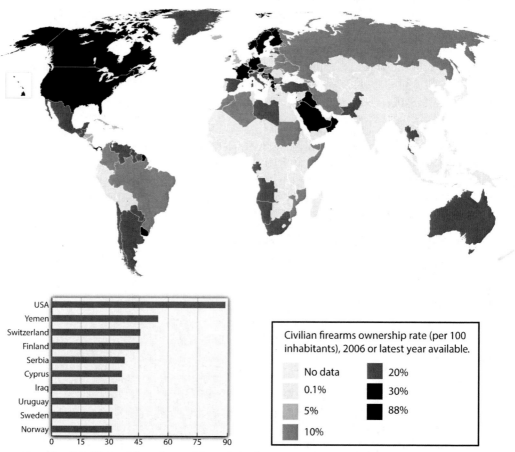

Source: Adapted from United Nations Office on Drugs and Crime Civilian firearms ownership, 2006 or latest year available (Figure 119).

Transnational Organized Crime Threat Assessment Report: Firearms. Available at: http://www.unodc.org/documents/data-and-analysis/tocta/

6.Firearms.pdf. Originally published in Karp A. Completing the count: civilian firearms. Small Arms Survey 2007: Guns and the City. Cambridge

University Press.

2.2   Guns and Violence

According to a report from the United Nations Office on Drugs and Crime, Americans owned 270 million private firearms in 2006.[48] Compare that to 3 million firearms in England and Wales. (Even British police are unarmed.[49]) Just under half of American men and 10 percent of women own a gun.[50] Out of the top 10 countries for civilian firearm ownership, the United States came in first.

Each year, nearly 100,000 Americans are shot—an average of about 270 people a day.[51] According to National Center for Injury Prevention and Control data for 2010, gun violence killed over 31,500 people and injured over 66,700.[52] Most of those deaths are suicides (over 19,000). Firearm-related homicides topped 11,000. Approximately 600 gun-related deaths were unintentional.

Women and children are more often injured or killed by guns in the home. Men are more often murdered outside of the home. In the case of battered women (and their children), their gun-owning male partners often use guns to scare, intimate, harm, and kill.

Currently, it's easy to buy a gun. Background checks at gun stores take mere minutes for people without criminal records. Other avenues (e.g., gun shows and private sales through classified ads) for buying guns require no background check.[53] A national survey of high school students found that almost 17 percent had carried some kind of weapon (gun, knife, or club) to school.

However, four mass shootings in 2012—at a movie theater in Aurora, Colorado; a Sikh temple in Oak Creek, Wisconsin; a mall in Portland, Oregon; and an elementary school in Newtown, Connecticut—have revived discussions of stricter gun regulations, including more rigorous background checks and bans on assault weapons (automatic and semiautomatic firearms, which are capable or discharging many bullets in rapid succession). Until 2004, there was a federal ban against assault weapons. Unfortunately, in April 2013, the United States Senate defeated a bill that would have required expanded background checks and a ban on military-style semiautomatic weapons.[54]

At the time of this writing, lawmakers are discussing changes in gun laws such as reinstating a ban on assault weapons. Powerful organizations such as the National Rifle Association (NRA) counter that the Second Amendment of the US Bill of Rights guarantees our right to bear arms. Others counter that this amendment refers to "a well-armed Militia," which is part of the organized armed forces.

Even if gun laws tightened, many guns remain in circulation. Australia solved that issue when, in 1996, the government passed the National Firearms Agreement. In addition to banning assault weapons, the law created a compulsory buyback program. The government bought back over 650,000 weapons. The percentage of households owning guns was nearly halved. Gun massacres ground to a halt. The homicide rate declined by 42 percent and the suicide rate declined by 58 percent.[55]

In the wake of the December 2012 elementary school shooting in Connecticut, nearly 600 guns were handed over at buyback programs in Oakland and San Francisco, California.[56] A buyback program in Los Angeles the previous May led to the collection of 1,650 firearms.[57] In counterpoint, the NRA's solution is not to change gun regulations but to install armed guards at schools.[58]

Granted, the majority of people who own guns aren't murderers. Compared to the handgun homicides that so commonly occur, mass murders are rare. Tougher regulations of firearm sales would not make the privately owned guns already in circulation vanish.

But what about the potential benefits of civilians owning firearms? Civilians typically buy rifles and shotguns to hunt or for target shootings and handguns for protection against crime. However, repeated studies fail to prove that gun ownership reduces crime.[59] Instead, gun ownership and violence rise in tandem. Gun owners actually increase the risk of violent death. Assaults, robberies, and other crimes become more deadly. In a moment of uncontrollable rage, a gun can become a deadly object. Laws restricting firearms result in a decline in suicides, homicides, and other violent acts.[60]

Audio Link 12.2

"I Just Wish Guns Were Harder to Come By"

In this Youth Radio segment, Davina La'Shay shares her intimate knowledge of gun violence in Oakland, California.

http://www.npr.org/2012/12/20/167739908/commentary-i-just-wish-guns-were-harder-to-come-by

Davina La'Shay. I just wish guns were harder to come by. National Public Radio, Youth Radio. 2012.

2.3   Child Maltreatment

Every day, older children and adults mistreat those younger, smaller, and more vulnerable. According to the CDC, state and local agencies receive three million reports of child maltreatment each year—about six reports a minute.[61] Children are neglected and abused emotionally, physically, and sexually.

Child neglect means that basic needs—food, clothing, shelter, education, safety, medical care, and emotional warmth—are withheld. Sometimes the responsible adults don't intend harm but rather can simply not provide for all the needs. For instance, a single parent may feel she has little choice but to leave a child alone while she works.

With **child abuse**, words or actions deliberately harm the child. Some people underestimate harsh words and relentless criticism. As you learned in Chapter 3, the resultant psychological distress can ultimately lead to biological changes that adversely affect mental, emotional, psychological, and physical health. Likewise, sexual and physical abuse injures more than the body.

Consequences are dire, particularly for small children. In addition to broken bones, burns, and brain injury, these kids are more at risk for substance abuse; depression; anxiety; posttraumatic stress disorder (PTSD); eating disorders; behavioral problems (aggression, conduct disorder); suicide; and difficulties with learning, attention, and memory.[62] Largely due to increased reactivity of the stress response, abused children are more likely to become adults with chronic conditions such as cardiovascular disease, obesity, metabolic syndrome, and diabetes.[63]

Kids who grow up in an environment where important adults betrayed them often have difficulty establishing trusting, intimate relationships of their own. When children witness partner violence, they may repeat the cycle in adulthood. And for lack of positive role models, they may lack the skills to parent their own children. In short, both quality of life and overall longevity decline. Remarkably, these ills don't befall all maltreated children. Some resilient individuals manage to survive with their humanity intact and grow into wise, loving, and productive adults.

Comprehensive programs aimed at preventing child maltreatment exist. Such programs provide education and support to disadvantaged parents and their children. For example, nurses can make home visits to new parents to encourage good child-rearing skills. A program funded by the CDC called the Triple P (positive parenting program) has been shown to improve parenting skills and benefit children.[64]

2.4   Youth Violence

The Globe Town Massive Bengali or Bangladeshi youth gang in east London.

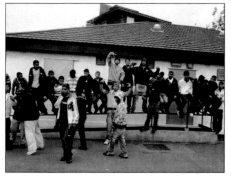

Source: http://commons.wikimedia.org/wiki/File:GTM.JPG.

Youth violence refers to harmful acts occurring during childhood and adolescence. The violent acts can include bullying, hitting, robbing, and destroying property. Kids may use weapons to threaten or inflict injury. Violence can occur in the home, at school, and in the greater community. Regardless of whether young people are victims, offenders, or witnesses, the ill effects can persist. Young offenders often grow up to be violent adults.

Youth gangs can become enticing. They offer a sense of belonging, identity, purpose, protection, and safety in numbers. Although gangs are more prevalent in larger cities, they also occur in small cities, suburbs, and rural communities, taking root in neighborhoods marked by poverty and poorly functioning families and schools. According to the National Gang Center at the Bureau of Justice Assistance, gangs became more numerous in the 1980s and 1990s, declined in the early 2000s, then proliferated over more recent years.[65] Between 2002 and 2007, youth gangs increased 25 percent in many areas.

These associations often attempt to control a neighborhood. To exert and maintain control, other gangs can't be tolerated. Fights among gangs, especially when members have weapons, have maimed and killed gang members and innocent bystanders. Drug trafficking creates additional risks. Juvenile offenders can end up in prison or other correctional facilities.

Bullying

Unwanted, repeated aggressive behavior can be used with the express purpose of creating or perpetuating a perceived imbalance of power. A child bully may use physical strength or social status to coerce another child into doing something. As with other forms of violence, the underlying pathology seems to be a perverse desire for power and control, or simply a sadistic enjoyment of causing suffering.

Bullying can be verbal, social, and physical.[66] Verbal bullying includes teasing; taunting; name-calling; making inappropriate sexual remarks; threatening to harm; and using derogatory terms aimed at undermining a person's race, gender, or perceived sexual preference.

Bullies may also socially ostracize other kids. They deliberately exclude the victim from activities, create social alliances against him or her, spread vicious rumors, and attempt to publicly humiliate the victim. Physical bullying can include physical blows, shoving, tripping, spitting, and stealing or breaking possessions.

A lot of bullying occurs on or near school grounds and on school buses. A Massachusetts study found that about 44 percent of middle school students and over 30 percent of high school students had been either been victims of bullying or had bullied others or both.[67]

Cyberbullying involves the use of electronic technology. Rumors can quickly go viral. It's also difficult to escape the 24-7 onslaught of electronic abuse.

A survey of American high school seniors revealed than one in six had been bullied in e-mail, texts, chat rooms, and social media websites.[68] One in five had been bullied on school grounds. The highest risk group overall was white, ninth-grade girls. On a more cheerful note, bullying declines with age. This survey did not specifically examine bullying of lesbian, gay, bisexual, and transgendered (LGBT) youth.

The consequences are great. Victims may avoid going to school. Academic performance falls, substance use rises, and mental health deteriorates. Middle school and high school can challenge self-esteem—even if no one deliberately torments you. When others seemingly make it their mission to convince you of your low worth, it can be tough not to buy the lie.

Furthermore, bullies and their victims were more at risk for intentional self-injury and suicidal thoughts. Victims may eventually retaliate. An extreme example is the massacre at Columbine High School in Colorado in 1999. Allegedly, the two shooters had been bullied and socially marginalized.

Increasingly, schools have begun to adopt zero-tolerance policies for violent behaviors and for bringing weapons or guns to school. Bullying and other acts of violence need to be reported. The bullies often threaten to further harm the victim (or someone he or she loves) if the victim tells an authority figure of the violent act. Nevertheless, reporting can stop the problem.

Young bullies can grow into adults who continue to intimidate and hurt. If you're a victim, gather evidence. Record dates and times of cyberbullying and real-time aggression. Report cyberbullying to social media sites. Contact campus police for other acts of aggression. If you or someone else is at immediate risk, call 911. For more information, go to http://www.stopbullying.gov.

 Video Clip 12.6

Ellen DeGeneres Speaks Out against Bullying
Actor Ellen DeGeneres addresses the epidemic of bullying in this country. She cites recent deaths of teens and young adults, focusing on those singled out for their sexual orientation. She wants kids to know there is hope.

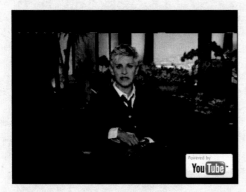

View the video online at: http://www.youtube.com/v/ddg-1v2esjM

Violence and Sexual Orientation

Lesbians, gays, bisexuals, and transgendered (LGBT) people are too often the victims of discrimination and violence. Violent acts include teasing, bullying, and verbal and physical harassment. A 2009 survey showed that 80 percent of LGBT middle- and high-school students experienced verbal harassment and 40 percent experienced physical harassment at school.[69] Although many LGBT youth remain happy and well-adjusted, persecution can drive others to depression, substance use, and suicidal thoughts and behaviors.

Video Clip 12.7

It Gets Better

Stephen Colbert talks about bullying of LGBT youth. The video is part of the larger It Gets Better Project, which was created to let LGBT teens know that the torment does come to an end. For more information, go to http://www.itgetsbetterproject.com.

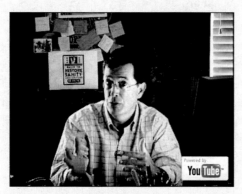

View the video online at: http://www.youtube.com/v/BThRZbCs-p8

Violence on College Campuses

Many college campuses seem downright idyllic—red bricks, ivy, manicured gardens. The ambiance can instill a false sense of security. As you may have noticed, the environment of a college or university differs vastly from a high school. The campus may spread over many acres. No teachers or parents are keeping track of your whereabouts. Anyone can stroll onto a college campus. Newly emancipated youth may overindulge in alcohol and drugs, which increases the likelihood of being the perpetrator or victim of violence.

Higher education institutions are required to track and report crimes on campus. Between 2005 and 2008, almost 75 percent of campus crimes were burglaries and motor vehicle thefts. More than 9 percent are *aggravated assaults* (attempts to cause or causing bodily injury, often with a weapon), 8.4 percent with robberies, and almost 6 percent were sexual offences involving physical force. Homicides represented only 0.1 percent of crimes, with 220 deaths reported in that time period.[70]

Higher education institutions actively work to ensure the safety of millions of people on their campuses. It's a daunting job. The Virginia Tech massacre of 2007 showed that a single psychologically disturbed individual with a gun can quickly kill and injure scores of people.

Types of Campus Violence

hazing

Actions taken by members of a group upon initiation that produce mental or physical discomfort or harm to new members.

Hazing, according to StopHazing.org, "refers to any activity expected of someone joining a group (or to maintain full status in a group) that humiliates, degrades or risks emotional and/or physical harm, regardless of the person's willingness to participate." In order to join, new gang members often have to endure hazing. Hazing occurs in military academies and in the military proper.

On college campuses, activities most commonly occur as an initiation rite into fraternities, sororities, athletic teams, marching bands, secret societies, and other clubs. The 2008 National Study of Student Hazing found that 55 percent of college students in such organizations experienced hazing.[71] Moreover, 47 percent of students surveyed had been hazed during high school.

The activities range from embarrassing to abusive. Ordeals may include verbal abuse, scavenger hunts, servitude, social isolation, embarrassing attire, chugging alcohol, forced feedings (usually of something vile), kidnappings, forced stripping, head shaving, performing calisthenics to the point of exhaustion, sexual assault, and beatings. Students have died.

Hazing is not a series of harmless pranks. It represents an abuse of perceived power, is morally wrong, and, in most states, is illegal. Refuse to take part in it. Report it. If you're a new member of an athletic team, contact the coach or someone in the athletic office. Otherwise, if you're unsure whom to speak to, contact the student affairs office. Other resources include faculty, staff, and residence assistants.

Video Clip 12.8

Fraternity Hazing
This news profile discusses the closure of a University of Nebraska fraternity after reports of hazing and underage drinking.

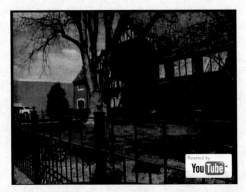

View the video online at: http://www.youtube.com/v/HywO1tF3KV4

Hate crimes occur on and off campus. The US Congress has defined **hate crime** as a "criminal offense against a person or property motivated in whole or in part by an offender's bias against a race, religion, disability, ethnic origin or sexual orientation."[72] These crimes include assault, homicide, arson, and vandalism.

Hate speech is communication—verbal, written, or symbolic—that expresses hatred toward a group. The intent is usually to intimidate and/or incite violence. Like hate crimes, the offenders assail and harass their victims based on race, gender, sexual orientation, ethnicity, religion, or disability. This information may be conveyed in graffiti, on posters, on fliers, in e-mails, in chat groups, on social media sites, and on clothing.

While the First Amendment guarantees free speech, hate speech has no purpose other than to harm. We have a fundamental right to express our thoughts, but not to the extent that such expression tramples another person's dignity. Many higher education institutions have adopted conduct codes calling for civil discourse and prohibiting hate speech. Courts have struck down some codes as violating the First Amendment.

Stalking is repetitive, unwanted harassment or threatening behavior. Stalkers may follow; spy on (in real time and on social media sites); or repeatedly talk to, write, phone, text, or e-mail a victim. They may also send gifts. In most cases, stalking is a form of sexual harassment.[73] Stalkers may be strangers, acquaintances, or current or former intimate partners. In a national survey of college students, 7 percent of women and 3.8 percent of men had been stalked.[74]

If you are stalked, gather evidence. Keep a log, take photos, and save texts, e-mails, phone messages, and letters. Get witnesses. Contact the police. You may need to change your phone number and e-mail address and remove yourself from social networking sites. Travel with a buddy. Most college campuses offer a number you can call to have someone walk you back to the dorm at night.

Sexual harassment, sexual assault, and intimate partner violence are all forms of gender-based violence. These crimes do occur on college campuses. We'll discuss them in the section titled "Gender-Based Violence."

hate crime

Any crime motivated by the offender's bias race, religion, sexual orientation, or disability.

hate speech

Communication with no other purpose than to express hatred toward some group.

stalking

Repetitive, unwanted harassment or threatening behavior.

Staying Safe on Campus

As you've seen, crime occurs on college campuses. You can, however, take a number of precautions to protect yourself.

- Travel in groups, especially at night. At night, stay on well-lit, well-traveled routes. Take earbuds out of your ears.
- Program into your phone the number for campus security and the number for escorts when traveling across campus alone at night. Most campuses also have call boxes.
- Don't prop open the door to your residence so a friend can get in. Don't give out your key or your electronic fob. Instead, have your friend phone you when he or she arrives.
- Keep the door to your room locked.

- Keep valuables in a locked drawer. Use a cable to lock your laptop to your desk.
- Don't give or accept rides from strangers.
- Have your keys in your hand as you head for your car. Lock the doors after you get in. Don't linger in an unlocked, parked car checking your e-mail or texting or doing anything else that makes you unaware of your surroundings.
- Report suspicious activity and crime.
- Form a buddy system. Tell your roommate or a friend where you're going at night.
- Stay safe when drinking. You need to remain aware of what's going on around you. Watch out for your friends at parties too.
- Get to know people gradually. Be careful about divulging intimate information (including your phone number) too quickly. Meet with strangers in public places during the daytime. If someone you meet makes you uncomfortable, trust your instincts and leave. If someone in your residence is bothering you, contact your resident assistance.

If you ever feel in danger, call campus security immediately. If you don't know that number, dial 911.

2.5 Gender-Based Violence

gender-based violence

Any unwanted act on the basis of gender that produces physical, sexual, or psychological harm and that result from power inequities.

Gender-based violence is any unwanted act on the basis of gender that produces physical, sexual, or psychological harm and that results from power inequities. Because of their subordinate status in many cultures, women are most often the victims and men are usually the perpetrators.[75] When women assail male partners, it's usually in self-defense.

The WHO notes that violence against women can include genital mutilation, forced or early marriage, deprivation of liberty, sexual exploitation and abuse, and intimate-partner violence.

Other at-risk groups include those who are under age 24, LGBT, mentally disabled, poor, homeless, institutionalized, immigrants, and drug and alcohol abusers.[76] College students are at risk because of their age, relative lack of supervision, rampant use of intoxicating substances, and a false perception of safety. Men, particularly those who don't conform to traditional ideals about masculinity, can also become victims. Ethnicity figures in, with the highest rates of abuse directed at American Indian and Alaska Native women. Prisons, jails, and juvenile detention centers are risky places for men and women.[77] The military isn't exactly a safe haven.[78]

Types of Gender-Based Violence

The following acts—all of which violate human rights and US law—fall under the umbrella of gender-based violence:

sexual harassment

Any form of unwelcome sexual advance.

Sexual harassment is any form of unwelcome sexual advance. It can include unwanted sexual touching or gestures; repeated requests for a person's phone number, a date, or sexual favors; and verbal or written sexual or derogatory comments and jokes. As with sexual assault, the harasser may wrongfully use his or her power and authority at work, at school, or on the playing field to pressure the victim. In addition to occurring on college campuses, this crime may happen in the workplace or anywhere else that people congregate. As with stalking, it's important to gather evidence and report the behavior to police or other authorities.

sexual assault

Any unwanted sexual touching (regardless of whether the person touched is fully clothed), child molestation, incest, rape, and attempted rape.

Sexual assault is any unwanted sexual touching (regardless of whether the person touched is fully clothed), child molestation, incest, rape, and attempted rape. It can also include being forced to view or participate in pornography.

rape

A type of sexual assault involving unwanted penetration of a body orifice (mouth, vagina, or anus) accomplished by physical force, threat of harm, or incapacitation.

Rape, which falls under the umbrella of sexual assault, refers to unwanted penetration of a body orifice (mouth, vagina, or anus) accomplished by physical force, threat of harm, or incapacitation. From a legal standpoint, people considered incapable of giving consent are those who are very young or old and intoxicated with drugs or alcohol.

Intimate-partner violence is defined by a pattern of activity wherein one partner gains and maintains power and control over the other through coercion, intimidation, isolation, and brute force. Violence occurs within heterosexual and homosexual relationships. Aggression against intimate partners often begins in junior high school. For that reason, prevention strategies are increasingly targeting younger populations.

intimate-partner violence

A pattern of activity wherein one partner gains and maintains power and control over the other through coercion, intimidation, isolation, and brute force.

Statistics about Gender-Based Violence

Underreporting of these crimes makes them difficult to quantify precisely. Violence affecting the LGBT community may be particularly underreported.[79] Nevertheless, the statistics are grim. A 2013 WHO report found that approximately 35 percent of women worldwide experience physical or sexual violence—most often violence at the hands of an intimate partner. In addition, 38 percent of murdered women were killed by intimate partners.[80]

At some point in their lives, about 20 percent of women are raped.[81] In a single year, rape strikes over 300,000 women and nearly 93,000 men.[82] Many victims are minors. Most victims of sexual assault know their assailants.[83] Unfortunately, most rapes and sexual assaults are not reported and not medically treated.[84]

College students are particularly vulnerable. A study of college women found that over 11 percent had been raped.[85] More than half of these rapes occur on dates.[86] On college campuses, acquaintances commit about 85 percent of rapes or attempted rapes.

Causes and Consequences of Gender-Based Violence

A key element in gender-based violence is unequal power relationships. A major reason that women and girls are so often the victims is that, in many cultures, women and children have less power than men. Assailants use violence to gain or maintain power and control. Around the world, such violence continues because of prevailing cultural attitudes that such violence is somehow acceptable, lack of legal prohibition, and justice systems that fail to punish perpetrators.

Aside from physical force, assailants may use psychological measures. For instance, the abuser may threaten job loss, academic failure, the loss of status on an athletic team, or violence to the victim or someone dear to him or her. Or the abuser may promise promotion, academic/athletic success, and so on. He or she may deceive, humiliate, insult, or otherwise manipulate and intimidate the victim. Any of these means of forcing or attempting to force someone to engage in sexual acts count as *coercion*.

The consequences of gender-based violence are both psychological and physical. When the attacker is someone previously trusted (parent, teacher, coach, clergy), the devastation tunnels to the spiritual level. A study in women found that those who experienced at least one form of gender-based violence faced a threefold increased risk of anxiety, depression, PTSD, and substance abuse.[87] Repeated abuse increases the likelihood of those ill effects.

Violent acts can have physical consequences: unplanned pregnancy, sexually transmitted infection, bodily harm, and, worst of all, death. In the United States in 2005, 1,181 women (more than 3 women a day) and 329 men died at the hands of their intimate partners (spouses, ex-spouses, boyfriends, girlfriends).[88] On a brighter note, the numbers of reported cases of both fatal and nonfatal partner violence have steadily declined over the past three decades.

While support services exist, women don't often access these resources. For victims who are socially and economically disadvantaged, escape can seem impossible. Victims stay with their abusers out of fear, financial dependence, and even love. In some countries, laws and religious beliefs may restrict a woman's ability to leave her husband.

In the United States, at best one-third of rape victims report the crime to law enforcement or to their doctor. Men are more likely to report the physical rather than the sexual component of an assault. A study of male and female college students identified age-old barriers to reporting sexual assault and rape such as shame, embarrassment, guilt, concerns about confidentiality, fears for their safety, and worries about not being believed.[89]

Prevention of Gender-Based Violence

Gender-based violence is a global public health problem with multiple causes. Putting an end to it will require major cultural and societal shifts. Nevertheless, you can act to keep yourself safe and to protect others. (For more ideas, explore the website of author and activist Jackson Katz, PhD, including the downloadable poster on this page: http://www.jacksonkatz.com/wmcd.html.)

- **Treat everyone with respect.** Doing so promotes gender equality and peace.
- **Examine your attitudes about sexism and gender-based violence.** No one—even if he or she grew up around violence—is destined to be a perpetrator or victim. Paying for dinner (or anything else) doesn't entitle anyone to sexual favors.

- **Don't take the absence of a "no" as a "yes."** If you aren't sure about someone's sexual desires, ask. Healthy sex is consensual.

- **Assert your rights.** Your body belongs to you. You have the right to say no—even to someone you love. You should not put up with sexual harassment or submit to sex out of guilt, fear, or shame.

- **Speak up.** Confront peers who verbally or physically abuse women, people perceived as being LGBT, or any other vulnerable individuals. Doing this takes courage, especially if the abusers are friends or relatives. Turning a blind eye makes you part of the problem. If confrontation is not safe, contact someone with the authority to intervene. If violence seems likely or is in progress, call 911 and speak to the police.

- **Learn self-protection strategies.** Find out if your college has a program that teaches ways to establish boundaries and means of physical, verbal, and psychological self-defense. The majority of studies suggest that women who verbally or physically resist unwanted sexual advances are more likely to avoid rape without increasing their risk of injury.[90]

- **Stay sober.** Alcohol and sedating drugs increase vulnerability to sexual assault, particularly among teens and college students.[91] All central nervous system depressants impair judgment and interfere with a person's ability to respond to an attack. Potential perpetrators may become more aggressive and less concerned about consequences when drunk. While intoxication does not justify violence, refraining from becoming incapacitated with drink is a reasonable preventive strategy and has other benefits.

- **Avoid unsafe situations.** If you begin to feel uneasy at a party, on a date, or anywhere else, leave. Call a friend, taxi, or the campus escort service to fetch you. If danger seems imminent, dial 911.

- **Get help** if you have suffered violence or if you have committed violent acts in the past or fear that you might in the future. If you have a history of physical or sexual aggression, contact a mental health specialist. A good place to start might be the campus health center.

What to Do If You Are Sexually Assaulted

If you have a rape crisis hotline in your area, call. The person answering will, at your request, provide information on what to do, who to call, and where to get help. Typically, you will proceed immediately to the emergency room (ER). ER staff will contact the police. Do not shower or change your clothes before you go.

Many ERs have sexual assault response teams that include a doctor, a sexual assault examiner, and a social worker or rape crisis counselor. With your permission, medical professionals will examine you, treat any physical injuries, and perform forensic tests (including DNA evidence). You will be offered emergency contraception to prevent pregnancy and antimicrobial drugs to prevent bacterial STDs and possibly HIV. Because an assailant's HIV status is often unknown, you may be offered anti-HIV medications. The counselors will support you and your loved ones through the process and connect you with community resources. You have the right to refuse any of these services.

If you're attacked, recognize that it's not your fault. People attacked while intoxicated are particularly likely to feel guilt and shame. These feelings will prevent you from getting the help you need and deserve.

2.6 Elder Maltreatment

As life expectancy continues to rise, the number and proportion of older people increases rapidly. Like children, debilitated elders are vulnerable. Usually the offender is a caretaker or otherwise known to the elder. Older Americans may be neglected; abandoned; and emotionally, physically, and sexually abused. Care providers may steal or otherwise financially exploit the elder.

Because elders may not report these crimes, the exact number of maltreated elders is uncertain. According to the National Institute of Justice, a 2007 survey estimated that 1 in 10 elders had been maltreated in the previous year.[92]

Risk factors that caregivers will harm an elder are similar to those for maltreating children. Caregivers who lack training (a particular problem for people with dementia and other chronic, high-need illnesses), social support, and financial resources can become stressed, desperate, and short-tempered. In addition, mental health challenges and substance abuse compromise one's ability to care compassionately for an elder.

Care providers need support from friends and family and local groups, such as those that provide adult day care. Hotlines exist to find help and to report abuse (1-800-677-1116). Other resources include the National Center on Elder Abuse (http://www.ncea.aoa.gov) and the National Institute of Justice (http://www.nij.gov/topics/crime/elder-abuse/welcome.htm).

2.7 Homicide

Each year, homicide claims 16,799 American lives.[93] Overall, it's the 15th most common cause of death. However, for Americans ages 15 to 24, homicide prematurely kills more than 8,500 young people[94] and follows unintentional injury as the second leading cause of death. Worse, for African American men under age 35, homicide is the number one cause of death. In general, men are six times more likely to be victims in homicides than women.[95] But the chance of being a homicide victim is 1 in 30 for black men, compared to 1 in 179 for white men.[96] Whereas homicides rates have generally fallen, the rates have increased in black males.[97] Usually homicide victims die at the hands of people of their own race and ethnicity.

As discussed earlier, the alarmingly high homicide rates stem largely from availability of firearms. Compared to other high-income countries, the overall homicide rate in the United States is nearly 7 times higher; firearm homicides are almost 20 times higher.[98] For the 15- to 24-year-old age group, firearm homicides were 42.7 times that of other wealthy countries.

Murder in America

This interactive *Wall Street Journal* website allows you to explore statistics on homicides occurring between 2000 and 2010. Available at: http://projects.wsj.com/murderdata/?mg=inert-wsj#view=all.

2.8 Suicide

Chapter 5 discusses suicide. Because it's a tragically common cause of fatal intentional injury, the topic bears repeating. For all ages combined, suicides occur at nearly double the rate of homicides. For teens and young adults, suicide is the third leading cause of death. Each year, about 4,140 young people take their own lives.[99] Access to firearms greatly increases the odds of completing a suicide. In the United States, the suicide rate overall is below that of other high-income nation, though firearm suicides are 5.8 times higher.[100]

Key risk factors include untreated psychiatric disorders (e.g., depression, bipolar disorder, and PTSD), substance abuse, and extreme situational stress.

As with homicide, there's a marked gender disparity. Although women more often attempt suicide, five times more men actually take their own lives.[101] Culture often discourages men from discussing and seeking help for emotional distress. Health care providers are less likely to suspect depression in men.[102] Lastly, more men than women own firearms, giving them the means to inflict fatal self-injury.

Another high-risk group for suicide is LGBT youth. For them, suicide is the number one cause of death.[103] During high school, the risk of suicide for LGBT teens is at least double that of heterosexuals. Social stigma, marginalization, bullying, and harassment may lead to depression and suicidal thoughts.

It turns out that a rebellious attitude about one's life and expectation of dying young can prove all too true. A study found that teens who expected to die young were more likely to take risks—including abusing substances—and to contemplate and attempt suicide.[104]

Efforts to prevent suicide include heightened recognition of warning signs, improving mental health services (including closer monitoring of people at risk for suicide), and restricting access to opioid and sedative drugs (to prevent overdoses) and firearms.

2.9 Terrorism

The September 11, 2001, terrorist attacks on the World Trade Center and Pentagon woke Americans up to their vulnerability. In the aftermath, the United States became involved in wars in Afghanistan and Iraq. Security measures and travel restrictions tightened. Politicians and the media fueled collective fear. The federal government created the Department of Homeland Security to prevent and respond to terrorist attacks, as well as human-caused accidents and natural disasters.

The CDC has created an Emergency Preparedness and Response website to keep the public informed and to marshal resources. At http://emergency.cdc.gov, you can find information on natural and man-made disasters.

Government efforts and community awareness have foiled terrorist plots, such as the 2010 plan to ignite a car bomb in front of Times Square in New York. However, in 2013 two bombs exploded near the finish line of the Boston Marathon, killing three people and injuring 264.[105]

2.10 Preventing Violence

Violent crime is on the decline in the United States. That trend shows we can become progressively more peaceful. Prevention has to start early. All children deserve responsible, kind, and compassionate parents—parents who teach them how to regulate their emotions, respect others, tolerate differences, and resolve disagreements peacefully. Kids should learn that they're not better than anyone else simply because of their sex, race, social or financial status, educational level, religion, or sexual preference. We should not tolerate cruelty in any form.

Close-knit communities where people greet one another cordially and look out for one another are safer. Schools can adopt zero-tolerance policies for bullying and fighting. Narrowing disparities between rich and poor for educational and economic opportunities would improve quality of life for all.

Perpetrators need to be held accountable. They also need to be rehabilitated to prevent repeat offenses. Greater access to resources for victims can maximize healing and also avoid recurrences. Doing so will require expansion of support services and trained staff.

In 2000, the WHO created the Department of Injuries and Violence Prevention (http://www.who.int/violence_injury_prevention/en/). The CDC's Division of Violence Prevention has funded a number of programs to avert violence. For more information, go to http://www.cdc.gov/ViolencePrevention/FundedPrograms/index.html.

Dr. Martin Luther King Jr. said, "We must build dikes of courage to hold back the flood of fear…The time is always right to do the right thing…Peace is not merely a distant goal that we seek, but a means by which we arrive at that goal."

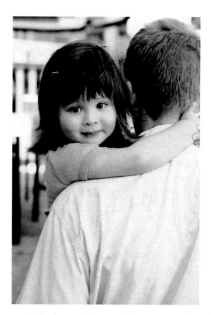

© *Thinkstock*

KEY TAKEAWAYS

- Violent crime has been declining in the United States. However, we still have a ways to go. Homicide and suicide are, respectively, the second and third leading causes of death in young Americans.
- Intentional injuries include bullying, hazing, hate crimes, gender-based violence, homicide, and suicide. All occur on college campuses. Substance abuse makes many of these injuries more common.
- Factors contributing to violence include poor parenting, cultural and religious beliefs that condone intentional injury (usually of certain groups), poverty, gangs, alcohol and illicit drugs, and availability of firearms.
- Men, particularly young African American men, face a higher risk of violent death than women.
- Gender-based violence is a worldwide public health threat. Power inequalities are thought to underlie these events. Women are most often the victims and men the perpetrators. Men, however, can also suffer from violent acts based on gender.
- In order to curtail violence, we need to start early to educate children. We also need to provide resources to reduce the inequalities that promote violence.

DISCUSSION QUESTIONS

1. What (or who) have had the most influence on your attitudes about violence? Consider parents, siblings, your school environment, your neighborhood, and the media.

2. Discuss your perception of the safety of your campus. Do you walk the campus alone at night? How easy is it for visitors to enter your residence? Does your campus have a night escort service and do you have the number? How often do you notice campus security officers on campus?

3. Have you experienced or witnessed hazing? If so, what happened? How did you feel about the experience? Did you report it? If you didn't (or wouldn't), what are your reasons?

4. Over a decade ago, the Southern Poverty Law Center started a program called Mix it Up at Lunch Day. On that day, American schoolchildren were encouraged to spend time with someone outside their usual social sphere.

    In 2012, an evangelical group known as the American Family Association urged families and school to boycott the event on the grounds that it "promoted a homosexual lifestyle."

    Read the *New York Times* news story at http://www.nytimes.com/2012/10/15/us/seeing-a-homosexual-agenda-christian-group-protests-an-anti-bullying-program.html?_r=1&. Now write your opinion of this development.

5. Examine your lifestyle habits, beliefs, and values. What factors put you at risk for being a victim or a perpetrator of gender-based violence? How can you reduce your risk?

3. RECOMMENDED RESOURCES

3.1 Book

Katz J. *The Macho Paradox: Why Some Men Hurt Women and How All Men Can Help.* Naperville, IL: Sourcebooks; 2006.

3.2 Organizations and Websites

Centers for Disease Control and Prevention, Injury Center: Violence Prevention. http://www.cdc.gov/ViolencePrevention.

Futures Without Violence. http://www.futureswithoutviolence.org.

National Safety Council. http://www.nsc.org.

Guns on Campus. Brady Campaign to Prevent Gun Violence. http://www.bradycampaign.org/stategunlaws/publicplaces/gunsoncampus.

Society for Public Health Education (SOPHE), Unintentional Injury and Violence Prevention. http://www.sophe.org/ui/Injury_Prevention_PublicHealth.cfm.

Stop Bullying, US Department of Health and Human Services. http://www.stopbullying.gov.

Stop Hazing. http://www.stophazing.org.

Teaching Tolerance: A Project of the Southern Poverty Law Center. http://www.tolerance.org.

Veto Violence. http://www.vetoviolence.org/index.html.

ENDNOTES

1. NCIPC: Web-based injury statistics query and reporting system (WISQARS). http://www.cdc.gov/injury/wisqars. As cited in: Injury: the leading cause of death among persons 1–44. Centers for Disease Control and Prevention. Available at: http://www.cdc.gov/injury/overview/leading_cod.html. Accessed October 13, 2012.

2. Miniño AM. *Mortality among Teenagers Aged 12–19 Years: United States, 1999–2006.* Hyattsville, MD: National Center for Health Statistics; 2010. NCHS Data Brief, no. 37. Available at: http://www.cdc.gov/nchs/data/hus/hus10.pdf. Accessed October 6, 2012.

3. Bergen G, Chen LH, Warner M. Injury in United States: 2007 chartbook. National Center for Health Statistics Office of Analysis and Epidemiology. Available at: http://www.cdc.gov/nchs/data/misc/injury2007.pdf. Accessed October 13, 2012.

4. Murphy SL, Xu J, Kochanek KD. Deaths: preliminary data for 2010. *Natl Vital Stat Rep.* 2012;60(4). Available at: http://www.cdc.gov/nchs/data/nvsr/nvsr60/nvsr60_04.pdf. Accessed October 5, 2012.

5. Blueprint for men's health. Men's Health Network website. Available at: http://www.menshealthnetwork.org/library/blueprint.pdf#page=65. Accessed September 1, 2011.

6. Injury facts. 2011 edition. National Safety Council. Available at: http://www.nsc.org/safety_work/Resources/Documents/IF_pgs52-83.pdf. Accessed October 13, 2012.

7. Harris CR, Jenkins M. Gender differences in risk assessment: why do women take fewer risks than men. *Judgm Decis Mak.* 2006;1(1):48–63. Available at: http://journal.sjdm.org/jdm06016.pdf. Accessed October 13, 2012.

8. Motor vehicle crash deaths in metropolitan areas—United States, 2009. *MMWR Morb Mortal Wkly Rep.* 2012;61(28):523–528. Available at: http://www.cdc.gov/mmwr/preview/mmwrhtml/mm6128a2.htm?s_cid=mm6128a2_w. Accessed October 5, 2012.

9. Vital signs: teen drinking and driving. Centers for Disease Control and Prevention. Available at: http://www.cdc.gov/Features/VitalSigns/TeenDrinkingAndDriving. Accessed October 6, 2012.

10. Mulye TP, Park MJ, Nelson CD, et al. Trends in adolescent and young adult health in the United States. *J Adolesc Health.* 2009 Jul;45(1):8–24.

11. US Department of Transportation, National Highway Traffic Safety Administration (NHTSA). *Traffic Safety Facts 2010: Alcohol-Impaired Driving.* Washington, DC: National Highway Traffic Safety Administration; 2012. Available at: http://www-nrd.nhtsa.dot.gov/Pubs/811606.PDF.

12. National Highway Traffic Safety Administration. *Traffic Safety Facts: Distracted Driving 2009.* DOT HS 811 379. Available at: http://www.distraction.gov/research/PDF-Files/Distracted-Driving-2009.pdf. Accessed October 6, 2012.

13. Mobile device use while driving: United States and seven European countries, 2011. *MMWR Morb Mortal Wkly Rep.* 2013 Mar 15;62(10):177–182. Available at: http://www.cdc.gov/mmwr/preview/mmwrhtml/mm6210a1.htm. Accessed May 31, 2013

14. CDC: majority of older teens text while driving. CBS News. June 7, 2012. Available at: http://www.cbsnews.com/8301-504763_162-57449111-10391704/cdc-majority-of-older-teens-text-while-driving/. Accessed October 6, 2012.

15. Wilson FA, Stimpson JP. Trends in fatalities from distracted driving in the United States, 1999 to 2008. *Am J Public Health.* 2010 Nov;100(11):2213–2219.

16. Schlehofer MM, Thompson SC, Ting S, et al. Psychological predictors of college students' cell phone use while driving. *Accid Anal Prev.* 2010 Jul;42(4):1107–1112.

17. Cell phone and texting laws. Governors Highway Safety Association. Available at: http://www.ghsa.org/html/stateinfo/laws/cellphone_laws.html. Accessed October 6, 2012.

18. Ishigami Y, Klein RM. Is a hands-free phone safer than a handheld phone? *J Safety Res.* 2009;40(2):157–164.

19. Naumann RB, Shults RA. Helmet use among motorcyclists who died in crashes and economic cost savings associated with state motorcycle helmet laws—United States, 2008–2010. *MMWR Morb Mortal Wkly Rep.* 2012;61(23):425–430. Available at: http://www.cdc.gov/mmwr/preview/mmwrhtml/mm6123a1.htm?s_cid=mm6123a1_w. Accessed October 7, 2012.

20. Motorcycle safety guide: prevention that works. Centers for Disease Control and Prevention. Available at: http://www.cdc.gov/motorvehiclesafety/mc/guide/prevention.html. Accessed October 7, 2012.

21. Reference group executive summary, spring 2011. American College Health Association, National College Health Assessment. Available at: http://www.achancha.org/docs/ACHA-NCHA-II_ReferenceGroup_ExecutiveSummary_Spring2011.pdf. Accessed October 17, 2012.

22. Persaud N, Coleman E, Zwolakowski BA, et al. Nonuse of bicycle helmets and risk of fatal head injury: a proportional mortality, case-control study. *CMAJ.* 2012. doi:10.1503/cmaj.120988. Available at: http://www.cmaj.ca/content/early/2012/10/15/cmaj.120988.full.pdf. Accessed October 24, 2012.

23. Bicycles. National Highway Traffic Safety Administration. Available at: http://www.nhtsa.gov/Bicycles. Accessed October 7, 2012.

24. Head injuries and bicycle safety. Resources of Entertainment Education Content Developments. Gateway to Health Communication & Social Marketing Practice. Centers for Disease Control and Prevention. Available at: http://www.cdc.gov/healthcommunication/ToolsTemplates/EntertainmentEd/Tips/HeadInjuries.html. Accessed October 7, 2012.

25. All-terrain vehicle safety. US Consumer Product Safety Commission. Available at: http://www.cpsc.gov/cpscpub/pubs/540.html. Accessed October 17, 2012.

26. Pedestrians. Traffic Safety Facts: 2008 Data. National Highway Traffic Safety Administration. DOT HS 811 163. Available at: http://www-nrd.nhtsa.dot.gov/Pubs/811163.PDF. Accessed October 7, 2012.

27. Poisoning in the United States: fact sheet. Centers for Disease Control and Prevention. Available at: http://www.cdc.gov/HomeandRecreationalSafety/Poisoning/poisoning-factsheet.htm. Accessed October 14, 2012.

28. Poisoning in the United States: fact sheet. Centers for Disease Control and Prevention. Available at: http://www.cdc.gov/HomeandRecreationalSafety/Poisoning/poisoning-factsheet.htm. Accessed October 14, 2012.

29. Acetaminophen toxicity. Medscape. Available at: http://emedicine.medscape.com/article/820200-overview. Accessed October 14, 2012.

30. Unintentional drug poisoning in the United States. Centers for Disease Control and Prevention. July 2010. Available at: http://www.cdc.gov/homeandrecreationalsafety/pdf/poison-issue-brief.pdf. Accessed May 31, 2013.

31. Preventing carbon monoxide problems. Colorado State University Extension. Available at: http://www.ext.colostate.edu/pubs/consumer/09939.html. Accessed October 14, 2012.

32. Accidents or unintentional injuries. National Center for Health Statistics. Centers for Disease Control and Prevention. Available at: http://www.cdc.gov/nchs/fastats/acc-inj.htm. Accessed October 13, 2012.

33. Fire deaths and injuries: fact sheet. Centers for Disease Control and Prevention. Available at: http://www.cdc.gov/HomeandRecreationalSafety/Fire-Prevention/fires-factsheet.html. Accessed October 14, 2012.

34. Unintentional drowning: get the facts. Centers for Disease Control and Prevention. Available at: http://www.cdc.gov/HomeAndRecreationalSafety/Water-Safety/waterinjuries-factsheet.html. Accessed October 15, 2012.

35. Choking and suffocation prevention fact sheet. Safe Kids. Available at: http://www.safekids.org/our-work/research/fact-sheets/choking-and-suffocation-prevention-fact-sheet.html. Accessed October 15, 2012.

36. Richardson EG, Hemenway D. Homicide, suicide, and unintentional firearm fatality: comparing the United States with other high-income countries, 2003. *J Trauma.* 2011 Jan;70(1):238–243.

37. MacInnis L. U.S. most armed country with 90 guns per 100 people. Reuters. August 28, 2007. Available at: http://www.reuters.com/article/2007/08/28/us-world-firearms-idUSL2834893820070828. Accessed October 24, 2012.

38. National SAFE KIDS Campaign (NSKC). *Unintentional Firearm Injury Fact Sheet.* Washington, DC: NSKC; 2004. Available at: http://www.preventinjury.org/PDFs/UNINTENTIONAL_FIREARM_INJURY.pdf. Accessed October 15, 2012.

39. Richardson EG, Hemenway D. Homicide, suicide, and unintentional firearm fatality: comparing the United States with other high-income countries, 2003. *J Trauma.* 2011 Jan;70(1):238–243.

40. Definition and typology of violence. Violence Prevention Alliance. Global Campaign for Violence Prevention. World Health Organization. Available at: http://www.who.int/violenceprevention/approach/definition/en/index.html.

41. FBI releases preliminary annual crime statistics for 2011. FBI National Press Office, Washington, DC. 2012. Available at: http://www.fbi.gov/news/pressrel/press-releases/fbi-releases-preliminary-annual-crime-statistics-for-2011. Accessed October 19, 2012.

42. Boutwell BB, Franklin CA, Barnes JC, Beaver KM. Physical punishment and childhood aggression: the role of gender and gene-environment interplay. *Aggressive Behav.* 2011 Nov–Dec;37(6):559–568. doi:10.1002/ab.20409.

43. Taylor CA, Manganello JA, Lee SJ, Rice JC. Mothers' spanking of 3-year-old children and subsequent risk of children's aggressive behavior. *Pediatrics.* 2010 May;125(5):e1057–e1065.

44. Anderson CA, Sakamoto A, Gentile DA, et al. Longitudinal effects of violent video games on aggression in Japan and the United States. *Pediatrics.* 2008 Nov;122(5):e1067–e1072.

45. Gentile DA, Stone W. Violent video game effects on children and adolescents: a review of the literature. *Minerva Pediatr.* 2005 Dec;57(6):337–358.

46. Browne KD, Hamilton-Giachritsis C. The influence of violent media on children and adolescents: a public-health approach. *Lancet.* 2005 Feb 19–25;365(9460):702–710.

47. Leading causes of death by age group, black males. United States, 2004. Centers for Disease Control and Prevention. Available at: http://www.cdc.gov/men/lcod/2004/04black.pdf. Accessed October 24, 2012.

48. Firearms. United Nations Office of Drugs and Crime. Available at: http://www.unodc.org/documents/data-and-analysis/tocta/6.Firearms.pdf. Accessed August 13, 2012.

49. Younge G. America's deadly devotion to guns. *The Guardian.* April 16, 2012. Available at: http://www.guardian.co.uk/world/2012/apr/16/americas-deadly-devotion-guns. Accessed October 24, 2012.

50. Hemenway D. Risks and benefits of a gun in the home. *Am J Lifestyle Med.* 2011;5(6):502–511.

51. Gun violence facts. Brady Campaign to Prevent Gun Violence. Available at: http://www.bradycampaign.org/facts/gunviolence?s=2. Accessed August 13, 2012. Data extracted from the National Center for Injury Prevention and Control, Centers for Disease Control and Prevention, web-based injury statistics query and reporting system 2008 (deaths) and 2009 (injuries).

52. Miniño AM, Murphy SL. *Death in the United States, 2010.* CHS Data Brief. 2012 Jul; (99):1–8. Available at: http://www.cdc.gov/nchs/data/databriefs/db99.htm. Accessed May 31, 2013.

53. NPR staff. Breaking down gun violence: No "simple formula." National Public Radio. August 13, 2012. Available at: http://www.npr.org/2012/08/12/158659172/breaking-down-gun-violence-no-simple-formula. Accessed August 13, 2012.

54. Barrett T, Cohen T. Senate rejects expanded gun background checks. CNN. April 18, 2013. Available at: http://www.cnn.com/2013/04/17/politics/senate-guns-vote. Accessed May 31, 2013.

55. Harvard Injury Control Research Center. The Australian gun buyback. *Bulletins*. 2011;4. Available at: http://www.hsph.harvard.edu/research/hicrc/files/bulletins_australia_spring_2011.pdf. Accessed December 21, 2012.

56. SF, Oakland gun buybacks in wake of Connecticut Tragedy. The Post News Group. December 21, 2012. Available at: http://www.postnewsgroup.com/publishedcontent/2012/12/21/sf-oakland-gun-buybacks-in-wake-of-connecticut-tragedy. Accessed December 21, 2012.

57. Miller M. Buy back guns, boost the economy. *Washington Post*. December 18, 2012. Available at: http://www.washingtonpost.com/opinions/matt-miller-buy-back-guns-boost-the-economy/2012/12/18/c8bc457a-4938-11e2-b6f0-e851e741d196_story.html. Accessed December 21, 2012.

58. Cushman JH. N.R.A. calls for armed guards in schools to deter violence. *New York Times*. December 21, 2012. Available at: http://www.nytimes.com/2012/12/22/us/nra-calls-for-armed-guards-at-schools.html?hp&_r=0. Accessed December 21, 2012.

59. Hemenway D. Risks and benefits of a gun in the home. *Am J Lifestyle Med*. 2011;5(6):502–511.

60. Wintemute GJ. Guns, fear, the Constitution, and the public's health. *N Engl J Med*. 2008;358(14):1421–1424.

61. Child maltreatment prevention: data and statistics. Centers for Disease Control and Prevention. Available at: http://www.cdc.gov/ViolencePrevention/childmaltreatment/index.html. Accessed October 21, 2012.

62. Neigh GN, Gillespie CF, Nemeroff CB. The neurobiological toll of child abuse and neglect. *Trauma Violence Abuse*. 2009 Oct;10(4):389–410.

63. Danese A, Moffitt TE, Harrington H, et al. Adverse childhood experiences and adult risk factors for age-related disease: depression, inflammation, and clustering of metabolic risk markers. *Arch Pediatr Adolesc Med*. 2009 Dec;163(12):1135–1143.

64. Hahlweg K, Heinrichs N, Kuschel A, Bertram H, Naumann S. Long-term outcome of a randomized controlled intervention trial through a positive parenting program: is it worth the effort? *Child Adolesc Psychiatry Ment Health*. 2010 May 16;4:14.

65. Frequently asked questions about gangs. National Gang Center. Bureau of Justice Assistance, Office of Juvenile Justice and Delinquency Prevention, US Department of Justice. Available at: http://www.nationalgangcenter.gov/About/FAQ. Accessed October 21, 2012.

66. Bullying definition. Stopbullying.gov. Available at: http://www.stopbullying.gov/what-is-bullying/definition/index.html#types. Accessed October 21, 2012.

67. Centers for Disease Control and Prevention. Bullying among middle school and high school students—Massachusetts, 2009. *MMWR Morb Mortal Wkly Rep*. 2011;60:465–471.

68. Youth risk behavior surveillance—United States, 2011. *MMWR Morb Mortal Wkly Rep*. 2012;61(4). Available at: http://www.cdc.gov/mmwr/pdf/ss/ss6104.pdf. Accessed October 6, 2012.

69. Experiences with violence. Lesbian, Gay, Bisexual and Transgender Health. Centers for Disease Control and Prevention. Available at: http://www.cdc.gov/lgbthealth/youth.htm. Accessed October 6, 2012.

70. Simons AB. *Campus Attacks: Targeted Violence Affecting Institutions of Higher Learning*. Washington, DC: United States Secret Service, US Department of Education, Federal Bureau of Investigation; 2010. Available at: http://www2.ed.gov/admins/lead/safety/campus-attacks.pdf. Accessed October 21, 2012.

71. Allan EJ, Madden M. Hazing in view: college students at risk. Initial Findings from the National Study of Student Hazing. Available at: http://www.hazingstudy.org/publications/hazing_in_view_web.pdf. Accessed October 22, 2012.

72. Hate crime: overview. Federal Bureau of Investigation. Available at: http://www.fbi.gov/about-us/investigate/civilrights/hate_crimes/overview. Accessed October 22, 2012.

73. Mechanic M. Fact sheet on stalking. National Violence against Women Prevent Research Center. University of Missouri at St. Louis. Available at: http://www.musc.edu/vawprevention/research/stalking.shtml. Accessed August 14, 2011.

74. Reference group executive summary, spring 2011. American College Health Association, National College Health Assessment. Available at: http://www.achancha.org/docs/ACHA-NCHA-II_ReferenceGroup_ExecutiveSummary_Spring2011.pdf. Accessed October 22, 2012.

75. Maston CT. *Bureau of Justice Statistics (BJS) Criminal Victimization in the United States, 2007—Statistical Tables, National Crime Victimization Survey*. Washington, DC: US Department of Justice; 2010. JCJ 227669. Available at: http://bjs.ojp.usdoj.gov/index.cfm?ty=pbdetail&iid=1743. Accessed August 12, 2011.

76. Linden JA. Care of the adult patient after sexual assault. *N Engl J Med*. 2011;365(9):834–841.

77. Sexual victimization in prisons and jails reported by inmates, 2008–2009. Bureau of Justice Statistics. August 26, 2010. NCJ 231169. Available at: http://bjs.ojp.usdoj.gov/index.cfm?ty=pbdetail&iid=2202. Accessed August 14, 2011.

78. Parker A. Lawsuit says military is rife with sexual abuse. *New York Times*. February 15, 2011. Available at: http://www.nytimes.com/2011/02/16/us/16military.html. Accessed August 14, 2011.

79. Lesbian, gay, bisexual, and transgender domestic violence in the United States in 2007. National Coalition of Anti-Violence Programs. Available at: http://avp.org/documents/2007NCAVPDVREPORT.pdf. Accessed August 14, 2011.

80. WHO. Global and regional estimates of violence against women: Prevalence and health effects of intimate partner violence and non-partner sexual violence. Executive Summary. World Health Organization, 2013. Available at: http://apps.who.int/iris/bitstream/10665/85241/1/WHO_RHR_HRP_13.06_eng.pdf. Accessed July 15, 2013.

81. Black MC, Basile KC, Breiding MJ, et al. The National Intimate Partner and Sexual Violence Survey (NISVS): 2010 summary report. National Center for Injury Prevention and Control, Centers for Disease Control and Prevention. 2011. Available at: http://www.cdc.gov/violenceprevention/nisvs. Accessed October 22, 2012.

82. Extent, nature, and consequences of rape victimization: findings from the national violence against women survey. January 2006. Available at: http://www.nij.gov/pubs-sum/210346.htm. Accessed September 7, 2011.

83. Maston CT. *Bureau of Justice Statistics (BJS) Criminal Victimization in the United States, 2007—Statistical Tables, National Crime Victimization Survey*. Washington, DC: US Department of Justice; 2010. JCJ 227669. Available at: http://bjs.ojp.usdoj.gov/index.cfm?ty=pbdetail&iid=1743. Accessed August 12, 2011.

84. Rennison CM. Rape and Sexual Assault: Reporting to Police and Medical Attention, 1992–2000. Washington, DC: US Department of Justice; 2002. NCJ 194530. Available at: http://www.bjs.ojp.usdoj.gov/content/pub/pdf/rsarp00.pdf. Accessed October 7, 2011.

85. McCauley J, Ruggiero KJ, Resnick HS, Conoscenti LM, Kilpatrick DG. Forcible, drug-facilitated, and incapacitated rape in relation to substance use problems: results from a national sample of college women. *Addict Behavs*. 2009 May;34(5):458–462.

86. Walsh JF, Devellis BM, Devellis RF. Date and acquaintance rape: development and validation of a set of scales. *Violence against Women*. 1997 Feb;3(1):46–58.

87. Rees S, Silove D, Chey T, et al. Lifetime prevalence of gender-based violence in women and the relationship with mental disorders and psychosocial function. *JAMA*. 2011;306(5): 513–521.

88. Homicide trends in the U.S., 2005. Bureau of Justice Statistics. Available at: http://bjs.ojp.usdoj.gov/content/homicide/intimates.cfm. Accessed August 12, 2011.

89. Sable MR, Danis F, Mauzy DL, Gallagher SK. Barriers to reporting sexual assault for women and men: perspectives of college students. *J Am Coll Health*. 2006 Nov–Dec;55(3):157–162.

90. Rheingold AA, Kilpatrick DG. Self-defense training: a brief overview. National Violence against Women Prevention Research Center. Medical University of South Carolina. Available at: http://www.musc.edu/vawprevention. Accessed August 14, 2011.

91. Testa M, Livingston JA. Alcohol consumption and women's vulnerability to sexual victimization: can reducing women's drinking prevent rape? *Subst Use Misuse*. 2009;44(9–10):1349–1376. Available at: http://www.ncbi.nlm.nih.gov/pmc/articles/PMC2784921/?tool=pubmed. Accessed August 12, 2011.

92. Extent of elder abuse victimization. National Institute of Justice. Available at: http://www.nij.gov/nij/topics/crime/elder-abuse/extent.htm. Accessed October 24, 2012.

93. Assault or homicide. Centers for Disease Control and Prevention. Available at: http://www.cdc.gov/nchs/fastats/homicide.htm. Accessed October 5, 2012.

94. Injuries and violence are leading causes of death: key data & statistics. National Center for Injury Prevention and Control, Centers for Disease Control and Prevention. Available at: http://www.cdc.gov/injury/overview/data.html. Accessed October 13, 2012.

95. Xu JQ, Kochanek KD, Murphy SL, Tejada-Vera B. Deaths among persons 15–24 years of age. *Deaths: Final Data for 2007. Natl Vital Stat Rep*. 2010;58(19):58. Available at: http://www.cdc.gov/nchs/data/hus/hus10.pdf. Accessed October 6, 2012.

96. US Department of Justice. Bureau of Justice Statistics data report, 1990. Available at: https://www.ncjrs.gov/App/Publications/abstract.aspx?ID=121514. Accessed September 21, 2011.

97. McWhirter C, Fields G. Communities struggle to break a grim cycle of killing. *Wall Street Journal*. August 8, 2012. Available at: http://online.wsj.com/article/SB10001424052702304830704577496501048197464.html. Accessed October 24, 2012.

98. Richardson EG, Hemenway D. Homicide, suicide, and unintentional firearm fatality: comparing the United States with other high-income countries, 2003. *J Trauma*. 2011 Jan;70(1):238–243.

99. Injuries and Violence Are Leading Causes of Death: Key Data & Statistics. National Center for Injury Prevention and Control, Centers for Disease Control and Prevention. Available at: http://www.cdc.gov/injury/overview/data.html. Accessed October 13, 2012.

100. Richardson EG, Hemenway D. Homicide, suicide, and unintentional firearm fatality: comparing the United States with other high-income countries, 2003. *J Trauma*. 2011 Jan;70(1):238–243.

101. Xu JQ, Kochanek KD, Murphy SL, Tejada-Vera B. Deaths among persons 15–24 years of age. *Deaths: Final Data for 2007. Natl Vital Stat Rep*. 2010;58(19):58. Available at: http://www.cdc.gov/nchs/data/hus/hus10.pdf. Accessed October 6, 2012.

102. Nolen-Hoeksema S. Sex differences in unipolar depression: evidence and theory. *Psychol Bull*. 1987;101(2):259.

103. Suicide risk and prevention for lesbian, gay, bisexual, and transgender youth. Suicide Prevention Resource Center. 2008. Available at: http://www.sprc.org/sites/sprc.org/files/library/SPRC_LGBT_Youth.pdf. Accessed October 6, 2012.

104. Nguyen QC, Villaveces A, Marshall SW, et al. Adolescent expectations of early death predict adult risk behaviors. *PLoS One*. 2012;7(8):e41905.

105. Bidgood J. Two groups in grief refuse to stand still. *New York Times*. April 23, 2013. Available at: http://www.nytimes.com/2013/04/24/us/boston-marathon-deaths-reinforce-community-bonds.html?pagewanted=all. Accessed May 31, 2013.

CHAPTER 13
Immune System Health

DANGERS WITHIN AND WITHOUT

Microscopic living organisms are everywhere. Soil, beach sand, and lake water teem with invisible life. Known as **microorganisms**, or microbes for short, they cling to doorknobs and shopping carts. They carpet the linings of our airways and intestinal tract. Like tiny bronco riders, they're gamely hugging my fingers as I type. It's probably a good thing we can't see these creatures with the naked eye. Fortunately, most of them are harmless, and some actually benefit us.

Other agents invisible to the naked eye threaten homeostasis. Examples include ultraviolet light, radiation, and toxic chemicals. All have the potential to damage cells and trigger cancer.

What keeps us from succumbing to overwhelming infection and cancer at tender ages? The immune system. This chapter provides an overview of **immunology**, the study of the organs, cells, and molecules involved in immunity. We start with a discussion of **immunity**, the recognition and removal of material that the immune system determines is "nonself" and therefore foreign. Next, we cover the ways in which immune system responses can actually do us harm. The chapter concludes with tips for keeping your immune system in optimal shape.

microorganisms

Microscopic living organisms such as bacteria, viruses, protozoa, and fungi.

immunology

The study of the organs, cells, and molecules involved in immunity; a medical specialty concerned with the body's distinction of self from nonself, defenses against infectious diseases, and hypersensitivity to foreign substances.

immunity

The recognition and removal of foreign material from the body; the state of being resistant to an infectious disease.

1. IMMUNE SYSTEM OVERVIEW

LEARNING OBJECTIVES

1. Identify the main functions of the immune system.
2. Explain the importance of recognition of self versus nonself.
3. Differentiate between the innate and adaptive immune systems.
4. Explain how the immune system responds to pathogenic microorganisms.
5. Differentiate between passive and active immunity and provide examples of each.

1.1 Key Functions

The immune system's main purpose is to protect against **pathogens** (disease-causing microorganisms), cancer, and anything else foreign (e.g., transplanted cells, toxins, splinters). In order to carry out that important function, immune system cells must be able to distinguish the good guys (normal bodily cells and molecules) from the bad guys. To do so, they have special cell surface receptors (molecules that bind in a specific way to other molecules). Receptors for unique molecules protruding from the surfaces of normal cells allow the immune cells to recognize self and prevent attacks against your own cells—unless they have become altered by infection or cancer. On the other hand, receptors for foreign molecules, when they encounter antigens, initiate warfare. (**Antigens** are organisms, molecules, or parts of molecules that immune cells recognize as foreign.) The immune system also has a housekeeping function, removing debris to keep tissues tidy and, after an infection, promoting healing.

pathogen

A disease-causing agent, usually an infectious organism.

antigen

A substance capable of stimulating an immune system response.

cytokines

Small protein molecules that regulate cellular activity within the immune system and also influence other organ systems.

In addition, research shows that **cytokines**, small protein molecules that regulate cellular activity, affect cells outside the immune system. Some experts liken the immune system to a sensory organ, one of the surveillance systems that sends the brain information from distant tissues.[1] As we discuss later, that interaction is bidirectional. The brain and its response to the outside environment also influence the immune system.

Cytokines provide the immune system the means to affect brain and behavior. Under normal situations, the immune system facilitates learning and memory.[2] However, chronic elevations in inflammatory cytokines not only disrupt learning and memory but also generate feelings of fatigue, malaise, anxiety, and depression.[3] A steady rise in inflammatory cytokines over the course of the day contributes to your feelings of sleepiness at night.[4] The next morning, you feel refreshed because sleep reduced levels of these chemicals. If you have an infection such as the common cold or influenza, inflammatory cytokines signal the brain that it's time to lie low and sleep. They make you feel tired, lacking in appetite, and perhaps feverish.

When persistently elevated, these inflammatory chemicals accelerate the aging process. Increasingly, scientists have recognized the role of inflammation in promoting a host of chronic diseases, including heart disease, atherosclerosis, Alzheimer's disease, arthritis, osteoporosis (brittle bones), type 2 diabetes, gum disease, certain cancers, and possibly depression.[5],[6]

1.2 The Two Divisions of the Immune System

FIGURE 13.1 Tissues of the Immune System

All blood cells are derived from stem cells (cells that can continuously divide and develop into more specialized cells) in the bone marrow. A special kind of cell called a T lymphocyte matures in the thymus gland, which lies just behind the breastbone. Other immune tissues are stationed at likely portals of entry for microbial pathogens: the adenoids and tonsils in the throat, the spleen in the abdomen, Peyer's patches in the intestines and appendix, and lymph nodes concentrated in the neck, armpits, abdomen, and groin.

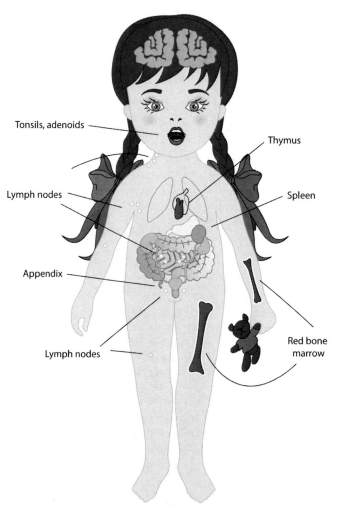

© *Shutterstock*

A diffuse, complex, interacting network of cells and chemicals belong to the immune system. This system includes the thymus, spleen, lymph nodes, bone marrow, white blood cells (leukocytes), and a variety of molecules secreted by cells. The immune system has two main divisions: the **innate immune system**, which requires no previous experience with intruders to dispatch them swiftly, and the **adaptive immune system**, which requires time and experience in order to develop a specific response to a particular pathogen. Both systems have humoral (molecules that float in bodily fluids) and cellular elements. The two systems are intricately linked.

The Innate Immune System: The Fortress and the Foot Soldiers

This system is in place at birth and represents your first line of defense against microbes. It reacts quickly and in a generalized fashion to anything foreign. Components include physical and chemical barriers to invasion, friendly microbes, and certain immune system cells and chemicals.

Our largest **physical barriers** are the skin and the mucous membranes. You can liken them to the fortress walls. Layers of cells in the skin envelop us to keep microbes and toxins out and bodily fluids in. People who suffer burns or abrasions that destroy large swaths of skin risk infection and dehydration.

The mucous membranes are the moist linings of bodily cavities that come into contact with the outside world such as the digestive, respiratory, urinary, and genital tracts. Cells in the mucous membranes produce a productive coat of slimy mucus, which acts like fly paper for microbes.

Organ systems can have specialized defenses. Eyelids, eyelashes, and tears protect the eyes. Earwax defends the ear canals. In the lower urinary tract, the act of urination flushes out any microbes trying to infect cells lining the bladder.

In the respiratory tract, sneeze, cough, gag, and swallow reflexes protect the airways from noxious substances.

Nostril hairs create air turbulence, which causes inhaled particles to become stuck in the mucus. Hair-like cilia jutting out from the airway linings move in a whip-like fashion to propel mucus (and the microbes and cells trapped in it) away from the lung's fragile air sacs. Chemicals in tobacco smoke and alcohol paralyze the cilia, which is one reason alcoholics and smokers tend to get respiratory infections.

Various chemicals in our outer defenses create an environment inhospitable to microbes. The acidic pH of the skin, stomach, and vagina discourage microbes, as do digestive enzymes in the intestinal tract. Small proteins called defensins protect against bacteria and fungi. Lysozyme, an enzyme that digests bacterial cell walls, is secreted by mucous membranes, the lacrimal glands (tear ducts) in the eyes, and phagocytic cells.

We also have allies in the microbial world. Hundreds of bacteria and fungi maintain a mutually beneficial relationship within us. They colonize the skin, the outer surface of the eye, upper respiratory tract, digestive tract, lower urinary tract, and vagina.[7] The intestines alone are home to up to 500 different bacterial species. These "gut flora" outnumber our own cells by a factor of 10.[8] Each of us is like a well-colonized planet.

In addition to other health benefits, these friendly microbes promote immune health in several ways. They out-compete pathogenic bacteria much as a well-planted garden leaves little room for weeds. They also shape the immune system response, boosting immune cells, antibodies, and chemicals that amplify the immune system response. A few days after birth, microbes colonize a newborn's intestinal tract. That's a good thing. Animals bred in a germ-free environment have less immune tissue in the gut, reduced antibody levels in the blood, and a heightened vulnerability to infection.[9],[10]

Last but not least are the cells of the innate immune system, which recognize and respond to foreign antigens. Cells in both branches of the immune system are types of **leukocytes**, all of which derive from stem cells in the bone marrow.

Cells in the innate immune system include the following:

- **Natural killer cells (NK cells)** are a type of lymphocyte with a nonspecific ability to kill virus-infected cells and some cancer cells.

- **Granulocytes** (also called granular leukocytes) have a speckled appearance under the microscope due to small sacs containing microbe-destroying enzymes and other chemicals. This group includes *neutrophils* (phagocytic cells that kill bacteria), *basophils* (which can develop into mast cells and contribute to inflammatory and allergic reactions), and *eosinophils* (involved in allergic reactions and defense against larger parasites such as worms).

- **Monocytes** can move from the blood into the tissues to mature into **macrophages** (Greek for "big eaters") or **dendritic cells**. Dendritic cells patrol likely entry points for microbes such as the skin and gastrointestinal tract. In a process called *phagocytosis*, macrophages and dendritic cells engulf and degrade cellular debris and foreign material. They can "present" foreign antigens on their cell surfaces to cells in the adaptive system called T lymphocytes, thereby activating that system. That's why these cells are also called **antigen-presenting cells**.

innate immune system

Nonspecific, first-line defense against infection mediated by physical barriers, chemicals, and cells.

adaptive immune system

Composed of T and B lymphocytes and their cytokines, which orchestrate a specialized response against a particular pathogen and develop immunologic memory; takes time to develop.

leukocytes

White blood cells.

Video Clip 13.1

Natural Killer Cells

This animated video depicts a natural killer (NK) cell attacking a virus (the green object injecting its genetic material into a cell), cancer cells, and sheep red blood cells, which a human's immune system would consider foreign.

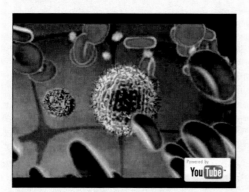

View the video online at: http://www.youtube.com/v/HNP1EAYLhOs

 Video Clip 13.2

White Blood Cell Chasing a Bacterium

In this video, a neutrophil bends and slithers around red blood cells in pursuit of a bacterium. In a perfect illustration of phagocytosis, the cell finally engulfs the microbe.

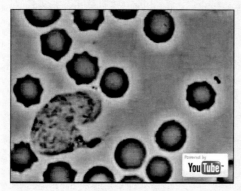

View the video online at: http://www.youtube.com/v/JnlULOjUhSQ

Video Clip 13.3

Defenses against Infection
This animated video reviews the key nonspecific defenses against infection—skin, neutrophils, and macrophages.

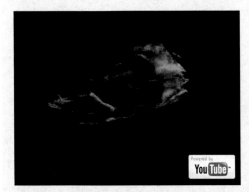

View the video online at: http://www.youtube.com/v/5DpNtMMuYUA

The innate system also has **humoral** components that float in bodily fluids: complement and cytokines.

Complement consists of more than 30 proteins. In a process called the complement cascade, each protein activates the next. Functions include attracting leukocytes to the site, enhancing antibody formation and effectiveness, neutralizing viruses, and killing bacteria.

FIGURE 13.2   Cells in the Blood

This image depicts the main types of cells in the blood. Erythrocytes (red blood cells) transport oxygen to the tissues. Platelets are involved in blood clotting. The bottom row lines up the major players in the immune system. Monocytes can mature into macrophages and dendritic cells, which digest material and present foreign antigens to lymphocytes. The granular cells in the middle (basophils, eosinophils, and neutrophils) belong to the innate immune system. Lymphocytes belong to the acquired immune system.

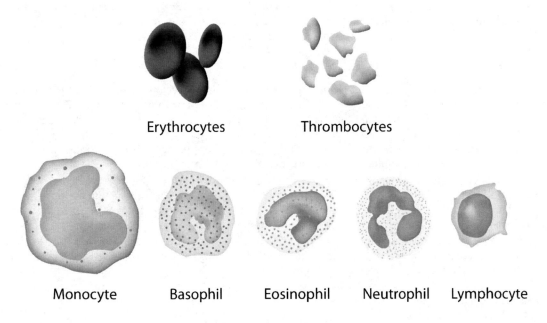

© Shutterstock

FIGURE 13.3 Antigen-Presenting Cell at Work

Action of antigen-presenting cell in human immune response.

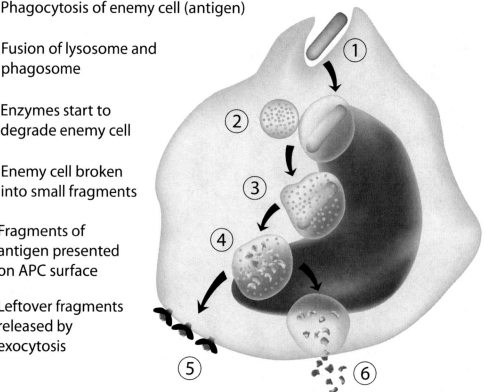

(1) Phagocytosis of enemy cell (antigen)

(2) Fusion of lysosome and phagosome

(3) Enzymes start to degrade enemy cell

(4) Enemy cell broken into small fragments

(5) Fragments of antigen presented on APC surface

(6) Leftover fragments released by exocytosis

© *Shutterstock*

Cytokines are chemical messengers. Leukocytes and other cells secrete them. There are many different cytokines, some with opposing actions. Two examples include *interleukins* and *interferons*. Their functions include attracting leukocytes, stimulating or inhibiting activity of immune system cells, interfering with viral replication (interferons), and communicating with the brain.

The Adaptive Immune System: The A-Team

This system, also called the *acquired immune system*, takes time to develop because takes time to develop because it responds selectively to each microbe. During those three to five days that specialized cells are gearing up, your innate system does its best to defend you, at the expense of some damage to your tissues. Once cells in the adaptive system learn to recognize a specific antigen, they retain an enduring memory. They can also generate millions of different receptors to match specific antigens. The response to subsequent encounters with the same microbe is quick and precise.

In other words, you have immune system cells that identify and respond to a particular strain of influenza virus and nothing else. The first time you're exposed to that virus, your innate immune system does its best to contain the infection. You get sick but survive. During that time, cells in the adaptive system learn to recognize this virus and mount an initial albeit puny response against it. At the end, a clone of identical cells has receptors for the virus and maintains **immunologic memory** for it. If your roommate later gets the same brand of influenza virus, your adaptive immune system springs into action so quickly you don't develop any symptoms.

The white blood cells of this system are called **lymphocytes**. There are two main types: B lymphocytes and T lymphocytes.

immunologic memory

The ability of the immune system to recall a previous exposure to an antigen and, thanks to the creation of memory T and B cells, mount an even stronger, swifter response upon subsequent encounters.

B lymphocytes (B cells) manufacture antibodies. (The B now stands for "bone-marrow de-rived," though the letter originally came from knowledge that these cells matured in a structure in birds called the bursa of Fabricius.) **Antibodies**, also called immunoglobulins, are protein molecules that interact with specific antigens. Each B cell line produces antibodies against one specific antigen. Once activated by a helper T cell, B cells mature into plasma cells and hunker down in the bone marrow or spleen to do nothing but secrete antibodies. Because antibodies can travel in tissue fluids, they are considered part of *humoral immunity*. You can think of B cells as archers releasing arrow-like antibodies.

T lymphocytes (T cells) are cells that arise from stem cells in the bone marrow and mature in the thymus gland. (The "T" stands for thymus-derived.) There are three main types of T cells: helper T cells, cytotoxic T cells, and regulatory T cells.

Helper T cells, sometimes called CD4+ T cells because of a cell surface marker, orchestrate many other aspects of the immune system. Once activated by antigen-presenting cells, helper T cells secrete cytokines that direct the activity of other immune cells, particularly the cytotoxic T cells and B cells. Human immunodeficiency viruses (HIV) infect these pivotal cells, bringing the immune system to its knees.

Cytotoxic T cells kill cells that express specific antigens. To do so, they must come into contact with an infected cell or cancer-ridden cell. You can think of them like soldiers in hand-to-hand combat. This approach is called *cell-mediated immunity*.

Regulatory T cells, as their name implies, regulate the immune system. They can suppress other immune cells to keep an immune response from spiraling out of control. They are key to making sure other immune cells tolerate rather than attack your own cells.

FIGURE 13.4 The Lymphatic System

This image depicts the lymphatic vessels that collect fluid from the tissues and return it to major veins in the vascular system. Lymph nodes are stationed at key locations to filter the lymph.

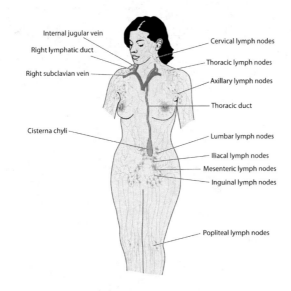

© Shutterstock

The lymphocytes and other white blood cells congregate in lymphoid organs such as the lymph nodes, spleen, thymus, and bone marrow, as well as lymphoid tissues in the gut and throat (tonsils and adenoids). They can move from these lymphoid tissues into the lymphatic vessels, which connect to the blood vessels. The lymphatic vessels collect tissue fluid, which then passes through the filter-like lymph nodes. An infection activates nearby lymph nodes. That's why you can feel tender swollen lymph nodes in your neck when you have a sore throat. (If enlarged lymph nodes persist, see your doctor, as other, more serious conditions can be responsible.)

B lymphocytes (B cells)

Lymphocytes that produce antibodies against a specific antigen.

antibodies

Also called immunoglobulins, these proteins are released from mature B cells to combine with specific antigens. Each B cell (and its clones) releases only one type of antibody.

T lymphocytes (T cells)

Type of lymphocyte that matures in the thymus gland.

In this image, cytotoxic T cells (blue) attack a cancer cell (orange).

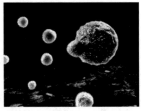

© Shutterstock

helper T cells

Lymphocytes that, once activated by antigen-presenting cells, secrete cytokines that direct the activity of other immune cells, particularly the cytotoxic T cells and B cells.

cytotoxic T cells

Lymphocytes that kill cells recognized as foreign (transplanted cells, cells infected by viruses or bacteria, or cells transformed by cancer).

regulatory T cells

Regulate other cells in the immune system, mainly by suppressing their activity. They maintain tolerance to "self" cells and otherwise keep the immune system from getting out of control.

1.3   When Pathogens Invade

FIGURE 13.5   Anatomy of a Lymph Node

In this image, you can see how the lymphatic vessels drain into and out of the lymph nodes. Tiny arteries and veins circulate blood and lymphocytes to the lymph nodes.

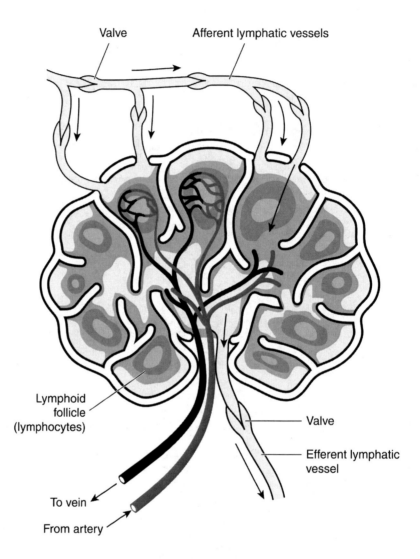

© Legger | Dreamstime.com

When microbes breach our physical and chemical barriers, phagocytic cells will attempt to dispose of them. In the immunologic equivalent of shouting "Intruder! Intruder!," antigen-presenting cells bring the foreign antigens (now protruding from their cell surfaces) to T lymphocytes, particularly the helper T cells. Helper T cells can then activate phagocytic cells, cytotoxic T cells, and B cells. The activated T and B cells clone themselves, and the B cells manufacture antibodies.

Cells in the innate and adaptive systems churn out *cytokines*, chemicals that regulate immune cells and signal cells in other organ systems. In response to viral infection, many cells release antiviral proteins called *interferons*. Activation of *complement*, a group of proteins floating in the blood, promotes the destruction of bacteria and causes inflammation.

Inflammation initiates healing but also produces collateral damage. The cardinal signs of inflammation are redness, heat, swelling, pain, and loss of function. Here's why. Inflammatory chemicals such as histamine dilate small arteries, which increases local blood circulation, generates redness and heat, and transports leukocytes to the area. The blood vessels also become leaky, allowing leukocytes to slip into the surrounding tissues. Fluid also seeps from the blood vessels into the tissues, causing swelling. Enzymes and other chemicals released from phagocytic cells can damage tissue. The swollen, damaged tissues cause discomfort. Meanwhile, *cortisol*, an adrenal gland hormone central to the stress response, is released to counter inflammation.

inflammation

The protective, nonspecific immune response of tissues to injury, infection, or irritation; characterized by local heat, redness, swelling, and pain.

Persistent infections, allergies, and other irritants can lead to chronic inflammation. In addition to unpleasant symptoms, chronic inflammation can, as mentioned earlier, raise the risk for a number of diseases.

The role of leukocytes from the innate system in the inflammatory response.

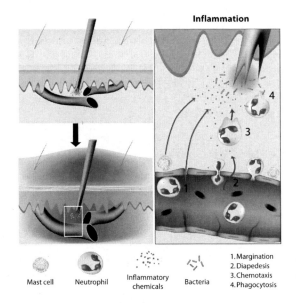

© *Shutterstock*

 Video Clip 13.4

The Inflammatory Response
These narrated images briefly describe the events occurring between the time of injury and the healing of the wound. The narrator discusses chemokines, which are a type of cytokine that mobilize and activate various leukocytes. Some of the viewers' comments below the video also add relevant information. (I'm not referring to comments such as, "cheers dude.")

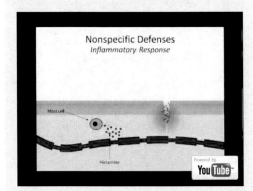

View the video online at: http://www.youtube.com/v/_bNN95sA6-8

1.4   Acquisition of Immunity

You can acquire immunity in one of two main ways: actively and passively. In **passive immunity**, you receive antibodies from a person (or animal) who was exposed to the foreign antigen. If, for instance, you go to a party and later learn the caterer had hepatitis A, your health care practitioner can inject you with antibodies (immunoglobulins) against this virus. Immunoglobulin injections are also used to protect people after bites from rabid animals and venomous snakes and spiders. Generally, passive immunity only lasts a few months.

Passive immunity is also transferred naturally from mothers to infants. During intrauterine life, fetuses receive maternal antibodies across the placenta. Breast milk contains antibodies and other components of the innate immune system. Breast-feeding also promotes the establishment of beneficial

passive immunity

Short-term immunity derived from the passive transfer of antibodies (immunoglobulins).

bacteria in the infant's intestines.[11] It may also protect against hereditary allergic conditions such as asthma, eczema, and hay fever.[12]

In **active immunity**, you develop B cells and T cells with memory for an antigen to which you were exposed. That exposure comes from actually having the infection or from an immunization. The immunity generated from an actual infection usually endures for long periods of time.

In **immunization** (also called vaccination), you receive a small amount of weakened or inactivated microbe, a fragment of the microbe, purified antigen, or inactivated bacteria toxin (e.g., tetanus toxin). These antigens are strong enough to activate the acquired immune system but too weak to cause illness. Vaccines may be given as injections and nasal sprays or taken by mouth. Booster vaccinations may be required at intervals to maintain immunity.

Universal immunizations stand with other public health measures—such as clean drinking water, sanitation, and basic hygiene—as our most effective means of preventing infectious diseases. As a result, many serious infections have dramatically declined.

Smallpox and the History of Vaccination

Hundreds of years ago, humans developed the art of vaccination against smallpox.[13] This viral infection caused a flu-like illness, followed by a pustular skin rash and ulcerated lesions within the mouth and nose. The more severe form of the illness killed 30 percent of its victims.[14]

Those who survived smallpox, while scarred, never contracted the illness again. Recognizing this phenomenon, 17th-century healers in the Middle East, Africa, India, and China introduced material from smallpox scabs into the noses or skin of healthy people. Many of those inoculated people were protected, although a small percentage died of smallpox infection.

Meanwhile, Europeans observed that milkmaids, regularly exposed to the relatively mild cowpox, were often immune to smallpox. (Much later scientists identified cowpox and smallpox as similar viruses.) In 1796, English scientist Edward Jenner inoculated his gardener's eight-year-old son with pus taken from the cowpox blisters on a milkmaid's hands. The boy developed a mild illness. When Jenner later exposed the boy to smallpox, the boy remained well. Jenner published his results, which precipitated mainly criticism and skepticism from colleagues. Nevertheless, other English physicians vaccinated people, confirming Jenner's findings. Vaccination caught on in Europe and America. In 1980, the World Health Organization declared the eradication of smallpox.

The bacterium *Corynebacterium diphtheriae* causes diphtheria. According to the World Health Organization, between 5 and 10 percent of infected people die. While the infection is now rare, epidemics continue to occur in other parts of the world.

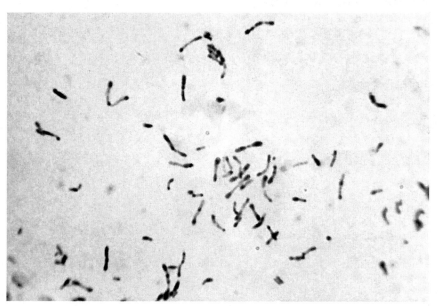

Source: Centers for Disease Control and Prevention. 1995. ID# 5325. Public Health Image Library (PHIL). Available at: http://www.cdc.gov/vaccines/ vpd-vac/diphtheria/photos.htm.

active immunity

The process of developing immunologic memory for a pathogen; results from fighting an infection or receiving an immunization.

immunization

Also called vaccination, the process of stimulating active immunity by exposing a person to a weakened form of a pathogen microbe or its toxin.

Immunizations benefit us in two main ways: (1) they protect individuals from infectious diseases, and (2) they protect entire populations by reducing the reservoir of microbial pathogens. This latter action, known as *herd immunity*, has stamped out a number of life-threatening pathogens. Even if the microbe remains in circulation, mass immunization protects vulnerable people such as pregnant women, infants, and people rendered immunodeficient by cancer treatment, HIV, or chronic illness.

Immunizations start in infancy because this age group is vulnerable to infection and because a vaccination should be given *before exposure to that particular microbe*. The Centers for Disease Control and Prevention provides a wealth of information about immunizations (CDC). For instance, you can find immunization schedules for different age groups and a downloadable blank vaccine record you can use to keep track of your vaccinations (http://www.cdc.gov/vaccines/schedules/index.html).

To learn about the diseases childhood immunizations prevent, go to http://www.cdc.gov/vaccines/vac-gen/10-shouldknow.htm. For instance, in diphtheria (the "D" in the DPT vaccine), the bacterial infection causes fever, chills, sore throat, swollen tonsils, and the formation of a membrane across the throat that obstructs breathing. The P stands for pertussis, or whooping cough, which causes such severe coughing the child (or adult) has trouble eating, drinking, and breathing. The T stands for tetanus, or lockjaw, so named because this bacterial toxin produces severe muscle spasms that hinder swallowing and breathing.

What about vaccine safety? While vaccinations can cause side effects (mainly soreness at the injection site and low-grade fever), the consequences of having these infections are far worse. Nevertheless, myths and erroneous beliefs about vaccinations abound. The CDC debunks six common misconceptions at http://www.cdc.gov/vaccines/vac-gen/6mishome.htm.

While the CDC provides fact-based information, other sources have propagated misinformation. A prime example is a 1998 article published in the venerable scientific journal *The Lancet*. British physician Andrew Wakefield and colleagues claimed an association between symptoms of autism and the MMR (measles, mumps, rubella) vaccination in 12 children. The report, quickly picked up by the popular media, generated mass hysteria, led to countless lawsuits against vaccine manufacturers, and caused alarmed parents in the United Kingdom and United States to forego vaccinating their children. Measles outbreaks followed. Between 1999 and 2000 in Ireland alone, a recorded 1,407 children came down with measles. Of 355 severely ill children attending a Dublin hospital, 111 were hospitalized and 3 died.[15]

Subsequent large-scale trials have failed to show any causal relationship between the MMR vaccine and autism,[16] though many parents and lawyers remained unconvinced. As it turns out, Wakefield's "research study" was fraudulent and unethical. In 2010, *The Lancet* retracted that paper.[17]

MMR is not the only vaccine to have been maligned by irresponsible reports in the media, legal action, and antivaccination groups. The result has been lower childhood vaccination rates and outbreaks of vaccine-preventable infections such as measles and pertussis, particularly among infants.[18],[19]

This coughing young boy has pertussis. Caused by bacterium *Bordetella pertussis*, the vaccine-preventable disease is highly communicable and can last many weeks. It's also called whooping cough because of the sound made when a person finally catches his breath at the end of a coughing fit. Vomiting may also follow coughing. The cough is so intense that children have trouble breathing and eating. Teens and adults may have fractured ribs.

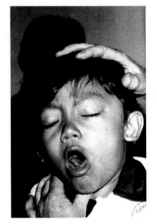

Source: Centers for Disease Control and Prevention. 1995. ID#: 6378. Public Health Image Library (PHIL). Available at: http://commons.wikimedia.org/wiki/File:Pertussis.jpg.

KEY TAKEAWAYS

- Scientists have long understood that the immune system guards against infection and cancer. Newer research shows that the influences are much broader than that. Cytokines contribute to fatigue, fever, mood, behavior, learning and memory, inflammation, and a number of chronic diseases.

- The immune system consists of several types of leukocytes and numerous chemicals.

    - The innate immune system offers you immediate, nonspecific protection against pathogens. Physical barriers keep pathogens out. Chemicals inhibit microbes, activate other immune system cells, and generate inflammation. Phagocytic cells patrol the perimeters, digest and attempt to eliminate debris and pathogens, and present antigens to lymphocytes.

    - The acquired immune system is specific but takes time to develop. After the first exposure to a foreign antigen, B cells and T cells develop immunologic memory. Upon subsequent exposures, B cells generate antibodies, and cytotoxic T cells combat infected cells.

    - The two systems interact. Microbes that penetrate physical and chemical barriers activate the innate and acquired immune systems. The process of combating an infection generates inflammation, which allows leukocytes to reach the trouble spot and contributes to healing but also produces some discomfort.

- We acquire immunity actively and passively.

    - Active immunity occurs when our immune systems encounter antigens either from exposure to the pathogen or from vaccinations.

    - Passive immunity occurs naturally when antibodies and other small immune chemicals cross the placenta or infuse breast milk and artificially when they enter from immunoglobulin injections.

2. WHEN THE IMMUNE SYSTEM GOES AWRY

LEARNING OBJECTIVES

1. **Discuss the three main types of immune system dysfunction: immunodeficiency, hypersensitivity, and autoimmunity.**

2. **Explore risk factors for immune dysfunction.**

3. **Explain how some of these conditions are treated.**

Considering the complexity of the immune system, it's not surprising that problems can arise. Abnormalities in immune function fall into three main camps: immunodeficiency, autoimmunity, and hypersensitivity.

2.1 Immunodeficiency

immunodeficiency

Failure of the immune system to protect the body from microbial pathogens and cancer.

As the word suggests, **immunodeficiency** means the system fails to fulfill its functions, putting the person at risk for overwhelming infection and cancer. Any part of the immune system can be affected: stem cells, lymphocytes, phagocytes, complement, or antibodies. The deficiency can be either present at birth or acquired later from environmental exposures, malnutrition, or chronic illness. Sometimes the treatment for a chronic illnesses can suppress the immune system, as when someone with cancer receives chemotherapy. Viruses can also impair immune function. A prime example is human immunodeficiency virus (HIV), which can lead to the *acquired immunodeficiency syndrome (AIDS)*.

2.2 Autoimmunity

autoimmunity

A condition in which the immune system attacks the person's own tissues.

In **autoimmunity**, the immune system mistakenly recognizes its own cells as foreign and attacks them. Genetics and environmental factors can both come into play. Here's a partial list of autoimmune diseases with the type of tissue attacked in parenthesis: type 1 diabetes (pancreas), multiple sclerosis (central nervous system), celiac disease (small intestine), systemic lupus erythematosus (multiple organs), Hashimoto's thyroiditis and Grave's disease (thyroid), and rheumatoid arthritis (joints). Several theories exist about how some agents (viruses, bacteria, drugs, foods) and shifts in immune function generate autoimmunity.

2.3 Hypersensitivity

In **hypersensitivity**, the immune system response is either excessive or inappropriate. The innate immune system, which is nonspecific in its approach, is largely responsible for the excess. Compared to the sniper-like specificity of the acquired system, the innate immune system deals with challenges by lobbing hand grenades, which causes collateral damage to normal tissues.

Inappropriate responses arise when the immune system attacks harmless material such as ragweed pollen, penicillin, and peanuts or excessively responds to irritants like bee venom. These normally harmless substances, when they trigger an allergic (hypersensitivity) reaction, are called **allergens**.

Four types of hypersensitivity reactions correspond to four different mechanisms whereby the immune system causes harm. Responses can be immediate or delayed. Most hypersensitivity reactions are immediate. Examples include most food allergies and bee stings. An example of delayed hypersensitivity is not developing a skin rash until one to three days after a brush against poison ivy.

In **atopy**, people are genetically susceptible to allergic conditions such as allergic rhinitis (hay fever), atopic dermatitis (eczema), and asthma. Usually symptoms become apparent in childhood and wane with age. Atopic conditions have been on the rise in industrialized countries, where as many as one in three people suffer symptoms.[20] Experts blame dietary habits, food additives, environmental pollutants, obesity, indoor lifestyles, and not having been breast-fed.[21]

Allergy tests can help identify the offenders. People can then take steps to avoid repeated exposures. Alternatively, they can try **allergen** desensitization (also called immunotherapy), which involves repeated injections of small amounts of the allergen ("allergy shots"). Successive doses of allergens can also be placed under the tongue. The goal is to increase a person's tolerance for the allergen.

Diet can also be improved, emphasizing fruits and vegetables and anti-inflammatory fatty acids such as those found in cold-water fish.[22] Some research has supported supplemental use of certain strains of probiotics (the beneficial microbes colonizing the gut). They may help prevent (if started in infancy), or ameliorate, atopic conditions.[23]

Now let's explore the three atopic conditions—allergic rhinitis, atopic dermatitis, and asthma—in more detail. **Allergic rhinitis**, more commonly called hay fever, results from exposure to airborne allergens such as pollen. Nearly 8 percent of adults and 10 percent of children have seasonal allergies.[24] Symptoms include a runny nose, sneezing, itchy skin, and watery, irritated eyes.

Drug treatment includes antihistamines, intranasal corticosteroids, and intranasal cromolyn. Allergy shots are one option for desensitization. Another technique is using preparations of particular allergens (e.g., timothy grass) given under the tongue over a period of several months to three years.[25] ,[26]

Nasal irrigation with salt water is also used to reduce symptoms.[27] To learn how to do this at home, go to the American Academy of Allergy, Asthma, and Immunology website (http://www.aaaai.org/patients/publicedmat/sinusitis/rinse.stm) or the National Jewish Hospital website (http://www.nationaljewish.org/healthinfo/medications/lung-diseases/alternative/nasal-wash-treatment). The University of Michigan Health System provides an instructional video (http://www.youtube.com/watch?v=62vm1Mb0T38&feature=related). Hygiene is key: wash your hands first, and only use water that has been boiled, bottled, or distilled.

In several studies, an herb called butterbur (*Petasites hybridus*) reduced hay fever symptoms in children and adults. In two of them, the herbal extract worked on par with the nonsedating antihistamines cetirizine (Zyrtec)[28] and fexofenadine (Allegra).[29] Special extracts that remove potentially liver-damaging chemicals must be used.

Dermatitis means skin inflammation. *Contact dermatitis* involves a delayed reaction to an allergen such as poison ivy, nickel, sheep's lanolin, and the antibiotic neomycin. **Atopic dermatitis**, more commonly called *eczema*, tends to run in families. In this case, the provoking allergens may never be identified. Up to 17 percent of school-aged kids have it, with 40–60 percent of cases persisting into adulthood.[30]

For both types of dermatitis, the affected patches of skin are red, itchy, scaly, and thickened, plus or minus oozing and crusting. Known allergens should be avoided. For eczema, management includes avoiding harsh soaps, keeping skin hydrated with soaks in water and moisturizing creams, and when necessary, using topical corticosteroids and other immunosuppressive drugs.

hypersensitivity

An exaggerated response of the immune system to an antigen.

atopy

A hereditary predisposition to develop hypersensitivity reactions such as allergic rhinitis, atopic dermatitis, and asthma.

allergen

A harmless substance that causes an allergic (hypersensitivity) reaction.

This image shows patches of redness and swelling after an allergy skin patch test, one of the common diagnostic tests to identify allergens.

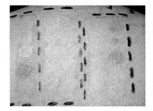

© Shutterstock

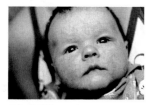

This newborn has eczema on his face. Note the patches of roughened, reddened skin.

© Radist | Dreamstime.com.

Preliminary research suggests that supplementation with certain probiotic strains can reduce eczema symptoms.[31],[32] Some herbs, applied topically, can soothe dermatitis. Aloe (*Aloe vera*) gel can promote healing and reduce inflammation in eczema.[33] Preliminary research has shown benefits from creams made from St. John's wort,[34] chamomile,[35] and licorice.[36]

Asthma is an inflammatory airway disease that affects nearly 8 percent of adults and 10 percent of children, making it the most common chronic childhood disease.[37] Allergens and other triggers cause symptoms such as chest tightness, wheezing, shortness of breath, and cough. During an asthma attack, the airways become inflamed, swollen, and constricted. Triggers can include tobacco smoke, dust mites, cockroaches, household molds, viral respiratory infections, cold air, psychological stress, exercise, and some medications.

People with asthma can learn to avoid triggers and use inhaled medications to reduce inflammation and maintain airway diameter. Oral and intravenous drugs are used short term to control severe attacks. For more information about asthma, go to the National Heart Lung and Blood Institute's web page on lung diseases (http://www.nhlbi.nih.gov/health/public/lung/index.htm) and click on "asthma." Use the form called "Asthma Action Plan" to help outline the appropriate action to take based on your symptoms.

A few studies suggest that a diet higher in the omega-3 fatty acids found in fish oil may improve asthma.[38],[39] Some studies show yoga and progressive muscle relaxation improve asthma.[40],[41] Some studies also suggest benefits from acupuncture.[42]

Another type of hypersensitivity reaction is **food allergies**. Like atopic conditions, they have become more common, with an 18 percent increase between 1997 and 2007.[43] In the United States, up to 8 percent of children and 3–4 percent of adults have allergic reactions to foods, and many of these reactions are severe.[44] Explanatory theories include the hygiene hypothesis (see the sidebar "The Hygiene Hypothesis: Get Dirty"), changes in infant feeding schedules, agricultural and food-processing practices, and insufficiency of certain dietary micronutrients.[45]

True food allergies involve an immediate or delayed immune system reaction to ingested material. Furthermore, food allergies can worsen atopic conditions. The most common offenders are cow's milk, soy, wheat, eggs, peanuts, tree nuts (e.g., almonds, walnuts, pecans, cashews), shellfish, and some fish. Symptoms can include gastrointestinal problems such as nausea, stomach pain, diarrhea, as well as hives and airway swelling. While allergic reactions to some foods are outgrown, others, such as to peanuts, can pose lifelong threats.

Some people confuse food allergies and *food intolerances*. The latter term is applied to foods an individual has trouble digesting but to which he or she is not allergic. In other words, the immune system is not involved. For instance, you can have a bad response to cow's milk because you're lactose intolerant and lack the enzyme to digest milk sugar or because you're allergic to proteins in the milk. Food intolerances cause nausea, gas, bloating, diarrhea, headache—but no skin rash or respiratory symptoms. Whereas a tiny amount of allergen can cause food allergies, it takes larger amounts and/or frequent exposures to elicit symptoms of intolerance.[46] Elimination diets can identify problem foods. Basically, you eat only foods that don't cause intolerance for several days, thereafter reintroducing one potential culprit every three days. Do not reintroduce known allergens unless under medical supervision. You don't want to risk anaphylaxis.

Anaphylaxis is a sudden, severe, widespread, and life-threatening allergic reaction. Causes include foods, insect stings, medications such as penicillin, the contrast material used in radiology studies, and latex (often used in rubber gloves). Up to 15 percent of Americans may be affected, with 500 to 1,000 deaths each year.[47]

An anaphylactic reaction may be heralded by feelings of uneasiness, dizziness, and tingling sensations. Soon thereafter, symptoms progress to itching, hives, rapid heart rate, gastrointestinal upset, swelling of the lips and mouth, hoarseness, runny nose, difficulty breathing, wheezing, confusion, and collapse.[48] Emergency treatment is needed. People with known severe allergies can inject themselves with epinephrine and head to the emergency room if symptoms persist.

anaphylaxis

A severe hypersensitivity reaction in which tissues in the mouth and throat swell and interfere with breathing; other symptoms include hives, itching, gastrointestinal upset, rapid heartbeat, and wheezing.

The Hygiene Hypothesis: Get Dirty

In response to the increase in allergic, autoimmune, and inflammatory conditions, some scientists have theorized that our immune systems were designed to cope with a pathogen-filled world. Unless you live on a farm, modern living can be relatively sterile. According to the hygiene hypothesis, decreased exposure to microbes and helminths (parasitic worms) early in life alters immune system development such that it favors chronic inflammation.[49] In a 2010 scientific article in *Microbes and Infection*, Italian researchers Manuela Sironi and Mario Clerici sum it up this way: "Too much cleanliness prevents the development of a well-balanced immune response; a touch of microbes is good for your health."[50]

In support of that theory, children who grow up in larger families (blessed with germy siblings) and around dogs, live in the country (around barnyard animals), or attend daycare early in life have a lower rate of atopic diseases. Exposure to infectious microbes can shift the balance of immune cells toward those that deal with important matters like combating tuberculosis, rather than those that go crazy over a little ragweed pollen. The development of healthy gut bacteria also seems to be another critical step toward shaping the immune system.

On the other hand, improved hygiene and sanitation (along with vaccinations and antibiotics) decreased the death rate from infections and lengthened our lives. Infections, however, continue to challenge us. Interestingly, use of antibiotics in the first year of life correlates with an increased risk of atopic conditions,[51],[52] suggesting that overuse of these drugs for minor infections may thwart immune maturation. Paradoxically, certain respiratory viral infections correlate with an increased risk of asthma.[53] Despite such inconsistencies, the hygiene hypothesis remains a hot topic in immunology circles.

In the meantime, go ahead—plunge your hands into dirt. Plant a garden. Muck out a barn. Take care of a dog. Afterward, wash your hands with plain soap and water.

If you already have an atopic condition, it's important to avoid triggers. For instance, dust mites and cockroaches can provoke atopic conditions such as asthma and eczema. In that case, it's important to keep a clean house and enclose pillows and mattresses in airtight covers.

According to the hygiene hypothesis, the child with the horse is less likely to have an atopic condition than the children on the couch.

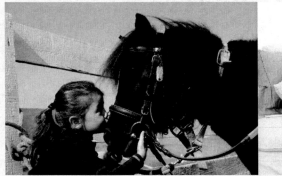 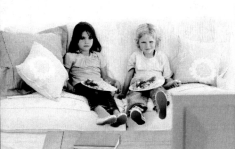

© Shutterstock

KEY TAKEAWAYS

Harmful immunity can take several forms:

- In immunodeficiency, the immune response is insufficient.
- In autoimmunity, the response involves an inappropriate attack of normal cells.
- In hypersensitivity, the response is excessive or unnecessary.
- Atopic conditions (atopic dermatitis, allergic rhinitis, and asthma) are hypersensitivity reactions in genetically susceptible people.

3. FORTIFYING IMMUNE FUNCTION

Keeping your immune system in tip-top shape involves two strategies: minimizing your exposure to things that weaken it and maximizing the factors that strengthen it.

3.1 Reducing Risk Factors for Infection

Some factors that raise the risk of infection are beyond your control; others you can eliminate or minimize.

- Age—the very young and the very old are most vulnerable
- Overcrowded, impoverished living conditions
- Lack of access to clean drinking water and inadequate public sanitation
- Frequent contact with small children (because they typically have frequent acute infections)
- Exposure to immunosuppressive agents (gamma radiation, drugs used to treat cancer, etc.)
- Undergoing a surgical procedure or other physical trauma (e.g., burns or abrasions over a large surface of skin) that breaches your physical barriers to infection
- Having an immunodeficiency disorder or a chronic disease that undermines immune function (e.g., diabetes, cancer, cystic fibrosis, depression)
- Alcohol in excess (binge drinking and chronic heavy consumption) impairs immune function.[54]
- Tobacco contains chemicals that unfavorably alter both humoral and cellular immunity. Tobacco smoke—whether you smoke or spend time in smoky environments—thickens the respiratory mucus and paralyzes the cilia, making it harder to expel microbes trapped in the mucus.
- Malnutrition can deplete your body of nutrients critical to proper immune function. Stay away from added sugar, which impairs phagocytosis by neutrophils.[55]
- Chronic stress overload depresses the ability to combat infections. By altering the balance of immune cells, allergies and autoimmunity can become more likely.
- Sleep deprivation activates the stress response. Chronic sleep deprivation takes a toll on immune function. Some but not all studies show transient dips in immune function after even one night of insufficient sleep.[56] People who habitually undersleep are more likely to get sick after exposure to cold viruses.[57]
- The perception of being socially isolated activates the stress response, generates inflammatory cytokines, and impairs some aspects of immune function.[58]

Your Head Affects Your Immune System

Our thoughts and feelings influence the immune system, and vice versa. Depression and anxiety can aggravate allergies and asthma and dampen immune function.[59],[60] Infection and inflammation can also sour mood. On the other hand, positive emotions and laughter buoy immunity.

Several decades ago, scientists documented that looking at pictures of hay could make some people with hay fever sniffle and sneeze. In the mid-1970s, Robert Ader and Nicholas Cohen at the University of Rochester coined psychoneuroimmunology, the study of how nervous, hormone, and immune systems interact. Their research included simultaneously giving lab animals saccharin-flavored water and an injection of a drug that suppressed the immune system. After three days of repeating this association, the sweet taste of the water coupled with an injection of harmless salt water depressed immune function.

The opposite—conditioned immune enhancement—is also possible. For instance, pairing the smell of camphor with an injection of a drug that activates immune cells can eventually lead to immune enhancement from the smell of camphor—even if the injection only contains salt water.[61]

Similar results have occurred in humans. For instance, after two weeks of using a placebo (dummy) inhaler while simultaneously smelling vanilla, children with asthma breathed more easily when they smelled vanilla, just as they would when using a real inhaler to dilate their airways.[62] While scientists don't understand precisely how this conditioning works, it's clear that our perceptions and expectations shape our health.

Chronic stress is not good for immune function.

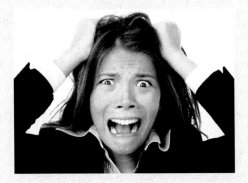

© Shutterstock

The Role of Stress in Immune Function

Stress overload is such a pervasive risk factor for immune dysfunction that it deserves a longer discussion. Having an infection is stressful. Any acute stressor activates the sympathetic nervous system (fight or flight), which boosts immune function.[63] Infection also produces inflammatory cytokines that trigger increases of the stress hormone cortisol,[64] which has short-term immune benefits. Specifically, cortisol counters inflammation, gets rid of old lymphocytes, and sends healthy lymphocytes into the tissues to combat the infection.[65] Bottom line: Moderate, acute stress enhances the immune system.

Too much stress, however, impairs the immune system. As discussed in Chapter 3, Hans Selye's chronically stressed laboratory rats had shriveled thymus glands and reduced lymphocyte counts and were susceptible to infection. A key reason is that persistently high cortisol levels suppress immune function. That's why people who have diseases that elevate cortisol (Cushing syndrome), take corticosteroid drugs, or endure excessive stress are vulnerable to infections. They're more likely to develop colds[66] and reactivations of latent viruses like herpes simplex.[67] Those already infected with HIV can worsen.[68] Antibody responses to vaccinations are less robust.[69]

Less often, chronic stress can promote a hypersensitive immune system and aggravate conditions such as allergies, asthma, and autoimmune disease.[70],[71],[72]

Stress reduction techniques repair the damage. Relaxation training improves atopic conditions such as eczema and asthma.[73] Activities that relieve stress—yoga, meditation, massage, listening to quiet music—and social support improve immune function.[74],[75],[76],[77],[78]

3.2 Maximizing Protective Factors

A whole foods diet that emphasizes vegetables, fruits, nuts, and leans meats (especially fish rich in omega-3 fatty acids) provides the nutrients the immune system needs.

© *Shutterstock*

Exercising outside and with a buddy benefits the immune system. The social stimulation, physical activity, sun-induced production of vitamin D, and stress relief all help. In addition, some plants release calming, immune-boosting scents.[83]
[84]

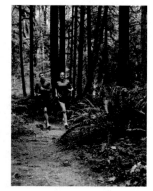

© *Shutterstock*

Fortunately, you can do a number of things to promote immune function.

- **Eat well.** Proper immune system function depends on a number of macronutrients and micronutrients. You can get most of them with a diet full of fruits, vegetables, and nuts. The needed protein can come from plants or animals. Cold-water fish and some plants (olives, walnuts, and the seeds of chia, flax, pumpkin, and hemp) supply anti-inflammatory oils. One study showed that simply increasing fruit and vegetable consumption to at least five portions a day for 12 weeks improved some immune markers.[79]

  Dietary antioxidants such as vitamin C, vitamin E, carotenes, zinc, and selenium play a protective role against infections and can help prevent cell damage caused during the immune response.[80] Unless you're deficient, supplements aren't necessary. Your best bet is to consume plenty of fruits, vegetables, and nuts, which are naturally rich in these nutrients.

- **Keep up to date on immunizations.** The Centers for Disease Control and Prevention posts immunization schedules (http://www.cdc.gov/vaccines/schedules/index.html). Keep a shot record handy. If in doubt about your immunization status, ask your primary care doctor.

- **Stay physically active.** Regular, moderate exercise appears to benefit immune function and have an anti-inflammatory effect.[81] Activities with a meditative component such as tai chi, qigong, and yoga also promote healthy immune systems.[82]

- **Spend time outdoors.** A Japanese research group has shown that spending time in forested areas increases immune markers such as NK cell activity.[85] One study found that neighborhoods with higher densities of trees had fewer asthmatic kids.[86] Perhaps the additional greenery helped remove air pollutants, relieved stress, or encouraged kids to play outside. Furthermore, sunlight activates the skin's production of vitamin D (which the immune system needs).

- **Wash your hands.** At least do so before eating and after going to the bathroom. You've heard this advice since childhood. Yet when researchers spied on people in public bathrooms, they found that about 30 percent of men and 12 percent of women didn't wash their hands.[87]

  Simple soap and water or alcohol-based hand sanitizers can reduce the transmission of many viruses, bacteria, and parasites.[88] Antibacterial soaps and gels containing substances such as triclosan and triclocarban are unnecessary, foster antibiotic-resistant bacteria, and harm the environment. Those two chemicals, which now pollute our surface water and soil, alter hormone regulation in animals.[89],[90]

- **Be water wise.** Adequate hydration ensures that you urinate often (which flushes away bacteria attempting to ascend the urinary system) and that your mucus is thin enough to easily clear. Americans have the luxury of safe tap water. In fact, commercially bottled water may have more bacteria than tap water.[91] However, water fountains can contain microbes, particularly if users spit into the basin. Water coolers can also harbor "bugs."

- **Be social.** Meaningful relationships have immune system perks.[92] Social support improves outcomes in serious immunological challenges such as cancer and HIV infection and may also protect against more mundane infections. For example, when researchers blew rhinoviruses (one of the causes of the common cold) up volunteers' noses, those with more social ties were less likely to get sick and, if they did, they had fewer symptoms for a shorter period of time.[93] Also, if you're an animal lover, contact with four-footed friends can also boost immune function.[94]

- **Laugh.** Having a sense of humor relieves stress, makes life more enjoyable, and stimulates the immune system. Watching a funny video can enhance immune activity for up to 12 hours.[95] Positive emotions such as happiness generally correlate with more robust immune health.[96]

Assess Yourself: Immune System Health

Do your health behaviors promote or undermine your immune system's ability to protect you from infectious diseases? To find out, complete the following checklist. Consider an unchecked space in the left-hand column a risk factor. Ideally, you have checked all of the spaces in the left-hand column and none of the spaces in the right-hand column. If not, create a plan for changing them for the better. You can find tips for success in other chapters in this book.

Protective Factors	Risk Factors
■ ____I exercise for at least 30 minutes most days of the week. ■ ____I belong to a network of supportive friends and family. ■ ____I eat a whole-foods, plant-based diet. ■ ____I usually awaken feeling refreshed. ■ ____I take time to relax and enjoy nature. ■ ____I'm up to date on my immunizations. ■ ____I wash my hands after using the bathroom and before handling food.	■ ____I smoke and/or hang out with smokers. ■ ____I often consume more than three alcoholic drinks within four hours. ■ ____I consume sugary beverages and snacks most days of the week. ■ ____I feel sleepy much of the day. ■ ____I feel stressed out most of the time.

Immune-Enhancing Herbs

Herbal immune tonics: ginseng roots, astragalus roots, garlic, and shiitake mushrooms.

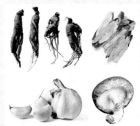

© Elenaray; Lcc54613; Johnfoto; Chiyacat | Dreamstime.com

If you're the type of person to catch every "bug" that's going around, herbal immune tonics may help. Traditional Chinese medicine practitioners have long used **astragalus** (*Astragalus membranaceous*) to build resistance to infection in people with weakened immune function. Root extracts promote a number of white blood cells and cytokines[97] that help counter the immunosuppressive effects of drugs used to treat cancer.[98] This nontoxic herb can be taken as a tincture or tea. The mild-tasting sliced roots (which look like tongue depressors) can also be added to soups and removed before serving.

Another Asian favorite is **ginseng** (*Panax ginseng*). The Native Americans made similar use of American ginseng (*Panax quinquefolius*). Like astragalus, ginseng enhances several types of immune cells and cytokines. Preliminary research indicates that ginseng extracts may help prevent respiratory infections and reduce the incidence of some cancers.[99],[100]

Garlic (*Allium sativum*) is cheap, versatile, readily available, and easy to grow. In addition to boosting the immune system, it has anticancer and antimicrobial activity against a variety of bacteria, viruses, fungi, and parasites. In one study, people taking a garlic supplement for 12 weeks developed fewer colds than those taking a placebo.[101] Because key ingredients are broken down by heat and stomach acid, researchers typically give volunteers tablets coated to increase absorption from the small intestine. You can also try adding a clove or two of minced garlic to meals just before serving.

Many edible **mushrooms** enhance immunity. One of the better-researched species is **shiitake** (*Lentinus edodes*),[102] which many grocery stores stock. While modern research uses concentrated, purified extracts, it won't hurt to consume shiitake and other mushrooms as food.

KEY TAKEAWAYS

- A number of factors, some of which you can control, undermine immune function.
  - Advancing age results in a diminution of some aspects of immune function, a process accelerated by modifiable risk factors such as smoking and stress overload.
  - A two-way relationship exists between thoughts and emotions and immune system function.
  - Acute stress produces a transient enhancement of immunity; chronic stress depresses immune function.
- Healthy lifestyle habits—eating whole foods, getting recommended vaccinations, sleeping enough, reducing stress, exercising regularly, enjoying friends, and basic hygiene—safeguard immune function.
  - Herbal immune tonics may have benefits for people with compromised immune function.

DISCUSSION QUESTIONS

1. Explain why smoking cigarettes impairs immune function.
2. Give an example of how thoughts and emotions affect immune function and how the immune system affects psychological state.
3. Think about the type of stressor our ancestors encountered. From the standpoint of survival, why does the effect of acute stress on immune function make sense?
4. In the face of chronic stress, what types of illnesses become more likely? Have you ever gotten sick during finals week, or just afterward? Give an example.
5. Explain the ways in which spending time in nature might improve immune function. (Presume the environment is safe and peaceful.) Do you think it's possible that just imagining you're in a pleasant natural environment might improve immune function? Defend your answer.

4. RECOMMENDED RESOURCES

4.1 Books

Doan T, Melvold R, Viselli S, Waltenbaugh C. *Lippincott's Illustrated Reviews: Immunology*. Philadelphia, PA: Lippincott Williams & Wilkins; 2007.

Playfair JHL, Chain BM. *Immunology at a Glance*. 9th ed. West Sussex, UK: Wiley-Blackwell; 2009.

Delves PJ, Martin SJ, Burton DR, Roitt IM. *Roitt's Essential Immunology*. 12th ed. London, UK: Wiley-Blackwell; 2011.

4.2 Organizations and Websites

American Academy of Allergy, Asthma and Immunology. Provides information on immunizations, food allergies, atopic conditions, and immunodeficiency diseases. http://www.aaaai.org/patients.stm.

Centers for Disease Control and Prevention. Provides an A to Z index with information on conditions discussed in this chapter, as well as immunizations. http://www.cdc.gov.

Mayo Clinic. Provides information on diseases and conditions discussed in this chapter. http://www.mayoclinic.com.

National Jewish Health. This highly ranked research and treatment center offers information on hypersensitivity disorders such as asthma, allergic rhinitis, and atopic dermatitis. http://www.nationaljewish.org.

ENDNOTES

1. Rabin BR. *Stress, Immune Function, and Health: The Connection.* New York, NY: Wiley-Liss; 1999.

2. Yirmiya R, Goshen I. Immune modulation of learning, memory, neural plasticity and neurogenesis. *Brain Behav Immun.* 2011 Feb;25(2):181–213.

3. Capuron L, Miller AH. Immune system to brain signaling: neuropsychopharmacological implications. *Pharmacol Ther.* 2011 May;130(2):226–238.

4. Lorton D, Lubahn CL, Estus C, et al. Bidirectional communication between the brain and the immune system: implications for physiological sleep and disorders with disrupted sleep. *Neuroimmunomodulation.* 2006;13(5–6):357–374.

5. Grippo AJ, Johnson AK. Stress, depression, and cardiovascular dysregulation: a review of neurobiological mechanisms and the integration of research from preclinical disease models. *Stress.* 2009;12(1):1–21. doi:10.1080/10253890802046281.

6. Kiecolt-Glaser JK, Glaser R. Depression and immune function: central pathways to morbidity and mortality. *J Psychosom Res.* 2002;53(4):873–876.

7. Doan T, Melvold R, Viselli S, Waltenbaugh C. *Lippincott's Illustrated Reviews: Immunology.* Philadelphia, PA: Lippincott Williams & Wilkins; 2008:30.

8. Bengmark S. Ecological control of the gastrointestinal tract: the role of probiotic flora. *Gut.* 1998;42(1):2–7. As cited in Guarner F, Malagelada JR. Gut flora in health and diseases. *Lancet.* 2003;61(9371):512–519.

9. Guarner F, Malagelada JR. Gut flora in health and disease. *Lancet.* 2003;61(9371):512–519.

10. Dong P, Yang Y, Wang WP. The role of intestinal bifidobacteria on immune system development in young rats [Epub ahead of print]. *Early Hum Dev.* 2010 Jan 25;86(1):51–58.

11. Yoshioka H, Iseki K, Fujita K. Development and differences of intestinal flora in the neonatal period in breast-fed and bottle-fed infants. *Pediatr.* 1983 Sep;72(3):317–321.

12. Halken S. Prevention of allergic disease in childhood: clinical and epidemiological aspects of primary and secondary allergy prevention. *Pediatr Allergy Immunol.* 2004 Jun;15(16)(suppl):4–5, 9–32.

13. Barquet N, Domingo P. Smallpox: the triumph over the most terrible of the ministers of death. *Ann Intern Med.* 1997 Oct 15;127(8 Pt 1):635–642.

14. Smallpox. World Health Organization. Available at: http://www.who.int/mediacentre/factsheets/smallpox/en. Accessed June 12, 2012.

15. McBrien J, Murphy J, Gill D, Cronin M, O'Donovan C, Cafferkey MT. Measles outbreak in Dublin, 2000. *Pediatr Infect Dis J.* 2003 Jul;22(7):580–584.

16. Madsen KM, Hviid A, Vestergaard M, et al. A population-based study of measles, mumps, and rubella vaccination and autism. *N Engl J Med.* 2002;347(19):1477–1482.

17. Eggertson L. *Lancet* retracts 12-year-old article linking autism to MMR vaccines. *Can Med Assoc J.* 2010;182(4):E199–200. doi:10.1503/cmaj.109–3179. Available at: http://www.ncbi.nlm.nih.gov/pmc/articles/PMC2831678/?tool=pubmed. Accessed June 9, 2011.

18. Poland GA, Jacobson RM. The age-old struggle against the antivaccinationists. *N Engl J Med.* 2011;364(2):97–101.

19. Roehr B. Whooping cough outbreak hits several US states. *BMJ.* 2010 Aug 24;341:c4627. doi:10.1136/bmj.c4627.

20. Asher M, Montefort S, Bjorksten B, et al.; ISAAC Phase Three Study Group. Worldwide time trends in the prevalence of symptoms of asthma, allergic rhinoconjunctivitis, and eczema in childhood: ISAAC phases one and three repeat multicountry cross-sectional surveys. *Lancet.* 2006;368:733–743.

21. Sehgal VN, Srivastava G, Dogra S. Atopic dermatitis: current options and treatment plan. *Skinmed.* 2010 Nov–Dec;8(6):335–344.

22. Kremmyda LS, Vlachava M, Noakes PS, Diaper ND, Miles EA, Calder PC. Atopy risk in infants and children in relation to early exposure to fish, oily fish, or long-chain omega-3 fatty acids: a systematic review. *Clin Rev Allergy Immunol.* 2009 Dec 9. doi 10.1007/s12016-009-8186-2. Available at: http://www.naturopatia-sanatum.pl/alergia.pdf. Accessed June 7, 2011.

23. Betsi GI, Papadavid E, Falagas ME. Probiotics for the treatment or prevention of atopic dermatitis: a review of the evidence from randomized controlled trials. *Am J Clin Dermatol.* 2008;9(2):93–103.

24. Centers for Disease Control and Prevention. FastStats: allergies and hay fever. National Center for Health Statistics. Available at: http://www.cdc.gov/nchs/fastats/allergies.htm. Accessed June 6, 2011.

25. Kay AB. An extract of Timothy-grass pollen used as sublingual immunotherapy for summer hay fever. *Drugs Today (Barc).* 2007 Dec;43(12):841–848.

26. Alesina R, Milani M, Pecora S. A multicenter, randomized, parallel-group trial assessing compliance, tolerability, safety, and efficacy to treatment with grass allergy tablets in 261 patients with grass pollen rhinoconjunctivitis. *J Allergy.* 2012. doi:10.1155/2012/673502.

27. Garavello W, Somigliana E, Acaia B, Gaini L, Pignataro L, Gaini RM. Nasal lavage in pregnant women with seasonal allergic rhinitis: a randomized study. *Int Arch Allergy Immunol.* 2010;151(2):137–141.

28. Schapowal A; Petasites Study Group. Randomised controlled trial of butterbur and cetirizine for treating seasonal allergic rhinitis. *BMJ.* 2002 Jan 19;324(7330):144–146. Available at: http://www.ncbi.nlm.nih.gov/pmc/articles/PMC64514/?tool=pubmed. Accessed June 6, 2011.

29. Schapowal A; Study Group. Treating intermittent allergic rhinitis: a prospective, randomized, placebo and antihistamine-controlled study of butterbur extract Ze 339. *Phytother Res.* 2005 Jun;19(6):530–537.

30. Shaw TE, Currie GP, Koudelka CW, Simpson EL. Eczema prevalence in the United States: data from the 2003 National Survey of Children's Health. *J Invest Dermatol.* 2011 Jan;131(1):67–73.

31. Isolauri E, Arvola T, Sutas Y, et al. Probiotics in the management of atopic eczema. *Clin Exp Allergy.* 2000;30:1604–1610.

32. Rosenfeldt V, Benfeldt E, Nielsen SD, et al. Effect of probiotic lactobacillus strains in children with atopic dermatitis. *J Allergy Clin Immunol.* 2003;111:389–395.

33. Kim J, Lee I, Park S, Choue R. Effects of Scutellariae radix and Aloe vera gel extracts on immunoglobulin E and cytokine levels in atopic dermatitis NC/Nga mice. *J Ethnopharmacol.* 2010 Nov 11;132(2):529–532.

34. Schempp CM, Hezel S, Simon JC. Topical treatment of atopic dermatitis with Hypericum cream. A randomised, placebo-controlled, double-blind half-side comparison study. *Hautarzt.* 2003 Mar;54(3):248–253.

35. Patzelt-Wenczler R, Ponce-Pöschl E. Proof of efficacy of Kamillosan cream in atopic eczema. *Eur J Med Res.* 2000 Apr 19;5(4):171–175.

36. Saeedi M, Morteza-Semnani K, Ghoreishi MR. The treatment of atopic dermatitis with licorice gel. *J Dermatolog Treat.* 2003 Sep;14(3):153–157.

37. Centers for Disease Control and Prevention. FastStats: Asthma. National Center for Health Statistics. Available at: http://www.cdc.gov/nchs/fastats/asthma.htm. Accessed June 6, 2011.

38. Schubert R, Kitz R, Beermann C, et al. Effect of n-3 polyunsaturated fatty acids in asthma after low-dose allergen challenge. *Int Arch Allergy Immunol.* 2009;148:321–329.

39. Peat JK, Mihrshahi S, Kemp AS, et al. Three-year outcomes of dietary fatty acid modification and house dust mite reduction in the Childhood Asthma Prevention Study. *J Allergy Clin Immunol.* 2004;114:807–813.

40. Posadzki P, Ernst E. Yoga for asthma? A systematic review of randomized Clin Trials [Epub ahead of print 2011 May 31]. *J Asthma.* 2011 Aug;48(6):632–639. Available at: http://www.ncbi.nlm.nih.gov/pubmed/21627405.

41. Huntley A, White AR, Ernst E. Relaxation therapies for asthma: a systematic review. *Thorax.* 2002 Feb;57(2):127–131. Available at: http://www.ncbi.nlm.nih.gov/pmc/articles/PMC1746244/?tool=pubmed.

42. Yu L, Zhang Y, Chen C, Cui HF, Yan XK. Meta-analysis on randomized controlled Clin Trials of acupuncture for asthma. *Zhongguo Zhen Jiu.* 2010 Sep;30(9):787–792. Article in Chinese. English abstract available at: http://www.ncbi.nlm.nih.gov/pubmed/20886804.

43. Branum AM, Lukacs SL. Food allergy among children in the United States. *Pediatrics.* 2009;124:1549–1555.

44. Gupta RS, Springston BA, Warrier MR, et al. The prevalence, severity, and distribution of childhood food allergy in the United States. *Pediatrics* [Published online ahead of print]. 2011 June 20. doi:10.1542/peds.2011–0204.

45. Leonard SA. Food allergy: what you need to know. Medscape. October 15, 2010. Available at: http://www.clontarfclinic.com/allergy/index.php/educational/2012-01-12-08-19-15/86-food-allergy-what-you-need-to-know. Accessed June 12, 2011.

46. Is it a food allergy or intolerance? Allergies Health Center. WebMD. Available at: http://www.webmd.com/allergies/foods-allergy-intolerance. Accessed June 3, 2011.

47. Neugut AI, Ghatak AT, Miller RL. Anaphylaxis in the United States: an investigation into its epidemiology. *Arch Intern Med.* 2001 Jan 8;161(1):15–21. Available at: http://www.ncbi.nlm.nih.gov/pubmed/11146694. Accessed June 14, 2011.

48. Merch & Co. Anaphylactic reactions. *The Merck Manual.* Whitehouse Station, NJ: Merck & Co., Inc; 2009–2010. Available at: http://www.merckmanuals.com/home/sec16/ch185/ch185i.html. Accessed June 3, 2011.

49. Flohr C, Yeo L. Atopic dermatitis and the hygiene hypothesis revisited. *Curr Probl Dermatol.* 2011;41:1–34.

50. Sironi M, Clerici, M. The hygiene hypothesis: an evolutionary perspective. *Microbes Infect.* 2010 Jun;12(6):421–427, doi:10.1016/j.micinf.2010.02.002.

51. Marra F, Lynd L, Coombes M, et al. Does antibiotic exposure during infancy lead to development of asthma?: a systematic review and metaanalysis. *Chest.* 2006 Mar;129(3):610–618. Available at: http://chestjournal.chestpubs.org/content/129/3/610.long. Accessed June 6, 2011.

52. Mullooly JP, Schuler R, Barrett M, Maher JE. Vaccines, antibiotics, and atopy. *Pharmacoepidemiol Drug Saf.* 2007 Mar;16(3):275–288.

53. Rautava S, Ruuskanen O, Ouwehand A, Salminen S, Isolauri E. The hygiene hypothesis of atopic disease—an extended version. *J Pediatr Gastroenterol Nutr.* 2004 Apr;38(4):378–388.

54. Kovaks EJ, Messingham K. Influence of alcohol and gender on immune response. National Institute of Alcohol Abuse and Alcoholism. Available at: http://pubs.niaaa.nih.gov/publications/arh26-4/257-263.htm. Accessed February 9, 2012.

55. Sanchez A, Reeser JL, Lau HS, et al. Role of sugars in human neutrophilic phagocytosis. *Am J Clin Nutr.* 1973 Nov;26(11):1180–1184.

56. Irwin M, McClintick J, Costlow C, Fortner M, White J, Gillin JC. Partial night sleep deprivation reduces natural killer and cellular immune responses in humans. *FASEB J.* 1996 Apr;10(5):643–653.

57. Cohen S, Doyle WJ, Alper CM, Janicki-Deverts D, Turner RB. Sleep habits and susceptibility to the common cold. *Arch Intern Med.* 2009 Jan 12;169(1):62–67.

58. Hawkley LC, Cacioppo JT. Loneliness matters: a theoretical and empirical review of consequences and mechanisms. *Ann Behav Med.* 2010 Oct;40(2):218–227.

59. Dave ND, Xiang L, Rehm KE, Marshall GD Jr. Stress and allergic diseases. *Immunol Allergy Clin North Am.* 2011 Feb;31(1):55–68. Available at: http://www.ncbi.nlm.nih.gov/pmc/articles/PMC3264048/?tool=pubmed. Accessed February 10, 2012.

60. Di Marco F, Santus P, Centanni S. Anxiety and depression in asthma. *Curr Opin Pulm Med.* 2011 Jan;17(1):39–44.

61. Ader R, Cohen N. Conditioning and immunity. In: Ader R, Felten DL, Cohen H, eds. *Psychoneuroimmunology.* Vol 2. 3rd ed. San Diego,CA: Academic Press;2001:3–39.

62. Castes M, Palenque M, Canelones P, Hagel I, Lynch N. Classic conditioning and placebo effects in the bronchodilator response of asthmatic children. *Neuroimmunomodulation.* 1998;5:70. As cited in Ader R. Conditioned immunomodulation: research needs and directions. *Brain Behav Immun.* 2003;17:S51–S57. Available at: http://www.sciencedirect.com/science/article/pii/S0889159102000673. Accessed June 2, 2011.

63. Dhabhar FS, McEwen BS. Enhancing versus suppressive effects of stress hormones on skin immune function. *PNAS (Proceedings of the Natural Academy of the Sciences).* 1999;96(3):1059–1064. doi:10.1073/pnas.96.3.1059.

64. Webster JI, Tonelli L, Sternberg EM. Neuroendocrine regulation of immunity. *Annu Rev Immunol.* 2002;20:125–163.

65. Dunn AJ. Interactions between the nervous system and the immune system: implications for psychopharmacology. *Am Coll Neuropsychopharmacol.* Available at: http://www.acnp.org/g4/gn401000069/ch069.html. Published 2000. Accessed June 3, 2011.

66. Cohen S, Tyrrell DA, Smith AP. Psychological stress and susceptibility to the common cold. *N Engl J Med.* 1991 Aug 29;325(9):606–612.

67. Sainz B, Loutsch JM, Marquart ME, Hill JM. Stress-associated immunomodulation and herpes simplex virus infections. *Med Hypotheses.* 2001 Mar;56(3):348–356.

68. Leserman J, Petitto JM, Gu H, et al. Progression to AIDS, a clinical AIDS condition and mortality: psychosocial and physiological predictors. *Psychol Med.* 2002 Aug;32(6):1059–1073.

69. Pedersen AF, Zachariae R, Bovbjerg DH. Psychological stress and antibody response to influenza vaccination: a meta-analysis. *Brain Behav Immun.* 2009 May;23(4):427–433.

70. Montoro J, Mullol J, Jáuregui I, et al. Stress and allergy. *J Investig Allergol Clin Immunol.* 2009;19(1)(suppl):40–47.

71. Stojanovich L. Stress and autoimmunity. *Autoimmun Rev.* 2010 Mar;9(5):A271–A276.

72. Chida Y, Hamer M, Steptoe A. A bidirectional relationship between psychosocial factors and atopic disorders: a systematic review and meta-analysis. *Psychosom Med.* 2008 Jan;70(1):102–116. Available at: http://www.ncbi.nlm.nih.gov/pubmed/18158379. Accessed June 4, 2011.

73. Chida Y, Steptoe A, Hirakawa N, Sudo N, Kubo C. The effects of psychological intervention on atopic dermatitis. A systematic review and meta-analysis. *Int Arch Allergy Immunol.* 2007;144(1):1–9.

74. Davidson R, Kabat-Zinn J, Schumacher J, et al. Alterations in brain and immune function produced by mindfulness meditation. *Psychosom Med.* 2003;65:564–570.

75. Hirokawa E, Ohira H. The effects of music listening after a stressful task on immune functions, neuroendocrine responses, and emotional states in college students. *J Music Ther.* 2003 Fall;40(3):189–211.

76. Spiegel D, Bloom JR, Kraemer HC, Gottheil E. Effect of psychosocial treatment on survival of patients with metastatic breast cancer. *Lancet.* 1989;2:888–891.

77. Ironson G, Hayward H. Do positive psychosocial factors predict disease progression in HIV-1? A review of the evidence. *Psychosom Med.* 2008 Jun;70(5):546–554. Available at: http://www.ncbi.nlm.nih.gov/pmc/articles/PMC2614870/?tool=pubmed.

78. Shor-Posner G, Hernandez-Reif M, Miguez MJ, et al. Impact of a massage therapy clinical trial on immune status in young Dominican children infected with HIV-1. *J Altern Complement Med.* 2006 Jul–Aug;12(6):511–516.

79. Sanderson P, Elsom RL, Kirpatrick V, et al. UK food standards agency workshop report: diet and immune function [Epub ahead of print 2010 Mar 9]. *Br J Nutr.* 2010 Jun;103(11):1684–1687. doi:1-1017/20007111409993692.

80. Puertollano MA, Puertollano E, de Cienfuegos GA, de Pablo MA. Dietary antioxidants: immunity and host defense [Epub ahead of print 2011 Apr 21]. *Curr Topics Med Chem.* 2011;11(14):1752–1766.

81. Walsh NP, Gleeson M, Shephard RJ, et al. Position statement. Part one: immune function and exercise. *Exerc Immunol Rev.* 2011;17:6–63. Available at: http://www.ncbi.nlm.nih.gov/pubmed/21446352.

82. Jahnke R, Larkey L, Rogers C, Etnier J, Lin F. A comprehensive review of health benefits of qigong and tai chi. *Am J Health Promot.* 2010;24(6):e1–e25.

83. Li Q, Kobayashi M, Wakayama Y, et al. Effect of phytoncide from trees on human natural killer cell function. *Int J Immunopathol Pharmacol.* 2009 Oct–Dec;22(4):951–959.

84. Sadlon AE, Lamson DW. Immune-modifying and antimicrobial effects of eucalyptus oil and simple inhalation devices. *Altern Med Rev.* 2010 Apr;15(1):33–47.

85. Li Q, Kawada T. Effect of forest environments on human natural killer (NK) activity. *Int J Immunopathol Pharmacol.* 2011 Jan–Mar;24(1)(suppl):39S–44S.

86. Lovasi G S, Quinn JW, Neckerman KM, Perzanowski M S, Rundle A. Children living in areas with more street trees have lower prevalence of asthma. *J Epidemiol Community Health.* 2008;62(7):647–649.

87. One in three men don't wash after bathroom visit. *Associated Press.* September 17, 2007. Available at: http://www.msnbc.msn.com/id/20823288. Accessed June 6, 2011.

88. Aiello AE, Murray GF, Perez V, et al. Mask use, hand hygiene, and seasonal influenza-like illness among young adults: a randomized intervention trial. *J Infect Dis.* 2010 Feb 15;201(4):491–498.

89. Triclosan: what consumers should know. Food and Drug Administration. April 8, 2010. Available at: http://www.fda.gov/forconsumers/consumerupdates/ucm205999.htm. Accessed June 6, 2011.

90. Hinther A, Bromba CM, Wulff JE, Helbing CC. Effects of triclocarban, triclosan, and methyl triclosan on thyroid hormone action and stress in frog and mammalian culture systems [Epub ahead of print 2011 May 16]. *Environ Sci Technol.* 2011 Jun 15;45(12):5395–5402. Available at: http://www.ncbi.nlm.nih.gov/pubmed/21574574.

91. Case Western Reserve University. Study finds some bottled water has more bacteria and less fluoride than tap water. *ScienceDaily.* March 22, 2000. Available at: http://www.sciencedaily.com/releases/2000/03/000322090356.htm. Accessed February 10, 2012.

92. Miyazaki T, Ishikawa T, Iimori, H, et al. Relationship between perceived social support and immune function. *Stress Health.* 2003;19(1):3–7.

93. Cohen S, Doyle WJ, Skoner DP, Rabin BS, Gwaltney JM Jr. Social ties and susceptibility to the common cold. *JAMA.* 1997 Jun 25;277(24):1940–1944.

94. Charnetski CJ, Riggers S, Brennan FX. Effect of petting a dog on immune system function. *Psychol Rep.* 2004 Dec;95(3 Pt 2):1087–1091.

95. Berk L, Felten D, Tan S, Bittman B, Westengard J. Modulation of neuroimmune parameters during the eustress of humor-associated mirthful laughter. *Altern Ther Health Med.* 2001;7(2):62–72, 74–76.

96. Barak Y. The immune system and happiness. *Autoimmun Rev.* 2006 Oct;5(8):523–527.

97. Astragalus membranaceus. Monograph. *Altern Med Rev.* 2003 Feb;8(1):72–77. Available at: http://www.ncbi.nlm.nih.gov/pubmed/12611564.

98. Duan P, Wang ZM. Clinical study on effect of Astragalus in efficacy enhancing and toxicity reducing of chemotherapy in patients of malignant tumor. *Zhongguo Zhong Xi Yi Jie He Za Zhi* [Article in Chinese]. 2002 Jul;22(7):515–517.

99. McElhaney JE, Gravenstein S, Cole SK, et al. A placebo-controlled trial of a proprietary extract of North American ginseng (CVT–E002) to prevent acute respiratory illness in institutionalized older adults. *J Am Geriatr Soc.* 2004 Jan;52(1):13–19.

100. Yun TK, Choi SY, Yun HY. Epidemiological study on cancer prevention by ginseng: are all kinds of cancers preventable by ginseng? *J Korean Med Sci.* 2001 Dec;16 Suppl:S19–27.

101. Josling P. Preventing the common cold with a garlic supplement: a double-blind, placebo-controlled survey. *Adv Ther.* 2001 Jul–Aug;18(4):189–193.

102. Bisen PS, Baghel RK, Sanodiya BS, Thakur GS, Prasad GB. Lentinus edodes: a macrofungus with pharmacological activities. *Curr Med Chem.* 2010;17(22):2419–2430.

CHAPTER 14
Coping with Common Infections

Microorganisms can be friends or foes. Some organisms are so virulent they sicken even the hardiest people. But many microbes harmlessly coexist with us, causing diseases only if our immune systems weaken. The human body harbors between 10^{13} and 10^{14} bacterial, fungal, and protozoan cells.[1] Many improve our health. The bacteria colonizing on our skin and mucous membranes contribute to nonspecific immune defenses. In the intestinal tract, they make certain vitamins, help digest our food, and break down dietary toxins and carcinogens (cancer-causing substances).

After a brief history of microbiology, this chapter reviews the main types of infectious agents, the methods of transmission, and stages of infection. The rest of the chapter covers the major infectious diseases in the respiratory, digestive, nervous, and urinary systems, as well as skin infections. You learn which types of microbes cause them, signs and symptoms of infection, and approaches to treatment and prevention.

1. UNDERSTANDING INFECTIONS

LEARNING OBJECTIVES

1. Discuss the advances in science and public health that have reduced the risk of death from infectious diseases.
2. Distinguish key features that differentiate the main types of microorganisms.
3. Identify common species and the types of illnesses they cause.
4. Define criteria necessary for an infection to occur.
5. Describe the stages of infection.

1.1 A Historical Perspective

Before the 20th century, infectious diseases were the main cause of illness and death. For instance, in the mid-1800s in America, infectious diseases such as tuberculosis, infectious diarrhea, and pneumonia most commonly caused death, and life expectancy was about 44 years.[2] Now, thanks to improvements in public sanitation, immunizations, and antibiotics, life expectancy has risen to 78.5 years.[3] Compared to influenza and pneumonia, which have fallen to the number eight cause of death, heart disease kills nearly 12 times more people.[4]

In order to avoid and treat infections, we humans had to first understand their origins. For millennia, we didn't. Ancient Egyptians thought angry gods sickened humans.[5] Hippocrates, a forward-thinking ancient Greek physician, blamed some sort of environmental factor. Unfortunately, his rational approach took time to catch on. In the meantime, infectious diseases were blamed on witches, vapors, and other mystical agents.

During the 1700s, scientists spied microorganisms under the microscope but didn't link them to disease. In 1854, London physician John Snow traced the source of a cholera outbreak to a contaminated water pump. Soon thereafter, French scientist Louis Pasteur determined that microscopic organisms caused infectious illnesses. He introduced pasteurization, a process of gently heating foods and beverages to kill microbes. He also worked to develop vaccines and encourage surgeons to wash their hands and equipment. Other scientists contributed to the germ theory of disease. The 1930s saw the development of antibiotics.

FIGURE 14.1 Louis Pasteur

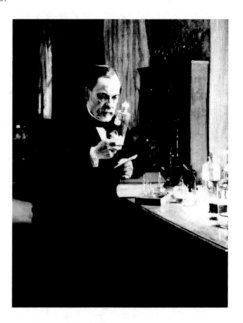

© *Thinkstock*

In the grand scheme of infectious disease control, the innovations that saved the most lives were the introduction of sewers, flush toilets, and water sanitation. While we take such amenities for granted, about 1.1 billion people lack access to clean water, and 2.6 billion do not have toilets.[6] Each year, some 12 million people—many of them children in developing countries—die of infectious illnesses that are largely preventable and treatable.[7]

Microbes, however, challenge even the most privileged. Some bacteria have become resistant to multiple antibiotics, and new infectious agents continually emerge, their dissemination hastened by globe-trotting travelers. Global warming has nudged tropical diseases northward.[8] For instance, mosquitoes carrying West Nile virus, which can infect the nervous system, arrived in North America in 1999 and spread quickly.[9] Despite these ever-present threats, you have many options decreasing your risk of infectious disease.

1.2 How Infections Develop

Types of Infectious Agents

In an **infection**, an organism has invaded to reproduce, multiply, and cause disease. A similar term is **infestation**, which means the organism has taken up residence within you to live off your energy resources. Seven classes of organisms cause infection or infestation: bacteria, viruses, protozoa, fungi, helminths, ectoparasites, and prions.

Strictly speaking, **microorganisms** (microbes for short) are life forms too small to see with the naked eye. Examples include bacteria and protozoa. While individual fungi are microscopic, they can group to form readily visible colonies. Furthermore, microbiologists also study viruses and prions—which are not living cells—and helminths and ectoparasites, which are visible without the aid of a microscope.

infection

The process by which microorganisms invade bodily tissues to reproduce, multiply, and cause disease.

infestation

The process by which a parasitic organism invades its host to live off its energy resources.

microorganisms

Microscopic organisms such as a bacterium, virus, or protozoa.

Bacteria are single-celled microorganisms. Unlike our cells, bacteria lack a nucleus and other organelles (structures within the cell that perform specific functions). Another difference is that they're surrounded by a rigid cell wall. They can move using tail-like flagella and other mechanisms. They have different shapes. *Cocci* are round; *bacilli* are long, thin, and rod-like; and *spirochetes* have a spiral shape. Other characteristics, such as whether they can survive without oxygen, classify them. Antibiotic drugs are used to treat *pathogenic* (disease-causing) bacteria.

bacterium

A unicellular organism that lacks organelles and an organized nucleus (*pl.* bacteria).

Video Clip 14.1

How Bacteria Cause Disease
The narrated images depict the ways bacteria infect us, as well as our immune system's response to these microbes.

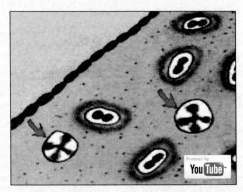

View the video online at: http://www.youtube.com/v/KM1DcGOY-tA

Viruses are nonliving microscopic particles that contain only DNA or RNA within a protein capsule. They can't multiply outside of a host cell. They operate by docking their protein coats onto a cell and injecting their genetic material inside. From there, the viral DNA or RNA takes over the cell's machinery to make more viruses. Once released from the host cell, these newly minted viruses infect other cells, replicate, and infect other cells, unless and until the immune system stops the chain reaction.

viruses

Tiny microbes that cannot reproduce outside a host cell; consist of DNA or RNA within a protein capsule.

Because viruses aren't alive outside of cells, they're difficult to kill. High heat and chlorine do destroy them. Rubbing alcohol (the active ingredient in most hand sanitizers) inactivates some but not all viruses.[10] None of the aforementioned agents can be used once the virus invades the body. (Rubbing alcohol and chlorine are poisonous to consume; chlorine shouldn't be applied to skin.)

Antibiotics don't touch viruses. Relatively few drugs have been developed to interfere with various stages of the viral infection cycle. Some viruses are contained by such medications, but many aren't. Synthetic interferons can be injected to augment the body's immune response to viral infections such as hepatitis B and C, though they cause flu-like side effects. An experimental approach is to synthesize antibodies against the virus and give these by injection.

Protozoa are unicellular organisms. Most are motile. Many are *parasites*, meaning they can't live outside of a nutrient-providing host. They are often transmitted via contaminated water, food, or feces. A few can travel by air to infect the lungs. Some require a **vector**, an agent (usually an invertebrate animal such as a tick) capable of transferring an infectious organism from one host to another. For instance, mosquitoes can carry malaria protozoa. In the developing world, protozoan infections cause much illness and death. Infections such as giardiasis (a diarrheal illness caused by *Giardia lamblia*) can be treated with drugs. Others, such as malaria, can be difficult to eliminate. Several species of *Plasmodium* cause it, and some have developed resistance to multiple drugs.

protozoa

A large group of unicellular organisms that contain an organized nucleus. Singular is protozoon.

vector

A carrier that transfers an infective organism from reservoir to host or from one host to another; usually an arthropod such as a mosquito or tick.

Fungi can be unicellular or multicellular and include mushrooms, yeasts, and molds. In a mutually beneficial relationship, some fungi live on our bodily surfaces. We also eat mushrooms, use yeasts to culture foods (bread, coleslaw, alcoholic beverages), and derive from them drugs such as the antibiotic penicillin.

Fungi reproduce by budding or by making spores that are tiny enough to be inhaled into the lungs, where they may cause pneumonia. Some infect the skin. The yeast *Candida*, a normal resident in the mouth, intestine, and vagina, can grow out of control in people who take antibiotics or have immunodeficiencies. With the exception of some fungal skin infections, most fungi aren't contagious.

fungi

Unicellular or multicellular. Includes mushrooms, yeasts, and molds.

helminths

Parasitic worms.

Helminths are parasitic worms that can infest us. They include roundworms, flatworms, and tapeworms. We acquire them by ingesting, inhaling, or contacting their eggs, which can contaminate food, water, air, feces, and inanimate objects. Most enter through our mouths and grow to maturity in our intestines. Depending on the type of helminth, symptoms and signs can be absent or include malaise, decreased appetite, weight loss, abdominal discomfort, nausea, diarrhea, anemia, and anal itching. Helminth infestations stunt the growth of millions of children in the developing world.[11] Drugs called anthelmintics help expel worms.

ectoparasites

Parasitic organisms such as a flea or tick that lives on its host surface.

More complicated organisms called **ectoparasites** can attach to our skin and hair to generate disease. Lice, which are in the arachnid (spider) family, fasten to hair shafts. Mites, also tiny arachnids, can burrow under the skin to cause scabies. Bedbugs are small insects whose nighttime feasts on the blood of slumbering humans can cause skin rashes and allergic symptoms. Other bloodsucking ectoparasites, such as mosquitoes, ticks, and fleas can act as vectors. For instance, mosquitoes can inject us with West Nile virus and malaria. Tick bites can give us the bacterial illnesses Rocky Mountain spotted fever and Lyme disease. Fleas can carry the bacterium that causes plague.

prions

Microscopic, abnormally folded proteins thought to cause nerve-degenerating diseases such as bovine spongiform encephalopathy ("mad cow disease").

Prions are the weirdest infectious agent. Like viruses, they aren't alive. Unlike viruses, they don't even contain genetic material—just a bit of misfolded protein. Prions are thought to cause conditions of severe brain degeneration such as bovine spongiform encephalopathy (BSE or "mad cow disease") and Creutzfeldt-Jakob disease. *Encephalopathy* means brain disease, and *spongiform* describes the sponge-like holes in the brain. Prions are transmitted through contaminated products derived from brain, blood, and other tissues. New research suggests the prion disease scrapie (which normally affects sheep) may be transmitted to mice via airborne exposure.[12] In BSE, prions enter meat during the slaughter process. They become deposited in the host's brain, where they can make other proteins misfold. Unfortunately, no known treatment exists for prions.

FIGURE 14.2

1) *E. coli* bacteria. 2) Influenza virus. 3) protozoa causing amoebiasis. 4) *Candida* yeast. 5) Tapeworm, a kind of helminth. 6) *Bedbug*, a type of ectoparasite.

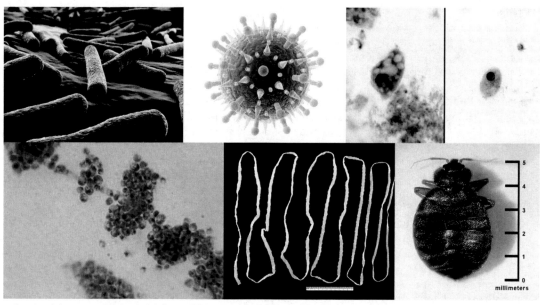

© *Shutterstock (images 1 and 2); http://phil.cdc.gov/phil/details.asp (6666) (image 3); http://phil.cdc.gov/phil/details.asp (2918) (image 4); http://phil.cdc.gov/phil/details.asp (5260) (image 5); http://phil.cdc.gov/phil/details.asp (12704) (image 6).*

TABLE 14.1 Common Microbial Pathogens

Type of pathogen	Species name	Diseases caused
Bacteria	*Staphyloccocus aureus*	skin infections, pneumonia, meningitis, and more methicillin-resistant strains are most feared
	Streptococcus pyogenes	strep throat, some skin infections
	Streptococcus pneumoniae	pneumonia, middle ear infection, meningitis, blood infection (bacteremia)
	Chlamydia trachomatis	sexually transmitted; can infect the urethra, rectum, prostate, and female reproductive organs (pelvic inflammatory disease)
	Neisseria meningitidis	meningitis
	Neisseria gonorrhoeae	gonorrhea (a sexually transmitted infection)
	Mycobacterium tuberculosis	tuberculosis
	Helicobacter pylori	peptic ulcers
Virus	corona virus, rhinovirus	common cold
	influenza viruses	influenza
	herpes simplex virus	cold sores, genital lesions
	varicella-zoster virus	chickenpox
	human papillomaviruses	warts, genital lesions, cervical cancer
	hepatitis viruses	hepatitis
	human immunodeficiency virus	HIV, acquired immunodeficiency syndrome (AIDS)
	Epstein-Barr virus	mononucleosis
Fungi	*Candida* species	overgrowth can affect the vagina, intestines, mouth
	dermatophytes	athlete's foot, ringworm, jock itch
	Coccidioides immitis, C. posadasii	coccidiomycosis ("valley fever"); rash, flu-like symptoms, possibly pneumonia
	Cryptococus neoformans	pneumonia, meningitis
	Histoplasma capsulatum	histoplasmosis ("Cave disease," "Spelunker's Lung")
Protozoa	*Entamoeba histolytica*	amoebiasis (diarrhea and other gastrointestinal symptoms); can cause abscesses in lung, liver, and brain
	Giardia lambila	giardiasis (diarrhea)
	Cryptosporidium	cryptosporidiosis (diarrhea)
	Plasmodium species	malaria
	Trichomonas vaginalis	trichomoniasis (a sexually transmitted infection of the urethra and vagina)
Helminths	*Ascaris lumbricoides*	a roundworm that competes for nutrients in the intestines
	Necator americanis	a hookworm that competes for intestinal nutrients
	Taenia solium, T. saginata	a tapeworm transmitted from undercooked pork and beef; can grow to great lengths within the intestines and cause abdominal discomfort, diarrhea, anemia, loss of appetite

1.3 Transmission of Infectious Diseases

Infectious diseases are illnesses caused by infectious agents or toxins produced by them. In this process, microorganisms invade the body, reproduce, and multiply. Some are also **communicable diseases**, meaning they spread from one person to another. In other words, they're contagious. The term *noncommunicable illness* refers to a condition that lacks an infectious cause, such as heart disease, stroke, diabetes, and cancer.

Sometimes communicable diseases become **epidemic**, meaning the infection spreads rapidly to affect many people. The term *epidemic* more broadly refers to any abnormal condition with a widespread distribution. For instance, cardiovascular disease and diabetes have swelled to epidemic proportions in the United States. **Pandemic** means an epidemic has gone global.

Pathogenic microorganisms are widespread, yet most people remain healthy. Clearly, certain requirements must be met in order for infection to occur.

1. The host must be susceptible. Some pathogens don't cause illness unless the person's immune system is compromised. Infants and elderly people are vulnerable because, in the first case, the immune system is immature and, in the second, it's weaker. Immunodeficiency diseases, cancer treatment, and some chronic conditions also put people at particular risk.

2. The microbe must be **virulent**, or capable of causing disease. Highly virulent microbes can attack even those with healthy immune systems.

3. The microbe also requires a *reservoir*, an environment—human, other animal, soil, water, food—in which it can survive. Normally the microbe does not adversely affect living reservoirs. In other words, the host is asymptomatic (without symptoms). Here are some examples of reservoirs: humans (tuberculosis); mice (hantaviruses); ticks (the Lyme disease bacterium); soil (tetanus bacteria); water (*Giardia lamblia*), and food (*E. coli*).

4. The microbe has a *route of transmission*, a means of migrating from its reservoir to its host. Sometimes the route occurs by direct *horizontal transmission* (spread from one person to the next). You kiss someone infected with Epstein-Barr virus (mononucleosis). Sometimes the route is indirect. You push the shopping cart recently used by someone with the common cold, then inoculate yourself with viruses by touching the inside of your nose. Or an animal or insect vector brings you the microbe, as happens when a tick carrying the Lyme disease bacterium bites you. Other pathogens can be *airborne* (influenza viruses), *waterborne* (cholera bacteria), or *food borne* (salmonella bacteria). *Vertical transmission* can occur between a pregnant woman and her developing fetus and between a mother and her breast-feeding baby.

5. The microbe requires a *portal of entry*, a means of entering the body. A break in the skin allows *Staphylococcus aureus*, which can be carried on the skin, to cause an infection. Inhalation of influenza viruses allows them to dock onto cells in respiratory passages. Microbes contaminating food or water latch onto the intestinal lining. Sometimes pathogens penetrate deeper, entering the bloodstream to cause systemic (widespread) infection.

6. To continue infecting other people, the microbe must find a *portal of exit*. Microbes such as respiratory viruses may be excreted from sputum (mucus brought up from the lungs) and nasal phlegm. Others exit the body in saliva, blood, and feces. Still others depend on direct contact with infected skin or mucous membranes (such as most sexually transmitted agents).

FIGURE 14.3 Chain of Infection

Possible illustration of chain of infection with *Giardia*.

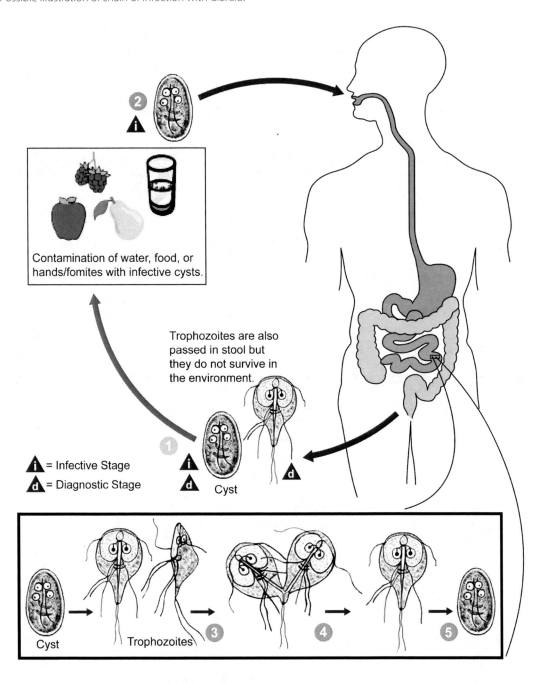

Contamination of water, food, or hands/fomites with infective cysts.

Trophozoites are also passed in stool but they do not survive in the environment.

▲i = Infective Stage
▲d = Diagnostic Stage

Cyst

Cyst   Trophozoites

Source: CDC/Alexander J. da Silva, PhD/Melanie Moser. ID# 3394. Public Health Image Library (PHIL). Available at: http://phil.cdc.gov/phil/ details.asp.

Interruptions anywhere in this **chain of infection** can prevent its spread. For instance, sleeping under a mosquito net and wearing insect repellent blocks malaria transmission. Sanitizing drinking water prevents cholera. Staying home if you have influenza hinders contagion. Washing your hands reduces the risk that you'll transfer pathogens to your food, nostrils, or any open wounds.

1.4 Stages of Infection

Once the pathogen has gained a foothold in your body, you don't immediately feel sick. This symptomless interlude is called the *incubation period*. Meanwhile, the microbe reproduces and attracts the attention of the innate immune system. Vague malaise signals the start of the *prodromal period*. You might attribute the symptoms to not getting enough sleep, hitting the books too hard, or exercising too vigorously the day before. Those misapprehensions vanish once the *period of illness* grips you. During that time, microbial and immune system warfare damages tissue and releases inflammatory cytokines into the circulation. Finally, the illness peaks, the immune system triumphs, and you enter what's called the *period of decline*, which means the illness is declining, not your health. Next comes the *convalescence period*. You crawl out of bed, taking it easy for some days while you recover. Soon, your body has repaired the damage, and you're back to life as usual.

Severe infections can produce persistent symptoms or signs, such as permanent hearing loss after meningitis or a damaged heart valve after strep throat. The length of these stages of infection and the severity of symptoms depend on things such as the **virulence** of the pathogen (its ability to infect the host), the efficiency of the immune system's response, and the body's overall recuperative power.

virulence

The degree to which a microorganism is capable of causing disease; the intensity and speed at which a microbial pathogen sickens its host.

KEY TAKEAWAYS

- Multiple advances—improved sanitation, better living conditions, heightened hospital hygiene standards, immunization programs, antimicrobial drugs—dramatically reduced the toll of microbial pathogens on us humans.
- Infectious agents include bacteria, viruses, protozoa, fungi, helminths, ectoparasites, and prions. Some can live independently of their host; some cannot. Many can't be seen by the naked eye. Some are not even, technically speaking, alive.
- In order for an infection to occur, the host has to be vulnerable, and the microbe must be sufficiently virulent and have a means of entering and exiting the host. Reservoirs for infection allow the microbe to persist in the environment. Routes of transmission allow it to move between reservoir and host.
- Infections follow a series of stages from the incubation period through the recovery from the illness.

DISCUSSION QUESTIONS

1. How have medical advances over the past century altered longevity? What types of diseases cause the most deaths in Americans? (Go to http://who.int/mediacentre/factsheets/fs310/en/index1.html for World Health Organization tables of the leading causes of death in high-income versus low-income countries.)

2. Name the main types of infection-causing pathogens and give an example of each.

3. What types of disease do prions cause?

4. How do ticks cause disease?

5. Give an example of a route of transmission for an infectious agent.

6. During what stage of infection is a person not yet feeling any symptoms? Can you think of any public health concerns related to asymptomatic (symptomless) illness?

2. COMMON RESPIRATORY INFECTIONS

LEARNING OBJECTIVES

1. Explain why, year after year, we remain vulnerable to the common cold and influenza.
2. Identify key signs and symptoms of upper and lower respiratory infection.
3. Discuss self-care for mild infections.
4. Identify warning signs for seeking prompt medical attention.

FIGURE 14.4 The Respiratory System

This image shows a virus entering the respiratory system.

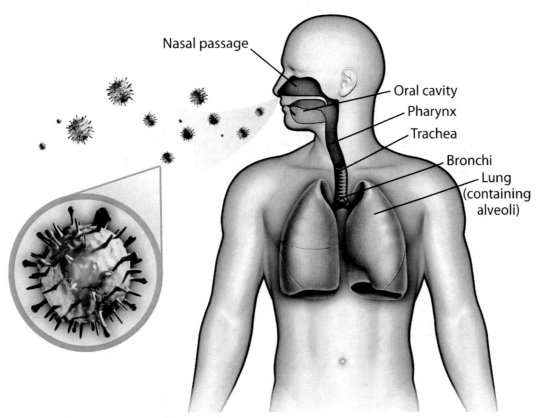

© Andreus | Dreamstime.com.

As is the case with all illnesses, infectious illnesses can be *acute* (coming on quickly and resolving within days) or *chronic* (persisting for months or more). Acute infections are generally self-limiting, meaning they resolve without medical intervention. Sometimes an antimicrobial drug is needed to reduce suffering, hasten recovery, prevent complications, and even avert death. Chronic conditions require long-term medical support. This section focuses on acute respiratory infections, which are exceedingly common.

All of the components of the respiratory system can become infected—the nose (**rhinitis**), sinuses (*sinusitis*), throat (*pharyngitis*), lower airways (*bronchitis*), and lungs (*pneumonia*). Some respiratory microbes can also infect the eyes' outer lining (*conjunctivitis*) and the middle ear (*otitis media*), which has a tube that opens into the pharynx. (Note: The ending "-itis" means inflammation. In addition to microbial pathogens, a number of other agents can cause the inflammation: allergens, chemicals, and excessive heat or cold.)

Health practitioners often lump respiratory infections into upper and lower. Upper respiratory infections affect you from the neck up—nose, sinuses, throat, larynx, and trachea. Lower respiratory infections involve the lower airways (bronchi and bronchioles) and alveoli (air sacs) of the lungs.

rhinitis

Inflammation of the nose, usually due to allergies or viruses.

Most of the time, the causative agents are viruses. In fact, viral respiratory infections are the most common illness we humans endure.[13] Bacteria are the next most common pathogen. Less often, fungi and protozoa are the culprits. Even helminths can make their way to the lungs, though that's uncommon in the United States.

Many respiratory infections, notably viral upper respiratory infections, plague us during the late fall and winter. There are several reasons for this seasonal variation. Though the viruses don't disappear in sunnier months, they're more abundant in winter. Contrary to myth, cold weather doesn't make you sick—not unless prolonged exposure taxes your immune system. Another theory is that, during the winter in higher latitudes, the sun's ultraviolet rays aren't sufficiently intense to generate production of vitamin D in the skin. Indeed, vitamin D insufficiency is much more common in winter.[14] Furthermore, deficiency correlates with an increased risk of respiratory tract infections.[15]

2.1 Common Cold

common cold

An acute, self-limiting, upper respiratory infection caused by multiple viruses.

No one is immune from the **common cold**, an acute, self-limiting, viral upper respiratory infection. The average adult catches two to four colds a year; children may have six to eight.[16] Several factors explain recurrences. One, more than 200 types of viruses cause the condition. Rhinoviruses account for up to 50 percent of colds. Other cold viruses include coronavirus, adenovirus, and parainfluenza virus. Two, these viruses undergo constant genetic alterations such that, each winter, they're sufficiently different to require a fresh immune response. Three, they survive for hours on nonporous surfaces such as pens, computer keyboards, and doorknobs. They also become airborne with sneezes or coughs, allowing bystanders to inhale them into their respiratory systems.

After a two- to three-day incubation period, the all-too-familiar symptoms and signs develop: runny nose, nasal stuffiness, sneezing, watery eyes, hoarseness, cough, fatigue, and diminished appetite. Sinus congestion can produce headaches. Antibiotics are useless against viruses and only serve to wipe out the "good" bacteria that contribute to immune health in your mucous membranes.

Uncomplicated colds should be over within a week and don't require medical intervention. Rest, fluids, and good nutrition are recommended. Complications include middle ear infections (more often in children than adults), sinusitis, and pneumonia.

Dietary Supplements and Respiratory Infections

Should you take extra vitamins, minerals, or herbs if you develop cold symptoms? Inconsistencies in the research make a straight answer difficult.

- **Vitamin C** used to be a popular remedy. However, the cumulative scientific data doesn't justify mega-dosing this vitamin to prevent or treat the common cold.[17] Some studies, however, support the use of supplements (600 to 1,000 milligrams/day) in people undergoing physical stress (prolonged, intense exercise) who have a history of frequent upper respiratory infections.[18]

- **Vitamin D** plays a role in regulating the immune system and may have direct antiviral effects.[19] Exposure to ultraviolet light and consumption of cod liver oil (a vitamin D source) and other vitamin D supplements have been linked to reduced viral respiratory infections.[20]

- Some research shows **zinc** supplementation has therapeutic benefits in infectious conditions such as acute respiratory tract infections, infectious diarrhea, and chronic hepatitis C.[21] Most studies use zinc gluconate or zinc acetate lozenges containing at least 13 milligrams of elemental zinc, one lozenge every two hours while awake starting when symptoms begin and stopping when they decline.[22] Side effects of the lozenges include an unpleasant taste and nausea. Prolonged intake of high amounts of zinc (150 milligrams/day and up) can depress immune function.[23]

  A number of herbs have been used traditionally to manage respiratory infections. Several have undergone scientific scrutiny.

- The best-researched herb for managing cold symptoms is immune-enhancing **echinacea**. Most studies show that when good products are taken frequently soon after symptoms begin, they *modestly* reduce symptom severity and duration of the common colds.[24] Products with the strongest research support are those made from the preserved juice of the aboveground parts of *Echinacea purpurea* or the alcoholic extracts ("tinctures") of the roots of *E. angustifolia* or *E. purpurea*. This herb belongs to the same plant family as ragweed and may provoke allergic skin rashes in sensitive people.

- Another herbal combination product has emerged as possibly more effective than echinacea in nipping viral respiratory infections in the bud—Kan Jang, which contains **eleuthero**, also called Siberian ginseng and **andrographis**.[25]

- **Garlic** is antimicrobial and immune-enhancing.[26] One study showed that a commercial product, taken for 12 weeks of winter, reduced the frequency of colds by 64 percent, as well as the severity and duration of those that did occur.[27]

- **Ginseng** also boosts immune function. While no studies have evaluated its usefulness in treating respiratory infections, three studies have shown that a proprietary extract of American ginseng called COLD-fX helps prevent respiratory infections in seniors.[28] One study showed better antibody responses to influenza vaccines and protection against the common cold for an Asian ginseng extract called Ginsana.[29]

- A traditional European remedy is elder flowers or berries made into tea, plus or minus peppermint. Research shows that the **elderberries** have immune-enhancing actions against influenza and other respiratory viruses.[30],[31] Three small studies have demonstrated rapid recovery from influenza with special elderberry extracts.[32],[33],[34]

1) Echinacea. 2) Eucalyptus. 3) Elderberry. 4) Garlic.

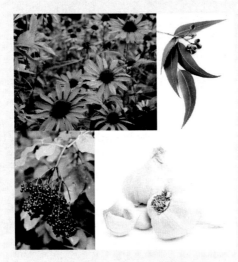

© Shutterstock

2.2   Influenza

Influenza, or flu, is a highly contagious viral respiratory illness. The virus spreads easily from person to person via respiratory droplets—tiny drops of moisture released into the air when an infected person talks, coughs, and sneezes. In an average year, 5 to 20 percent of Americans will develop influenza, more than 200,000 will wind up in the hospital, and more than 36,000 will die.[35] Those most vulnerable to severe disease are people over the age of 65 and under the age of 2, as well as people with chronic medical conditions.

influenza

A viral infection that can affect both the upper and lower respiratory tract. More virulent influenza viruses can cause severe disease and spawn pandemics. In addition to influenza viruses, other viruses can produce similar symptoms.

Video Clip 14.2

How Influenza Viruses Invade the Respiratory Tract
This National Public Radio video briefly explains how influenza viruses infect and replicate within respiratory cells. The narrator refers to "yellow knobby things" (the virus's hemagglutinin) and "noodly" things (the virus's genetic material).

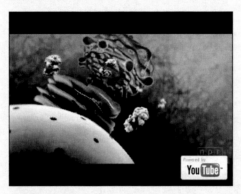

View the video online at: http://www.youtube.com/v/RpjOemEGShQ

While other viruses can cause flu-like illness, influenza is caused by one of three types of influenza viruses: A, B, and C. The last infrequently causes illness. Only influenza A viruses have produced pandemics. The viruses are subtyped based on characteristics of two surface proteins: hemagglutinin (H) and neuraminidase (N). For instance, the 2009 pandemic involved H1N1 viruses. Antibodies protect us against particular hemagglutinin antigens (substances that trigger the production of antibodies).

These antigens alter constantly. As far as our acquired immune system is concerned, each winter brings fresh enemies. Unless you've been vaccinated against that particular virus strain, you're vulnerable. The antigens change either through subtle, gradual modifications called *antigenic drift* or through more radical transformations called *antigenic shift*. Antigenic drifts in influenza viruses are common and contribute to most cases of seasonal influenza. You may get sick, but the illness isn't severe due to at least partial immune recognition.

Antigenic shifts give rise to viruses against which we have little or no immunity, thereby spawning pandemics. You may have noticed that some influenza viruses are named after animals (swine flu, avian flu). Normally, pathogenic microbes, including influenza, only torment a single species. Pigs, birds, and humans each have their own pool of viruses. Occasionally, humans working in close contact with infected pig and domesticated fowl pick up a swine or avian virus. That's bad for the infected human, but normally other humans don't get sick—not until that novel virus becomes capable of human-to-human transmission. Pigs can become infected with swine, avian, and human influenza viruses.[36] If genetic reassortment occurs, genes are swapped among viruses, producing an antigenic shift. With a critical roll of the dice, you can get a brand-new virus with enough human genetic material that it can spread person to person.

Global travel has increased the risk of pandemics. Let's say a tourist goes to Southeast Asia, visits a market full of caged chickens and ducks, and picks up an avian virus—one that has just developed the ability to travel person to person. Two days later, he and his family board a plane back to Los Angeles. During the flight, he talks, laughs, and snores, releasing viruses into the air. By the time the plane touches down, he feels lousy but chalks it up to jet lag. On the way home, he stops by his busy office. By morning, he has a fever and a cough. His wife sends the tired, cranky kids off to school. The pandemic is off and running.

Influenza pandemics vary in severity. The 2009 H1N1 virus produced relatively mild symptoms. On the other hand, the 1918 pandemic killed 20 to 40 million people—mortality on par with a world war.[37]

These highly contagious viruses are spread primarily through respiratory droplets. Direct contact and self-inoculation can also lead to infection. After an incubation period of 2 days, symptoms develop abruptly with fever, chills, malaise, muscle aches, headache, sore throat, runny nose, and nonproductive cough (little to no sputum). Even though influenza is a respiratory illness, vomiting and diarrhea may occur. The common cold is, in comparison, a cakewalk. The period of contagion begins the day before symptoms and continues for another 5 to 10 days.[38]

Uncomplicated infections usually resolve within 3 to 7 days. Fatigue and cough may linger. Complications include viral pneumonia, worsening of chronic lung and heart conditions, and secondary bacterial infections such as sinusitis, middle ear infection, and bacterial pneumonia. ("Secondary" refers to the fact that the primary viral infection weakened the host, making him or her vulnerable to a bacterial infection.) People at elevated risk for complications include very young children, pregnant women, people over the age of 65, and those with chronic conditions such as asthma, heart disease, chronic obstructive lung disease, diabetes, and immunodeficiency diseases.

Usually, a diagnosis is made based on symptoms. If confirmation of influenza virus is needed, the health care provider swabs the inside of your nose or the back of your throat. Rapid viral tests provide results within 30 minutes but may miss some cases. For more sensitive testing, specimens are sent to specialized diagnostic laboratories.

What should you do if you suspect influenza? Stay home! (See sidebar "Self-Care for Viral Respiratory Infections" for tips on self-care.) If your symptoms are severe or you are at risk for complications, contact your health care provider. Antiviral medications can be used both to prevent infection and to reduce illness severity. Amantadine is active only against type A influenza viruses. Oseltamivir (Tamiflu) and zanamivir (Relenza) are active against both type A and B viruses and also produce fewer side effects. However, viruses can become resistant to antiviral medications. Severe, complicated illness usually requires hospitalization. Your best strategy for preventing influenza is to get an annual influenza vaccine, which is designed to target prominent viral strains for the season.

Is It a Cold or the Flu?

Many people with common colds continue their usual activities. If you have influenza, it's a good idea to stay home and avoid spreading the infection. Also, influenza usually makes most people want to stay in bed. If you have any doubt or are at high risk for complications from influenza, contact your doctor.

Circle any symptoms you have in these three columns.		
sneezing	dry cough	nausea
nasal congestion	muscle aches	vomiting
sore throat	headache	diarrhea
watery eyes	fever	fatigue
mild, wet cough	chills	

If you only circled items in column one, you have an upper respiratory infection, most likely the common cold. If you circled sore throat, nasal congestion, and most of the items in column two, you may a respiratory infection caused by influenza or a similar virus. Notice that symptoms are more widespread and more disabling. If you only circled items in column three, you may have gastroenteritis (inflammation of the stomach and intestines). See the Gastroenteritis section for its causes. People often call gastroenteritis "the flu." However, influenza is a respiratory condition.

Self-Care for Viral Respiratory Infections

Stay home, particularly if you have influenza-like symptoms, and stay hydrated. Dehydration drives up body temperature and causes headaches. Drink lots of clear fluids—water, herbal tea, broth—to keep respiratory mucus thin and easier to expel. If you live in a dry climate, run a humidifier, but keep the machine clean. The last thing you want to do is spew fungi and viruses into the air.

Inhaling hot, moist air is a time-honored home remedy. It won't kill cold viruses—not without enough heat to hurt you. Studies are mixed as to whether steam inhalation relieves symptoms. You be the judge: boil a pot of water, carefully remove the pot from the stove, lean over the pot (but not so close that the steam feels too hot), and drape a towel over your head to corral the vapors. Breathe through your nose to decrease nasal congestion and through your mouth to bring the steam into your lower airways.

You can add to the pot two to three drops of essential oils from plants with decongesting, antimicrobial herbs such as eucalyptus, rosemary, or peppermint. Close your eyes and gradually lean over the pot to make sure the essential oils don't trigger coughing, a particular problem for people with asthma. Warm baths relieve muscle aches. Before you climb in, you can add five to eight drops of essential oils from the aforementioned plants and disperse with your hand.

Another water-based therapy is gargling. Add one half teaspoon of salt to one cup warm water. You can also add lemon juice or one drop of essential oil of lemon. Shake well before taking a mouthful. The last hydrotherapy is nasal irrigation. Putting water up your nose may seem counterintuitive, but it helps. Studies show that salt-water nasal irrigation improves sinusitis symptoms.[39],[40] For a description of making your own saltwater nasal rinse, go to http://www.webmd.com/cold-and-flu/cold-guide/cold-remedies.

What about exercise? If you have a cold, moderate exercise may help. It can help with decongestion, expulsion of mucus, and enhancement of immune function. On the other hand, if you have fever, body aches, or a bad cough, you're better off taking it easy.

2.3 Pharyngitis

Pharyngitis is the medical term for sore throat. A number of agents can inflame the throat: hot liquids, chemicals, smoke, allergies, postnasal drip from sinusitis, and even sleeping with your mouth open at night. Microbial pathogens are the most common cause. Of these, respiratory viruses generate the vast majority of sore throats. Normally, other respiratory symptoms such as runny nose and sneezing accompany the throat pain.

The Epstein-Barr virus (EBV) produces severe sore throat as part of the constellation of symptoms and signs associated with **mononucleosis ("mono")**—extreme fatigue, malaise, decreased appetite, sore throat, chills, fever, body aches, swollen lymph nodes in the neck, enlarged spleen, and sensitivity to light. The name derives from the characteristic increase in unusual-looking lymphocytes seen upon examination of the blood. It's also called "the kissing disease," because the disease spreads from close contact with infected saliva or respiratory mucus.

EBV belongs to the herpes virus family, along with herpes simplex viruses and varicella zoster (chickenpox virus). By adulthood, most people have antibodies against this ubiquitous virus, even if they've never developed noticeable symptoms. If illness does develop, it's usually during adolescence and young adulthood.

Diagnosis is confirmed with blood tests. No treatment is usually necessary, aside from lots of rest. Contact sports should be avoided because of the risk of rupturing the swollen spleen. Unfortunately, the fatigue can persist for months. Complications are rare, although liver inflammation (hepatitis) can occur. EBV has rarely been associated with some cancers, such as certain types of lymphoma (cancer of the lymphatic tissue).

Bacteria can also infect the throat. The most common culprit is *Streptococcus pyogenes*, the cause of strep throat. The onset of sore throat is sudden, with pain on swallowing, tender and swollen lymph nodes in the neck, fever, headache, and possibly nausea and vomiting (especially in children). Runny nose, sneezing, and cough are absent, unless a respiratory viral infection coincides. The throat and tonsils have a characteristic appearance. To confirm the diagnosis, throat swabs are submitted to rapid strep tests and possibly culture. Because this contagious illness can cause significant illness and has the potential for complications, doctors treat it with antibiotics.

Complications can include invasion of nearby structures to produce sinusitis, middle ear infection, and abscesses in the tonsils.[41] Some strains produce toxins that cause **scarlet fever**, a condition marked by sore throat, fever, and a fine, sandpapery red rash. The tongue appears first white and coated, then red. The advent of antibiotics ended the era of deadly epidemics of scarlet fever.

A serious complication of strep pharyngitis is **rheumatic fever**, an autoimmune response wherein antibodies against some bacterial strains cross-react with tissue in the heart, joints, skin, and brain. Permanent heart damage can occur. Antibiotic treatment of the initial strep pharyngitis prevents the development of rheumatic fever.

2.4 Sinusitis

The sinuses are air-filled spaces within the skull. Mucous membranes line their surfaces. Tiny openings about the diameter of pencil lead connect the sinuses with the nasal cavities. Here's how **sinusitis** (sinus inflammation) develops. Allergies, microbes, or air pollutants such as tobacco smoke trigger swelling of the mucous membranes in the nose and sinuses, augment mucus secretion, and impair the cilia that clear the mucus. Boggy mucous membranes block drainage from the sinuses into the nose. Mucus accumulates, generating a sense of pressure and allowing microbes trapped there to multiply.

Respiratory viruses cause most acute sinus infections and can continue to inflame the sinuses for a couple weeks. Bacteria may complicate the acute infection and linger for up to 12 weeks. Sinusitis lasting longer than that is termed chronic. Fungi can be involved in this condition.

Sinusitis symptoms include pressure and pain (which may be worse when leaning over), fatigue, fever, bad breath, and green or brownish nasal discharge. Postnasal drip can irritate the throat and cause a mild cough that worsens at night. Note that changes in respiratory secretions from clear to

---

pharyngitis

Inflammation of the pharynx, the tube that delivers air to the larynx ("voice box") and trachea ("windpipe") and food to the esophagus. The main symptom is sore throat. Most of the time, viruses produce pharyngitis, although strep bacteria and other bacteria can also infect the throat.

mononucleosis ("mono")

An infection caused by the Epstein-Barr virus that results in throat pain, swollen lymph nodes, fever, and fatigue.

FIGURE 14.5 Main Symptoms of Infectious Mononucleosis

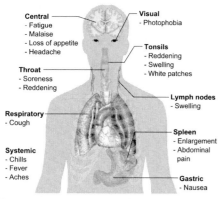

Source: Häggström M. 2009. Available at:

http://commons.wikimedia.org/wiki/

File:Main_symptoms_of_Infectious_mononucleosis.png.

sinusitis

Inflammation of the sinuses, the air spaces within the bones of the face. Viruses cause most cases of acute sinusitis, though bacteria can complicate the infection. Because the nose is usually simultaneously involved, the term *rhinosinusitis* is often used.

yellow are normal. The yellow indicates your white blood cells are doing their work and doesn't mean a bacterial infection has taken root.

Acute sinusitis usually resolves without treatment. To relieve symptoms, you can inhale steam, apply warm compresses, and irrigate your nose with salt water. If the pain bothers you, try an over-the-counter analgesic such as acetaminophen or ibuprofen. Decongestants may relieve some stuffiness. Antibiotics don't seem to result in significant improvements in symptoms.[42]

When should you worry about sinus symptoms? Normally, viral infection of the nose and sinuses resolves within 10 days. Persistent symptoms, especially if you feel worse rather than better, may indicate it's time to check in with your health practitioner. Seek help immediately if you notice swelling over the sinus or around the eye.

Fear Not Fever

Normal body temperature runs about 98.6°F. Exercise, overbundling, hot weather, and warm food or beverages mildly elevate body temperature. Fever is defined as a significant elevation, starting at an oral temperature of more than 100°F (37.8°C). Your palm, by the way, is not an accurate temperature gauge. Fever usually causes no symptoms until it reaches 102°F to 103°F.

Many people reflexively reach for a fever-reducing drug. However, fever represents a normal immune response and has benefits. Some viruses and bacteria can't survive in a hotter climate. In animals, blocking a fever with medications can increase the risk of death from infectious agents such as influenza viruses.[43] Preliminary research suggests fever-reducers may also prolong infectious illnesses in humans.[44]

Most medical experts advise against taking a medication such as acetaminophen (Tylenol) or ibuprofen (Motrin, Advil)—unless the fever causes discomfort. (Aspirin, though it reduces fever, is not recommended for children and adolescents during a viral infection because of the risk of Reye's syndrome, a dangerous illness involving the brain and liver.) Do drink plenty of clear liquids. Dehydration can drive the fever higher.

When should you worry? Fever does not cause permanent damage to the brain or other tissues until it crests 107°F. However, high fever (over 103°F) can be a sign of serious illness. How you feel is more important than your temperature. Worrisome signs include lethargy, confusion, unsteady gait, stiff neck, unusual skin rash, difficulty breathing, discomfort with urination, and flank pain. A persistent or recurring fever can be a sign of an infection such as malaria or tuberculosis. When in doubt, call your health care provider.

2.5 Acute Bronchitis

Bronchitis is an inflammation of mucous membranes of the bronchi (tubes that conduct air into the lungs). Acute bronchitis is a common condition, particularly in fall and winter. About 90 percent of the time, the causative agent is a virus such as rhinovirus, influenza virus, parainfluenza virus, and respiratory syncytial virus (RSV).[45] Bacteria can also infect the bronchi.

The main symptom is a cough, usually with the production of mucus. Sore throat and nasal congestion are often also present at the start of the illness. Coughs, however, linger as long as three to four weeks. Chest muscles can become sore. Severe infection can also produce shortness of breath and fever.

Acute bronchitis usually resolves without treatment within three or four weeks. Because the illness is usually viral, experts don't recommend antibiotics. Cough medications don't alter the course of the infection. (See the sidebars "Over-the-Counter Drugs for Colds and Coughs" and "Self-Care for Viral Respiratory Infections".) Bronchitis becomes chronic when it lasts for at least three months. Tobacco smoke usually causes chronic bronchitis, though other irritants such as marijuana smoke can be to blame.

bronchitis

Inflammation of the lower airways (bronchi) that causes cough and excess mucus production. Cold and flu viruses cause most cases of acute bronchitis, though bacteria can complicate the infection. The main cause of chronic bronchitis is tobacco smoke.

Over-the-Counter Drugs for Colds and Coughs

While over-the-counter cough and cold remedies generate a lot of money for manufacturers, most don't improve respiratory infections, and some can do harm.

Decongestants such as pseudoephedrine (Sudafed) and phenylephrine (Neosynephrine) constrict blood vessels, which shrink boggy mucous membranes, to decrease stuffiness. Beware that nasal sprays produce relief, followed by rebound congestion. As tolerance rises, the relief periods diminish. People can actually become hooked on their decongestant sprays. Don't use them for more than three days. Side effects for oral medications include elevated heart rate, palpitations, nervousness, and insomnia.

Antihistamines dry secretions. If your nose is running, that action may sound like a good idea. However, watery respiratory secretions represent an immune system defense, a means to flush out the pathogens. Drier, thicker mucus is harder to expel, possibly increasing the risk of sinusitis. Side effects, particularly for the old-fashioned, "first generation" antihistamines include drowsiness, dry mouth, difficulty urinating, and constipation.

Cough suppressants such as dextromethorphan (the DM in cough syrups) create a dilemma. One, research reviews conclude that none of the over-the-counter drugs (cough suppressants, the expectorant guaifenesin [Mucinex], antihistamines, or decongestants) significantly improve coughs.[46] Two, their use can be dangerous for children under the age of four. Three, coughing, which propels infected mucus away from delicate lung tissue, is part of your nonspecific immune defense. On the other hand, you can't cough without waking up, even if the arousal is so brief as not to be remembered in the morning. And sleep promotes healthy immune function. For that reason, health care practitioners may support nighttime use of cough suppressants.

Analgesics (pain relievers) such as acetaminophen (Tylenol) and ibuprofen (Motrin, Advil) can relieve headaches, body aches, and fevers. While providing some symptom relief, these drugs may prolong illness.[47] ,[48] ,[49] A more serious problem is unintentional poisoning. Because many cough and cold remedies and analgesics contain acetaminophen, people who combine these products may consume too much, leading to liver damage. The usual dosage is 650 milligrams (two 325-milligram tablets) every 4 to 6 hours with a maximum of 4,000 milligrams (4 grams) in 24 hours. Ibuprofen has its own risks, most notably gastrointestinal irritation and bleeding. The usual dosage is 200 to 400 milligrams every four to six hours, with a maximum of 1.2 grams (1,200 milligrams) in 24 hours.

Healthy alveoli (air sacs) contain air and nothing else. In pneumonia, infected mucus fills the alveoli. Alveolar walls are permanently destroyed in emphysema.

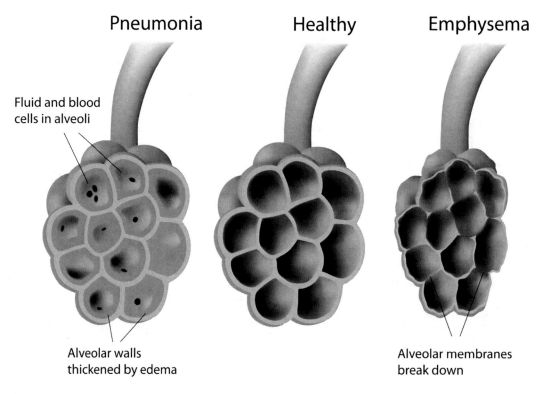

Pneumonia   Healthy   Emphysema

Fluid and blood cells in alveoli

Alveolar walls thickened by edema

Alveolar membranes break down

© Shutterstock

2.6 Pneumonia

pneumonia

Inflammation of alveoli (air sacs) in the lung. Microbial causes include viruses, bacteria, and fungi.

Pneumonia is an infection of the alveoli, the delicate air sacs where gas exchange occurs. Our immune defenses try hard to prevent this end-of-the-line infection. In the United States, pneumonia is the leading cause of death due to infectious disease.[50] In terms of death from any cause, influenza and pneumonia rank number eight. Influenza virus usually kills by causing pneumonia. According to the Centers for Disease Control and Prevention (CDC), pneumonia put 1.2 million Americans in the hospital in 2007 and killed more than 52,000 people.[51]

The cause is usually viral or bacterial. In some regions of the United States, fungi can cause pneumonia. Regardless of the pathogen, the infected alveoli become filled with fluid, which interferes with the normal exchange of oxygen and carbon dioxide. Symptoms include coughing, shortness of breath, chest pain, fever, weakness, and lethargy. The cough may produce yellow, green, or brown sputum. Compared to viral pneumonia, bacterial pneumonia tends to come on suddenly and produce more severe symptoms. Drug treatment depends on the underlying cause. If the illness is severe, hospitalization is required.

The image on the left is a normal chest X-ray. The lungs appear black. In the center, the heart (and large blood vessels entering and leaving it) appear white. In the right-hand image, the lungs have a diffusely hazy appearance characteristic of viral pneumonia.

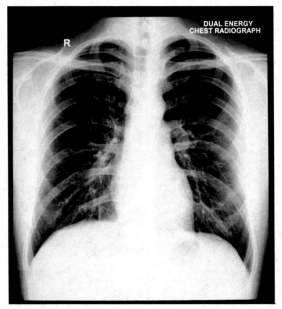 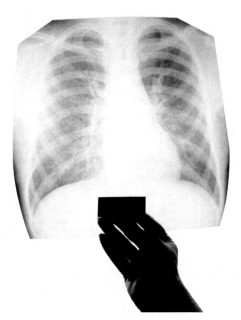

© Shutterstock; Nomadsoul1 | Dreamstime.com

When to Seek Help for Respiratory Infections

In otherwise healthy people, most respiratory infections produce mild symptoms that resolve without treatment within a few days. People at higher risk for severe, complicated illness should stay in touch with their health care providers.

The following are signs indicating that you should seek medical attention:

- You haven't gotten better after three to five days or seem to be getting worse
- Fever persists beyond two to three days
- Sinusitis symptoms persist more than two weeks or have worsened
- A cough lasts more than three or four weeks or seems to be getting worse
- Coughing produces rust-colored or dark-green sputum
- You have chest pain with coughing
- You have any other concerns about your health

Signs to call for emergency assistance include

- Difficulty breathing, rapid respiratory rate at rest, or shortness of breath
- Blue tinge to lips or nail beds

2.7 Tuberculosis

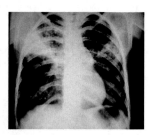

© *Drpluton | Dreamstime.com.*

Tuberculosis (TB) is caused by *Mycobacterium tuberculosis* bacteria. According to the World Health Organization, one third of the population is infected.[52] Though it most commonly affects the lungs, the bacteria can spread via the bloodstream to infect many organs. Symptoms include malaise, cough, blood-tinged sputum, weight loss, fever, and night sweats. The weight loss can be so severe that the illness used to be called "consumption." Without treatment, the infection can be fatal.

The bacteria become airborne when an infected person laughs, coughs, sings, shouts, or sneezes. Spitting the infected sputum also spreads the disease. Many infected people have latent TB. What happens is, after inoculation, the immune system succeeds in walling off the bacteria in one area of the lungs but fails to kill them. In this way, tuberculosis bacteria can be held in check for years, until the immune system declines. If the infection becomes active again, bacteria can be spread, even before the person develops symptoms.

Although the illness is contagious, it usually takes prolonged exposure to acquire the bacterium. Risk factors include crowded conditions (including prisons), being very young or very old, and immunodeficiency. People infected with HIV are particularly at risk for TB. And TB accelerates the progression of HIV infection. Otherwise, a common situation used to be that grandma (an asymptomatic carrier) would immigrate from the mother country and move into the crowded apartment with her kids and grandkids. Young, susceptible children would then become infected.

TB skin tests screen for latent and active disease. Diagnosis is confirmed with chest X-rays and analysis of sputum samples. Treatment centers on taking antibiotic drugs for up to two years. Because antibiotic resistance is common, often more than one drug is needed.

Preventing Respiratory Infections

Viruses are the most common cause of respiratory infection and the hardest to avoid, particularly when coughs and sneezes project them into your airspace. Plus, viruses such as influenza are released by normal breathing[53] and start to be shed into respiratory secretions the day before symptoms begin.

You are not, however, completely defenseless. Here's what you can do.

1. **Practice good hygiene.** Washing your hands with soap and water reduces the spread of respiratory viruses.[54] You can also refrain from sharing glasses, forks, and kisses with obviously sick friends. If you become ill, protect others by sneezing and coughing into a tissue or the crook of your arm (rather than into your hand), and, when feasible, staying home.

2. **Keep your immune system hardy.** Some people stay well, even after exposure to viruses. In one experiment, researchers inoculated more than 100 volunteers with various cold viruses. Twenty percent of them didn't become infected.[55] Among the rest of the people, viruses began to multiply but only caused significant symptoms in less than half. See Chapter 13 for more lifestyle strategies for keeping your protective armor in shining shape. In addition, research, most of which has involved children, indicates that taking *probiotics* (live microorganisms similar to those that normally colonize mucous membranes) may strengthen the immune system and thereby protect against respiratory infections.[56] ,[57] ,[58]

3. **Stay away from tobacco smoke.** It increases respiratory mucus and paralyzes the hair-like cilia that normally clear the mucus. One study found that exposure to secondhand smoke suppressed nasal antiviral responses to influenza viruses.[59] Whether you're a smoker or an innocent bystander, inhaling cigarette smoke increases the risk of respiratory infections and, particularly in children, middle ear infections. It also increases the severity of these infections and the likelihood of needing hospitalization. Smokers are more at risk for tuberculosis.[60]

4. **Maintain your mellow.** Chronic stress increases susceptibility to the common cold.[61] ,[62] See Chapter 3 for tips about managing your stress.

5. **Get vaccinated.** Several childhood immunizations protect against respiratory infections: the vaccines against pertussis (whooping cough), varicella (chickenpox), *Haemophilus influenzae* type b, and measles. In addition, seasonal influenza vaccines are recommended.

DISCUSSION QUESTIONS

1. Why are we vulnerable to influenza year after year?
2. What are the key signs of sinusitis? Are antibiotics usually necessary to treat an infection?
3. Samantha visits the campus health clinic with a nasal discharge, sore throat, and a mild cold. When the doctor diagnoses the common cold and recommends rest and fluids, Samantha insists the doctor write a prescription for antibiotics. For what reasons should the doctor refuse?
4. Even if you're not extremely ill, why might your doctor nevertheless encourage you take a course of antibiotics for pharyngitis caused by *Streptococcus pyogenes*?
5. What are the pros and cons of suppressing a fever with over-the-counter drugs such as Tylenol and Motrin?
6. Why does tobacco smoke increase the risk of respiratory infections? Is secondhand smoke a risk?

3.   GASTROINTESTINAL INFECTIONS

LEARNING OBJECTIVES

1. Define and discuss the causes of gastroenteritis, hepatitis, and peptic ulcers.
2. Identify warning signs that it's time to seek medical attention for vomiting and diarrhea.
3. Discuss self-care for mild gastrointestinal infections.
4. List strategies for reducing the risk of developing hepatitis.

3.1   Gastroenteritis

Gastroenteritis means inflammation of the stomach and intestines. Noninfectious agents such as aspirin and alcohol can inflame the digestive tract. The causes of infectious gastroenteritis include viruses (norovirus, rotatvirus), bacteria (*Escherichia coli*, *Salmonella*, *Shigella*), and protozoa (*Giardia*, *Cryptosporidium*).

gastroenteritis

Inflammation of the stomach and intestines, usually caused by viruses or bacteria and, less often, protozoa. The main symptoms are nausea, vomiting, diarrhea, and abdominal discomfort.

FIGURE 14.6 The Gastrointestinal System

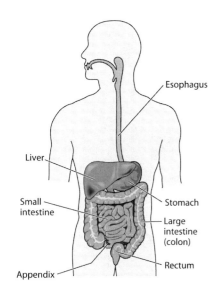

Esophagus

Liver

Small intestine

Stomach

Large intestine (colon)

Appendix

Rectum

© Shutterstock

These conditions are very contagious. You acquire the organisms either from having close contact with an infected person or from consuming contaminated food or beverages. Depending on the microbe, illness usually begins one to two days after exposure. The main symptoms are diarrhea, nausea, and vomiting. Others include fever, loss of appetite, headache, and crampy abdominal pain. Fever and blood in the stools indicate serious infection.

Children under the age of 5 are the most vulnerable to infectious gastroenteritis. Their small body size makes them at the highest risk for dehydration. According to the World Health Organization, diarrheal illnesses kill 1.5 million children each year and are the second-leading cause of death in low-income countries.[63] In the United States, people over the age of 60 face the highest risk of hospitalization and death.

Contaminated food and water are particularly problematic in the developing world. However, the United States has its share of foodborne illnesses. Each year, there are 48 million such illnesses, 128,000 hospitalizations, and 3,000 deaths.[64],[65] The major microbial pathogens cause 9.4 million of these illnesses and nearly 56 million hospitalizations and 1,351 deaths. Other culprits include metals, toxins from mushrooms, and shellfish contaminated with phytoplankton.

Fortunately, the Food Safety Modernization Act of 2010 enhanced the Food and Drug Administration's authority to regulate food safety and the CDC's surveillance and investigation of foodborne infection outbreaks. To learn more, check out the following websites from the CDC (http://www.cdc.gov/winnablebattles/foodsafety/index.html), the President's Food Safety Working Group (http://www.foodsafetyworkinggroup.gov), FoodSafety.gov (http://www.foodsafety.gov), and the Partnership for Food Safety Education (http://www.fightbac.org).

You can reduce your risks of infectious gastroenteritis by washing your hands and disinfecting surfaces that contact raw eggs, meats, and seafood, as well as surfaces contaminated by someone with such an infection. Cook meats thoroughly. If you're camping, filter your drinking water with a device designed to eliminate microbes. If you're traveling outside the country, check with a health care authority about food and water safety. A good resource is the CDC's website on traveler's health (http://wwwnc.cdc.gov/travel/page/safe-food-water.htm). Chapter 8 also contains tips on reducing foodborne illnesses.

Your best strategy for weathering a bout of gastroenteritis is to stay hydrated. Consume lots of clear liquids: herbal tea, soup broth, and sports rehydration drinks. You can make your own rehydration solution by adding six teaspoons of sugar and a half teaspoon salt to one liter (about a quart) of clean water.[66] If your main problem is vomiting, health professionals usually recommend taking frequent small sips (a tablespoon or so) of liquid rather than big gulps. When your appetite returns, start with bland, easy-to-digest foods such as bananas, cooked carrots, boiled or baked chicken, rice, and soda crackers.

Probiotics are live microorganisms such as bacteria and yeast that normally colonize your mucous membranes. While fermented foods (yogurt, kefir, sauerkraut, kimchi, miso, tempeh) have health benefits, most of the research has focused on supplements derived from strains of *Lactobacillus* species. Some treat and prevent certain types of infectious diarrhea (mainly rotavirus in children), including traveler's diarrhea.[67] Probiotics may also improve symptoms associated with **irritable bowel syndrome**, a condition characterized by abdominal pain, bloating, diarrhea, and/or constipation.[68]

When to Seek Help for Vomiting and Diarrhea

Call your health provider if you have the following symptoms or other concerns:

- Vomiting that continues more than 48 hours
- Diarrhea that hasn't improved within 72 hours
- Fever higher than 101°F that lasts more than 24 hours
- Significant abdominal pain
- Blood or lots of mucus in the stool; Black bowel movements, which can be a sign of bleeding higher in the gastrointestinal tract; (Note: Taking Pepto-Bismol can also turn the stool black, which is normal)
- Vomiting blood
- Signs of dehydration: light-headedness, decreased urination, lack of sweat, and dry mouth, lips, and eyes

Oral Hygiene

A lot of people overlook the importance of regularly brushing and flossing of teeth. Bacteria are normally found in the mouth. The problem is plaque, a sticky film that allows bacteria to proliferate and form tissue-damaging acids. The result is dental caries (tooth decay) and *gingivitis* (gum inflammation). Signs of gingivitis include tenderness, swelling, and bleeding of the gums, as well as bad breath. The infection can go deeper, to involve underlying tissues and bone (*periodontitis*). Gingivitis and periodontitis generate more widespread inflammation that contributes to diseases elsewhere in the body, such as cardiovascular disease.[69]

To keep your mouth healthy, brush your teeth after meals at least twice a day, floss daily, replace your toothbrush at least every three months (and at the end of any infectious illness), keep sweet foods and drinks to a minimum, quit smoking, and see your dentist regularly. For more information, go to the American Dental Association website (http://www.ada.org).

3.2   Viral Hepatitis

Hepatitis means inflammation of the liver. This vital organ, tucked neatly under your right ribs, carries out several functions, including detoxification. Causes of hepatitis include microbes, toxins (alcohol, some medications, poisonous mushrooms), and certain medical conditions. Hepatitis viruses are the most common cause.

Signs and symptoms of acute hepatitis can be so mild as to go unnoticed or include fatigue, decreased appetite, malaise, nausea, vomiting, low-grade fever, skin rashes, brownish urine, pale stools, enlargement and tenderness of the liver, and *jaundice* (a yellowing of the skin and whites of the eyes). Chronic hepatitis lasts more than six months. The ongoing inflammation leads to *cirrhosis*, the term for scarring of the liver.

If you suspect you have hepatitis, see your health care provider. Blood tests can determine how well your liver is functioning and can detect the presence of infection with some of the hepatitis viruses.

An alphabet of hepatitis viruses—hepatitis A, B, C, D, and E—cause this disease.

> **hepatitis**
>
> Inflammation of the liver. Microbial causes are usually hepatitis viruses.

- **Hepatitis A** is fairly common, tends to cause mild disease, and heals without become chronic. A two-dose vaccine series prevents it. It's contracted from eating food or beverages contaminated with feces from an infected human. (This means transmission is called fecal-oral.) The incubation period is nearly a month. Infected people then start shedding the virus into their feces a week or two before symptoms begin. If you've been exposed to someone infected with hepatitis A and haven't already had the hepatitis A vaccine, contact your health care provider.[70] He or she may give you the vaccine or an immune globulin injection. The former illustrates active immunity; the latter, passive immunity.

The person in this photograph has hepatitis A. Note the jaundice, the yellow discoloration of skin and the whites of the eyes.

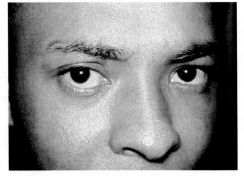

Source: CDC/Dr. Thomas F. Sellers/Emory University. 1963. ID# 2860. Public Health Image Library (PHIL). Available at:

http://commons.wikimedia.org/wiki/File:Jaundice_eye.jpg.

- **Hepatitis B** virus is transmitted when infected bodily fluids (blood, saliva, semen, vaginal fluid, urine) enter the body. In the United States, the virus is most often acquired during sex with an infected partner.[71] Infection can also occur from needle sharing in drug users, accidental punctures by needles, scalpels or other sharp objects in health care workers, and sharing razors and toothbrushes with an infected person. An infected pregnant woman can also transmit the virus to her unborn child. Piercing and tattooing are generally not a risk in licensed, commercial enterprises.

The incubation period averages around three months. Most adults recover without developing chronic hepatitis B. Unfortunately, the risk is much higher for infected children.[72] Chronic hepatitis B is treated with synthetic interferons and antiviral drugs.

Hepatitis B vaccination prevents the disease. It can also be given to unvaccinated people immediately after a known exposure to hepatitis B. Since routine vaccination of children began in 1990, the incidence of hepatitis B has decreased dramatically.

- **Hepatitis C** virus is transmitted via exposure to infected blood. The main risk is illicit drug injection. Others include having blood transfusions or organ transplants before 1992 (when adequate screening tests became available), multiple sexual partners, and accidental needle-sticks in health care workers.[73] Infected pregnant women can pass the virus to their unborn children.

  This virus has become the most common blood-borne infection in America.[74] Unfortunately, much of the time, the viral infection persists, leading to chronic hepatitis, cirrhosis, liver failure, and liver cancer. According to the CDC, an estimated 3.2 million Americans have chronic hepatitis C. Like hepatitis B, it's treated with interferon-based and antiviral drugs.

- **Hepatitis D** is uncommon and requires coinfection with hepatitis B virus. Like hepatitis B, it's acquired when infected blood enters the body through a nick in the skin or from contact with mucous membranes.

- **Hepatitis E** causes a serious, acute infection but does not become chronic. It's uncommon in the United States. Like hepatitis A, it follows a fecal-oral transmission, mainly from contaminated water in countries without good sanitation measures.

3.3 Peptic Ulcers

peptic ulcers

Open sores in the lining of the stomach and the first part of the small intestine (duodenum). The main cause is the bacterium *Helicobacter pylori*.

Peptic ulcers are erosions of the mucous membrane lining the stomach and first part of the small intestine (duodenum). Not long ago, doctors blamed ulcers on stress, spicy foods, and other dietary factors. Stress does play a role in the generation of ulcers. For a long time, no one suspected an infectious cause. The stomach is acidic, which aids in digestion and kills most microbial pathogens. "Most" is the operative word. It turns out that a bacterium called *Helicobacter pylori* not only survives but replicates in this hostile environment. The resultant inflammation causes *gastritis* (stomach inflammation) and, eventually, ulcers. The ulcers can erode into blood vessels (resulting in bleeding) and clear through the stomach wall (perforation).

Peptic ulcers erode the lining of the stomach and duodenum.

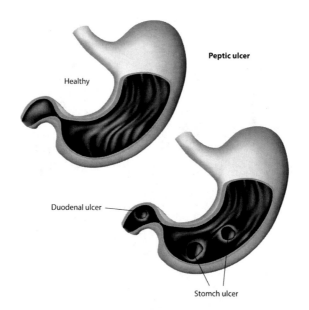

© *Shutterstock*

Nonsteroidal anti-inflammatory drugs (NSAIDs) such as aspirin and excessive alcohol intake can also cause gastritis and ulcers. Stress contributes to ulcers through several mechanisms such as decreasing blood flow to the stomach, reducing the mucus that protects stomach cells from the acid, and impairing immune function.

Because the main cause is now recognized as *H. pylori*, the main treatment is antibiotics. Infection with the bacteria can be confirmed by tests like breath tests and culture of biopsy specimens.

KEY TAKEAWAYS

- Gastroenteritis continues to cause much morbidity and mortality (illness and death), particularly among children in the developing world.
- While most Americans have ready access to clean drinking water, foodborne infections continue to be a problem.
- Five known hepatitis viruses cause hepatitis. In the United States, hepatitis A, B, and C are most common.
- Peptic ulcers are open sores in the stomach and/or duodenum.

DISCUSSION QUESTIONS

1. What are the most common causes of gastroenteritis?
2. What's the biggest risk with having protracted vomiting and/or diarrhea? Which age group is most vulnerable?
3. When should you seek medical attention for vomiting and diarrhea?
4. Review the information on hepatitis A, B, and C. Which is mainly transmitted by a fecal-oral route? Which is often sexually transmitted? Which can you be immunized against? Which most commonly causes chronic hepatitis?
5. What can you do to reduce your risk of contracting hepatitis?
6. What is the main cause of peptic ulcer?

4. CENTRAL NERVOUS SYSTEM INFECTIONS

LEARNING OBJECTIVES

1. Define meningitis and encephalitis.
2. Identify the most common microbial pathogens that infect the central nervous system.
3. List warning signs of such infections.
4. Discuss methods to reduce the risk of some of these potentially deadly infections.

Many of us fear injuries and illnesses that threaten the ivory tower—the brain and spinal cord, which together form the central nervous system (CNS). Microbial pathogens can infect and inflame the membranes and spinal fluid enveloping the CNS (**meningitis**) and also the brain (**encephalitis**). Other agents, such as certain drugs and cancer, can produce meningitis and encephalitis.

The protective membranes surrounding the brain and spinal cord are called meninges. Infectious causes include a variety of viruses, bacteria, and fungi. Noninfectious causes include cancer, physical injury, and certain drugs. Bacteria and viruses are the most common agents. Fungal meningitis is rare, except among people with AIDS (acquired immunodeficiency syndrome).

Bacterial meningitis is usually more severe and more likely to result in long-term consequences such as hearing loss and learning disabilities. The onset is usually sudden and dramatic with fever, headache, stiff neck, nausea, vomiting, sensitivity to light, confusion, and disorientation. The bacteria can be transmitted to other close contacts.

Each year there are about 4,100 cases of bacterial meningitis and 500 deaths.[75] Between 1998 and 2007, the incidence of meningitis cases dropped 31 percent, but the fatality rate didn't change much. About 15 percent of people developing this dreaded infection died. People at greatest risk were children under the age of two months and African Americans of any age.

Vaccines protect against three meningitis-causing bacteria: *Streptococcus pneumoniae*, *Hemophilus influenzae*, and *Neisseria meningitidis* (meningococcus). Meningococcus is the most common cause of bacterial meningitis among college students. The bacterium can also infect the blood, producing a rash that looks like tiny bruises. According to the CDC, between 1,000 and 2,600 Americans develop

meningitis

Inflammation of the membranes surround the central nervous system (meninges); caused by infectious agents, certain drugs, trauma, and cancer.

encephalitis

Inflammation of the brain caused by infectious agents such as bacteria and viruses, as well as certain drugs, chronic diseases, and cancer.

meningococcal disease each year.[76] Even when treated with antibiotics, 10–15 percent die, often within one to two days. Survivors can have permanent problems such as deafness, seizures, strokes, mental retardation, kidney failure, and limb amputations. For that reason, the meningococcal conjugate vaccine (which prevents four types of meningococcal infection) is recommended at age 11 or 12, with a booster dose at ages 16 to 18.

In this image, you can see that the meninges have three layers. They envelop both the brain and spinal cord. In meningitis, viruses or bacteria inflame the meninges.

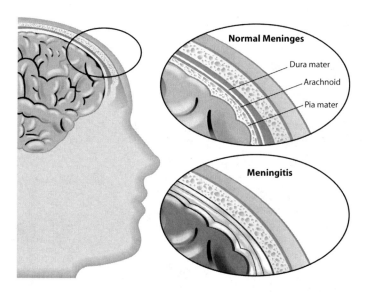

© Rob3000 | Dreamstime.com.

Compared to bacterial meningitis, **viral meningitis** is less severe. The disease usually resolves completely, which is a good thing, considering that no drugs exist to combat many of these viruses. Viruses that cause meningitis include those that cause measles, mumps, and rubella; herpes simplex viruses; Epstein-Barr virus; influenza viruses; and viruses spread by mosquitoes and other insects.

 Video Clip 14.3

Meningitis on College Campuses
This news video explains why college students are at risk for meningitis, how the infection spreads, signs and symptoms, and ways to reduce risks.

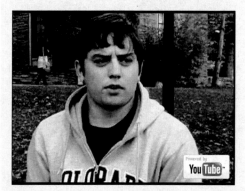

View the video online at: http://www.youtube.com/v/5x8XqyGg7Cs

Encephalitis is most often caused by viruses. Bacteria, fungi, and protozoa can also infect the brain. People with AIDS are particularly vulnerable. Viral culprits include those that cause childhood illnesses such as measles, mumps, and rubella (prevented by the MMR vaccine); poliovirus (also prevented by a vaccine); herpes simplex viruses; Epstein-Barr virus; rabies virus (transmitted from a rabid animal bite); and mosquito-borne viruses such as St. Louis encephalitis, West Nile virus, and western and eastern equine encephalitis. You can reduce your risk of infection from mosquito and tick-borne microbes by staying indoors the times of day mosquitoes are most active, wearing protective clothing, and using insect repellent.

With some infectious agents, symptoms may be relatively mild with fever, fatigue, and headache. Other infections progress to disorientation, confusion, unsteady gait, numbness, muscle paralysis, seizures (convulsions), coma, and death.

Signs and symptoms of meningitis and encephalitis warrant emergency medical treatment.

KEY TAKEAWAYS

- Encephalitis and meningitis are two of the more dreaded infections.
- Warning signs include fever, severe headache, stiff neck, a rash that resembles tiny bruises, confusion, seizure, and trouble moving.
- *Neisseria meningitidis* (meningococcus) is the most common cause of bacterial meningitis in teens and young adults. Routine vaccination is recommended, particularly for college students.

DISCUSSION QUESTIONS

1. Which types of microorganisms usually cause meningitis?
2. What are the warning signs of meningitis? Of encephalitis?
3. How can college students reduce their risk of developing bacterial meningitis?

---

5. SKIN INFECTIONS

LEARNING OBJECTIVES

1. Discuss the main microbial pathogens that infect the skin.
2. Explore the reasons for restraint in using antibiotics.

Viruses, fungi, and bacteria can infect the skin. The main viral offenders are *human papillomavirus* (HPV) and *herpes simplex virus* (HSV). Because both can infect the genitalia, these viruses are discussed in greater detail in Chapter 7. In addition to producing genital warts, human papillomaviruses cause warts on the skin. They will often spontaneously regress, though that process can take many months. If warts spread or create discomfort (physical or psychological), they can be removed with topical agents, cryotherapy (freezing), and other means.

HSV can cause both oral ("fever blisters" or "cold sores") and genital mucous membrane lesions. The first oral infection may occur without symptoms or with painful sores, fever, swollen lymph nodes in the neck, muscle aches, and general malaise. Afterward, the virus remains in the body in a latent state. A tingling on the lips often heralds a recurrence.

A number of fungal species can superficially infect the skin, causing conditions such as ringworm, athlete's foot, and jock itch. They can also affect the scalp, fingernails, and toenails. The appearance of the skin varies based on the fungal species and location on the body. Often the fungus grows centrifugally to form round plaques. The skin may become more or less pigmented, scaly, and itchy. Invasion into the hair shaft causes hair on the scalp to break. The most common treatment is with topical antifungal agents. Essential oil of tea tree (*Melaleuca alternifolia*) in various dilutions may cure some of these infections, though skin irritation has been reported.[77] Fungal infections of the nail are very difficult to eradicate.

This photograph from the CDC shows ringworm on the scalp caused by the dermatophyte *Trichophyton tonsurans*.

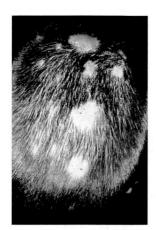

Source: CDC/Dr. Lucille K. Georg. 1968. ID# 12546. Public Health Image Library (PHIL). Available at: http://phil.cdc.gov/phil/details.asp.

methicillin-resistant
Staphylococcus aureus
(MRSA)

Infection caused by a strain of *Staphylococcus aureus* that's resistant to multiple antibiotics.

Bacterial skin infections generate redness, warmth, swelling, pain, and pus. *Streptococcus pyogenes* and *Staphylococcus aureus* can infect the skin. Both can cause *impetigo*, which is very contagious. The lesions begin as tiny blisters or pustules. When they burst, a honey-colored crust forms. Topical antibiotic ointments treat mild infection; oral antibiotics are used for more severe cases. Hygiene (hand washing, washing bedclothes and towels in hot water) is key to preventing the bacteria from spreading.

You've probably heard of infections caused by **methicillin-resistant** *Staphylococcus aureus* **(MRSA)**. The bacterium is resistant not just to methicillin but to a number of other antibiotics. About a third of people carry staph bacteria in the nose, though about 2 percent harbor MRSA. Most of the infections are of the skin, initially appearing like an infected pimple or hair follicle. If untreated, the bacterium may invade deeper tissues, enter the blood, and spread to vital organs.

MRSA emerged as a big problem in the 1990s. Between 1993 and 2005, visits to emergency rooms for soft tissue infections (involving the skin and tissues underneath it) nearly tripled.[78] It can be spread by direct contact with people carrying the bacteria or indirectly from contaminated surfaces. Risk factors include crowding, skin-to-skin contact, sharing soap bars and towels, having broken areas of skin, and poor hygiene. One study found MRSA on surfaces in the locker rooms of college athletes, the wrestling pit, and weight room, as well as from some athletes' noses and skin.[79]

Prevention of skin infections includes keeping your hands and the rest of your body reasonably clean. Avoid sharing razors, towels, gym clothes, and other personal affects that directly contact your skin. In your personal space, wipe down frequently used surfaces such as computer keyboards. When you go to the gym, wipe down equipment with a disinfectant, and shower (or at least wash your hands) when you're finished working out. Shower before entering swimming pools and whirlpools. If you use the steam room, sit on a towel. Clean wounds well and cover with a clean, dry bandage until healed. If you're concerned that you have a skin infection, contact your health care practitioner.

Video Link 14.1

Staph Infections

This video from WebMD discusses infections by *Staphylococcus aureus*.

http://www.webmd.com/video/preventing-staph-infections

Wise Use of Antimicrobial Drugs

Antimicrobial drugs can save lives in the face of overwhelming infection. Unfortunately, microbes can quickly evolve to become resistant to these drugs. While drug-resistance is inevitable, overuse and misuse of antibiotics have accelerated the rise of bacteria that no longer respond to them. Viruses and parasites can also develop resistance to the drugs used against them.

The obvious consequence is that antimicrobial drugs may fail when they're most needed. Microbial drug resistance has become a public health crisis. Some strains of viruses and bacteria are now resistant to all but one drug. MRSA (methicillin-resistant *Staphylococcus aureus*) represents only one example.

Another issue is that antibiotics injure the friendly bacteria that form part of innate immune defense. Common adverse effects are diarrhea and yeast overgrowth in the vagina and mouth. Allergic reactions can also occur. A 2010 report raised questions about "whether antibiotic-induced damage to the human microbiota might underlie four recent and detrimental health trends: increasing rates of obesity, autism, asthma, and atopy, such as peanut allergy."[80] As of yet, no one has proven that repeated rounds of antibiotics cause any of these conditions. And clearly, the benefit of treating a serious bacterial infection outweighs these side effects.

Antibiotic overuse stems from two main sources: the health care system and agriculture. In outpatient settings, nearly 50 million antibiotic prescriptions are written a year.[81] A leading reason for antibiotics is acute upper respiratory tract infections, most of which have viral origins or otherwise resolve without treatment. Also, doctors may prescribe more expensive, broad-spectrum antibiotics when older, cheaper, and more specific drugs would do. Education of both physicians and patients has dampened the rate of use. Nevertheless, overprescription continues. For instance, about 40 percent of patients with the common cold walk out of the doctor's office clutching a prescription.

Another misuse is not completing a course of antibiotics and saving the remaining pills for an infection you self-diagnose as bacterial. That's unwise on at least two accounts. One, you may not adequately fight infection number one. Two, the second infection may not have a bacterial cause. Even if it is, you don't know whether the bacteria in question will respond to the particular antibiotic pills left in the bottle.

Many antibiotics used to treat human infections are also given to food animals—cows, pigs, poultry, goats, rabbits, sheep, and farmed fish—as well as honey bees. Often the drugs are added to feed to prevent infection and, in theory, to promote growth in healthy animals, rather than to treat an actual infection. The unfortunate result is an increase in resistant bacteria that can infect humans, including an increase in foodborne diseases that don't respond well to drug treatment. Antifungal drugs are also applied to some crops and antibiotics may be sprayed on some fruit trees.

Here's what you can do to help contain the emergence of antimicrobial-resistant bacteria.

- If your health provider says your infection isn't bacterial, don't beg for an antibiotic prescription. If your condition worsens, you can always return to the clinic for a reassessment.
- If you're diagnosed with a bacterial infection, take the antibiotics as prescribed.
- Wash your hands with soap and water, rather than antibacterial solutions.
- Buy organic eggs, meats, and dairy.

When Antibiotics Are Needed: Reducing Adverse Effects

Sometimes antibiotics are needed to reduce suffering, prevent complications, and halt the spread of contagious bacteria to other people. They have saved many lives. But they can cause side effects. Here's what you can do to reduce them.

If you've had an allergic reaction to an antibiotic in the past, be sure to tell your health provider. That information should be in your medical chart.

To repair antibiotic-induced disruption of beneficial intestinal microbes and decrease the risk of diarrhea, take **probiotics** during the course of the antibiotics and for two weeks afterward. According to one analysis, a specific strain of *Lactobacillus rhamnosus* (Lactobacillus GG) may decrease the risk of antibiotic-associated diarrhea by nearly 60 percent.[82] Yogurt drinks containing live cultures may also help.[83] Preliminary research has failed to show that oral probiotics prevent vaginal yeast overgrowth after antibiotics. However, intravaginal suppositories of Lactobacillus GG twice a day for seven days may have reduced symptoms.[84]

KEY TAKEAWAYS

- Viruses, fungi, and bacteria can infect the skin.
- Methicillin-resistant *Staphylococcus aureus* (MRSA) is feared because it's resistant to many antibiotics.
- Overuse of antibiotics in healthcare and agriculture have increased the development of antimicrobial resistance.

DISCUSSION QUESTIONS

1. You can get warts on your feet, hands, face, and genitals. Are they caused by different viruses? Explain your answer.
2. What are warning signs that you have a bacterial skin infection? Should you seek medical attention if you notice these signs?
3. How can you reduce your risk of getting skin infections? What extra precautions should student athletes (or anyone who works out in a gym) take? Two websites to consult before answering these questions are WebMD's Fungus among Us Slideshow (http://www.webmd.com/skin-problems-and-treatments/ss/slideshow-fungus-infection) and Stop MRSA Now (http://www.stopmrsanow.org/locker-room-or-gym.html).
4. What are common side effects of using antibiotics?
5. How have humans increased the development of antibiotic resistance among many bacteria?

6. URINARY TRACT INFECTIONS

LEARNING OBJECTIVES

1. Discuss the types of infections that occur in the urinary system.
2. Explain risk factors for bladder infections.
3. Explain the reasons medical treatment is important.
4. Describe strategies to reduce the risk of urinary tract infections.

FIGURE 14.7 The Urinary System

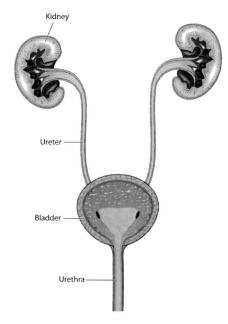

© *Shutterstock*

cystitis

Inflammation of the bladder, usually caused by a bacterial infection.

pyelonephritis

Inflammation of the kidneys, usually caused by a bacterial infection.

urethritis

Inflammation of the urethra; can be caused by sexually transmitted microbes.

The urinary system starts with the kidneys, which continually filter the plasma (the fluid component of blood)—at the rate of about 180 liters (about 48 gallons) a day. They return precious nutrients such as glucose to the circulation. Waste products, other chemicals, and some body water end up as urine. It's a huge, delicate operation. The urine trickles down the ureters into the holding tank of your bladder. Eventually the pressure builds enough to activate the nerves that notify your brain it's time to seek a publicly acceptable location to discharge the fluid out the final bit of tubing—the urethra. Infection can occur in any of these anatomical parts. While the term *urinary tract infection* (UTI) technically includes the entire system, most health care practitioners use it to refer to bladder infections.

The bladder is a common site of infection. The medical term is **cystitis**. Women have many more bladder infections than men, presumably because the female urethra is shorter and placed between the anus and vagina—the two sources for bacteria such as *Escherichia coli*. An estimated one in three women will have at least one bout of cystitis by the age of 24, and half experience one during their lives.[85] About 30 percent of women have one or more recurrences after antibiotic treatment. On the other hand, the condition is rare in men, unless they have a congenital abnormality of the urinary tract or unless age-associated enlargement of the prostate gland significantly hinders the outflow of urine.

In addition to female sex, other risk factors include age (infants and elders), pregnancy, diabetes, obesity, sexual activity, poor hygiene, and having a urinary catheter (a tube into the bladder). Also, the spermicide Nonoxynol-9 (used with or without a diaphragm) kills some species of bacteria that normally inhabit and protect the vagina but doesn't have much impact on yeast and pathogenic bacteria.[86] Immunodeficiency (HIV infection/AIDS) and neurologic conditions that make it difficult to empty the bladder are less common risks.

The most common symptoms of cystitis are urgent, frequent, painful, or difficult urination. It may hurt to press just above the pubic bone. Fever and blood in the urine indicate more severe infection. Interstitial cystitis is a chronic inflammatory condition of unknown cause that also produces pain in the area of the bladder and urgent, frequent urination.

Health care practitioners can often diagnose cystitis based on symptoms. Urine analysis confirms the diagnosis. Prompt antibiotic treatment quickly eradicates the bacteria, relieving symptoms and preventing the microbes from ascending to the kidneys.

Kidney infection (**pyelonephritis**) is serious and can lead to permanent damage. Signs and symptoms include flank pain, fever, chills, blood in the urine, weakness, malaise, appetite loss, nausea, and vomiting. If you have such symptoms, call your health care provider.

Urethritis, or inflammation of the urethra, can have multiple causes, most commonly, sexually transmitted bacteria. In women, chemical irritants such as bubble bath can also irritate the urethra. As with cystitis, urination is difficult and painful.

Preventing Urinary Tract Infections

Some women are vulnerable to recurrent cystitis. Preventive strategies can minimize repeat infections.

- **Stay hydrated.** Drinking lots of fluids increases the volume of diluted urine.

- **Drink cranberry juice.** Most research shows that taking cranberry as a juice or concentrated solid extracts (capsules) helps prevent recurrent UTIs. It works mainly by preventing bacteria from sticking to bladder cells rather than by acidifying the urine or directly killing the bacteria. That's why, once the bacteria have infected the bladder, cranberry isn't an effective treatment. For prevention, drink 10 to 16 ounces a day of cranberry cocktail, about 8 ounces a day of straight cranberry juice (it's tart!), or 800 milligrams twice a day of encapsulated cranberry concentrate.[87]
- **Urinate often.** Women should urinate after sexual intercourse. Urination flushes out any bacteria making the ascent up the urethra.
- **Practice good bathroom hygiene.** After you go to the bathroom, wipe from front to back to avoid swabbing bowel bacteria toward the urethra.
- **Don't douche.** Doing so disrupts the vaginal ecology. A healthy vagina contains predominantly lactobacilli bacteria, which protect against organisms that cause UTIs and some vaginal infections.
- **Consider probiotics.** While the research on oral probiotics is mixed, several studies support intravaginal use of *Lactobacillus* species that normally colonize the intestinal tract and vagina.[88] ,[89] ,[90]

KEY TAKEAWAYS

- Cystitis (bladder infections) is particularly common among women.
- The main risk of untreated cystitis is the development of pyelonephritis, which can permanently damage the kidneys.
- Men and women can develop urethritis from sexually transmitted bacteria.

DISCUSSION QUESTIONS

1. Why are women more at risk for cystitis?
2. How do health care practitioners usually treat cystitis? Why is such treatment recommended?
3. How can women reduce their risk for recurrent cystitis?

7. RECOMMENDED RESOURCES

7.1 Books

Barry JM. *The Great Influenza: The Epic Story of the Deadliest Plague in History*. New York, NY: Penguin Books; 2005.

Crawford DH. *Deadly Companions: How Microbes Shaped Our History*. Oxford, UK: Oxford University Press; 2009.

Drexler M. *Emerging Epidemics: The Menace of New Infections*. New York, NY: Penguin Books; 2009.

Kelly J. *The Great Mortality: An Intimate History of the Black Death, the Most Devastating Plague of All Time*. New York, NY: Harper Perennial; 2006.

Tortora GJ, Funke BR, Case CL. *Microbiology: An Introduction*. 11th ed. Boston, MA: Benjamin Cummings; 2012.

7.2 Organizations and Websites

Alliance for Prudent Use of Antibiotics, Tufts University. http://www.tufts.edu/med/apua.

American Society for Microbiology. http://www.asm.org.

National Center for Infectious Diseases, Centers for Disease Control and Prevention (CDC). http://www.cdc.gov/ncidod/diseases/eid.

Office of Infectious Diseases: Infectious Disease Information, Centers for Disease Control and Prevention. http://www.cdc.gov/oid.

World Health Organization: Antimicrobial Resistance. http://www.who.int/drugresistance/en.

World Health Organization: Infectious Diseases. http://www.who.int/topics/infectious_diseases/en.

ENDNOTES

1. Theriot J. The world within us: microbes that help and harm. Stanford University lecture. February 18, 2010. Available at: http://www.youtube.com/watch?v=dedlL8l0YIM. Accessed June 24, 2011.

2. Haines M. Fertility and mortality in the United States. *Economic History Association*. Published February 4, 2011. Available at: http://eh.net/encyclopedia/article/haines.demography. Accessed May 24, 2011.

3. Health, United States, 2011. National Centers for Health Statistics. Centers for Disease Control and Prevention. Available at: http://www.cdc.gov/nchs/data/hus/hus11.pdf. Accessed December 20, 2012.

4. Leading causes of death. National Centers for Health Statistics. Centers for Disease Control and Prevention. Available at: http://www.cdc.gov/nchs/fastats/lcod.htm. Accessed December 18, 2012.

5. *What Is Ancient Egyptian Medicine? A History of Medicine.* Medical News Today. Available at: http://www.medicalnewstoday.com/info/medicine/ancient-egyptian-medicine.php#.UNNEx6Wc8yE. Accessed December 20, 2012.

6. Meeting the MDG drinking water and sanitation target: the urban and rural challenge of the decade. World Health Organization and UNICEF. 2006. Available at: http://www.who.int/water_sanitation_health/monitoring/jmpfinal.pdf. Accessed July 20, 2011.

7. World Health Organization. The global burden of disease: 2004 update. Available at: http://www.who.int/healthinfo/global_burden_disease/2004_report_update/en/index.html. Accessed June 24, 2011.

8. Shuman EK. Global climate change and infectious diseases. *N Engl J Med.* 2010;326:1061–1063. Available at: http://www.nejm.org/doi/full/10.1056/NEJMp0912931. Accessed July 20, 2011.

9. Harrigan RJ, Thomassen HA, Buermann W, Cummings RF, Kahn ME, Smith TB. Economic conditions predict prevalence of West Nile virus. *PLoS One.* 2010 Nov 12;5(11):e15437.

10. Steinmann J, Becker B, Bischoff B, et al. Virucidal activity of 2 alcohol-based formulations proposed as hand rubs by the World Health Organization. *Am J Infect Control.* 2010 Feb;38(1):66–68.

11. Crompton DWT, Montresor A, Nesheim MC, Savioli L, eds. Controlling diseases due to helminth infections. World Health Organization. 2003. Available at: http://www.who.int/wormcontrol/documents/en/Controlling%20Helminths.pdf. Accessed June 24, 2011.

12. Haybaeck J, Heikenwalder M, Klevenz B, et al. Aerosols transmit prions to immunocompetent and immunodeficient mice. *PLoS Pathog.* 2011;7(1):e1001257. doi:10.1371/journal.ppat.1001257. Available at: http://www.plospathogens.org/article/info%3Adoi%2F10.1371%2Fjournal.ppat.1001257. Accessed June 24, 2011.

13. Fendrick AM, Monto AS, Nightengale B, Sarnes M. The economic burden of non-influenza-related viral respiratory tract infection in the United States. *Arch Intern Med.* 2003 Feb 24;163(4):487–494. Available at: http://archinte.ama-assn.org/cgi/content/full/163/4/487. Accessed June 29, 2011.

14. Hypponen E, Power C. Hypovitaminosis D in British adults at age 45 y: nationwide cohort study of dietary and lifestyle predictors. *Am J Clin Nutr.* 2007 Mar;85(3):860–868.

15. Sabetta JR, DePetrillo P, Cipriani RJ, Smardin J, Burns LA, Landry ML. Serum 25-hydroxyvitamin d and the incidence of acute viral respiratory infections in healthy adults. *PLoS One.* 2010 Jun 14;5(6):e11088. Available at: http://www.ncbi.nlm.nih.gov/pmc/articles/PMC2885414/?tool=pubmed. Accessed June 27, 2011.

16. Monto AS. Epidemiology of viral respiratory infections. *Am J Med.* 2002;112(suppl 6A):4S–12S.

17. Douglas RM, Hemila H, Chalker E, et al. Vitamin C for preventing and treating the common cold. *Cochrane Database Syst Rev.* 2004 Oct 18;(4):CD000980.

18. Peters EM. Exercise, immunology and upper respiratory tract infections. *Int J Sports Med.* 1997 Mar;18(suppl 1):S69–77.

19. Beard JA, Bearden A, Striker R. Vitamin D and the anti-viral state. *J Clin Virol.* 2011 Mar;50(3):194–200.

20. Cannell JJ, Vieth R, Umhau JC, et al. Epidemic influenza and vitamin D. *Epidemiol Infect.* 2006 Dec;134(6):1129–1140.

21. Prasad AS. Zinc: role in immunity, oxidative stress and chronic inflammation. *Curr Opin Clin Nutr Metab Care.* 2009 Nov;12(6):646–652.

22. Singh M, Das RR. Zinc for the common cold. *Cochrane Database Syst Rev.* 2011;16(2):CD001364. doi:10.1002/14651858.

23. Murray MT. *Encyclopedia of Nutritional Supplements.* Rocklin, CA: Prima; 1996:188–189.

24. Barrett B, Vohmann M, Calabrese C. Echinacea for upper respiratory tract infection. *J Fam Pract.* 1999;48(8):628–635.

25. Coon JT, Ernst E. Andrographis paniculata in the treatment of upper respiratory tract infections: a systematic review of safety and efficacy. *Planta Med.* 2004 Apr;70(4):293–298.

26. Tsai Y, Cole LL, Davis LE, et al. Antiviral properties of garlic: in vitro effects on influenza B, herpes simplex and coxsackie viruses. *Planta Med.* 1985 Oct;(5):460–461.

27. Josling P. Preventing the common cold with a garlic supplement: a double-blind, placebo-controlled survey. *Adv Ther.* 2001 Jul-Aug;18(4):189–193.

28. McElhaney JE, Goel V, Toane B, Hooten J, Shan JJ. Efficacy of COLD-fX in the prevention of respiratory symptoms in community-dwelling adults: a randomized, double-blinded, placebo controlled trial. *J Altern Complement Med.* 2006 Mar;12(2):153–157.

29. Scaglione F, Cattaneo G, Alessandria M, Cogo R. Efficacy and safety of the standardised ginseng extract G115 for potentiating vaccination against the influenza syndrome and protection against the common cold [corrected]. *Drug Exp Clin Res.* 1996;22(2):65–72.

30. Barak V, Halperin T, Kalickman I. The effect of Sambucol, a black elderberry-based, natural product, on the production of human cytokines: I. inflammatory cytokines. *Eur Cytokine Netw.* 2001;12(2):290–296.

31. Krawitz C, Mraheil MA, Stein M, et al. Inhibitory activity of a standardized elderberry liquid extract against clinically-relevant human respiratory bacterial pathogens and influenza A and B viruses. *BMC Complement Altern Med.* 2011 Feb 25;11:16.

32. Zakay-Rones Z, Varsano N, Zlotnik M, et al. Inhibition of several strains of influenza virus in vitro and reduction of symptoms by an elderberry extract (Sambucus nigra L.) during an outbreak of influenza B Panama. *J Altern Complement Med.* 1995;1(4):361–369.

33. Zakay-Rones Z, Thom E, Wollan T, Wadstein J. Randomized study of the efficacy and safety of oral elderberry extract in the treatment of influenza A and B virus infections. *J Int Med Res.* 2004;32(2):132–140.

34. Kong F. Pilot clinical study on a proprietary elderberry extract: efficacy in addressing influenza symptoms. *Online J Pharmacol PharmacoKinetics.* 2009;5:32–43. Available at: http://omicron-pharma.com/pdfs/ElderberryClinicalOJPK_Published.pdf. Accessed February 15, 2012.

35. Santibañez S, Fiore AE, Merlin TL, Redd S. A primer on strategies for prevention and control of seasonal and pandemic influenza. *Am J Public Health.* 2009;99(suppl 2):S216–S223.

36. Key facts about swine influenza (swine flu). Centers for Disease Control and Prevention. Available at: http://www.cdc.gov/flu/swineflu/key_facts.htm. Accessed July 1, 2011.

37. The influenza pandemic of 1918. Human Virology at Stanford. Stanford University. 2005. Available at: http://virus.stanford.edu/uda. Accessed February 18, 2012.

38. Leekha S, Zitterkopf NL, Espy MJ, Smith TF, Thompson RL, Sampathkumar P. Duration of influenza A virus shedding in hospitalized patients and implications for infection control. *Infect Control Hosp Epidemiol.* 2007 Sep;28(9):1071–1076.

39. Jurkiewicz D, Rapiejko P. Use of isotonic NaCl solution in patients with acute rhinosinusitis. *Otolaryngol Pol.* 2011 Jan–Feb;65(1):47–53.

40. Rabago D, Zgierska A, Mundt M, Barrett B, Bobula J, Maberry R. Efficacy of daily hypertonic saline nasal irrigation among patients with sinusitis: a randomized controlled trial. *J Fam Pract.* 2002 Dec;51(12):1049–1055.

41. Halsey ES, Burke AC. Bacterial pharyngitis. Medscape. 2009. Available at: http://emedicine.medscape.com/article/225243-overview. Accessed July 4, 1011.

42. Garbutt JM, Banister C, Spitznagel E, Piccirillo JF. Amoxicillin for acute rhinosinusitis: a randomized controlled trial. *JAMA.* 2012;307(7):685–692.

43. Eyers S, Weatherall M, Shirtcliffe P, Perrin K, Beasley R. The effect on mortality of antipyretics in the treatment of influenza infection: systematic review and meta-analysis. *J R Soc Med.* 2010 Oct;103(10):403–411.

44. Carey JV. Literature review: should antipyretic therapies routinely be administered to patients with [corrected] fever? *J Clin Nurs.* 2010 Sep;19(17–18):2377–2393. doi:10.1111/j.1365-2702.2010.03258.x.

45. Albert RH. Diagnosis and treatment of acute bronchitis. *Am Fam Physician.* 2010 Dec 1;82(11):1345–1350.

46. Smith SM, Schroeder K, Fahey T. Over-the-counter medications for acute cough in children and adults in ambulatory settings. *Cochrane Database Syst Rev.* 2008 Jan 23;(1):CD001831.

47. Goto M, Kawamura T, Shimbo T, et al.; Great Cold Investigators-II. Influence of loxoprofen use on recovery from naturally acquired upper respiratory tract infections: a randomized controlled trial. *Intern Med.* 2007;46(15):1179–1186.

48. Voiriot G, Dury S, Parrot A, Mayaud C, Fartoukh M. Nonsteroidal antiinflammatory drugs may affect the presentation and course of community-acquired pneumonia. *Chest.* 2011 Feb;139(2):387–394.

49. Doran TF, De Angelis C, Baumgardner RA, Mellits ED. Acetaminophen: more harm than good for chickenpox? *J Pediatr.* 1989 Jun;114(6):1045–1048.

50. Heron MP, Hoyert DL, Murphy SL, Xu J, Kochanek KD, Tejada-Vera B. Deaths: final data for 2006. *Natl Vital Stat Rep;* 2009;57(14). Available at: http://www.cdc.gov/nchs/data/nvsr/nvsr57/nvsr57_14.pdf. Accessed June 1, 2011.

51. Pneumonia can be prevented—vaccines can help. Centers for Disease Control and Prevention. Available at: http://www.cdc.gov/Features/Pneumonia. Accessed June 29, 2011.

52. Tuberculosis. World Health Organization. Fact sheet no. 104. November 2010. Available at: http://www.who.int/mediacentre/factsheets/fs104/en. Accessed June 29, 2011.

53. Fabian P, McDevitt JJ, DeHaan WH, et al. Influenza virus in human exhaled breath: an observational study. *PLoS One.* 2008 Jul 16;3(7):e2691.

54. Jefferson T, Del Mar C, Dooley L, et al. Physical interventions to interrupt or reduce the spread of respiratory viruses: a Cochrane review. *Health Technol Assess.* 2010 Jul;14(34):347–476.

55. Tyrrell DA, Cohen S, Schlarb JE. Signs and symptoms in common colds. *Epidemiology and Infection.* 1993 Aug;111(1):143–156. Available at: http://www.ncbi.nlm.nih.gov/pmc/articles/PMC2271186/?page=2. Accessed June 29, 2011.

56. Berggren A, Lazou Ahrén I, Larsson N, Onning G. Randomised, double-blind and placebo-controlled study using new probiotic lactobacilli for strengthening the body immune defence against viral infections. *Eur J Nutr.* 2011;50(3):203–210.

57. Pregliasco F, Anselmi G, Fonte L, Giussani F, Schieppati S, Soletti L. A new chance of preventing winter diseases by the administration of synbiotic formulations. *J Clin Gastroenterol*. 2008 Sep;42(suppl 3 pt 2):S224–33.

58. Winkler P, de Vrese M, Laue Ch, Schrezenmeir J. Effect of a dietary supplement containing probiotic bacteria plus vitamins and minerals on common cold infections and cellular immune parameters. *Int J Clin Pharmacol Ther*. 2005 Jul;43(7):318–326.

59. Noah TL, Zhou H, Monaco J, Horvath K, Herbst M, Jaspers I. Tobacco smoke exposure and altered nasal responses to live attenuated influenza virus. *Environ Health Perspect*. 2011 Jan;119(1):78–83. Available at: http://www.ncbi.nlm.nih.gov/pmc/articles/PMC3018504/?tool=pubmed. Accessed July 9, 2011.

60. Huttunen R, Heikkinen T, Syrjänen J. Smoking and the outcome of infection. *J Intern Med*. 2011 Mar;269(3):258–269. doi:10.1111/j.1365-2796.2010.02332.x.

61. Cohen S, Frank E, Doyle WJ, et al. Types of stressors that increase susceptibility to the common cold in healthy adults. *Health Psychol*. 1998 May;17(3):214–223.

62. Cohen S, Tyrrell DA, Smith AP. Psychological stress and susceptibility to the common cold. *N Engl J Med*. 1991 Aug 29;325(9):606–612.

63. The top 10 causes of death. World Health Organization. Fact sheet no. 310. Available at: http://www.who.int/mediacentre/factsheets/fs310/en. Updated June 2011. Accessed July 7, 2011.

64. Scallan E, Hoekstra RM, Angulo FJ, et al. Foodborne illness acquired in the United States—major pathogens. *Emerg Infect Dis*. 2011;17:7–15. Available at: http://www.cdc.gov/eid/content/17/1/7.htm. Accessed June 8, 2011.

65. Scallan E, Griffin PM, Angulo FJ, Tauxe RV, Hoekstra RM. Foodborne illness acquired in the United States—unspecified agents. *Emerg Infect Dis*. 2011;17:16–22. Available at: http://www.cdc.gov/eid/content/17/1/16.htm. Accessed June 8, 2011.

66. Oral rehydration solutions: made at home. Rehydration Project. Available at: http://rehydrate.org/solutions/homemade.htm. Accessed July 7, 2011.

67. Hilton E, Kolakowski P, Singer C, et al. Efficacy of lactobacillus GG as a diarrheal preventative in travelers. *J Travel Med*. 1997;4:41–3.

68. Kim HJ, Camilleri M, McKinzie S, et al. A randomized controlled trial of a probiotic, VSL#3, on gut transit and symptoms in diarrhoea-predominant irritable bowel syndrome. *Aliment Pharmacol Ther*. 2003;17:895–904.

69. Teles R, Wang CY. Mechanisms involved in the association between peridontal diseases and cardiovascular disease. *Oral Dis*. 2011 Jul;17(5):450–461. doi:10.1111/j.1601-0825.2010.01784.x.

70. Hepatitis A FAQs for health professionals. Centers for Disease Control and Prevention. Available at: http://www.cdc.gov/hepatitis/HAV/HAVfaq.htm#protection. Accessed July 8, 2011.

71. Hepatitis B FAQs for the public. Centers for Disease Control and Prevention. Available at: http://www.cdc.gov/hepatitis/B/bFAQ.htm#overview. Accessed July 8, 2011.

72. Hepatitis B FAQs for health professionals. Centers for Disease Control and Prevention. Available at: http://www.cdc.gov/hepatitis/HBV/HBVfaq.htm#overview. Accessed July 8, 2011.

73. Rosen HR. Chronic hepatitis C infection. *N Engl J Med*. 2011;364(25):2429–2438.

74. Hepatitis C Information for health professionals. Centers for Disease Control and Prevention. Available at: http://www.cdc.gov/hepatitis/HCV/index.htm. Accessed July 8, 2011.

75. Thigpen MC, Whitney CG, Messonnier NE, et al.; Emerging Infections Programs Network. Bacterial meningitis in the United States, 1998–2007. *N Engl J Med*. 2011 May 26;364(21):2016–2025.

76. Meningococal vaccines: what you need to know. Centers for Disease Control and Prevention. Available at: http://www.cdc.gov/vaccines/pubs/vis/default.htm#mening. Accessed July 3, 2011.

77. Satchell AC, Saurajen A, Bell C, Barnetson RS. Treatment of interdigital tinea pedis with 25% and 50% tea tree oil solution: a randomized, placebo-controlled, blinded study. *Australas J Dermatol*. 2002 Aug;43(3):175–178.

78. Gorwitz RJ. Community-associated methicillin-resistant Staphylococcus aureus: epidemiology and update. *Pediatr Infect Dis J*. 2008 Oct;27(10):925–926.

79. Oller AR, Province L, Curless B. Staphylococcus aureus recovery from environmental and human locations in 2 collegiate athletic teams. *J Athl Train*. 2010 May–Jun;45(3):222–229. Available at: http://www.ncbi.nlm.nih.gov/pmc/articles/PMC2865959/?tool=pubmed. Accessed July 8, 2011.

80. Institute of Medicine (US) Forum on Microbial Threats. Antibiotic resistance: implications for global health and novel intervention strategies. National Academies Press (US); 2010:70. Bookshelf ID: NBK54255. Available at: http://www.ncbi.nlm.nih.gov/books/NBK54255. Accessed July 5, 2011.

81. Rutschmann OT, Domino ME. Antibiotics for upper respiratory tract infections in ambulatory practice in the United States, 1997–1999: does physician specialty matter? *J Am Board Fam Pract*. 2004;17(3):196–200. Available at: http://www.jabfm.org/cgi/content/full/17/3/196. Accessed July 5, 2011.

82. McFarland LV. Meta-analysis of probiotics for the prevention of antibiotic associated diarrhea and the treatment of Clostridium difficile disease. *Am J Gastroenterol*. 2006;101:812–822.

83. Hickson M, D'Souza AL, Muthu N, et al. Use of probiotic lactobacillus preparation to prevent diarrhoea associated with antibiotics: randomised double blind placebo controlled trial. *BMJ*. 2007;335(7610):80. Available at: http://www.ncbi.nlm.nih.gov/pmc/articles/PMC1914504/?tool=pubmed. Accessed July 6, 2011.

84. Hilton E, Rindos P, Isenberg HD. Lactobacillus GG vaginal suppositories and vaginitis. *J Clin Microbiol*. 1995 May;33(5):1433. Available at: http://www.ncbi.nlm.nih.gov/pmc/articles/PMC228189/?tool=pubmed. Accessed July 6, 2011.

85. Foxman B. Epidemiology of urinary tract infections: incidence, morbidity, and economic costs. *Dis Mon*. 2003;49(2):53–70.

86. Reid G, Bruce AW, McGroarty JA, Cheng KJ, Costerton JW. Is there a role for lactobacilli in prevention of urogenital and intestinal infections? *Clin Microbiol Rev*. 1990 Oct;3(4):335–344.

87. Cranberry. Natural Medicine Comprehensive Database. Available at: http://naturaldatabase.therapeuticresearch.com/home.aspx?cs=&s=ND. Accessed June 29, 2011.

88. Baerheim A, Larsen E, Digranes A. Vaginal application of lactobacilli in the prophylaxis of recurrent lower urinary tract infection in women. *Scand J Prim Health Care*. 1994;12:239–243.

89. Reid G, Bruce AW, Taylor M. Influence of three-day antimicrobial therapy and lactobacillus vaginal suppositories on recurrence of urinary tract infections. *Clin Ther*. 1992;14:11–16.

90. Uehara S, Monden K, Nomoto K, Seno Y, Kariyama R, Kumon H. A pilot study evaluating the safety and effectiveness of lactobacillus vaginal suppositories in patients with recurrent urinary tract infection. *Int J Antimicrob Agents*. 2006 Aug;28(suppl 1):S30–4.

CHAPTER 15

Preventing Diabetes and Cardiovascular Disease

CHRONIC DISEASES

Most of us don't lie awake at night worrying whether lions will attack, whether the rusty nail that punctured our foot contained tetanus spores, or whether the mushroom we ate for dinner was poisonous. Instead, most of us survive to middle age only to spend our last years on multiple medications for chronic diseases, hoping to dodge the fatal heart attack, the paralyzing stroke, the sight-robbing diabetes, or the devouring cancer. These all-too-common illnesses rank among the top 10 killers in America. In this chapter, you'll learn about diabetes and cardiovascular diseases, which include heart attack and stroke. Cancer, the second leading cause of death after heart disease, is covered in Chapter 16.

The "Western" lifestyle—too little physical activity, too much stress, too little sleep, too many calories—power most chronic illnesses. Healthy lifestyle choices can prevent or delay their onset. These diseases often take root in childhood or adolescence, though symptoms might not appear until much later in life. In other words, the sooner you take steps to prevent them the better.

Chronic diseases are the most common and costly of all health problems, but they are also the most preventable.

 - Centers for Disease Control and Prevention

1.   UNDERSTANDING DIABETES MELLITUS

LEARNING OBJECTIVES

1. Define the two types of diabetes mellitus.
2. Explore trends in the prevalence of diabetes.
3. Discuss risk factors, prevention strategies, and treatments for diabetes.

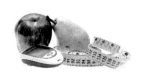

© Thinkstock

diabetes mellitus

A condition in which blood glucose is abnormally high due to defective production or action of insulin.

insulin

A hormone made by the pancreas that lowers blood glucose.

type 1 diabetes

An autoimmune condition with loss of insulin-producing pancreatic cells; also called insulin-dependent diabetes.

type 2 diabetes

A condition marked by insulin resistance; also called non-insulin-dependent diabetes.

gestational diabetes

Abnormally high blood sugar that develops during pregnancy.

Diabetes mellitus is categorized as a *metabolic disorder*, a condition that affects the way you process the energy from food. The problem in diabetes lies with **insulin**, a hormone that lowers blood glucose (sugar). After a meal, blood glucose rises, stimulating the pancreas—an organ that lies near the stomach—to release insulin. In the same way you can't enter a movie theater without a ticket, glucose can't enter cells such as muscle and fat cells without insulin. Glucose can pass inside other tissues without the aid of insulin. Once inside, glucose is either burned for energy or stored. In terms of blood glucose levels, the net result is that glucose returns to normal.

Insulin has other effects such as moving dietary amino acids into cells, stimulating the liver to store glucose as the polysaccharide glycogen, and increasing triglyceride (fat) stores in fat cells.

Two things can go wrong with insulin: (a) the pancreas doesn't make enough; and (b) the cells that require insulin no longer respond to it. There are hence two main types of diabetes: type 1 and type 2. Either way, blood glucose rises to unhealthy levels, a condition called *hyperglycemia*. Because glucose isn't entering fat and muscle, people with diabetes feel tired and hungry. Increased urination (because glucose "spills" into the urine) leads to increased thirst.

In **type 1 diabetes**, the body's immune system attacks insulin-producing cells in the pancreas. It's not yet known what triggers the autoimmune response in genetically susceptible people, though scientists suspect various viruses.[1] This condition usually appears in childhood or adolescence. The onset is fairly dramatic, with frequent urination, thirst, nausea, vomiting, and stomach pains. Treatment requires insulin replacement. Only about 5 percent of diabetes is type 1.

The other 95 percent of cases are **type 2 diabetes**. The pancreas makes plenty of insulin, but the liver, muscle, and fat become *insulin resistant*, meaning the cells fail to respond to this hormone. The main problem is that fat cells have taken in as much fat as they can hold. It's like showing up at the movie theater with your ticket (insulin) and being told, "Sorry, there are no empty seats." In addition, the ticket taker has become hard of hearing. The normal human response is to shout. The hormonal equivalent is to make more insulin. The cycle is that the cells become resistant to insulin, causing blood glucose to rise, which causes the pancreas to churn out more insulin. When insulin can't rise high enough to overcome insulin resistance, blood glucose becomes abnormally high, resulting in ill health.

Fortunately, type 2 diabetes is largely preventable. It's considered a multifactorial condition, one caused by genes and multiple environmental factors. Some races—particularly blacks, but also Hispanics and American Indians—are more at risk. Older age is also a factor. In fact, type 2 diabetes used to be called "adult-onset diabetes," a name that was dropped when the condition became common in children. Both under- and overnutrition during fetal life increases the child's insulin resistance.

Lifestyle changes are key to preventing and managing type 2 diabetes. Things that promote insulin resistance include being overweight or obese, chronically stressed, sleep deprived, and physically inactive. Doctors may also prescribe oral medications that increase pancreatic insulin production, make the cells more sensitive to insulin, or otherwise reduce blood glucose. Sometimes insulin replacement is ultimately needed.

A third type of diabetes, **gestational diabetes**, involves insulin resistance during pregnancy. About 18 percent of pregnant women develop diabetes during pregnancy (which is also called *gestation*).[2] Hormones made by the placenta, which nourishes the fetus, seem to cause insulin resistance. Gestational diabetes usually resolves after giving birth. However, the woman is at risk for developing type 2 diabetes later on. If the pregnant woman's blood glucose isn't controlled, and the fetus gains too much weight. After the birth, the newborn may experience abnormally low blood glucose and is at risk for developing obesity and type 2 diabetes later in life.

Video Clip 15.1

A Diabetes Primer
This video provides of brief overview of diabetes, including its consequences and management.

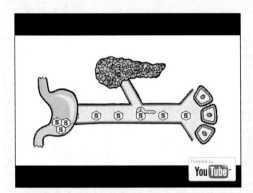

View the video online at: http://www.youtube.com/v/MGL6km1NBWE
Source: emedtv.

FIGURE 15.1 County-Level Estimates of Diagnosed Diabetes among Adults Aged ≥ 20 Years (2009)

Notice that diabetes hits the Southeastern and Appalachian regions of the United States harder than other areas. These regions also have a higher prevalence of obesity and physical inactivity.

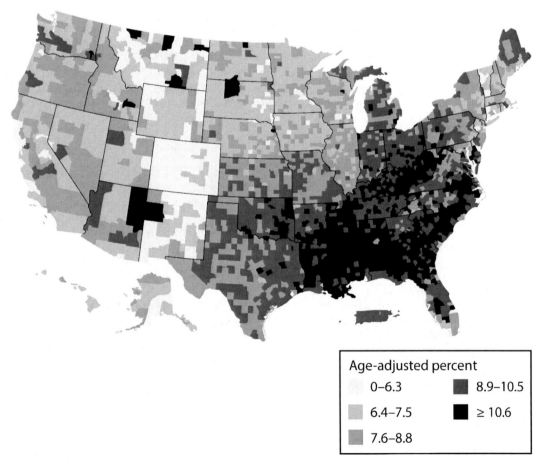

Source: Adapted from Centers for Disease Control and Prevention. County level estimates of diagnosed diabetes—US maps. Available at:
http://apps.nccd.cdc.gov/DDT_STRS2/NationalDiabetesPrevalenceEstimates.aspx?mode=DBT.

FIGURE 15.2 Diabetes on the Rise

This bar graph illustrates the burgeoning epidemic of diabetes.

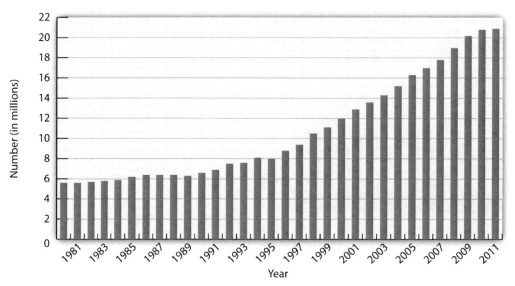

Source: Adapted from Centers for Disease Control and Prevention. Number (in millions) of civilian, noninstitutionalized persons with diagnosed diabetes, United States, 1980–2010. Available at: http://www.cdc.gov/diabetes/statistics/prev/national/figpersons.htm.

Worldwide, diabetes is one of the most common noncommunicable diseases. In developed countries, diabetes has reached epidemic proportions and is rapidly increasing in the developing world. This increase in type 2 diabetes has piggybacked the skyrocketing number of people becoming overweight and obese. In the United States, the number of people diagnosed with diabetes tripled between 1980 and 2010, when the number reached 20 million. According to the Centers for Disease Control and Prevention (CDC), nearly 10 percent of blacks have diabetes and about 6 percent of Asians and whites have diabetes. Worldwide, diabetes is expected to soar from 246 to 380 million people by 2025.[3] This condition has become alarmingly common in children, who have also become overweight and less physically active. The public health implications of a chronic disease affecting so many young people are ominous.

1.1 Signs and Symptoms of Diabetes

Normally, blood glucose doesn't end up in urine. However, with hyperglycemia, the kidneys can't recycle it all back into the blood and some "spills" into the urine, pulling extra water with it. Frequent urination and increased water loss leads to thirst. Because fat and muscle cells require insulin for glucose entry, those cells starve. Fatigue and weight loss ensue. Disease-causing microbes thrive on high glucose, which is why bladder infections and vaginal yeast infections become more common.

In type 1 diabetes, the signs and symptoms often develop quickly. In addition to increased thirst and urination and weight loss, people can develop **diabetic ketoacidosis**, a life-threatening condition related to the breakdown of fat and muscle for energy, which releases ketones and fatty acids. Signs include abdominal pain, vomiting, fruity breath, flushed and dry skin, rapid and deep breathing, drowsiness, and eventually coma. This condition requires emergency treatment.

In type 2 diabetes, early signs and symptoms are more subtle and vague. Meanwhile, high blood glucose damages many tissues, especially arteries and nerves. Some people don't know they have the condition until they have a heart attack or other calamity occurs.

Here's a summary of the signs and symptoms for both types of diabetes. If you are concerned about your diabetes risk, contact your doctor.

- fatigue
- increased thirst
- frequent urination
- dry mouth
- unexplained weight loss
- possibly increased hunger
- blurred vision

- recurrent bladder and vaginal infections
- yeast infections in skin folds
- poorly healing wounds
- numbness or tingling in hands and feet

1.2 Consequences of Unmanaged Diabetes

Type 1 and type 2 diabetes require long-term medical attention to limit the development of complications. Both diabetes and obesity increase levels of inflammatory chemicals, which aggravate insulin resistance and fuel other chronic diseases. Glucose can bind to proteins, disturbing their function. For instance, a structural protein called collagen becomes stiff. Stiffened collagen within blood vessels elevates blood pressure.

Arteries and nerves become damaged. Damaged arteries raise the risk of heart attack, *stroke* (loss of brain cells due to inadequate blood flow), *retinopathy* (a disease of the light-sensitive tissue in the eye, which can eventually lead to blindness), and kidney disease. Continued kidney damage can eventually lead to kidney failure. Nerve damage can cause tingling, numbness, and burning sensations in the hands and feet. Loss of nerve function also makes it harder to appreciate injuries. Wounds heal more slowly and are more at risk for infection, which is why diabetes is a common cause of amputations. Gums can more easily become infected. Women are more likely to develop vaginal yeast infections. Elevations in insulin and insulin-like growth factors may promote cancer. For all these reasons, diabetes is the seventh leading cause of death in the United States. On a positive note, people with diabetes who adopt recommended lifestyle and treatment are more likely to prevent or delay the onset of complications.

Complications of diabetes:

- heart attack
- stroke
- retinopathy
- kidney disease
- slow wound healing
- increased risk of infection
- amputation of limbs
- gum infection
- some cancers

1.3 Preventing and Managing Diabetes

The following strategies can help prevent diabetes.

Keep Up with Medical Check-Ups

If you're at risk for diabetes, particularly if you're overweight and have a family history of the condition, schedule regular exams. For most people, prediabetes—blood glucose levels above normal but yet high enough to meet criteria for diabetes—develops first. Prevention becomes critically important at that time. In fact, a large study called the Diabetes Prevention Program demonstrated that people predisposed to type 2 diabetes could prevent or delay its onset through modest weight loss (a 5 to 7 percent body weight loss), increased physical activity, and improved diet).[4] Specifically, lifestyle changes lowered their diabetes risk by 58 percent, which was nearly twice as effective as simply taking the medication metformin.

If you already have diabetes, healthy lifestyle goes a long way toward managing the condition. However, you still need to work closely with your health practitioner and dietitian to make sure blood glucose levels are under control.

Exercise

Physical activity increases insulin sensitivity, thereby countering any tendency for cells to become resistant to insulin's action. Regular exercise adds muscle mass and burns calories, which makes it easier to regulate blood sugar and to lose weight. Moving your body also relieves stress.

Achieve and Maintain a Normal Weight

Excess body fat is a big risk factor for diabetes, especially when it's added to the belly. Conversely, reducing body fat improves insulin sensitivity. It's easier said than done. See Chapter 10 for tips about losing weight and keeping it off. People with diabetes should work with their health practitioner or a registered dietitian to plan dietary changes.

Eat Right

Emphasize fruits, vegetables, legumes, and whole grains. The World Health Organization recommends at least five portions of fruit and vegetables a day to prevent diabetes. They contain fiber and many nutrients beneficial to overall health and to reducing diabetes risks. A study published in *Diabetes Care* found that people who ate a greater quantity and variety of fruits and vegetables had a much lower risk of developing type 2 diabetes.[5]

Plants—fruits, vegetables, and whole grains—contain carbohydrates, which increase blood glucose. However, some of the carbohydrate content is starch and fiber, which slows absorption of dietary sugars. On the other hand, simple sugars such as those found in fruit juice, sodas, alcoholic beverages, ice cream, sorbet, sweetened yogurt, candy, and many baked goods cause a rapid rise in glucose—something you don't want. In fact, a study showed that women who drank water rather than sweetened beverages such as juice and sodas had a lower risk of developing type 2 diabetes.[6]

Fats help satisfy appetite and serve valuable functions in the body. However, because they're high in calories, restricted intake helps achieve weight loss. Furthermore, diets high in saturated fats (found in meat and dairy) can increase insulin resistance, whereas consuming monounsaturated fats instead can enhance insulin sensitivity. A simple strategy is to choose fats that are liquid at room temperature. The American Diabetes Association recommends about 10 percent of daily calories come from monounsaturated and polyunsaturated fats, such as those found in avocados; cold-water fish; almonds; hazelnuts; filberts; and olive, sunflower, and safflower oil.

Because diabetes and cardiovascular disease go hand in hand, there's another reason to avoid saturated fat and trans fats (fats artificially created by the addition of hydrogen): both increase heart disease risk. Protein needs can be increased in diabetes. However, because most Americans normally consume more protein than they need, people with diabetes don't need more.

Stress Less

When you're stressed, cortisol, epinephrine, and glucagon (also made by the pancreas) go up. All three hormones antagonize insulin and drive glucose higher. Severe stress (as in enduring a serious injury or being sick enough to need intensive care) can result in hyperglycemia. For people who already have diabetes, moderate psychosocial stress can undermine glucose management. Furthermore, having diabetes can be distressing. People need to check their glucose sugar levels and readjust diet, activity, and medications as needed. Controlling stress, on the other hand, improves glucose levels. Preliminary research supports mindfulness-based stress reduction in diabetes.[7]

Sleep Well

Chronic sleep deprivation and poor quality sleep increase the risk of obesity and diabetes.[8] Contributors include severe insomnia, not scheduling enough time for sleep, and sleep disorders such as obstructive sleep apnea (repeated episodes of absent breathing during sleep). Inadequate sleep activates stress hormones and unbalances other chemicals related to appetite and metabolism. See Chapter 4 for tips on sleeping better. If, despite your best efforts, you still feel sleepy during the day, see your doctor.

KEY TAKEAWAYS

- Diabetes mellitus is a chronic disease marked by high blood glucose (hyperglycemia).
  - In type 1 diabetes, an autoimmune reaction destroys insulin-producing cells in the pancreas.
  - Insulin resistance causes type 2 diabetes, the most common type of diabetes and one that has become epidemic.
- Gestational diabetes occurs during pregnancy.
- While genes and several other uncontrollable factors raise the risk of type 2 diabetes, modifiable behaviors are more important.
- People with diabetes need to work closely with medical experts to control their blood glucose. Doing so can limit the possibility of serious complications.

2. CARDIOVASCULAR SYSTEM

LEARNING OBJECTIVES

1. Identify the main structures in the cardiovascular system.
2. Explain how blood circulates through the body.
3. List key risk factors for cardiovascular disease.
4. Differentiate between risk factors you cannot control versus those that you can.
5. Describe simple lifestyle changes that protect the cardiovascular system.

FIGURE 15.3 The Heart

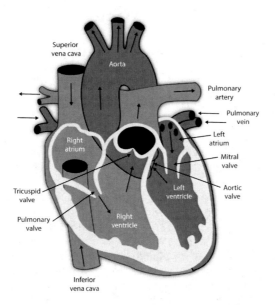

The cardiovascular system is basically a pump (the heart) connected to a closed circuit of tubes (the vascular system). While cardiologists (heart specialists) might object to this oversimplification, it works for our purposes. The main purpose of the cardiovascular system is twofold: (1) to deliver useful chemicals—oxygenated blood in the lungs, nutrients from the intestines, hormones, and other chemicals—to all the cells in the body and (2) to pick up waste product eliminated by the lungs, liver, kidneys, and intestines.

As you can see in Figure 15.3, the heart is a hollow muscular organ nestled slightly left of center in the chest, between the right and left lung. The heart also has a right side, which pumps blood through the lungs, and a left side, which pumps blood to the rest of the body. As you can imagine, the left side works harder than the right. Because of the lungs' critical role, the heart and lungs are sometimes lumped together as the *cardiorespiratory system*.

The heart is divided into four chambers: *right atrium*, *right ventricle*, *left atrium*, and *left ventricle*. Valves prevent the backward flow of blood. Two large veins, the *superior vena cava* and *inferior vena cava*, carry blood that's low in oxygen and high in carbon dioxide and other waste products to the right side of the heart.

The right atrium pumps blood to the right ventricle, which contracts, propelling the blood through the pulmonary veins. As blood passes though the vascular system in the lungs, carbon dioxide is exchanged for oxygen. The pulmonary arteries return oxygenated blood to the left atrium, pushing the blood into the left ventricle, which pumps the blood out a large artery called the *aorta*. From there, a network of branching arteries carries oxygen and nutrients to cells all over the body.

When the heart pumps, the muscles contract. The contraction phase is called **systole**. The relaxation phase, when the heart's chambers fill with blood, is called **diastole**.

 Video Clip 15.2

How the Cardiovascular System Works
This video shows you the basics of how the heart pumps and how the blood circulates in the body.

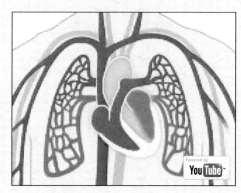

View the video online at: http://www.youtube.com/v/oE8tGkP5_tc

The vascular system has three types of blood vessels: (1) arteries, which carry oxygen-rich blood away from the heart and on to other tissues; (2) veins, which carry carbon dioxide and other wastes away from the tissues and return it to the heart; and (3) capillaries, the tiniest blood vessels, which connect the arteries and the veins.

The largest artery (the aorta) exits the left ventricle. It has to withstand the pressure waves coming from the heart. Protein fibers allow it to widen with systole and snap back with diastole. From the aorta, arteries fork into progressively smaller branches. Medium-sized arteries have more muscular walls, which allow them to regulate the flow of blood. When the muscles contract, the vessels narrows to restrict blood flow, a process called *vasoconstriction*. When the muscles relax, the vessel diameter widens, a process called *vasodilation*.

You can see this process at work. When you're cold, the small arteries in the skin vasoconstrict to conserve heat in your body's core, making you look paler. With heat, the arteries vasodilate to allow heat to radiate away from your body, creating a flushed appearance.

The arteries end in the tiny capillaries. Capillaries are only one-cell layer thick, thus allowing for an easy exchange of molecules like oxygen, carbon dioxide, and glucose (sugar).

Veins are relatively thin walled and have valves to prevent blood from flowing backward. Gravity, pressure differentials within the vascular system, and the massaging action of skeletal muscles propel the blood toward the heart. The deoxygenated blood they hold gives them a bluish hue.

Cells, fluids, and dissolved chemicals float within the vascular system. Red blood cells (*erythrocytes*) contain the oxygen-binding molecule *hemoglobin*. White blood cells (*leukocytes*) belong to the immune system. *Platelets* are fragments of a type of cell made in the bone marrow; their main job is to form blood clots when a blood vessel is injured. *Plasma*, the fluid portion of blood, is a watery substance that contains chemicals such as hormones, enzymes, antibodies, glucose, and minerals (sodium, chloride, potassium, and calcium).

systole

The contraction of the heart muscle, which pushes blood into the arteries.

diastole

The relaxation period of the heart, when the chambers become filled with blood.

FIGURE 15.4
The Cardiovascular System

Arteries (colored red) carry oxygenated blood from the left side heart to tissues throughout the body. The veins (colored blue) carry oxygen-poor, waste-laden blood back to the right side of the heart, which then pumps it to the lungs.

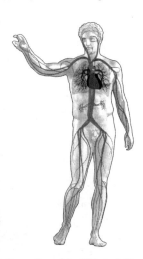

Source: Sansculotte. 2005. Available at: http://commons.wikimedia.org/ wiki/File:Grafik_blutkreislauf.jpg.

Blood also contains **lipids**, oily, waxy, fatty molecules that don't dissolve into water. The main lipids are **triglycerides** and **cholesterol**. Triglycerides are fat. They're carried in the blood and stored in fat cells and other tissues. Levels rise when you eat dietary fat from either plants or animals. No matter what you consume, the body stores any surplus of calories as triglycerides.

Though often maligned, cholesterol is essential to life. It's a building block for cell membranes, vitamin D, and steroid hormones such as estrogen, testosterone, progesterone, and cortisol. Cells in your body make it; your liver produces most of it. Diet influences blood levels in two ways.

1. All animal foods (dairy, red meat, poultry, and seafood) contain cholesterol. Although many texts say plants don't make cholesterol, they do contain small amounts.[9] At any rate, dietary cholesterol raises your blood cholesterol, though your body compensates to some extent by making less.

2. The type of fats you eat can raise or lower blood levels of cholesterol. You'll learn more about this relationship in the section on risk factors.

Cholesterol and triglycerides float in the bloodstream in spherical compounds made of protein and lipid called *lipoproteins*. These lipoproteins are stratified based on how dense they are: very low density, low density, and high density. The lower the density, the more fat (because fat is less dense than protein). **High-density lipoprotein (HDL)** is considered beneficial because it can pick up excess cholesterol and shuttle it to the liver to be recycled or excreted into the gut as bile. Very low–density lipoprotein (VLDL) and **low-density lipoprotein (LDL)** are considered undesirable because they're rich in triglycerides and cholesterol and damage the arteries. VLDL is loaded with triglycerides. LDL is the most abundant form of cholesterol in blood. When LDL oxidizes (the same process that makes butter go bad), it's particularly harmful.

 Video Clip 15.3

The Blood Vessels
This video explains the difference between arteries, veins, and capillaries.

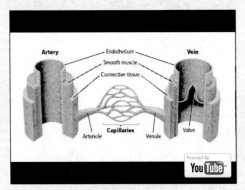

View the video online at: http://www.youtube.com/v/3ffSxq9iyB8

2.1   Risk Factors for Cardiovascular Disease

As mentioned earlier, cardiovascular disease is the number one cause of death in America. Although the death rate has steadily declined, the toll is still enormous. In 2008, 82.6 million men and women had cardiovascular disease and nearly 812,000 died as a result.[10] Every day, over 2,200 people die of cardiovascular disease—one every 39 seconds.

Most cardiovascular diseases, like type 2 diabetes, are multifactorial conditions. As always, some risks fall largely outside your control, some are well within your control, and some fall in between. Nevertheless, heart-healthy lifestyle choices cushion those nonnegotiable factors such as getting older day by day.

2.2   Risks Mainly Outside Your Control

1. **Family history.** Genetics influence your cholesterol levels and blood pressure. Some people have a genetic disorder (familial hypercholesterolemia) that leads to excessive cholesterol production. Genetic predisposition combined with poor diet, inactivity, smoking, stress-management styles,

lipids

Waxy, fatty molecules such as triglycerides and cholesterol.

triglycerides

Fat; dietary fat is carried in the blood as triglycerides.

cholesterol

A waxy substance found in all animals, including humans.

high-density lipoprotein (HDL)

A compound made of lipid and protein that carry cholesterol from tissue to the liver.

low-density lipoprotein (LDL)

A compound that contains more lipid (cholesterol and triglycerides) than protein; considered a risk factor for cardiovascular disease.

and other behavioral habits (most of which are also shaped by the family environment) can lead to cardiovascular disease.

2. **Increasing age.** The older you are, the greater your potential exposure to the modifiable risk factors listed later. Many of these factors produce small, cumulative changes that affect the cardiovascular system. Regardless of exposure to known risks, the cardiovascular system changes with time. Because maximum heart rate falls with age, older adults have a harder time meeting the challenge of physical exertion. For a variety of reasons, arteries become stiffer with age.

3. **Sex and gender.** The myth is that heart disease is a man's disease. For years, scientists thought that, compared with men, women's higher estrogen levels protected them from heart disease and that heart disease risk rose sharply after menopause. New research suggests that a woman's risk of life-threatening heart disease rises gradually with age. In contrast, men have a hastened risk of dying of heart disease at younger ages, though death rates stabilize around age 45.[11] Even though women tend to develop heart disease later than men, they are more likely to die of a heart attack.

4. **Race.** People of African ancestry carry the greatest burden of cardiovascular disease. In part because of a higher occurrence of diabetes and obesity, Mexican Americans, Native Americans, and native Hawaiians also have more heart and arterial disease than whites.

   Overall, the prevalence of cardiovascular disease is 47 percent for black women and nearly 45 percent for black men. Compare that to nearly 31 percent for Mexican Americans and almost 34 percent in white women and 37 percent in white men. Furthermore, the rate of cardiovascular death is highest for black men (390.4 per 100,000) and lowest for white women (200.5 per 100,000). High blood pressure is particularly high in the black community.

   Multiple factors contribute to these health disparities, including dietary influences, less education, lower income, more stress, and reduced access to recreational activities and health care. However, racial differences may affect biological processes, such as responses to dietary salt, an issue addressed in the discussion on high blood pressure.

5. **Your past.** The roots of cardiovascular disease originate in your personal history. A variety of prenatal (before birth) stressors, childhood trauma, and bad nutrition during your childhood can all increase your risk of developing problems later in life. But the past is past, and we humans are remarkably resilient creatures. There's plenty you can do to turn that ship toward healthier harbors. Section 4 tells you how.

2.3 Risks Factors You Can Control

Most of us know the pillars of healthy living, all of which protect the cardiovascular system. Large surveys show that few Americans—children included—meet the components of "ideal cardiovascular health": healthy diet, regular physical activity, no smoking, and normal body weight, blood pressure, cholesterol levels, and glucose levels.

Tobacco

Smoking tobacco, including secondhand smoke, damages your vascular system. The number one cause of death for smokers is cardiovascular disease, not lung disease. Smokers are two to four times more likely to develop heart disease and about twice as likely to have a stroke.[12] It damages the lining of your arteries, raises triglycerides, elevates LDL cholesterol and oxidizes it (which basically makes it go rancid), lowers HDL cholesterol, and increases blood pressure—all things that increase your risk of atherosclerosis. In addition, blood becomes more viscous (gelatinous), and the platelets tend to stick together to form a clot that can obstruct blood flow. Also, carbon dioxide in cigarette smoke lowers the oxygen-carrying capacity of blood, which makes you tired. Smokeless tobacco carries a lower risk of cardiovascular risk and stroke but is far from a safe habit. If you use tobacco, quit. It's not easy, but it's well worth the trouble. See Chapter 11 for locating resources to help you. If you don't use tobacco, stay away from other people's smoke.

High Blood Pressure

Also called hypertension, chronically elevated blood pressure can damage the arteries, overwork the heart, and lead to a number of cardiovascular diseases. This type of cardiovascular disease is discussed in detail in the Common Cardiovascular Diseases section.

Unhealthy Blood Lipids

As mentioned, high blood levels of total cholesterol, LDL cholesterol, and triglycerides correlate with an increased risk of cardiovascular disease. High HDL cholesterol, on the other hand, seems to offer protection, mainly by shuttling LDL cholesterol away from the arteries. A lipid panel or lipid profile is a blood test that measures cholesterol and triglycerides. It's usually done after a 9- to 12-hour fast.

TABLE 15.1   Interpreting Cholesterol and Triglyceride Levels

Total cholesterol—the total amount of blood cholesterol	
Optimal	Below 200 mg/dL
Borderline high	200–239 mg/dL
High	240 mg/dL and above
LDL cholesterol	
Optimal	Below 100 mg/dL
Normal	100–129 mg/dL
Borderline high	130–159 mg/dL
High	160–189 mg/dL
Very high	190 mg/dL and above
HDL cholesterol	
Optimal	60 mg/dL and above
Good	50–59 mg/dL
Poor	Below 40 mg/dL (men) and below 50 mg/dL (women)
Triglycerides	
Optimal	Under 150 mg/dL
Borderline high	151–200 mg/dL
High	201–499 mg/dL
Very high	500 mg/dL or higher
Note: Numbers are in milligrams per deciliter (mg/dL. 1 deciliter = 100 milliliters)	

Source: American Heart Association. What your cholesterol levels mean. 2012. Available at: http://www.heart.org/HEARTORG/Conditions/

Cholesterol/AboutCholesterol/What-Your-Cholesterol-Levels-Mean_UCM_305562_Article.jsp. Accessed July 1, 2012.

Slideshow 15.1.

AHA Slideshow on Cholesterol

http://watchlearnlive.heart.org/CVML_Player.php?moduleSelect=tisatk

Physical Inactivity

Sedentary people are at increased risk for cardiovascular disease, stroke, and diabetes. In the section on preventing cardiovascular disease, we'll examine the multiple benefits regular physical activity has on the cardiovascular system.

Unhealthy Diet

Certain dietary patterns stand out as bad news for the heart. Specifically, the American diet—too much processed and fatty meats, refined grains, fried and sugary foods, and high-fat dairy, as well as too few fruits, vegetables, and whole grains—injures the cardiovascular system. It also increases the risk for stroke and type 2 diabetes.[13],[14]

A study associated higher meat consumption with a greater risk of death from any cause. In terms of death from cardiovascular disease, each additional serving a day ramped up the risk by 16 percent.[15] All animal foods—meat, dairy, poultry, fish—contain cholesterol and saturated fats.

At this point, the relationship of particular foods to cardiovascular health becomes murky. Whether it comes from plants or animals, food is chemically complex. No one consumes a food or dietary supplement in isolation. Even when considering fats, any given food contains more than one kind. For instance, compared to corn-fed cattle, grass-fed cattle are leaner and yield meat and dairy products lower in fats linked to heart disease and higher in fats such as omega-3 fatty acids that reduce cardiovascular risk. While mono- and polyunsaturated fats (vegetable oils liquid at room temperature) are generally considered heart-healthy, they are vulnerable to oxidation, and oxidized fats promote tissue-damaging free radicals and inflammation.

Dietary **cholesterol** is another tricky topic. As noted earlier, your body makes plenty of it: enough so that you don't need to eat any. The body also regulates cholesterol levels. If you consume cholesterol, the body makes less. If you eat few cholesterol-containing foods, the body makes more. The bottom line is that your dietary intake of cholesterol has a relatively small impact on blood cholesterol levels.[16]

Nevertheless, health experts generally recommend that people at risk for cardiovascular disease restrict dietary cholesterol intake to less than 300 milligrams a day. If people already have heart disease or an LDL level equal to or above 100 mg/dL, they shouldn't consume more than 200 mg a day. The average American consumes more than that. One egg yolk contains 210 mg of cholesterol. (Egg whites contain no cholesterol.) A double cheeseburger contains 110 mg of cholesterol. A 3-ounce serving of meat or chicken contains about 60 to 70 mg of cholesterol. A cup of whole milk contains 33 mg.[17]

Animal foods and some plants (coconut, chocolate, cashews, Brazil nuts, macadamia nuts, and pine nuts) also contain **saturated fats**. For years, consumption of saturated fats has been linked to an increased risk of cardiovascular disease. Recent research has, however, challenged that belief. While dietary saturated fats do drive up LDL cholesterol, they also increase HDL cholesterol, which is good.[18] In other words, saturated fats may be more neutral for cardiovascular health than previously thought. Although some scientists contend that it's not necessary to restrict saturated fats,[19] many experts still recommend restricting saturated fat intake to less than 10 percent of daily calories—7 percent if LDL cholesterol exceeds 100 mg/dL.[20]

Trans fatty acids (also referred to as trans fats and hydrogenated fats) are one type of fat that health experts recognize as unequivocally unhealthy. Trans fats raise LDL cholesterol and oxidize it, lower HDL cholesterol, and make platelets "stickier." For a time, doctors encouraged patients to eat stick margarine, made from hydrogenated plant oils, rather than butter. It turned out that trans fats were much worse for heart health.

A critical issue is what type of food substitutes for saturated and trans fats. In the recent past, low-fat diets became the rage. "Low-fat" baked goods, chips, and ice creams lined grocery aisles. These foods were still high in calories, but the calories came from refined carbohydrates. Most Americans consume carbohydrates as sugar, refined starch (corn, white flour, white rice), and starch from potatoes.

It turns out that high-glycemic carbohydrates (those that quickly elevate blood glucose such as white bread, juice, sodas, and sweets) are *worse* for cardiovascular health than saturated fat, causing relatively more heart attacks.[21] Moreover, current research indicates that saturated fat may mainly promote arterial disease when consumed with high-glycemic carbohydrates. In addition to spiking blood glucose levels, high-glycemic foods increase blood levels of triglycerides and, when they replace fats, lower HDL cholesterol. On the other hand, substituting saturated fats with *complex*, low-glycemic carbohydrates slightly lowers the risk of heart attack. Foods lower on the glycemic index scale include most fruits and vegetables, legumes, and whole grains.

Sweetened beverages represent a significant source of extra sugar in the American diet. They increase triglycerides and inflammatory chemicals and promote weight gain—all cardiovascular disease risk factors. Routine consumption of regular and diet soda is linked to metabolic syndrome, diabetes, cardiovascular disease, hypertension, and stroke.[22],[23],[24] One study found that a single can of sugary soda a day increased the risk of heart disease by 20 percent.[25]

Another beverage to limit is **alcohol**. While moderate intake seems to protect the cardiovascular system, excessive amounts elevate triglycerides and blood pressure.

High levels of dietary **salt** (sodium chloride) cause fluid retention, which elevates blood pressure. Some people are "salt sensitive," meaning their kidneys don't efficiently eliminate excess sodium. African Americans are a vulnerable group. Recent research has shown that very low intakes of sodium may elevate cardiovascular risk.[26] Most Americans, however, consume more than enough salt.

Being Overweight and Obese

Obesity is also associated with depressed HDL cholesterol and elevated blood pressure, LDL cholesterol, and triglycerides. It's also linked with insulin resistance and diabetes. What's dangerous is not so much fat under the skin as fat in the belly. Abdominal fat creates the apple shape, a situation where waist circumference exceeds hip circumference. It releases inflammatory chemicals and hormones that promote cardiovascular disease and diabetes.

Insulin Resistance and Diabetes

As mentioned, people with diabetes have twice the risk of heart disease and stroke and tend to develop cardiovascular disease at earlier ages.

Metabolic Syndrome

People with **metabolic syndrome** have a cluster of risk factors—elevated blood pressure and blood glucose, low HDL cholesterol, high triglycerides, and central obesity (excess abdominal fat)—that pushes them closer to a diagnosis of hypertension and diabetes. Metabolic syndrome triples the risk of developing diabetes and doubles the cardiovascular disease risk.[27] It also increases the risk of stroke. Unfortunately, changes in the human environment and behaviors have increased the prevalence of metabolic syndrome worldwide. About a third of American adults have the condition.[28]

Stress Overload

Psychosocial stress has long been associated with cardiovascular disease. Scientists have begun to figure out why.[29] During the stress response, heightened sympathetic nervous system activation elevates heart rate and blood pressure.[30] The stress hormone cortisol also participates in these changes. A rise in another hormone (aldosterone) leads to retention of sodium (from salt) and water, which further increases blood pressure. Inflammatory chemicals rise, which lead to arterial dysfunction. Platelets become stickier. In vulnerable people, extreme stress can trigger heart attack, irregular heart rhythm, and sudden cardiac death.[31]

Personality Style

For a time, the type A personality was considered a risk for cardiovascular disease. It turns out that only the associated anger and hostility harm the cardiovascular system. The reasons are similar to those behind recurrent psychological stress. Anger and hostility also increase the risk of rapid, irregular heart rhythm called atrial fibrillation[32] and stroke.[33] In addition, hostility and the sense of time urgency characteristic of the type A personality increase the risk of high blood pressure.[34]

Sleep Deprivation

Insufficient sleep and a lack of deep, restorative, slow-wave sleep elevate the risk of high blood pressure and heart disease.[35] ,[36] Night-shift work is associated with metabolic syndrome, diabetes, and heart disease.[37] Obstructive sleep apnea represents a huge cardiovascular disease risk. It raises the chances of high blood pressure, heart disease, heart attack, abnormal heart rhythms, stroke, and overall cardiovascular mortality.[38]

Loneliness and Depression

Social isolation and depression are both stressful and stand as independent risk factors for cardiovascular disease. Depression increases the risk of heart attacks[39] and strokes.[40] It also increases the chance of death from cardiovascular disease. Conversely, depression is a common consequence of heart attack and stroke and worsens the outcome.[41] ,[42]

Inflammation and Oxidation

Inflammation is an immune system response to any injury or infection. Oxidation, from a chemistry standpoint, has to do with the addition of oxygen to a substance. You can see it happen when an apple slice goes brown. Oxidation and inflammation feed off each other. Too much of either stresses cells, accelerates aging, and promotes most diseases, including cardiovascular disease. Tobacco smoke, diets low in antioxidants (i.e., not enough fruits and vegetables), being overweight, sleep deprivation, psychological stress, metabolic syndrome, and diabetes increase the load.

Doctors often check blood levels of a substance called C-reactive protein, which generally indicates inflammation. A high level of C-reactive protein is a risk factor for cardiovascular disease.

metabolic syndrome

A condition marked by a group of risk factors (central obesity, low HDL cholesterol, and elevated blood pressure, triglycerides, and blood glucose) associated with heart disease, diabetes, and stroke.

KEY TAKEAWAYS

- The cardiovascular system is a closed loop that contains the heart, arteries, veins, and capillaries.
- The right side of the heart pumps blood to the lungs; the left side pumps blood to the other tissues in the body.
    - Arteries control the circulation of blood to tissues by vasodilating and vasoconstricting.
    - Blood contains erythrocytes, leukocytes, and plasma.
    - Plasma contains salts, lipids, hormones, and other chemicals.
- A number of factors can increase your risk of cardiovascular disease; some you can't change, but most are well within your control.
- Risk factors you can't control include your family history, age, sex, race, and early childhood environment.
- You can change many risk factors by altering your behaviors, getting medical treatment, or a combination of both. These include smoking, high blood pressure, unfavorable blood lipid levels, physical inactivity, an unhealthy diet, being overweight and obese, diabetes, metabolic syndrome, stress overload, sleep deprivation, and psychological factors (anger, hostility, depression). Many of these things contribute to excessive amounts of inflammation and oxidation in the body, which alone foster cardiovascular disease.

DISCUSSION QUESTIONS

1. Find a watch with a minute hand or a phone with a stopwatch function. Sit quietly. Turn one palm up and, using the finger pads of the other hand, find your pulse just below your wrist, on the same side as your thumb. (Don't take your pulse with your thumb as you may also feel the thumb's pulse.) Alternatively, you can feel the pulse in your neck, below the angle or your jaw.

    Count the pulse beats within 15 seconds and multiply it by 4. Write down the beats per minute. Time your respirations in 30 seconds and multiply by 2.

    The average heart rate for adults at rest is 80, but ranges between 60 to 100 beats a minute. People who regularly engage in aerobic exercise tend to have lower resting heart rates. Because their cardiorespiratory systems become more efficient, elite athletes can have heart rates as low as 40. The average respiratory rate at rest is 12 breaths per minute.

    Now exercise for one minute. Climb or run stairs, do pushups or sit-ups, jog around the building, hop, or any other kind of physical activity you're able to do. Immediately take your pulse and record the number. Pay attention to your breathing rate too and simply note the change from resting.

    Sit down. Take your pulse again at one minute and five minutes and record those numbers.

    What happened to your heart rate with exertion? Why did this happen? How long did it take for your heart rate to return to baseline? The fitter you are the more quickly your pulse returns to its resting rate. Compare your results to classmates or roommates.

2. Harvard University's School of Public Health has created an assessment tool on heart disease risk. Go to http://www.diseaseriskindex.harvard.edu/update/hccpquiz.pl?lang=english&func=home&quiz=heart and complete the questionnaire. What was your overall risk? What things are you doing to lower your risk? What factors put you at risk for cardiovascular disease? Which of these risk factors can you change? Of those, pick one risk factor that you can reduce right now.

3. Why is tobacco so bad for the cardiovascular system?

4. Which fat is considered bad for the cardiovascular system: saturated fat, trans fat, polyunsaturated fat? Explain your choice.

5. Why does dietary cholesterol have less impact on blood cholesterol levels than people often imagine?

3.   COMMON CARDIOVASCULAR DISEASES

LEARNING OBJECTIVES

1. Understand key pathological changes in cardiovascular structure and function for these diseases.
2. Identify warning signs and symptoms for the major cardiovascular diseases.
3. Discuss key diagnostic tests and treatment approaches for common cardiovascular diseases.

According to the American Heart Association (AHA), 82.6 million—more than one in three—Americans have at least one type of cardiovascular disease. These conditions affect the health of arteries and veins, blood pressure, heart rate and rhythm, heart valves, and the heart muscle. Most of the conditions become apparent with age, even though they may begin many years beforehand.

This section will focus on cardiovascular conditions that are largely prevention. Congenital cardiovascular defects (those present at birth) and those caused by infectious agents will not be covered. Suffice it to say that congenital defects can be multiple and complicated. Surgery is used to correct more severe abnormalities. Bacteria, fungi, and viruses that infect the heart are treated with medications and supportive therapy. Poor oral hygiene and intravenous drug use constitute risks for introducing microorganisms into the circulation.

3.1   Hypertension

Blood pressure is the force of blood against the arterial walls. It's a product of the strength of the heart's contraction, the volume of blood in the circulatory system, and relative narrowness and stiffness of the blood vessels.

Blood pressure is highest during systole and lowest during diastole. You can feel that pressure wave as the pulse in your wrist, neck, groin, and other places where arteries are near the surface. Blood pressure measurements have two numbers: systolic (the highest blood pressure with the heart's contraction) and diastolic (the lowest).

Blood pressure is measured with a *sphygmomanometer*. A cuff is wrapped around your arm and inflated with a hand pump until the pressure within the cuff is above your anticipated systolic pressure. That's enough pressure to close the artery in your upper arm. As the pressure is slowly released, the health practitioner listens through a stethoscope, whose bell-like end is placed on the skin above the artery at your inner elbow. The point at which blood first audibly whooshes through the partially closed artery is the *systolic pressure*; the point at which the sound becomes muffled (because the cuff is loose enough to allow blood through during diastole) is called the *diastolic pressure*. These numbers are measured in millimeters of mercury (abbreviated mm Hg). Systolic pressure is recorded first, then diastolic—for example, 115/75.

This image depicts a health practitioner using a sphygmomanometer to measure blood pressure.

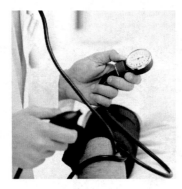

© *Thinkstock*

Hypertension means high blood pressure. Normal blood pressure is a systolic pressure under 120 and a diastolic pressure under 80 mm Hg. *Prehypertension* is defined as a systolic blood pressure between 120 and 139 mm Hg or diastolic blood pressure between 80 and 89 mm Hg. The threshold for hypertension is a systolic blood pressure of 140 mm Hg or diastolic blood pressure of 90 mm Hg.

hypertension

Abnormally high blood pressure.

According to the AHA, about 76.4 million (33.5 percent) adults age 20 and up have hypertension. Forty-four percent of African Americans have hypertension—the highest rate in the world. Hypertension occurs in kids, too. In fact, it's become more common over the last half century, an ominous trend that has something to do with the tripling in childhood obesity over the last generation.[43],[44] A 2011 study found that nearly one in five (9 percent) young adults aged 24 to 32 had hypertension.[45]

There are two main types of hypertension:

1. In *essential hypertension*, the cause isn't clear.

2. In *secondary hypertension*, another disease created the abnormally high blood pressure. Examples include a diseased kidney artery (the kidney helps regulate blood pressure) or an adrenal gland tumor that churns out the stress hormone epinephrine (a.k.a., adrenaline), which elevates blood pressure.

The majority of hypertension cases fall into the essential hypertension category.

Commonly recognized risk factors for hypertension are increasing age (which causes arteries to become stiffer), obesity, a high dietary intake of sodium, physical inactivity, smoking, psychological stress, chronic anger and hostility, sleep deprivation, and obstructive sleep apnea. Consumption of sugar-sweetened and artificially sweetened beverages, as well as excessive amounts of alcohol, raises the risk of hypertension.[46]

When pressure rises within the medium-sized arteries, they become more muscular, which narrows the diameter, further increasing blood pressure. Elevated blood pressure increases the heart's work, which causes the left ventricle to get more muscular, a condition called *left ventricular hypertrophy*.

Hypertension lacks telltale signs or symptoms. According to the AHA, about 20 percent of people have hypertension but don't know it. Less than half of those with diagnosed hypertension have their blood pressure under control. That's unfortunate, because elevated blood pressure can do great damage, elevating the risk for eye disease, kidney disease, heart failure, heart attack, and stroke. On average, hypertension decreases life expectancy by five years. Worldwide, this "silent killer" causes 7.6 million deaths a year.[47] A study found that having elevated blood pressure freshman year of college predicted a greater risk of death, heart disease, and vascular disease in middle age.[48]

Fortunately, hypertension is easy to detect and treat. Health practitioners routinely measure blood pressure. People at risk for hypertension can buy blood pressure monitors to use at home.

Treatment includes medications and lifestyle modifications such as regular exercise, achieving and maintaining a healthy weight, managing stress, avoiding tobacco smoke, restricting alcohol intake, limiting sodium to under 2,300 milligrams (one teaspoon of salt) a day, and eating a plant-based diet. However, getting people to commit to behavior changes and stay on their medications isn't always easy. There are two main reasons people don't follow medical advice: (1) hypertension causes no symptoms and (2) the medications, which aren't free, may produce side effects. Bottom line: treatment may not make a person with hypertension feel better, which diminishes perseverance.

 Video Clip 15.4

Consequences of Hypertension
This video explains the ill effects of hypertension on the arteries, heart, brain, kidneys, and eyes.

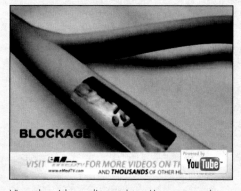

View the video online at: http://www.youtube.com/v/pPxnlh_WTb8

3.2   Atherosclerosis

Arteriosclerosis means hardening of the arteries. **Atherosclerosis** is a type of arteriosclerosis in which lipid-laden deposits build up inside the arteries. Damage to the arterial lining (*endothelium*) typically initiates the process. Hypertension, chemicals in tobacco smoke, and oxidized cholesterol can all injure the endothelium. In addition to elevating blood pressure and stiffening the arteries, chronic psychological stress can also promote inflammation in the arterial lining, which advances atherosclerosis.[49]

A prominent theory on the genesis of atherosclerosis is as follows: High blood levels of LDL cholesterol penetrate an injured *endothelium*. Once there, free radicals oxidize the LDL cholesterol, which accumulates. White blood cells called monocytes are attracted to the area, engulf the cholesterol and fat, and become *foam cells*. Smooth muscle cells in the middle layer of the artery build up. Eventually a fibrous cap covers the bulge. The whole thing is called an *atherosclerotic plaque*. As a result, arteries become narrower, weaker, and stiffer.

The process can begin early in life and progress silently, stealthily until obvious signs like chest pain develop. The beginning signs, called fatty streaks, have been seen in the arteries of children.[50] Like hypertension, symptoms don't develop until the disease is advanced. Unlike hypertension, atherosclerosis isn't as easy to detect.

 Video Clip 15.5

The Biology of Atherosclerosis
This video explains the process of atherosclerosis, focusing on their occurrence in the coronary arteries. The narrator mentions "MI." MI stands for myocardial infarction, the medical term for heart attack.

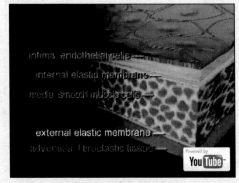

View the video online at: http://www.youtube.com/v/mCYAOeEe6-w

3.3   Coronary Heart Disease

Going back to the pump and hoses analogy, imagine that the heart continues to pump out the same volume of blood at the same rate. Nothing has changed except that atherosclerosis has made the hoses (arteries) stiffer and narrower. You already know that the result would be a rise in blood pressure. Now you can see that hypertension contributes to atherosclerosis, which contributes to hypertension.

You also already know the response of the left ventricle to the increased work of pumping blood through a narrow, inelastic, high-pressure arterial system: left ventricular hypertrophy. The problem is that adding muscle to the left ventricle increases the oxygen requirements of the heart. Unfortunately, atherosclerosis often affects the arteries that feed the heart (*coronary arteries*), thereby reducing blood flow to heart. This condition is called **coronary artery disease (CAD)** or coronary heart disease (CHD). It affects more than 16 million Americans[51] and is the leading cause of death, killing more than half a million Americans each year.[52]

Eventually the atherosclerotic coronary arteries can no longer supply the heart with enough blood, particularly when the cardiovascular system is taxed due to physical exertion or psychological distress. Whenever blood flow is insufficient, tissues don't receive enough oxygen. We feel that deprivation as pain. To experience that for yourself, wrap a rubber band around your finger. Notice the color change in the fingertip. As soon as discomfort begins, remove the rubber band.

arteriosclerosis

Hardening of the arteries.

atherosclerosis

A type of arteriosclerosis caused by the deposition of waxy plaques in the arteries.

FIGURE 15.5
Atherosclerosis

This illustration shows a cross section of three arteries. The top one is normal. The middle one has developed an atherosclerotic plaque. In the third, the plaque has progressed to the extent that blood flow is severely compromised.

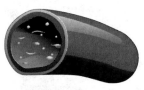
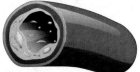
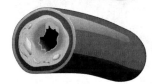

© *Thinkstock*

coronary artery disease (CAD)

A condition involving disease or damage to the coronary arteries (the blood vessels supplying the heart) usually caused by atherosclerosis; also called coronary heart disease (CHD).

angina pectoris

Chest pain due to insufficient blood supply to the heart.

Chest discomfort due to insufficient blood flow to the heart is called **angina pectoris**. Because atherosclerosis doesn't create symptoms until significant damage occurs, the first sign may be angina pectoris, or worse, heart attack.

Most people first experience angina with exertion. Once the exertions stops, the pain resolves. As the condition worsens, less and less exertion produces the chest discomfort. Medications such as nitroglycerin are taken to dilate the coronary arteries. Other drugs can help if the underlying problem is spasms in the coronary arteries.

3.4 Myocardial Infarction

thrombus

A blood clot that forms within a blood vessel (*pl.* thrombi).

embolus

A blood clot or clump of fat (after a bone breaks) or bacteria, air bubble, or other object travels in the bloodstream and lodges in a blood vessel to obstruct flow (*pl.* emboli).

myocardial infarction

Destruction of heart tissue resulting from obstruction of a coronary artery.

Let's return our attention to the atherosclerotic plaque. When the outer fibrous shell is thin and can easily rupture, the plaque is called "unstable." Rupture of the plaque creates a rough surface that attracts platelets, which form a clot at the site, further narrowing the artery's lumen (interior). A blood clot within a blood vessel is called a **thrombus** (*pl.* thrombi).

If a thrombus completely blocks blood flow, tissues downstream of it will die. If a thrombus breaks free, it will float in the blood until it reaches an artery so narrow it becomes lodged, again killing tissue supplied by that artery. A traveling thrombus is called an **embolus** (*pl.* emboli).

A blood clot that blocks the coronary arteries leads to **myocardial infarction** (heart attack). When thrombi that form in large veins in the legs *embolize* (break loose to become emboli) they often pass through the right side of the heart and become stuck in the pulmonary arteries. These pulmonary emboli lead to sudden shortness of breath due to low arterial oxygen and can threaten life. Thrombi and emboli in the arteries to the brain can cause a stroke.

 Video Clip 15.6

Myocardial Infarction
This animated video explains how atherosclerosis of the coronary arteries leads to heart attack.

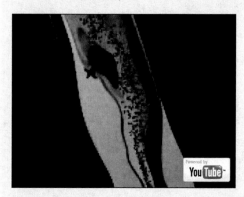

View the video online at: http://www.youtube.com/v/T_t-0cAP1C4

When Heart Attack Strikes

When the blood supply to heart tissue is cut off, a *myocardial infarction* (heart attack or MI) occurs. According to the AHA, each year about 785,000 Americans have a first heart attack and about 470,000 have a recurrent heart attack.[53]

Classic symptoms of a myocardial infarction are

- a feeling of pressure or pain in the chest;
- pain in the jaw, neck, shoulder, arm, or back;
- abdominal discomfort;
- shortness of breath;
- feeling faint or dizzy;
- nausea, vomiting;
- sweating;
- a sense of impending doom.

Heart attacks are more often fatal in women than in men. Within a year of a myocardial infarction, 42 percent of women and 24 percent of men die.[54] Several things account for this disparity.

A key problem is that public awareness about heart disease in women lags behind scientific facts. For instance, although women are much more likely to die of heart disease, they fear breast cancer more. Lack of awareness can delay prompt emergency treatment for a woman having symptoms, which leads to unnecessary deaths.

Not only may women and their doctors fail to recognize risk factors and symptoms of heart disease, but also women may not have many warning signs of cardiovascular disease. The majority of women have no history of chest pain before a myocardial infection.

Women also experience less typical and/or less severe symptoms during a heart attack. About 40 percent of women have no chest pain.[55] Instead, they're likely to have more subtle, vague symptoms such as discomfort in the abdomen (similar to indigestion), shoulder, and upper back; fatigue; sweating; dizziness; and nausea and vomiting.

Sudden cardiac death occurs more commonly in men. However, in women it's more often the first manifestation of heart disease.[56] For both sexes, the underlying process is usually coronary artery disease. Other risk factors include smoking, hypertension, diabetes, and a previous nonfatal heart attack. Low oxygen in the heart (due to a ruptured plaque or thrombus or other event) can trigger irregular heartbeats (arrhythmias). An arrhythmia called *ventricular fibrillation* makes the ventricles quiver so that blood is not pumped into the arteries. Death can quickly follow.

If you suspect someone is having a heart attack, call 911. Have the symptomatic person lie down with legs bent. Never let someone who might be having a heart attack drive to the emergency room. A number of conditions can mimic at least some heart attack symptoms—panic attacks, heartburn, chest wall pain from injury or exertion. But it's better to be safe than sorry.

Consider taking a CPR (cardiopulmonary resuscitation) training course. That way, you know what to do if someone's heart stops pumping. Your college campus may periodically offer CPR training. Otherwise, you can find your local Red Cross chapter at http://www.redcross.org.

Public places increasingly have AEDs (automated external defibrillation), portable devices that nonmedical people can use to deliver an electric shock to restore normal heart rhythm. For information go to this AHA page: http://www.heart.org/idc/groups/heart-public/@wcm/@hcm/documents/downloadable/ucm_300340.pdf.

 Video Clip 15.7

Hands-only CPR
The American Heart Association provides the following instructional video on performing hands-only CPR.

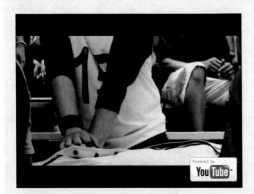

View the video online at: http://www.youtube.com/v/2J-oSj5lkEY

3.5   Arrhythmias

An **arrhythmia** is an abnormality with either the heart rate or rhythm. Normally, the heart beats regularly. Specialized tissue in the right atrium called the *sinoatrial node* acts as the heart's pacemaker. It sets a basic rhythm, which spreads over all the heart muscle, so that the atria and ventricles contract in an organized fashion. This is why a heart removed from the chest cavity continues beating.

Both branches of the parasympathetic system send nerve fibers to the heart. The parasympathetic nervous system slows the heart rate; the sympathetic nervous system hastens it.

arrhythmia

A heart beat that is too slow, too fast, or irregular.

Anything between 60 and 100 beats per minute is considered a normal resting heart rate. However, some experts have called for a reduction in that upper limit, making the ideal resting heart rate between 60 and 80. One study found that, for each increment of 10 beats per minute, the risk of heart disease mortality rose 18 percent in women under age 70 and 10 percent in men.[57] People with heart rates above 80 are also more likely to develop obesity and diabetes.[58] More physically active people have lower heart rates at rest.

There are many types of arrhythmias, most of which are harmless. An abnormally rapid heart rate is called *tachycardia*. One that is abnormally slow is called *bradycardia*. The heart rate can also be irregular. If the electrical signal travels in a disorganized fashion, the heart muscle can quiver ineffectively rather than contract. Such quivering of the atria is called *atrial fibrillation*. The same process occurring in the ventricles, *ventricular fibrillation*, is life threatening.

   Video Link 15.1

Arrhythmias

This webpage from the National Heart, Lung, and Blood Institute at the National Institutes of Health contains videos on three types of arrhythmias. Each begins with an explanation of how the electrical signal for contraction normally spreads across the heart.

http://www.nhlbi.nih.gov/health/health-topics/topics/arr/types.html

3.6 Congestive Heart Failure

congestive heart failure

Inability of the heart to pump enough blood to meet the body's needs.

In **congestive heart failure**, your heart can't pump enough blood to meet the body's demands. Common underlying causes are hypertension and atherosclerosis. As you've seen, arterial disease increases the work of the heart. Like any other muscle, the left ventricle hypertrophies (thickens), which increases its needs for oxygenated blood (needs that diseased coronary arteries can't meet). In another compensatory mechanism, the heart fills with more blood before contracting. In balloon-like fashion, the extra volume leads to a more vigorous expulsion of blood with each contraction. Eventually, the heart, like a worn-out balloon, becomes baggy and begins to fail.

Other conditions that can injure the heart include rheumatic heart disease (a complication of strep throat), infection of the heart muscle, heart attack, and some drugs. No matter the underlying cause, a failing heart can't circulate the blood fast enough.

Usually the left heart fails first. The result is increased pressure within the pulmonary vessels, which causes fluid to leak into the lungs. Shortness of breath follows. People with congestive heart failure may sleep propped up on a couple of pillows in order to breathe more easily. They may also need oxygen.

If the right side of the heart fails, fluid leaks into tissues in the legs and abdomen. Dependent areas such as the feet and ankles swell. Excess tissue fluid is called *edema*. The whole circulatory system, like a city highway, becomes congested, hence the name congestive heart failure.

3.7 Peripheral Arterial Disease

peripheral arterial disease

A condition in which narrowing of the arteries impairs circulation; also called peripheral artery disease.

Peripheral arterial disease (PAD, also called peripheral arterial occlusive disease and peripheral vascular disease) involves the arteries carrying blood to the limbs, head, and organs outside the heart. This condition affects up to 12 million Americans.[59] The underlying cause is usually atherosclerosis. The plaques reduce blood flow. Initially, symptoms such as numbness and pain result with activity but can eventually occur at rest. Reduced blood flow also impairs wound healing and raises the risk of infection.

A typical presentation is that physical activity provokes leg pain and rest resolves the discomfort. Though it can cause pain, walking is also therapeutic and can reduce the risk of subsequent heart attack and stroke. Specialized physical therapists normally supervise exercise in people with PAD.

Arterial Disease and Sexual Function

As with arteries anywhere in the body, those going to the genitals can become diseased. Male erections depend on healthy blood flow. *Erectile dysfunction* (difficulty maintaining an erectile during sex) is primarily a condition of arterial dysfunction. Key underlying causes are smoking, hypertension, high blood lipids, and diabetes. ED has become a recognized precursor to atherosclerosis and coronary artery disease.[60],[61] By age 50, 50 percent of diabetic men have ED[62] and 30 percent of hypertensive men complain of ED.[63] Furthermore, some of the medications to treat that condition interfere with sexual function. That diminishes the motivation to take the medications, which worsens management of hypertension.

While female sexual health is more complex, it nonetheless relies on good circulation. The same conditions that underlie ED (smoking, hypertension, high blood lipids, and diabetes) compromise female sexual function.[64]

3.8   Stroke

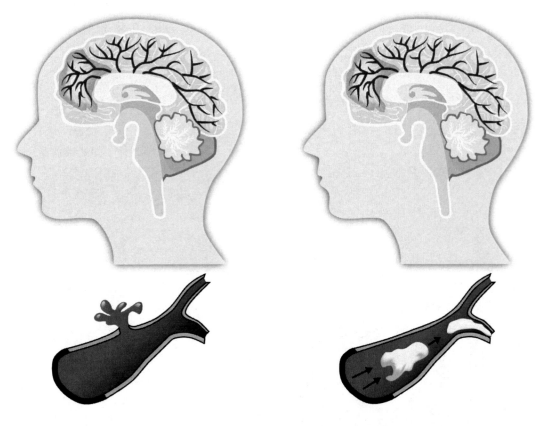

A hemorrhagic stroke occurs when a blood vessel bursts within the brain.

An ischemic stroke occurs when a blood clot blocks the blood flow in an artery within the brain.

Source: Adapted from Centers for Disease Control. Types of Stroke. 2010. Available at: http://www.cdc.gov/stroke/types_of_stroke.htm.

Each year, approximately 610,000 Americans have a **stroke**, a condition that occurs when an interruption in the blood supply damages the brain. Another 185,000 have a recurrent stroke. Altogether that means someone has a stroke every 40 seconds. It's the fourth leading cause of death in the United States, accounting for 1 in 18 deaths.[65]

Another name for stroke is *cerebrovascular accident*. That term suggests the cause—a problem with the vascular supply to the brain (cerebrum). There are two kinds of stroke: *ischemic* and *hemorrhagic*. Ischemia means inadequate blood supply. In ischemic stroke (a brain attack), the process is the same as in a heart attack: an atherosclerotic plaque and/or a blood clot obstructs the blood circulation. The clot can be a thrombus (one that forms in an artery in the brain) or an embolus that has traveled from elsewhere (usually the heart). About 80 percent of strokes are ischemic. The remaining 20 percent

stroke

Damage to brain tissue resulting from the interruption of blood circulation to a part of the brain due to a blood clot blocking or an artery bursting.

are hemorrhagic, caused by a leaky or ruptured blood vessel. A common underlying cause is an *aneurysm*, a weakened, bulging blood vessel that can burst under pressure.

Symptoms and signs of stroke depend on the area of the brain that is affected. Common manifestations are sudden numbness, weakness, or paralysis in one side of the face, one arm, or one leg. Others include difficulty speaking or understanding speech, confusion, dizziness, problems with vision, unsteady gait, loss of consciousness, and severe headache. Death may also result. Sometimes, however, a stroke damages such a tiny area as to be "silent." Over time, a number of small strokes can add up to significant neurologic problems, such as memory loss.

A stroke is a medical emergency. If you suspect someone has had one, the best thing you can do is call 911 immediately. Note the time the symptoms developed. Stay with the person until help arrives.

Recovery from a stroke depends on the location, extent, and severity of damage. A swift medical response can dramatically improve outcomes. Over the years, improvements in diagnostic and treatment options have lowered the death rate and enhanced recovery. For instance, clot-dissolving drugs, if given within three hours of an ischemic stroke, can decrease the extent of brain injury. Furthermore, the brain is an amazingly adaptable organ and can, with time, compensate. Various types of therapy can help people overcome disabilities resulting from the stroke.

Strokes can strike out of the blue or be preceded by a **transient ischemic attack (TIA)**, a condition caused by brief interruption to blood flow to an area of the brain. Symptoms, though similar to a stroke, are milder and resolve within minutes to a few hours. You may hear TIAs referred to as "ministrokes." That term, however, is incorrect, since a stroke, no matter how small, would result in brain cell death.

TIAs indicate a high risk of impending stroke and should be taken seriously. Treatment addresses underlying causes such as hypertension, atherosclerosis, diabetes, and tobacco smoking.

For more information, check the National Stroke Association (http://www.stroke.org) and the National Institute of Neurologic Disorders and Stroke (http://www.ninds.nih.gov/index.htm).

transient ischemic attack (TIA)

A condition caused by a brief interruption in blood flow to the brain.

Slideshow 15.2.

Transient Ischemic Attack

This is an American Heart Association slideshow: http://watchlearnlive.heart.org/CVML_Player.php?moduleSelect=tisatk

 Video Clip 15.8

Stroke
This video explains the two types of cerebrovascular accidents.

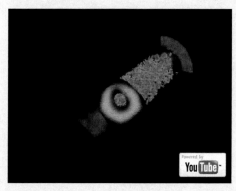

View the video online at: http://www.youtube.com/v/SQq_1oSBei0

3.9 Diagnosing Cardiovascular Disease

A number of tests can be used to evaluate the cardiovascular system. Some are done routinely (e.g., checking blood pressure, listening to the heart, and periodic blood tests for lipids and glucose). Otherwise, their use depends on the person's signs and symptoms and the physician's suspicion of the cause.

Auscultation. This time-honored examination involves listening to the heart and to sounds within some of the arteries with a *stethoscope. Cardiologists* are particularly well trained in recognizing sounds associated with arrhythmias and defects in the heart valves.

Blood tests can measure levels of cholesterol, triglycerides, insulin, glucose, and other substances that indicate risks for cardiovascular disease, metabolic syndrome, and diabetes. The other tests are done after eight or so hours of fasting.

Electrocardiogram (ECG or EKG). An ECG records the electrical activity of the heart by using electrodes attached to the skin of the chest and limbs. The recorded impulses are displayed as waves on a monitor or printed on paper. ECGs can help diagnose heart attacks, rhythm disturbances, and cardiac abnormalities. Portable ECGs can be used to make records for 24 hours or longer.

This image shows a normal ECG tracing.

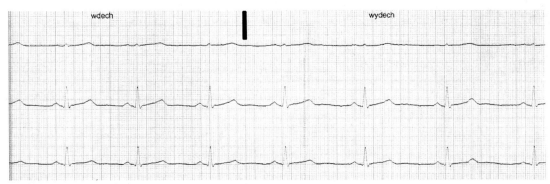

Source: novic84. 2005. Available at: http://commons.wikimedia.org/wiki/File:EKG.jpg.

This image shows the heart in ventricular fibrillation. The heart is quivering without effectively pumping blood.

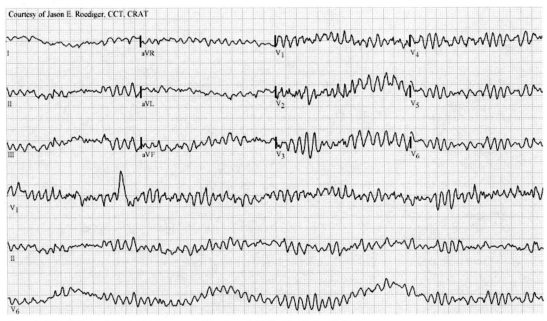

Source: Jer5150. 2012. Available at: http://commons.wikimedia.org/wiki/File:Ventricular_fibrillation.png.

Stress test. During this test, ECG recordings are made while the person pedals a stationary bike or walks or runs on a treadmill. The goal is to pick up problems such as coronary artery disease that only appear with exertion.

Echocardiogram. This test uses ultrasound waves to visualize the heart on a monitor. It allows a view of the systole and diastole in real time. The health practitioner can examine the heart valves, the thickness of the chamber walls, the diameter of the chambers, the amount of blood ejected with each systole (*ejection fraction*), and other things. In congestive heart failure, the ejection fraction declines. After a myocardial infarction, areas of dead tissue no longer contract. Ultrasound can also examine blood vessels.

This still photogram captures the four heart chambers during an echocardiogram.

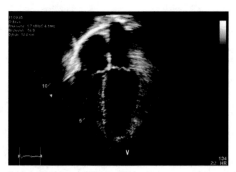

Source: Kjetil Lenes. 2005. Available at:
http://commons.wikimedia.org/wiki/
File:Echocardiogram_4chambers.jpg.

Angiogram. This type of study involves a study of the arteries by injecting contrast material (dye) that is visible on X-rays. In a cardiac catheterization, the doctor inserts a thin flexible tube (*catheter*) into a blood vessel in the groin or arm and maneuvers it into the heart. The catheter may be used to sample oxygen levels, measure blood flow patterns, and biopsy the heart. Taking X-rays after injecting contrast medium (dye) into the coronary arteries creates a coronary angiogram. In cerebral angiograms, a similar process provides images of blood vessels in the brain to help diagnose brain aneurysms and stroke.

Computerized tomography (CT) uses X-rays to collect serial images of the heart. **Magnetic resonance imaging (MRI)** uses a powerful magnet to create images of the heart. Both can also be used to provide images of the brain to diagnose stroke and other abnormalities.

Radionuclide testing involves the injection of radioactive substances. Certain substances provide images of the heart and can be used to evaluate function at rest and with exertion. Examples of radionuclide imaging include positron emission tomography (PET), single-photon emission computed tomography (SPECT), technetium, and thallium scans.

3.10   Treating Cardiovascular Diseases

As with diagnosis, treatment depends on each individual's presentation. Sometimes lifestyle changes (more fruits and vegetables, less junk food and alcohol, salt restriction, more physical activity, weight loss, and avoidance of tobacco smoke) are enough to control conditions such as hypertension, blood lipid abnormalities, and atherosclerosis.

Medications

A number of medications are used for cardiovascular conditions. Here are some examples:

- Low-dose aspirin is often used to reduce the risk of blood clots in people at risk for heart attack and stroke. Side effects include gastrointestinal irritation, ulcers, and bleeding abnormalities.

- Thrombolytic drugs are used immediately after a heart attack or ischemic stroke occurs to attempt to dissolve blood clots. Other drugs (often called "blood-thinners") may be taken long term to prevent clots from reoccurring in arteries and veins.

- Diuretics increase water loss with urination. They decrease the volume of blood, which reduces blood pressure. Hence these drugs are used to manage hypertension and congestive heart failure.

- Beta-blockers reduce blood pressure by competing with the hormone epinephrine. As a result, the heart beats more slowly and less forcefully. Alpha-blockers interfere with norepinephrine from the sympathetic nervous system, which keeps arteries more open and blood pressure lower. Several other classes of medication also lower blood pressure by blocking processes that affect heart function and blood vessel diameter.

- Digoxin (also called digitalis) and similar drugs were originally derived from the plant foxglove. The plant is poisonous. The purified drugs must be used with caution. They work by increasing the strength of the heart's contraction to counter heart failure.

- Statins (more properly called HMG-CoA reductase inhibitors) are a class of medication that block the liver's production of cholesterol. They also lower triglycerides, mildly raise HDL cholesterol, and reduce inflammation. Other medications can decrease intestinal absorption of dietary cholesterol. Cholesterol-lowering medication is particularly important for people genetically predisposed to high cholesterol levels.

- The B vitamin niacin reduces LDL cholesterol and triglycerides and elevates HDL cholesterol. Even though it's available as an over-the-counter supplement, side effects often occur. Some aren't serious (flushing of the skin, upset stomach, headaches, and dizziness); some are (liver damage). Physician monitoring is recommended.

High-Tech Treatments

FIGURE 15.6 Angioplasty

In the left-hand artery, the catheter is within the atherosclerotic plaque. In the middle artery, the balloon is inflated to open the lumen (the inside space). In the right-hand artery, a mesh-like stent is placed to hold the artery open.

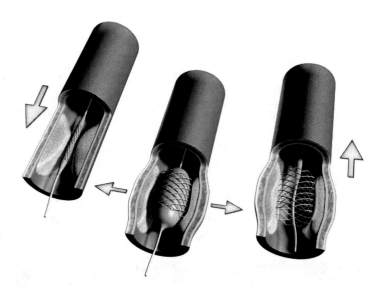

© Thinkstock

Several nondrug interventions are used to treat cardiovascular disease. Diseased arteries can be opened or bypassed to restore blood flow. In **angioplasty**, a catheter is inserted into an atherosclerotic artery. A balloon at the catheter's tip is inflated to widen the artery and a stent (a metal coil or mesh-like tube) is left in place to keep the artery open. Coronary angioplasty means the procedure addressed a blockage in a coronary artery. The procedure is also used in peripheral arterial disease. Unfortunately, stented arteries can become clogged again.

In **atherectomy**, a catheter tip is also advanced to an atherosclerotic artery. Once it's there, a cutting device or laser beam shaves down the plaque to improve blood flow. This procedure is more often used to treat peripheral arterial disease than coronary artery disease.

In **coronary bypass surgery (CABG)**, a blood vessel taken from elsewhere in the body (often a vein in the leg) is grafted on coronary arteries to allow blood to detour around a blockage. CABG may be needed when multiple coronary arteries are blocked or the blockage of a main artery is extensive. CABG is open-heart surgery, meaning the surgeon opens the chest to gain access to the heart.

KEY TAKEAWAYS

- While there are a number of cardiovascular diseases, they are all interrelated.
- Hypertension is abnormally high blood pressure. It increases the risk of the other cardiovascular diseases.
- Atherosclerosis is a type of arteriosclerosis (hardened arteries) characterized by deposits of lipid-laden plaques inside the arteries.
  - Atherosclerosis of the coronary arteries (which feed the heart muscle) leads to coronary artery disease.
  - Atherosclerosis elsewhere produces peripheral arterial disease.
  - Angina pectoris is the chest discomfort arising from coronary artery disease.
- Myocardial infarction, or heart attack, occurs when a ruptured plaque or blood clot obstructs blood flow within a coronary artery.
- Atherosclerosis, hypertension, myocardial infarction, and other conditions increase the risk of congestive heart failure.
- Cerebrovascular accidents, or strokes, come in two varieties: ischemic (caused by blood clots) and hemorrhagic. The former is much more common.
- Arrhythmias occur when the heart rate or rhythm is abnormal.
- A number of tests help diagnose cardiovascular disease.
- Treatment options include resolving underlying problems with lifestyle modifications, medications, and surgical interventions such as angioplasty and open-heart surgery.

DISCUSSION QUESTIONS

1. When you're stressed or exercising, the sympathetic nervous system becomes activated. That system causes your heart to beat faster and harder and constricts blood vessels in many organs (gastrointestinal tract, urinary system, skin). There's a key difference. Exercising warms up muscles and helps release waste products, which causes the small arteries servicing them to dilate. That reaction doesn't happen when you're sitting still and psychologically stressed.

   Imagine yourself in two situations: jogging and watching a scary movie. Considering that the cardiovascular system is a closed loop, what might happen to blood pressure (the pressure within the arteries) in these two situations? (In which situation is blood pressure higher?)

2. Imagine that you're at a dinner party. A 60-year-old woman seated beside you turns pale. Sweat beads form above her lip. When you ask if she's all right, she smiles weakly, points to her upper abdomen, and says, "Heartburn." If she doesn't quickly recover, what else could be going on? How should you respond?

3. Imagine you're visiting a 75-year-old relative. You don't know much about his medical history. In the midst of telling you an exciting story about the Vietnam War, he begins to slur his words. Before that, his speech had been crisp and he seemed completely sober. You ask him how he's feeling. He says very slowly that he'd like a glass of water. When you fetch it, he spills some on the table as he attempts to drink. He coughs. You pat his back. You're about to call 911 when he starts talking normally again. He says nothing like this has happened before. What do you think might have happened? What might you do next?

4. KEEPING YOUR CARDIOVASCULAR SYSTEM HEALTHY

LEARNING OBJECTIVE

1. Identify lifestyle habits and other strategies that maintain cardiovascular health and prevent disease.

Cardiovascular disease is largely preventable. Multiple studies show that the most important things you can do to prevent cardiovascular disease are to avoid tobacco, exercise regularly, eat a nutritious diet, and manage weight.[66] As you'll learn, a few other healthy habits can also lower your risk.

Preventive strategies work. A 2011 study found that women who maintained heart-healthy habits reduced their risk of sudden cardiac death by as much as 90 percent.[67]

4.1   Exercise

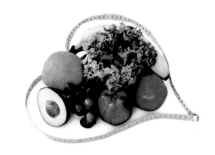

© Thinkstock

Multiple studies demonstrate that people who regularly engage in physical activity lower their risk of hypertension, atherosclerosis, stroke, and metabolic syndrome. Regular physical activity keeps the heart in shape, much as it does any other muscle. The heart becomes more efficient, pumping out more blood with each contraction. Because the heart doesn't need to beat as fast to circulate blood, resting heart rate falls. Heart rate also returns to baseline more quickly after exertion. Blood pressure declines, which decreases the heart's work. Blood triglycerides decline and cholesterol levels improve, mainly because HDL cholesterol rises. Physical activity also reduces the likelihood of (or helps manage) two other cardiovascular risks: diabetes and obesity.

Aerobic exercise is particularly helpful at any age and at any level of exertion. A study showed that the recommended 150 minutes (2.5 hours) a week of moderate-intensity physical activity reduced coronary heart disease 14 percent compared to the risk in sedentary people. Increasing the weekly time to 300 minutes reduced the risk by 20 percent.[68] The exercise needn't be extreme. Simply walking reduces the risk of stroke.[69] See Chapter 9 (Physical Fitness) for tips about becoming more physically active.

If you already have a cardiovascular condition and haven't yet started an exercise program, check with your doctor first.

4.2   Feed Your Heart

Plant-based diets protect the cardiovascular system because they're rich in fiber, vitamins, minerals, and other beneficial plant chemicals. People who follow a Mediterranean diet—one that emphasizes vegetables, fruits, legumes, nuts, and whole grains and includes fish and moderate amounts of alcohol—enjoy a reduced risk of metabolic syndrome, cardiovascular disease, and stroke.[70] ,[71] The diet also reduces risk of sudden cardiac death and heart failure among people who already have heart disease.[72]

The Dietary Approaches to Stop Hypertension (DASH) diet has been shown to lower blood pressure and reduce the risk of cardiovascular disease and stroke.[73] Like the Mediterranean diet, the DASH diet is heavy on fruits and vegetables. The daily recommendations are for 8 to 12 servings of fruit and vegetables, 6 to 8 servings of whole grains, 2 to 3 servings of low-fat or nonfat dairy, and 2 or fewer servings of lean meats, fish, or poultry. In addition, 4 to 5 servings of nuts, seeds, and legumes are recommended each week. Fats and sweets are restricted. The original plan called for a sodium cap at 2,300 milligrams a day. The National Heart, Lung, and Blood website notes that a sodium max of 1,500 milligrams a day is better for reducing blood pressure. For more information, go to http://www.nhlbi.nih.gov/health/public/heart/hbp/dash/new_dash.pdf.

Both of the diets mentioned contain plenty of fiber. Soluble fiber binds dietary cholesterol to inhibit its absorption from the intestines into the bloodstream. Sources include oats, flaxseeds, psyllium, lentils, carrots, cucumbers, apples, and several other fruits. Insoluble fiber lowers blood pressure. Sources include dark leafy greens, green beans, grapes, wheat bran, whole wheat, and several other whole grains.[74] ,[75]

Plant-based diets also contain vitamins and minerals essential to cardiovascular function, as well as antioxidant and anti-inflammatory chemicals such as flavonoids and carotenoids. Diets high in antioxidant-rich foods reduce cardiovascular disease and stroke risk.[76] ,[77] Potent antioxidant substances called polyphenols are found in a variety of plant-based foods and drinks, most notably red berries, blueberries, cherries, black currants, blood oranges, eggplant, red grapes, red wine, cocoa, and tea. These polyphenols protect the blood vessels and reduce hypertension and heart disease risk.[78] They protect against oxidation of LDL cholesterol, discourage clots from forming within the blood vessels, and promote the dilation of arteries, which lowers blood pressure.

A key component of the Mediterranean diet is olive oil, which has cardiovascular benefits and lowers stroke risk.[79] Compared to other plant oils, olive oil is relatively resistant to oxidation. Consider substituting olive oil (a monounsaturated fat) for butter and stick margarine. Butter contains cholesterol and saturated fat. Margarines are made of plant oil. Stick margarines remain solid at room temperature because plant oils were hydrogenated, creating trans fats. Tub margarines made of polyunsaturated fats are fine. Look for labels proclaiming the product trans-fat free.

Cold-water fish (e.g., salmon, tuna, sardines, anchovies, and herring) contains another kind of heart-healthy fat: omega-3 fatty acids. Omega-3s decrease inflammation and triglycerides, raise HDL cholesterol, inhibit blood clot formation, inhibit the growth of atherosclerotic plaques, stabilize heart rhythm to reduce the risk of sudden cardiac death, and may lower blood pressure.[80] Regular consumption of fish—about two servings a week—can cut the risk of heart disease. Remove the skin. Avoid fried fish, which has the opposite effect.[81] For years, experts have told people at risk for cardiovascular disease to shun shellfish such as shrimp and lobster, which are rich in cholesterol and omega-3 fatty acids. Recent research suggests that shellfish may not raise LDL cholesterol.[82],[83]

When eating meat, opt for lean cuts and limit consumption to three servings a week. Avoid duck, goose, marbled meats such as rib-eye steak, bacon, hot dogs, sausage, processed meats, and fatty luncheon meats such as bologna. Trim off visible fat and remove the skin from poultry. Limit egg yolks to three to four a week.[84] For all meats, cook them without frying. Instead bake, broil, steam, roast, or microwave.

Nuts are part of the DASH and Mediterranean diets and contain healthful oils, fiber, protein, and vitamins. Moderate consumption of nuts improves blood lipids. They're dense in both nutrients and calories. A handful a day is plenty.[85] You can use a serving of nuts as a meat substitute.

Give up sodas and other sweetened beverages. Drink water instead. You might also try drinking green tea. People who habitually drink tea, particularly green tea, are less likely to suffer heart attacks and strokes.[86] Green tea can reduce LDL cholesterol, and it also improves glucose tolerance.[87] Another tea to consider is hibiscus. Studies show that hibiscus tea can increase HDL cholesterol and decrease LDL cholesterol, blood glucose, and blood pressure.[88],[89],[90]

Coffee, which also contains flavonoids, has been linked to a reduced stroke risk.[91] Compared to green tea, coffee contains more caffeine, which increases heart rate and blood pressure, albeit only temporarily. Also coffee, particularly unfiltered coffee, can increase LDL cholesterol and triglycerides.[92] Some scientists note that long-term moderate consumption of coffee doesn't seem to have detrimental effects in healthy people and may even protect against the risk of developing type 2 diabetes.[93] Keep in mind that putting cream in your coffee and tea adds cholesterol and saturated fat.

Moderate amounts of alcohol seem to protect the cardiovascular system. Red wine contains a potent flavonoid called resveratrol. However, excessive amounts increase triglycerides and drive up blood pressure.

If you want sweets, choose chocolate. Dark chocolate, which is richer in polyphenols than milk chocolate, inhibits platelets from forming clots within blood vessels and lowers blood pressure, fasting glucose, and total cholesterol levels.[94],[95] A little goes a long way. Commercial chocolate bars contain calories in the form of sugar and fat (much of which is saturated). Dark chocolate has more flavonoids than milk chocolate. White chocolate contains no flavonoids.

4.3 Season Wisely

The AHA recommends people consume less than 1,500 mg of sodium (from salt) a day. Other experts contend that salt restriction isn't necessary for people without hypertension or other cardiovascular risk facts.[96] Common sodium sources include deli meats, pizza, pasta dishes, bread, snack foods, poultry, and cheese. Olives, seafood, and some legumes are naturally high in sodium. One teaspoon of table salt contains 2,300 mg of sodium.

Some people complain that food tastes bland without adding table salt. A good remedy is to use culinary herbs and spices in place of salt. Many of them have cardiovascular benefits. A standout culinary herb is *garlic*. It inhibits oxidation of LDL cholesterol, reduces atherosclerotic plaque size,[97] retards the deposition of calcium that hardens the arteries,[98] lowers blood pressure and triglycerides, hinders platelets from clotting, and reduces homocysteine (an amino acid that raises cardiovascular disease and stroke risk).[99]

Garlic's ability to reduce cholesterol was called into question by a 2007 Stanford University study, in which none of the previously successful garlic preparations (raw garlic as a sandwich spread, powdered garlic tablets, or aged garlic extract) significantly reduced cholesterol in people with moderately elevated levels.[100] Subsequent analyses of the many studies on garlic and blood lipids judged that garlic significantly reduced total cholesterol and triglycerides but had no significant effect on LDL and HDL cholesterol.[101],[102] Because cooking destroys some of garlic's active ingredients, it's better to add raw minced garlic to foods before serving.

4.4 Achieve and Maintain a Healthy Weight

Regular physical activity and a heart-healthy diet promote loss of excess body weight. For other ideas on weight loss, see Chapter 10.

4.5 Control Diabetes and Metabolic Syndrome

Both conditions greatly increase the risk of developing cardiovascular disease. All of the items on this list can help, but medications may also be necessary.

4.6 Express Emotions and Learn to Be Positive

Hostility and anger hurt the heart. Bottling up emotions isn't good either. Find healthy, socially acceptable ways to deflate those feelings. See Chapter 6 for ideas on constructive communication skills. Slow, deep breathing and meditation can also dissipate "hot" emotions. Discover outlets such as exercise, writing, gardening, dance, and playing and listening to music.

At the other end of the scale, people who are more upbeat, optimistic, and generally have a better sense of well-being tend to have a healthier body weight, levels of cholesterol, and blood pressure.[103] They're also more social and more likely to take care of themselves by eating well, exercising, getting enough sleep, and avoiding tobacco smoke. See Chapter 5 (Psychological Health) for ways to increase positive emotions.

4.7 Seek the Company of Others

Social support provides a buffer against other heart-harming factors such as stress and loneliness. High-quality relationships protect against cardiovascular disease and morbidity.[104] Plus, you can socialize while engaging in other heart-healthy activities. Sign up for dance classes or kick boxing with a friend. Invite friends over to cook and eat healthy meals. When a heart attack, stroke, or any other calamity strikes, social support improves outcomes.

Nonhuman companions also heal hearts. Studies show that interactions with domesticated animals can lower blood pressure.[105] Some evidence suggests that, compared to their dogless peers, people with dogs tend to get more physical activity; have lower blood pressure, blood cholesterol, and triglycerides; respond less intensely to stressful situations; and have greater odds of surviving a myocardial infarction.[106] That association only works if you like dogs or can easily and responsibly care for an animal that thrives on companionship.

4.8 Tame Stress

Meditation is one means to that end. A regular meditation practice has multiple benefits, including reducing stress and blood pressure. Two well-researched techniques are mindfulness meditation and Transcendental Meditation.[107] A study in prehypertensive African American teens found that Transcendental Meditation (which involves the silent repetition of a mantra) reduced early signs of left ventricular hypertrophy.[108] Spiritual practices, particularly prayer, have a meditative effect; spirituality has cardiovascular protective effects.[109] For more information on meditation techniques, see Chapter 2.

In addition to reducing psychological stress, soothing music positively affects heart rate and rhythm. At the other extreme, heavy metal and techno music can trigger stress and arrhythmias in vulnerable people.[110] Certain yogic breathing techniques may help stabilize heart rhythm in people with arrhythmias.[111]

4.9 Sleep Enough

Most people need around eight hours sleep a night. Keep a regular sleep-wake cycle. See Chapter 4 for strategies to improve your sleep. If you have persistent insomnia or suspect you have obstructive sleep apnea or any other sleep disorder, contact your doctor.

4.10 Spend Time in Nature

For most people, green spaces are relaxing, reduce stress, and encourage physical activity. Some research links access to green spaces to a reduced risk of cardiovascular disease.[112] It doesn't matter if you live miles from the ocean, mountains, grasslands, or woods. Most cities have parks and botanic gardens. Most college campuses have patches of green. Even if it's the dead of winter, a stroll through a snowy, leafless campus gets you outside. Pay attention. Look and listen for signs of wildlife.

4.11 Serve Others

Acts of kindness gladden your heart and the person you helped. Notice the feeling in your chest when you open the door for someone, particularly when he or she smiles and thanks you. Most college campuses offer a variety of service learning activities.

4.12 Stay in Touch with Your Doctor

Blood pressure measurement is part of a routine office visit. If yours is high or borderline high, you may need to monitor it more frequently. Testing for blood lipid (cholesterol and triglycerides) begins in your early 20s. If it's normal, the test is repeated every five years. People with diabetes need to take steps to manage their condition.

Assess Yourself: Cardiovascular Disease Prevention

The following list covers the main modifiable risks for cardiovascular disease. The more "yes" responses you have, the more you're protecting yourself from cardiovascular disease. "No" responses indicate a risk. If you have any concerns about your cardiovascular health, make an appointment with your doctor.

	Yes	No	Don't know
Total cholesterol is less than 200 mg/dL (without medication)	Yes	No	Don't know
Systolic blood pressure is less than 120 mg Hg and diastolic blood pressure is less than 80 mm Hg (untreated)	Yes	No	Don't know
Do not smoke (never or quit over a year ago)	Yes	No	
BMI is less than 25 hg/m^2 *	Yes	No	Don't know
Blood glucose is less than 100 mg/dL when fasting	Yes	No	Don't know
Engage in physical activity (at least 150 minutes of moderate-intensity aerobic activity each week)	Yes	No	
Four out of five dietary goals are met ■ Fruits and vegetables—at least 4.5 cups a day ■ Fish—2- to 3.5-ounce or more servings a week ■ Sodium—no more than 1,500 mg a day ■ Sugar-sweetened beverages—less than 450 calories/week ■ Whole grains—three or more one-ounce servings a day	Yes	No	
Stress levels under control; take time to relax	Yes	No	
Sleep eight hours a night most nights of the week	Yes	No	
Psychological health ■ Generally happy and optimistic ■ Rarely angry or hostile	Yes	No	
Social health ■ Have supportive friends	Yes	No	
Totals	**Yes**	**No**	

* **You can find a BMI calculator at** http://www.heart.org/HEARTORG/GettingHealthy/Weight Management/BodyMassIndex/Body-Mass-Index-BMI-Calculator_UCM_307849_Article.jsp.

Adapted from table 2.2 of Roger VL, Go AS, Lloyd-Jones DM, et al. Heart disease and stroke statistics—2012 update: a report from the American Heart Association. Circulation. 2012 Jan 3;125(1):188–97. Available at: http://circ.ahajournals.org/content/125/1/e2.full.pdf+html.

KEY TAKEAWAYS

- Cardiovascular disease is largely preventable.
- The pillars of a heart-healthy lifestyle are avoidance of tobacco smoking; regular physical activity; a diet rich in fruits, vegetables, whole grains, and nuts, with occasional fish and lean poultry and meat; healthy body weight; robust stress-management skills; positive psychological health; adequate sleep; and social support.
- Keep up with regular medical check-ups to monitor blood pressure, blood lipid levels, and other indicators of cardiovascular health.

DISCUSSION QUESTIONS

1. Examine your responses to the assessment of cardiovascular disease prevention. For each item to which you gave a "no" response, discuss four things:

    a. your willingness to change;

    b. your concrete, specific plans for making this change;

    c. any perceived barriers toward affecting positive behavioral change; and

    d. whether you plan on consulting a health professional for assistance. For instance, prescription medication may be needed to manage persistently high LDL cholesterol and blood pressure. You might need professional help to quit smoking, lose weight, improve sleep, manage stress, and resolve psychological issues.

---

5.   RECOMMENDED RESOURCES

5.1   Organizations and Websites

American Diabetes Association. http://www.diabetes.org.

American Heart Association. http://www.heart.org.

Centers for Disease Control and Prevention. http://www.cdc.gov.

National Diabetes Information Clearinghouse (NDIC). http://www.diabetes.niddk.nih.gov.

National Heart, Lung, and Blood Institute. http://www.nhlbi.nih.gov.

National Institute of Neurological Disorders and Stroke (NINDS). http://www.ninds.nih.gov.

ENDNOTES

1. Knip M, Veijola R, Virtanen SM, Hyoty H, Vaarala O, Akerblom HK. Environmental triggers and determinants of type 1 diabetes. *Diabetes*. 2005;54(2). doi:10.2337/diabetes.54.suppl_2.S125. Available at: http://diabetes.diabetesjournals.org/content/54/suppl_2/S125.full#sec-2. Accessed July 5, 2012.

2. American Diabetes Association. What is gestational diabetes. Available at: http://www.diabetes.org/diabetes-basics/gestational/what-is-gestational-diabetes.html. Accessed July 5, 2012.

3. Alberti G, Zimmet P, Shaw J, Bloomgarden Z, Kaufman F, Silink M; Consensus Workshop Group. Type 2 diabetes in the young: the evolving epidemic: the international diabetes federation consensus workshop. *Diabetes Care*. 2004;27(7):1798–1811.

4. Diabetes Prevention Program. National Diabetes Information Clearinghouse (NDIC). A service of the National Institute of Diabetes and Digestive and Kidney Diseases (NIDDK), National Institutes of Health (NIH). NIH publication no. 09-5099. October 2008. Available at: http://www.diabetes.niddk.nih.gov/dm/pubs/preventionprogram/index.aspx#result. Updated December 6, 2011. Accessed July 5, 2012.

5. Cooper AJ, Sharp SJ, Lentjes MA, et al. A prospective study of the association between quantity and variety of fruit and vegetable intake and incident type 2 diabetes. *Diabetes Care*. 2012 Jun;35(6):1293–1300. Available at: http://www.ncbi.nlm.nih.gov/pmc/articles/PMC3357245/?tool=pubmed. Accessed July 10, 2012.

6. Pan A, Malik VS, Schulze M, et al. Plain-water intake and risk of type 2 diabetes in young and middle-aged women. *Am J Clin Nutr*. 2012;95(6):1454–1460. doi:10.3945/ajcn.111.032698.

7. Rosenzweig S, Reibel DK, Greeson JM, et al. Mindfulness-based stress reduction is associated with improved glycemic control in type 2 diabetes mellitus: a pilot study. *Alternative Therapies in Health and Med*. 2007 Sep–Oct;13(5):36–38.

8. Hernandez A, Philippe J, Jornayvaz FR. Sleep and diabetes. *Rev Med Suisse*. 2012 Jun 6;8(344):1198–1200, 1202–1203.

9. Behrman EJ, Gopalan V. Cholesterol and plants. Concepts in biochemistry. *J Chem Educ*. 2005;82:1791–1793. Available at: http://chemistry.osu.edu/~gopalan.5/file/7B.PDF. Accessed July 17, 2012.

10. Roger VL, Go AS, Lloyd-Jones DM, et al. American Heart Association Statistics Committee and Stroke Statistics Subcommittee. Executive summary: heart disease and stroke statistics—2012 update: a report from the American Heart Association. *Circulation*. 2012 Jan 3;125(1):188–197. Summary available at: http://circ.ahajournals.org/content/125/1/188.full.pdf+html. Accessed July 10, 2012.

11. Vaidya D, Beck DM, Bittner V, Mathias RA, Ouyang P. Aging, menopause, and ischemic heart disease mortality in England, Wales, and the United States: modeling study of national mortality data. *BMJ*. 2011. doi:10.1136/bmj.d5170. Available at: http://www.bmj.com/content/343/bmj.d5170.long. Accessed September 9, 2011.

12. Centers for Disease Control and Prevention. Smoking and tobacco use: heart disease and stroke. Centers for Disease Control and Prevention. Available at: http://www.cdc.gov/tobacco/basic_information/health_effects/heart_disease/index.htm. Accessed July 11, 2012.

13. Fung TT, Schulze M, Manson JE, Willett WC, Hu FB. Dietary patterns, meat intake, and the risk of type 2 diabetes in women. *Arch Intern Med*. 2004 Nov 8;164(20):2235–2240.

14. Fung TT, Stampfer MJ, Manson JE, Rexrode KM, Willett WC, Hu FB. Prospective study of major dietary patterns and stroke risk in women. *Stroke*. 2004 Sep;35(9):2014–2019.

15. Pan A, Sun Q, Bernstein AM, et al. Red meat consumption and mortality. *Arch Intern Med*. 2012. doi:10.1001/archinternmed.2011.2287. Available at: http://www.archinternmed.com. Accessed June 19, 2012.

16. Kratz M. Dietary cholesterol, atherosclerosis and coronary heart disease. *Handb Exp Pharmacol*. 2005;(170):195–213.

17. Stadler KM, Thye FM. Heart healthy eating: cholesterol, fat, fiber, & sodium. Virginia State University. Available at: http://pubs.ext.vt.edu/348/348-898/348-898.html. Accessed July 11, 2012.

18. Baum SJ, Kris-Etherton PM, Willett WC, et al. Fatty acids in cardiovascular health and disease: a comprehensive update. *J Clin Lipidol*. 2012 May;6(3):216–234.

19. Volek JS, Forsythe. The case for not restricting saturated fat on a low carbohydrate diet. *Nutr Metab*. 2005;2:21.

20. American Diabetes Association. Evidence-based nutrition principles and recommendations for the treatment and prevention of diabetes and related complications. *Diabetes Care*. 2002;25(suppl 1):S50–S60. doi:10.2337/diacare.25.2007.S50. Available at: http://care.diabetesjournals.org/content/25/suppl_1/s50.full?loc=what-to-do-prediabetes. Accessed July 5, 2012.

21. Jakobsen MU, Dethlefsen C, Joensen AM, et al. Intake of carbohydrates compared with intake of saturated fatty acids and risk of myocardial infarction: importance of the glycemic index. *Am J Clin Nutr*. 2010 Jun;91(6):1764–1768.

22. Gardener H, Rundek T, Markert M, et al. Diet soft drink consumption is associated with an increased risk of vascular events in the northern Manhattan study. *J Gen Intern Med*. 2012. doi:10.1007/s11606-011-1968-2.

23. Nettleton JA, Lutsey PL, Wang Y, et al. Diet soda intake and risk of incident metabolic syndrome and type 2 diabetes in the Multi-Ethnic Study of Atherosclerosis (MESA). *Diabetes Care*. 2009;32(4):688–694. doi:10.2337/dc08-1799.

24. Bernstein AM, de Koning L, Flint AJ, Rexrode KM, Willett WC. Soda consumption and the risk of stroke in men and women. *Am J Clin Nutr*. 2012;95:1190–1199.

25. de Koning L, Malik VS, Kellogg MD, et al. Sweetened beverage consumption, incident coronary heart disease and biomarkers of risk in men. *Circulation* 2012. doi:10.1161/CIRCULATIONAHA.111.067017. Available at: http://circ.ahajournals.org.

26. Alderman MH, Cohen HW. Dietary sodium intake and cardiovascular mortality: controversy resolved? *Am J Hypertens*. 2012 Jul;25(7):727–734. doi:10.1038/ajh.2012.52.

27. Zimmet P, Magliano D, Matsuzawa Y, Alberti G, Shaw J. The metabolic syndrome: a global public health problem and a new definition. *J Atheroscler Thromb*. 2005;12(6):295–300.

28. Ervin RB. Prevalence of metabolic syndrome among adults 20 years of age and over, by sex, age, race and ethnicity, and body mass index: United States 2003–2006. *National Health Statistics Report*. 2009. No. 13. Centers for Disease Control and Prevention. Available at: http://www.cdc.gov/nchs/data/nhsr/nhsr013.pdf. Accessed July 17, 2012.

29. Ho RC, Neo LF, Chua AN, Cheak AA, Mak A. Research on psychoneuroimmunology: does stress influence immunity and cause coronary artery disease? *Ann Acad Med Singapore*. 2010 Mar;39(3):191–196.

30. Utsugi M, Saijo Y, Yoshioka E, et al. Relationship between two alternative occupational stress models and arterial stiffness: a cross-sectional study among Japanese workers. *Int Arch Occup Environ Health*. 2009 Jan;82(2):175–183.

31. Vale S. Psychosocial stress and cardiovascular diseases. *Postgrad Med J*. 2005 Jul;81(957):429–435.

32. Eaker ED, Sullivan LM, Kelly-Hayes M, D'Agostino RB Sr, Benjamin EJ. Anger and hostility predict the development of atrial fibrillation in men in the Framingham Offspring Study. *Circulation*. 2004 Mar 16;109(10):1267–1271.

33. Williams JE, Nieto FJ, Sanford CP, Couper DJ, Tyroler HA. The association between trait anger and incident stroke risk: the Atherosclerosis Risk in Communities (ARIC) Study. *Stroke*. 2002 Jan;33(1):13–19.

34. Yan LL, Liu K, Matthews KA, Daviglus ML, Ferguson TF, Kiefe CI. Psychosocial factors and risk of hypertension: the Coronary Artery Risk Development in Young Adults (CARDIA) study. *JAMA*. 2003 Oct 22;290(16):2138–2148.

35. Knutson KL. Sociodemographic and cultural determinants of sleep deficiency: implications for cardiometabolic disease risk. *Soc Sci Med*. 2012 May 26 [Epub ahead of print].

36. Fung MM, Peters K, Redine S, et al. Decreased slow wave sleep increases risk of developing hypertension in elderly men. *Hypertension*. 2011;58:596–603.

37. Pietroiusti A, Neri A, Somma G, et al. Incidence of metabolic syndrome among night-shift healthcare workers. *Occup Environ Med*. 2010 Jan;67(1):54–57.

38. Levy P, Tamisier R, Arnaud C, et al. Sleep deprivation, sleep apnea and cardiovascular diseases. *Front Biosci (Elite Ed)*. 2012 Jan 1;4:2007–2021.

39. Whang W, Kubzansky LD, Kawachi I, et al. Depression and risk of sudden cardiac death and coronary heart disease in women: results from the Nurses' Health Study. *J Am Coll Cardiol*. 2009;53:950–958. doi:10.1016/j.jacc.2008.10.060. Available at: http://www.ncbi.nlm.nih.gov/pmc/articles/PMC2664253/?tool=pubmed. Accessed August 12, 2011.

40. Pan A, Okereke OI, Sun Q, et al. Depression and incident stroke in women. *Stroke*. 2011. doi:10.1161/strokeaha.111.617043 [Published online ahead of print]. Available at: http://stroke.ahajournals.org/content/early/2011/08/11/STROKEAHA.111.617043.abstract. Accessed August 12, 2011.

41. Larsen KK, Vestergaard M, Søndergaard J, Christensen B. Screening for depression in patients with myocardial infarction by general practitioners. *Eur J Prev Cardiol*. 2012 Apr 10 [Epub ahead of print].

42. Taylor-Piliae RE, Hepworth JT, Coull BM. Predictors of depressive symptoms among community-dwelling stroke survivors. *J Cardiovasc Nurs*. 2012 Jun 15 [Epub ahead of print].

43. Samuels J. The increasing burden of pediatric hypertension. *Hypertension* 2012. doi:10.1161/HYPERTENSIONAHA.112.197624.

44. Flynn JT. Pediatric hypertension: recent trends and accomplishments, future challenges. *Am J Hypertens*. 2008 Jun;21(6):605–612.

45. Nguyen Q, Tabor JW, Entzel PP, et al. Discordance in national estimates of hypertension among young adults. *Epidemiology*. 2011;22:532–541. doi:10.1097/EDE.0b013e31821c79d2. Available at: Journals@Ovid LWW Total Access Collection. Accessed May 26, 2011.

46. Cohen L, Curhan G, Forman J. Association of sweetened beverage intake with incident hypertension. *J Gen Intern Med*. 2012 Apr 27 [Epub ahead of print].

47. Arima H, Barzi F, Chalmers J. Mortality patterns in hypertension. *J Hypertens*. 2011 Dec;29(Suppl 1):S3–7.

48. Gray L, Lee IM, Sesso HD, Batty GD. Blood pressure in early adulthood, hypertension in middle age, and future cardiovascular disease mortality: HAHS (Harvard Alumni Health Study). *J Am Coll Cardiol*. 2011;58:2396–2403.

49. Lu XT, Liu YF, Zhao L, et al. Chronic psychological stress induces vascular inflammation in rabbits. *Stress*. 2012 Apr 25 [Epub ahead of print].

50. Oliveira FL, Patin RV, Escrivão MA. Atherosclerosis prevention and treatment in children and adolescents. *Expert Rev Cardiovasc Ther*. 2010 Apr;8(4):513–528.

51. Roger VL, Go AS, Lloyd-Jones DM, et al. American Heart Association Statistics Committee and Stroke Statistics Subcommittee. Executive summary: heart disease and stroke statistics—2012 update: a report from the American Heart Association. *Circulation*. 2012 Jan 3;125(1):188–197. Available at: http://circ.ahajournals.org/content/125/1/188.full.pdf+html. Accessed July 10, 2012.

52. National Heart, Lung, and Blood Institute. Who is at risk for coronary artery disease? Available at: http://www.nhlbi.nih.gov/health/dci/Diseases/Cad/CAD_WhoIsAtRisk.html. Accessed May 26, 2011.

53. Roger VL, Go AS, Lloyd-Jones DM, et al. Heart disease and stroke statistics—2012 update: a report from the American Heart Association. *Circulation*. 2012 Jan 3;125(1):188–197. Available at: http://circ.ahajournals.org/content/125/1/e2.full.pdf+html. Accessed July 10, 2012.

54. Women and heat disease facts. Women's Heart Foundation. Available at: http://www.womensheart.org/content/heartdisease/heart_disease_facts.asp. Accessed May 30, 2013.

55. Canto JG, Rogers WJ, Goldberg RJ, et al. Association of age with sex with myocardial infarction symptom presentation and in-hospital mortality. *JAMA*. 2012;7:813–822.

56. Albert CM, Chae CU, Grodstein F, et al. Prospective study of sudden cardiac death among women in the United States. *Circulation*. 2003 Apr 29;107(16):2096–2101.

57. Nauman J, Nilsen TI, Wisløff U, Vatten LJ. Combined effect of resting heart rate and physical activity on ischaemic heart disease: mortality follow-up in a population study (the HUNT study, Norway). *J Epidemiol Community Health*. 2010 Feb;64(2):175–181.

58. Shigetoh Y, Adachi H, Yamagishi S, et al. Higher heart rate may predispose to obesity and diabetes mellitus: 20-year prospective study in a general population. *Am J Hypertens*. 2009 Feb;22(2):151–155.

59. Milani RV, Lavie CJ. The role of exercise training in peripheral arterial disease. *Vasc Med*. 2007 Nov;12(4):351–358.

60. Ganz P. Erectile dysfunction: pathophysiologic mechanisms pointing to underlying cardiovascular disease. *Am J Cardiol*. 2005 Dec 26;96(12B):8M–12M.

61. Vlachopoulos C, Ioakeimidis N, Terentes-Printzios D, Stefanadis C. The triad: erectile dysfunction—endothelial dysfunction—cardiovascular disease. *Curr Pharm Des*. 2008;14(35):3700–3714.

62. Chaiban JT, Azar ST. Erectile dysfunction in diabetic patients. *J Med Liban*. 2004 Oct–Dec;52(4):217–219.

63. Nunes KP, Labazi H, Webb RC. New insights into hypertension-associated erectile dysfunction. *Curr Opin Nephrol Hypertens*. 2012 Mar;21(2):163–170.

64. Miner M, Esposito K, Guay A, Montorsi P, Goldstein I. Cardiometabolic risk and female sexual health: the Princeton III summary. *J Sex Med*. 2012 Mar;9(3):641–651; quiz 652. doi:10.1111/j.1743-6109.2012.02649.x.

65. Roger VL, Go AS, Lloyd-Jones DM, et al. American Heart Association Statistics Committee and Stroke Statistics Subcommittee. Executive summary: heart disease and stroke statistics—2012 update: a report from the American Heart Association. *Circulation*. 2012 Jan 3;125(1):188–197. Available at: http://circ.ahajournals.org/content/125/1/188.full.pdf+html. Accessed July 10, 2012.

66. Chiuve SE, Fung TT, Rexrode KM, et al. Adherence to a low-risk, healthy lifestyle and risk of sudden cardiac death among women. *JAMA*. 2011;306:62–69. doi:10.1001/jama.2011.907.

67. Chiuve SE, Fung TT, Rexrode KM, et al. Adherence to a low-risk, healthy lifestyle and risk of sudden cardiac death among women. *JAMA*. 2011;306(1):62–69. doi:10.1001/jama.2011.907.

68. Sattelmair J, Pertman J, Ding E, et al. Dose response between physical activity and risk of coronary heart disease. A meta-analysis. *Circulation* 2011. doi:10.1161/CIRCULATIONAHA.110.010710.

69. Sattelmair JR, Kurth T, Buring JE, Lee IM. Physical activity and risk of stroke in women. *Stroke*. 2010 Jun;41(6):1243–1250.

70. de Lorgeril M, Salen P. The Mediterranean diet: rationale and evidence for its benefit. *Curr Atheroscler Rep*. 2008 Dec;10(6):518–522.

71. Kastorini CM, Milionis HJ, Kantas D, et al. Adherence to the Mediterranean diet in relation to ischemic stroke nonfatal events in nonhypercholesterolemic and hypercholesterolemic participants: results of a case/case-control study. *Angiology*. 2011 Dec 5 [Epub ahead of print]. doi:10.1177/0003319711427392.

72. de Lorgeril M, Salen P. Mediterranean diet in secondary prevention of CHD. *Public Health Nutr*. 2011 Dec;14(12A):2333–2337.

73. Fung TT, Chiuve SE, McCullough ML, et al. Adherence to a DASH-style diet and risk of coronary heart disease and stroke in women. *Arch Intern Med*. 2008 Apr 14;168(7):713–720.

74. Rondanelli M, Opizzi A, Monteferrario F, Klersy C, Cazzola R, Cestaro B. Beta-glucan- or rice bran-enriched foods: a comparative crossover clinical trial on lipidic pattern in mildly hypercholesterolemic men. *Eur J Clin Nutr*. 2011 Jul;65(7):864–871. doi:10.1038/ejcn.2011.48.

75. Harris KA, Kris-Etherton PM. Effects of whole grains on coronary heart disease risk. *Curr Atheroscler Rep*. 2010 Nov;12(6):368–376.

76. Rautiainen S, Larsson S, Virtamo J, Wolk A. Total antioxidant capacity of diet and risk of stroke: a population-based prospective cohort of women. *Stroke*. 2012 Feb;43(2):335–340.

77. Stoclet JC, Chataigneau T, Ndiaye M, et al. Vascular protection by dietary polyphenols. *Eur J Pharmacol*. 2004 Oct 1;500(1–3):299–313.

78. Cassidy A, O'Reilly EJ, Sampson L, et al. Habitual intake of flavonoid subclasses and incident hypertension in adults. *Am J Clin Nutr*. 2011;93(2):338–347. doi:10.3945/ajcn.110.006783.

79. Samieri C, Féart C, Proust-Lima C, et al. Olive oil consumption, plasma oleic acid, and stroke incidence: the three-city study. *Neurology*. 2011 Aug 2;77(5):418–425.

80. Cabo J, Alonso R, Mata P. Omega-3 fatty acids and blood pressure. *Br J Nutr*. 2012 Jun;107(suppl 2):S195–200.

81. Belin RJ, Greenland P, Martin L, et al. Fish intake and the risk of incident heart failure: the Women's Health Initiative. *Circ Heart Fail*. 2011;4:404–413.

82. Isherwood C, Wong M, Jones WS, Davies IG, Griffin BA. Lack of effect of cold water prawns on plasma cholesterol and lipoproteins in normo-lipidaemic men. *Cell Mol Biol (Noisy-le-grand)*. 2010 Feb 25;56(1):52–58.

83. Matheson EM, Mainous AG 3rd, Hill EG, Carnemolla MA. Shellfish consumption and risk of coronary heart disease. *Journal of the American Dietetic Association*. 2009 Aug;109(8):1422–1426.

84. Heart disease and diet. MedlinePlus. US National Library of Medicine, National Institutes of Health. Available at: http://www.nlm.nih.gov/medlineplus/ency/article/002436.htm. Accessed July 11, 2012.

85. Sabaté J, Oda K, Ros E. Nut consumption and blood lipid levels: a pooled analysis of 25 intervention trials. *Arch Intern Med*. 2010;170:821–827.

86. Mak JC. Potential role of green tea catechins in various disease therapies: progress and promise. *Clin Exp Pharmacol Physiol*. 2012 Mar;39(3):265–273. doi:10.1111/j.1440-1681.2012.05673.x.

87. Wu AH, Spicer D, Stanczyk FZ, Tseng CC, Yang CS, Pike MC. Effect of 2-month controlled green tea intervention on lipoprotein cholesterol, glucose, and hormone levels in healthy postmenopausal women. *Cancer Prev Res (Phila)*. 2012 Mar;5(3):393–402.

88. Mozaffari-Khosravi H, Jalali-Khanabadi BA, Afkhami-Ardekani M, et al. Effects of sour tea (Hibiscus sabdariffa) on lipid profile and lipoproteins in patients with type II diabetes. *J Altern Complement Med*. 2009 Aug;15(8):899–903.

89. Gurrola-Díaz CM, García-López PM, Sánchez-Enríquez S, et al. Effects of Hibiscus sabdariffa extract powder and preventive treatment (diet) on the lipid profiles of patients with metabolic syndrome (MeSy). *Phytomedicine*. 2010 Jun;17(7):500–505. Available at: http://www.ncbi.nlm.nih.gov/pubmed/19962289.

90. McKay DL, Chen CY, Saltzman E, Blumberg JB. Hibiscus sabdariffa L. tea (tisane) lowers blood pressure in prehypertensive and mildly hypertensive adults. *J Nutr*. 2010 Feb;140(2):298–303.

91. Larsson SC, Virtamo J, Wolk A. Coffee consumption and risk of stroke in women. *Stroke*. 2011;42:908–912.

92. Cai L, Ma D, Zhang Y, Liu Z, Wang P. The effect of coffee consumption on serum lipids: a meta-analysis of randomized controlled trials. *Eur J Clin Nutr*. 2012 Jun 20. doi:10.1038/ejcn.2012.68 [Epub ahead of print].

93. Bøhn SK, Ward NC, Hodgson JM, Croft KD. Effects of tea and coffee on cardiovascular disease risk. *Food Funct*. 2012 Mar 29 [Epub ahead of print].

94. Almoosawi S, Fyfe L, Ho C, Al-Dujaili E. The effect of polyphenol-rich dark chocolate on fasting capillary whole blood glucose, total cholesterol, blood pressure and glucocorticoids in healthy overweight and obese subjects. *Br J Nutr*. 2010 Mar;103(6):842–850.

95. Sudano I, Flammer AJ, Roas S, et al. Cocoa, blood pressure, and vascular function. *Curr Hypertens Rep*. 2012 Aug;14(4):279–284.

96. Nainggolan L. New salt paper causes controversy. Medscape.com. May 3, 2011. Available at: http://www.medscape.com/viewarticle/742034. Accessed July 12, 2012.

97. Gonen A, Harats D, Rabinkov A, et al. The antiatherogenic effect of allicin: possible mode of action. *Pathobiology*. 2005;72:325–334.

98. Budoff M. Aged garlic extract retards progression of coronary artery calcification. *J Nutr*. 2006;136(3)(suppl):741S–744S.

99. Rahman K, Lowe GM. Garlic and cardiovascular disease: a critical review. *J Nutr*. 2006;136:736S–740S; Borek C. Garlic reduces dementia and heart-disease risk. *J Nutr*. 2006;136:810S–812S.

100. Gardner CD, Lawson LD, Block E, et al. Effect of raw garlic vs commercial garlic supplements on plasma lipid concentrations in adults with moderate hypercholesterolemia. *Arch Intern Med*. 2007;167:346–353.

101. Reinhart K, Talati R, White C, et al. The impact of garlic on lipid parameters: a systematic review and meta-analysis. *Nutr Res Rev*. 2009;22:39–48.

102. Zeng T, Guo FF, Zhang CL, Song FY, Zhao XL, Xie KQ. A meta-analysis of randomized, double-blind, placebo-controlled trials for the effects of garlic on serum lipid profiles. *J Sci Food Agric*. 2012 Jul;92(9):1892–1902. doi:10.1002/jsfa.5557.

103. Boehm JK, Kubzansky LD. The heart's content: the association between positive psychological well-being and cardiovascular health. *Psychol Bull*. 2012 Jul;138(4):655–691.

104. Holt-Lunstad J, Smith TB, Layton JB. Social relationships and mortality risk: a meta-analytic review. *PLoS Med*. 2010 Jul 27;7(7):e1000316.

105. Stasi MF, Amati D, Costa C, et al. Pet-therapy: a trial for institutionalized frail elderly patients. *Arch Gerontol Geriat*. 2004;(9)(suppl):407–412.

106. Arhant-Sudhir K, Arhant-Sudhir R, Sudhir K. Pet ownership and cardiovascular risk reduction: supporting evidence, conflicting data and underlying mechanisms. *Clin Exp Pharmacol Physiol*. 2011 Nov;38(11):734–738. doi:10.1111/j.1440-1681.2011.05583.x.

107. Niazi AK, Niazi SK. Mindfulness-based stress reduction: a non-pharmacological approach for chronic illnesses. *N Am J Med Sci*. 2011 Jan;3(1):20–23.

108. Barnes VA, Kapuku GK, Treiber FA. Impact of Transcendental Meditation on left ventricular mass in African American adolescents. *Evid Based Complement Alternat Med*. 2012;2012:923153.

109. Lucchetti G, Lucchetti AL, Koenig HG. Impact of spirituality/religiosity on mortality: comparison with other health interventions. *Explore (NY)*. 2011 Jul–Aug;7(4):234–238.

110. Trappe HJ. The effects of music on the cardiovascular system and cardiovascular health. *Heart*. 2010 Dec;96(23):1868–1871.

111. Dabhade AM, Pawar BH, Ghunage MS, Ghunage VM. Effect of pranayama (breathing exercise) on arrhythmias in the human heart. *Explore (NY)*. 2012 Jan–Feb;8(1):12–15.

112. Richardson EA, Mitchell R. Gender differences in relationships between urban green space and health in the United Kingdom. *Soc Sci Med*. 2010 Aug;71(3):568–575.

CHAPTER 16
Cancer: Causes, Prevention, and Treatment

Cancer is the second leading cause of death in the United States, accounting for one in four deaths.[1] In 2008, 12 million Americans were living with this disease. The American Cancer Society (ACS) estimates in 2012 that nearly 1,634,000 people will receive a cancer diagnosis—a number that excludes skin cancers, which are so exceedingly common they're not reported to cancer registries. Over 577,000 will die this year, a rate of more than 1,500 people a day.

Survival rates, though they depend on the type of cancer, have steadily improved. In general, earlier detection and treatment improves the odds. As usual, prevention trumps treatment. Fortunately, experts now think that cancer is a largely preventable disease. Because cancer begins decades before it's diagnosed, the sooner you start to protect yourself the better.

By the time you finish reading this chapter, you'll know what cancer is and its possible causes, the major types of cancer, how cancer is detected and treated, and actions you can take to reduce your risk.

Cancer is a word, not a sentence.

- *John Diamond, British broadcaster and journalist*

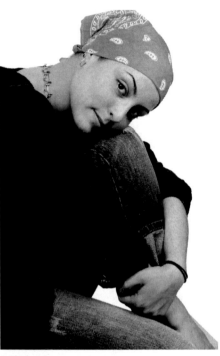

© *Thinkstock*

1. DEFINING CANCER

LEARNING OBJECTIVES

1. Define cancer.
2. Explain how cancer spreads.
3. List common causes of cancer.

Cancer is the uncontrolled division and spread of cells. Cell division is normal. In a process called *mitosis*, one cell splits into two. That's how we grow and replace worn-out cells. Some tissues divide quite rapidly—cells in the skin, along mucous membranes, the bone marrow.

The bone marrow and other tissues contain **stem cells**. These cells are undifferentiated, meaning they are nondescript, spherical cells that could become anything and can divide indefinitely. Adult stem cells are somewhat set in their ways. That is, stem cells from the bone marrow become one of the several types of blood cells, but not pancreatic cells or liver cells. Once a stem cell *differentiates* (becomes a specialized cell such as a nerve cell) there's no going back—unless a mutation occurs.

Normally, cellular growth and *proliferation* (a rapid increase in numbers) is a tightly regulated affair. Only so many divisions occur. *Tumor suppressor genes* monitor these events and squelch excessive replication. Also, cells belonging to the same type of tissue stick to one another and don't go wandering off. That's why hair doesn't start growing out of your eyeball and you don't have pancreatic cells taking up shop in the brain and secreting insulin and digestive enzymes.

cancer

The uncontrolled division and spread of cells.

However, the mere fact that cells divide creates opportunities for genetic errors. Recall from Chapter 1 that the cell's genetic material lies within the nucleus. Chromosomes contain the genes, each of which codes for a particular protein. Genes are made of DNA (deoxyribonucleic acid). When a cell divides, the double-stranded chromosomes split down the middle, then replicate. The process doesn't always go perfectly.

FIGURE 16.1 Loss of Normal Growth Control

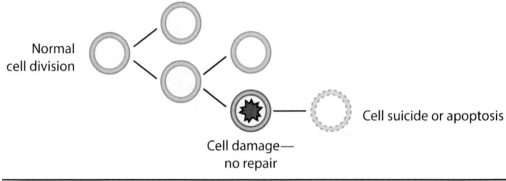

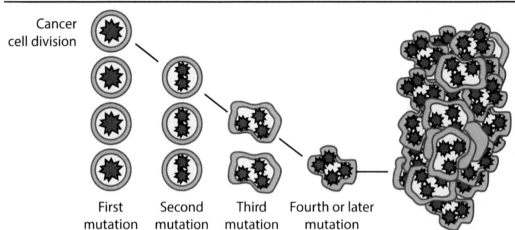

mutation

A permanent change in the DNA sequence.

mutagen

A substance that causes gene mutations.

apoptosis

Programmed cell death or cell suicide; this mechanism controls the number of cells and eliminates abnormal or unnecessary cells.

A **mutation** is any change in the DNA sequence. In addition to replication errors, environmental agents can cause them. A **mutagen** is any substance that causes a gene mutation. Sometimes mutations aren't of much consequence; sometimes they alter the gene—favorably or unfavorably. For example, mutations of tumor suppressor genes can remove the brake against cell division.

Normally, the body has ways of halting the division process in order to give cellular enzymes a chance to repair damaged DNA. Specialized structures within cells can get rid of defective parts by digesting them. Old or damaged cells self-destruct in a process called **apoptosis** (a type of programmed cell death). Failing those means, one of the immune system's jobs is to identify abnormal cells and destroy them. Loss of these regulatory control mechanisms and others can permit unbridled growth and proliferation.

Tumors, also called *neoplasms*, are abnormal masses or swellings. Causes include injury, inflammation, and an overgrowth of cells. For instance, if you bump your head, you can get a hematoma (i.e., bleeding under the scalp, more commonly referred to as an "egg"). Tumors caused by cellular overgrowth can be benign or malignant. A **benign tumor** does not invade and damage nearby tissue or spread to distant sites. A **malignant tumor** is capable of spreading and damaging tissue.

The term *cancer* refers to abnormal cells that grow out of control. Viewed under the microscope, cancer cells appear abnormal and less differentiated, looking more like stem cells than the specialized cells they were meant to be.

Cancer development (**carcinogenesis**) takes many years. **Carcinogens** are cancer-causing substances. Twenty to 30 years can elapse between the microscopic origins and diagnosis of a tumor. A host of events can conspire to initiate tumor growth. The process follows three main stages:

1. **Initiation.** The process of changing a normal cell to an abnormal one.
2. **Promotion.** The process of stimulating tumors to grow.
3. **Progression.** The process wherein tumor cells gain the ability to proliferate and spread.

All cells in the body need to be very close to a blood vessel, which supplies oxygen, glucose, and other energy substrates and removes carbon dioxide and other wastes. In order to enlarge, tumors must stimulate the formation of new blood vessels, a process called **angiogenesis**. Rather than stick together like normal cells, cancer cells also penetrate into neighboring tissues, which is called **invasion**. In a process called **metastasis**, cancer cells slip into the blood and lymphatic vessels and migrate to distant tissues. These cells can then establish colonies referred to as *secondary tumors* to distinguish them from the *primary tumor*, or original tumor.

1.1 Causes of Cancer

Cancer is considered a *multifactorial* disease, meaning that a number of factors contribute to the condition. In addition, it takes many years to become a diagnosable mass. For those two reasons, pinpointing the cause becomes difficult. Nevertheless, a number of factors stand out as contributing significantly to cancer risk.

Genetics accounts for only about 5 percent of cancer risk. Otherwise, experts attribute one-third of cancers to tobacco use; one-third to a combination of diet, physical activity, and body weight; and one-third to environmental exposures (infectious microorganisms, ultraviolet light, radiation, pollutants, and other toxins).[2],[3] In other words, the bulk of the causes have to do with lifestyle habits and environmental exposures. While we can't control genetics and past events, we do have the power to alter our lifestyles to eliminate or reduce many of the other risks.

Cancer Risk Factors

Nonmodifiable Risks

Although you can't control the following factors, assessing these risks can motivate you to get recommended screening tests and reduce modifiable risks.

- **Family history.** Some genes raise the risk of certain cancers. In general, however, genetics contribute to a small percentage of cancer risk. Family members also share health-related habits and environmental exposures. That's why a history of cancer among close relatives can indicate you're also at risk.

- **Race.** Some genetic risks are more common in certain races. For instance, Ashkenazi Jews (descendants of German, French, and Eastern European Jews) are more likely to carry certain genes predisposing to breast cancer. As with families, ethnic groups share cultural practices such as diet and substance use that may influence cancer risk. Furthermore, race creates disparities in socioeconomic status. Lower education and income correlate with worse health and too often limit access to health care services, including cancer screening tests and treatment. For instance, although cancer deaths have recently fallen among blacks, the survival for most cancers is worse than any other racial group.[4]

- **Advancing age.** Cancer risk rises with age for several reasons. The longer you live, the greater your exposure to carcinogens and tumor-promoting substances. Cellular repair systems and immune function both decline.

- **Sex.** Some cancers affect one sex more than the other. For instance, breast cancer can occur in men but more often strikes women—a difference largely due to greater production of estrogen in women. Reproductive system cancers differ based on anatomy: prostate and testicular cancers in men and uterine, cervical, and ovarian cancer in women. In addition, lifestyle habits and

---

tumor

An abnormal mass or swelling; also called a neoplasm.

benign tumor

A growth that does not invade nearby tissue or spread to distant sites; also called noncancerous tumor.

malignant tumor

A cancerous growth that invades and destroys nearby tissues and spreads to distant sites.

carcinogenesis

The process of developing cancer, which takes many years and follows a series of stages.

carcinogen

A substance that causes cancer (*adj.* carcinogenic).

angiogenesis

The creation of new blood vessels.

invasion

The process whereby cancer cells penetrate and destroy neighboring tissues.

metastasis

The process whereby cancer cells spread, via the blood and lymphatic vessels, and grow at sites distant from the primary site (*adj.* metastatic, *v.* metastasize).

occupational exposures to hazardous materials vary. For years, more men than women smoked, though women have been steadily catching up.

- **Reproductive history.** Estrogen promotes cell growth in sensitive organs. While men make estrogen, significant increases arise from obesity and hormone disorders rather than reproductive history. In women, cumulative lifetime exposure to estrogen influences cancer of the breast and female reproductive organs. Women who start menstruating early and enter menopause later in life (and/or use hormone replacement after menopause) have more years of estrogen exposure. Because pregnancy and breast-feeding suppress normal menstrual cycles, having children before age 35 and nursing those babies protects against female cancers.

Modifiable Risk Factors

You have some degree of control over your risk factors. Take full advantage of that. Eliminating or minimizing your exposure improves your odds against cancer and many other ills. Aside from substances that are directly carcinogenic, a common pathway of many cancer-promoting agents is inflammation and oxidative stress. Inflammation generates free radicals and other forms of oxidative stress, which can damage DNA. All toxins stir up inflammation and oxidation (free radical damage). So do most chronic diseases.

The following list highlights modifiable risk factors common to many cancers.

- **Tobacco** contributes more than any other single factor to cancer risk. Among other poisons, tobacco products contain more than 70 carcinogens.[5] The list includes arsenic, benzene, cadmium, formaldehyde, and tar (a mixture of chemicals that sticks to the airways). When the smoke is inhaled or tobacco is chewed, toxic chemicals enter the bloodstream and travel to all cells. One of the best things you can do to improve overall health, look and feel younger, lengthen your life, and reduce your risk of cancer and other chronic illnesses is to avoid all tobacco products. Smokeless tobacco products also cause cancer, especially of the mouth, lips, throat, and esophagus (the tube connecting the mouth to the stomach). Inhaling other people's smoke increases your risk.

- **Alcohol.** Excessive drinking clearly contributes to cancer of the mouth, throat, larynx (voice box), esophagus, liver, breast, and possibly the pancreas. Researchers have lately recognized that the threshold for risk for breast cancer in women is quite low. Regular consumption of as little as three alcoholic drinks a week can lead to a small but significant increase in invasive breast cancer. The risk rises with higher intakes and binge drinking. Compared to nondrinkers, women who habitually down two or more drinks a day increase their risk by 50 percent.[6]

- **Diet.** Eating more red meat, especially pan-fried, charcoal-grilled, and processed meats (bacon, sausages, bologna, deli meats, hot dogs), raises the risk of cancer deaths and deaths in general.[7] Some studies link low fiber intake with a greater risk of colon cancer. The effect of fiber is hard to distinguish from the clear benefits of the usual sources of dietary fiber—fruits, vegetables, legumes, whole grains—which more clearly protect against many cancers.

- **Sleep deprivation.** Studies have linked disruption in circadian rhythms with an increased risk of cancers.[8] Working the night shift is linked to an increase in breast[9] and prostate cancer.[10] Exposure to nighttime light suppresses melatonin. This hormone regulates many processes and has an antioxidant, anticancer, and immune-enhancing action. Night-shift workers often have trouble sleeping during the day, leading to chronic sleep deprivation, which suppresses immune function and increases inflammation.

- **Overweight and obesity.** Carrying excessive body fat raises the risk of some cancer and decreases the odds of surviving the disease.[11] Obesity and surplus calorie intake increases inflammatory chemicals, insulin (the hormone that moves sugar inside cells), estrogen, insulin-like growth factors (chemicals that stimulate cells growth), and other tumor-promoting factors.[12]

- **Diabetes.** While the most common complication of diabetes is cardiovascular disease, cancer has emerged as another leading cause of death.[13] People with diabetes have a greater risk of uterus, breast, colon, and bladder cancer. The reasons aren't clear. Those who have diabetes may be overweight, have excessive calorie intake, or be physically inactive. Oxidation, inflammation, elevations in insulin, and medications to treat the disease can influence cancer risk.

- **Electromagnetic radiation.** This energy form comes from man-made and natural sources. There are two main types of radiation: ionizing radiation (X-rays, radioactive substances, and radon) and nonionizing radiation (radio waves). Ionizing radiation is strong enough to dislodge electrons (the negatively charged particles that revolve around the nucleus of an atom). Examples include X-rays and radon (a naturally occurring radioactive gas that escapes from soil and rocks into the air or water). The energy of nonionizing radiation is lower in frequency and penetrates less deeply. Examples include radio waves, electromagnetic fields, microwaves, and ultraviolet (UV) light.

Although sunlight has many benefits, it also serves as an ever-present source of potentially carcinogenic radiation. UV light can cause sunburn, prematurely ages the skin (leading to wrinkles, blotches, and sagging), suppresses immunity, impairs DNA repair systems, and elevates skin cancer risk.[14] People with darker skin pigmentation are more protected from UV but are not immune to skin cancer.

There are two main types of UV light: UVA and UVB. Initially, scientists identified UVB, which damages DNA, as the cause of skin cancers. Sunscreens were developed that blocked UVB but had little effect on UVA. The vast majority of UV radiation reaching the earth's surface is UVA. Compared to UVB, UVA penetrates the skin more deeply (and can pass through clouds and window glass) and causes more harm. It ages the skin, suppresses immunity, generates free radicals and other chemicals that injure DNA, and degrades vitamin D, which has immune-enhancing and anticancer effects.[15],[16]

Compared to outdoor light, tanning beds and sunlamps have a higher ratio of UVA to UVB. Twenty tanning salon sessions can exceed the average yearly UVA exposure by a factor of 1.2.[17] Unfortunately indoor tanning has become all too popular in America, particularly among adolescents and young adults.

- **Toxic chemicals.** Exposure to environmental agents is not entirely within our control. Chemicals are variously able to stimulate cell division, cause mutations, promote cancer, and disrupt natural hormones. Most of these chemicals, called endocrine disrupters, have an estrogen-like effect, which has particular relevance for cancers of the reproductive organs. Suspect chemicals exist in cleaning products, personal care products, foods, building materials, water, air, and soil. Scientists typically use animal and cell studies to determine the tolerable levels of any one chemical. The idea is that the higher the dose, the greater the risk. However, the effects of repeated exposure to multiple chemicals in humans are much harder to establish.

  For most people, using tobacco threatens health more than any other environmental exposure. Otherwise, workers in industries that involve high levels of chemical exposures face the greatest risk from other toxic substances. For example, production of polymers is a big industry. Polymers are made into products such as plastic, rubber, fiberglass, food containers, plastic packaging, disposable cups, pipes, car parts, food containers, and carpet backing.[18]

  Formaldehyde is now mainly used to produce industrial resins, which are then made into adhesives and binders for plastics, wood and paper products, synthetic fibers, and some textiles.[19] It can also be used to preserve tissues. It's in tobacco smoke and automobile emissions.

  Some agricultural *pesticides* are linked to an increased risk of cancer.[20],[21] Farmers are the group at highest risk of exposure.

  Potentially carcinogenic *heavy metals* include arsenic (well water, wood preservatives), mercury (in fish), cadmium (in tobacco smoke, batteries), and lead (multiple sources, including soil, air, old plumbing, tobacco smoke, alcoholic beverages). Heavy metals, all of which are naturally occurring, can contaminate air, water, and soil. Edible plants grown on tainted soil absorb these metals. Although not carcinogenic, the aluminum used in underarm antiperspirants may promote proliferation of breast cancer cells.[22] So far, research on actual risk to women who use such products has yielded conflicting results.[23]

- **Microorganisms.** Some viruses, bacteria, parasites, and fungi can lead to cancer. Some strains of human papillomavirus (HPV), which can be sexually transmitted, cause cervical cancer, as well as cancers of the anus, penis, mouth, and throat.

  Chronic infection with hepatitis B and C viruses can result in liver cancer. Epstein-Barr virus infection can cause some types of lymphoma. People infected with human immunodeficiency virus (HIV) can develop acquired immunodeficiency syndrome (AIDS), which impairs the immune system's ability to fight cancer and lowers resistance to infection with other viruses that cause cancer.

  The bacterium *Helicobacter pylori* can infect the stomach, causing inflammation, ulcers, and cancer. A few parasites found in the developing world can increase specific cancers.

  Foods contaminated with fungi (mold) that make aflatoxin raise the risk of liver cancer. This toxin can form on peanuts, nuts, corn, and other grains. Safety guidelines in the United States limit aflatoxin in foods.

In Section 2, we will explore different types of cancer and the specific risk factors associated with them.

Cell Phones and Brain Cancer Risk

Instead of holding your phone to your head, try using a headset or the speaker function.

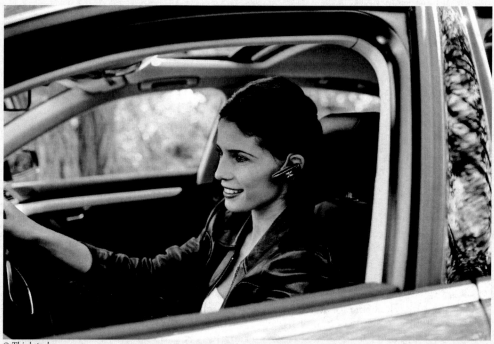

© *Thinkstock*

Cell phones have come under scrutiny because they emit radiofrequency energy, a form of electromagnetic radiation. Tissues nearest the phone's antenna absorb that energy. Many people now spend more time with a mobile phone clamped to the side of their heads. That energy heats tissues and increases brain metabolism (use of energy).[24] Most studies in people have not found a clear connection between cell phone use and brain tumors.[25],[26] Over the past decade, the incidence of brain cancer has not gone up. However, experts recognize the need for further research. A particular concern is early use of cell phones in children.

Most US government agencies state that there is no conclusive evidence linking cell phone use to cancer. However, the International Agency for Research on Cancer, a branch of the World Health Organization, classified "radiofrequency electromagnetic fields as possibly carcinogenic to humans."[27]

Until more is known, keep your phone away from your head. Use a headset or put the phone in speaker mode. If you can't, reserve your cell phone for short conversations. Keep in mind that the most dangerous thing you can do with your phone is use it while driving, cycling, and crossing busy streets on foot.

Assess Yourself: What's Your Cancer Risk?

The following items represent risk factors for cancer. Cancer-promoting factors can add up. While it's nearly impossible to reduce the odds to zero, we can all do our best to minimize potential, modifiable threats. The more boxes you have checked, the higher your risk. If you have concerns, discuss your cancer risk with your doctor. Learn more about risk assessment by visiting http://www.cancer.gov/cancertopics/wyntk/cancer/page3.

- __ Close family members (parents, siblings) have had cancer.
- __ I smoke and/or hang out with smokers.
- __ I grew up in a house where people smoked indoors.
- __ I drink more than one serving of alcohol a day (two if you're a man).
- __ I eat processed meat once a week or more.
- __ I often eat grilled or fried meat (red meat, poultry, fish).
- __ I usually eat less than two servings of fruits or vegetables a day.
- __ I am obese.
- __ I do not engage in regular physical activity.

- __ I work a night shift.
- __ I habitually sleep six hours or less a night.

KEY TAKEAWAYS

- Cell division is a tightly regulated process. A number of mechanisms hinder uncontrolled cell division, repair mutations to the DNA sequence, and eliminate abnormal cells.
- Tumors are swellings. Tumors caused by cellular overgrowth can be benign or malignant.
- Cancers are malignant tumors. The abnormal cells divide without control and spread by invasion and metastasis.
- Cancer is largely a preventable illness. Inherited genetic abnormalities account for only a small proportion of cancer. Lifestyle habits and environmental exposures cause the vast majority of cancers.

DISCUSSION QUESTIONS

1. Mutations happen frequently. Why doesn't cancer develop more often? How does the body control cell division, repair errors to DNA, and get rid of abnormal cells?
2. Of the modifiable risk factors you're exposed to, which one do you think you can change now? Explain your strategy for doing so.
3. What is the difference between a benign and a malignant tumor?

2. TYPES OF CANCER

LEARNING OBJECTIVES

1. Review the main categories of cancer based on tissue type.
2. Discuss the most common cancers, including risk factors, signs, and symptoms.

More than a hundred of types of cancer exist. Cancers are divided into the following five categories based on the type of tissue they arise from:

carcinoma

A cancer that arises from the skin and tissues that cover or line internal organs.

sarcoma

A cancer that arises from connective tissue (e.g., muscle, bone, cartilage, fat, blood vessels).

leukemia

A cancer of blood-forming tissue (e.g., bone marrow) resulting in numerous abnormal blood cells.

lymphoma

A lymphatic system cancer in which lymphocytes (a type of white blood cell) grow out of control.

myeloma

A cancer that develops in the bone marrow and affects plasma cells, an immune cell that makes antibodies.

central nervous system cancers

Cancers of the spinal cord and brain.

■ 1. **Carcinoma**: cancer that starts in the skin and tissues that cover or line internal organs.

■ 2. **Sarcoma**: cancer that arises from connective tissue (e.g., muscle, bone, cartilage, fat, blood vessels).

■ 3. **Leukemia**: cancer of blood-forming tissue (e.g., bone marrow) resulting in number abnormal blood cells.

■ 4. **Lymphoma** and **myeloma**: immune system cancers. Lymphomas begin in immune cells called lymphocytes in the lymphatic system, a network of slender tubes (lymphatic vessels) and lymph nodes. Myelomas begin in the bone marrow's plasma cells, which make antibodies.

■ 5. **Central nervous system cancers**: cancers of the spinal cord and brain.

Within those categories, particular cancers are named based on the tissue they start in. Examples include basal cell carcinoma (a type of skin cancer), myosarcoma (muscle cancer), osteosarcoma (bone cancer), acute lymphocytic leukemia (a rapidly progressive cancer of immature blood cells called lymphocytes), Hodgkin's lymphoma (a type of cancer of the lymphatic system), and meningioma (a tumor arising from the meninges, the membranes surrounding the central nervous system).

Skin cancers are by far the most commonly diagnosed cancers for both sexes. Next, the most commonly diagnosed cancer in men is prostate cancer; for women it is breast cancer. For men and women, lung cancer and colon cancer are, respectively, the second and third most common cancers. Lung cancer causes the most deaths.

TABLE 16.1 Cancer Incidence and Mortality (Excluding Skin Cancers) for Both Sexes

Most commonly diagnosed cancers (estimated new cases for 2012)	Most common causes of cancer deaths (estimated numbers for 2012)
Prostate (241,740)	Lung (160,340)
Breast (229,060–226,780 female + 2,190 male)	Colon and rectum (51,690)
Lung (226,160)	Breast (39,920–39,510 women + 410 men)
Colon and rectum (143,460)	Prostate (28,170)

Data source: Adapted from the National Cancer Institute at the National Institutes of Health. Common cancer types. 2013. Available at: http://www.cancer.gov/cancertopics/types/commoncancers. Also available at: http://www.cancer.org/acs/groups/content/@epidemiologysurveilance/documents/document/acspc-031941.pdf.

TABLE 16.2 Cancer in Women

The three most commonly diagnosed cancers	The three most common causes of cancer death
1. Breast	1. Lung
2. Lung	2. Breast
3. Colon and rectum	3. Colon and rectum

Source: US Cancer Statistics Working Group. United States Cancer Statistics: 1999–2009 Incidence and Mortality Web-based Report. Atlanta, GA: Department of Health and Human Services, Centers for Disease Control and Prevention, and National Cancer Institute; 2013. Available at: http://www.cdc.gov/cancer/dcpc/data.

TABLE 16.3 Cancer in Men

The three most commonly diagnosed cancers	The three most common causes of cancer death
1. Prostate	1. Lung
2. Lung	2. Prostate
3. Colon and rectum	3. Colon and rectum

Source: US Cancer Statistics Working Group. United States Cancer Statistics: 1999–2009 Incidence and Mortality Web-based Report. Atlanta, GA: Department of Health and Human Services, Centers for Disease Control and Prevention, and National Cancer Institute; 2013. Available at: http://www.cdc.gov/cancer/dcpc/data.

2.1 Common Cancers

Skin Cancer

This cancer is exceedingly common. There are three main types of skin cancer: *basal cell carcinoma*, *squamous cell carcinoma*, and *malignant melanoma*. Over the past three decades, the incidence of all three has risen. The number of newly diagnosed cases in a year is about 3.5 million basal and squamous cell carcinomas[28] and 76,250 melanomas.[29]

The primary risk factor for skin cancer is UV light exposure from sunlight, tanning beds, and sunlamps. Chronic exposure raises the risk of squamous cell carcinoma. Episodes of more intense exposure with blistering sunburns increase the risk of melanoma and basal cell carcinoma.[30] Light-skinned people, especially those who freckle and burn easily, are at particularly high risk. But skin cancer can occur in anyone. For instance, dark-skinned people typically develop melanomas on the palms, soles, and under the nails.

Basal cell carcinomas, the most common skin cancer, arise from cells called keratinocytes at the base of the epidermis (top layer of skin). Squamous cell carcinomas start in keratinocytes located closer to the surface. Melanoma is formed from skin cells called melanocytes, which produce the pigment melanin.

The good thing about skin cancer is you can see it. Basal cell and squamous cell carcinomas are relatively slow growing. As long as they're surgically removed in a timely fashion, they're rarely fatal. Melanoma is, by far, the deadliest of the three cancers. Even at a small size, the tumor readily metastasizes, making it difficult to treat.

Alarmingly, between 1970 and 2009, the incidence increased eightfold in young women and fourfold in young men.[31] Contributing factors include the rising popularity of tanning salons and the fact that, until recently, few sunscreens effectively filtered UVA rays but blocked the UVB rays that stimulate the skin's production of vitamin D. (See the sidebar "Making Sense of Sunscreens")

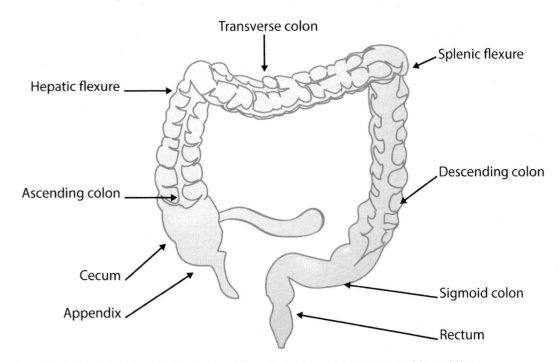

Source: Adapted from National Cancer Institute. Anatomy of colon and rectum (Figure 2). SEER Training Modules. Available at:

http://commons.wikimedia.org/wiki/File:Illu_colorectal_anatomy.jpg.

Colon Cancer

Large intestine, large bowel, and colon are synonymous. Researchers often refer to cancer of the colon and rectum (last part of the large intestine) as *colorectal cancer*. In this discussion, colon cancer refers to the entire large intestine.

Worldwide, colon cancer is the third most common cause of cancer. Over a lifetime, nearly 5 percent of Americans receive a diagnosis of colorectal cancer. Chances of survival are good if treatment begins before the cancer has spread outside the colon.[32]

Risk factors for colon cancer include tobacco, excessive alcohol intake, being overweight and obese, high intake of red and processed meat and fat, and a low intake of fruits, vegetables, and whole grains. Signs and symptoms don't occur until the tumor causes bleeding or becomes large enough to change bowel habits, resulting in persistent diarrhea, constipation, or narrow caliber stool. Other symptoms include belly pain, fatigue, weakness, and unintended weight loss.

This chest X-ray shows a lung cancer—the white mass outlined by the box.

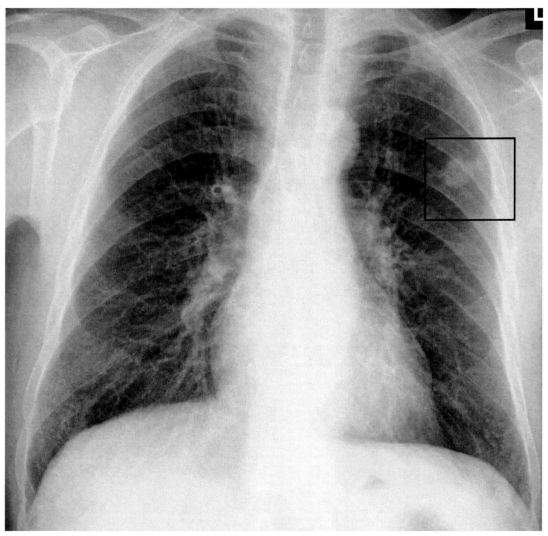

Source: Lange123. 2004. Available at: http://commons.wikimedia.org/wiki/File:Thorax_pa_peripheres_Bronchialcarcinom_li_OF_markiert.jpg.

Lung Cancer

This kind of cancer begins in the cells that line the airways (bronchi and bronchioles) and the tiny air sacs (alveoli). There are two main types: small cell and non–small cell lung cancer. The latter constitutes about 90 percent of lung cancers.

The main risk by far is smoking tobacco—both active and passive smoking (breathing other people's smoke). The other risks are radiation treatment to the chest and exposure to radon (a naturally occurring radioactive from rocks and soil), asbestos (a group of naturally occurring minerals used in some building materials [e.g., insulation] and motor vehicle breaks), and diesel exhaust. Public health efforts to discourage smoking have led to a decline in lung cancer rates.

Symptoms don't develop until the cancer has become advanced and include shortness of breath, wheezing, coughing up blood, and chest pain. No affordable screening tools diagnose the condition early. Chest X-rays can detect larger masses but do not reduce the risk of death. Newer imaging studies for lung cancer are in development. Despite the fact that prognosis is often poor at the time of diagnosis, some people do survive.

Breast Cancer

After skin cancer, breast cancer is the most commonly diagnosed cancer in women and the second leading cause of cancer death in women. About 12 percent of women born today will receive a breast cancer diagnosis sometime during their lives.[33] That's one in eight women. The average age of diagnosis is 61. The odds of survival are over 98 percent if the cancer hasn't yet spread.

Risks factors for breast cancer include a personal or family history of breast or ovarian cancer, especially if diagnosed in first-degree relatives (mother, sister, and daughter) before the age of 50. Greater lifetime exposure to estrogen contributes not just to breast cancer but also to tumors in the female reproductive organs. Estrogen is essential for the development, function, and maintenance of the breasts and reproductive organs. It also keeps bones strong and promotes a healthy cardiovascular system. The risk comes in stimulating cell division, including the division of cancers that are sensitive to estrogen.

Women who start menstruating early (before age 12) and enter menopause relatively late (after 55) generate more estrogen. Pregnancy before age 30 and breast-feeding protect women from breast cancer because they reduce the total number of menstrual cycles and therefore the total estrogen exposure. Studies vary as to whether oral contraceptives, which suppress the natural monthly peak in estrogen, cause a slight increased risk or actually protect women against breast cancer.[34] Estrogen replacement after menopause raises the risk. Being overweight and obese, especially just before and after menopause, is a risk because fat cells can make estrogen.

Diet affects breast cancer risk, in part by its effects on estrogen and other hormones that stimulate cell division. As mentioned, even moderate consumption of alcohol elevates breast cancer risk. So do high-fat diets and greater consumption of animal products.[35]

On the other hand, high-fiber, low-fat, plant-based diets appear protective. Consuming more phytoestrogens (plant estrogens) before menopause reduces risk. That's because phytoestrogens compete with more potent human estrogens in the body, thereby diminishing the effects of the latter. Sources include soybeans and other legumes, whole grains, flaxseeds, sesame seeds, and pomegranate seeds.

Physical activity is also protective. Women who exercise for about two hours a day, regardless of the intensity, are 30 percent less likely to develop breast cancer.[36] For more information on assessing your breast cancer risk, check out this tool on the National Cancer Institute's website: http://www.cancer.gov/bcrisktool.

While breast cancer mainly strikes women, the disease occurs in men too. According to the ACS, each year there are over 2,000 new cases of male breast cancer and 410 deaths.[37] Risk factors include a history of an undescended testicle or testicular disease, older age, significant radiation to the chest, obesity, heavy drinking, liver disease, use of estrogen-like drugs (a treatment for prostate cancer), and a family history of male or female breast cancer. Sadly, some men, upon noticing a breast mass, delay treatment due to feelings of shame about having a "female condition."

2.2 Female Reproductive Cancers

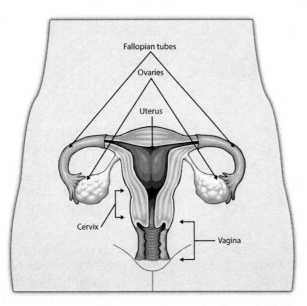

Source: Adapted from Centers for Disease Control. 2008. Available at: http://commons.wikimedia.org/wiki/File:Scheme_female_reproductive_system-en.svg.

The female reproductive tract includes the ovaries, fallopian tubes, uterus, and vagina. Although cancer can occur anywhere, the most affected areas are the cervix (opening to the vagina), uterus, and ovaries. As with breast cancer, greater lifetime exposure to estrogen increases the risk of these estrogen-sensitive organs.

Cervical Cancer

The cervix is the end of the uterus, where it opens into the vagina. Worldwide, cervical cancer ranks as the third most common cancer in women.[38] Each year in the United States, over 12,000 women receive a diagnosis of cervical cancer and over 4,000 women die. The main risk is sexual activity, with transmission of more aggressive strains of human papillomavirus (HPV). HPV, the most common sexually transmitted virus, is considered the cause of cervical cancers. Other risks include greater lifetime exposure to estrogen, multiple sexual partners, smoking, and immunosuppressive drugs or diseases. Regular screening tests can catch the disease early. When cervical cancer hasn't spread, the survival is excellent. The abnormal tissue is destroyed with intense heat or cold, laser, or surgery.

Ovarian Cancer

A woman's two ovaries contain ova (eggs) and manufacture estrogen and progesterone. Each year in the United States, over 22,000 new cases of ovarian cancer are diagnosed and 15,500 women die. Risks include a family history of breast or ovarian cancer. Some women carry genes (BRCA1 and BRCA2) that increase the risk of both cancers. Other risks include smoking, obesity, diabetes, having polycystic ovarian syndrome (which leads to abnormal hormone levels), not having or not breast-feeding children, and taking estrogen without progesterone after menopause. Oral contraceptives protect women against this cancer.[39]

Symptoms don't occur until the tumor becomes large enough to cause vague symptoms such as pressure in the lower abdomen, bloating, a full feeling soon after eating, pelvic or back pain, constipation or diarrhea, frequent urination, and fatigue. Regular pelvic exams are recommended, though they aren't sensitive at detecting this cancer. Women at high risk are recommended to have periodic ultrasound exams and bloods for the tumor marker cancer antigen 125 (CA 125).

Uterine Cancer

The uterus (womb) is the hollow, muscular organ inside of which the fetus develops. This cancer is more properly called endometrial cancer, because it begins in the endometrium or lining of the uterine cavity. According to the ACS, more than 47,000 cases of uterine cancer are diagnosed each year. Risks include advancing age, greater lifetime exposure to estrogen, and obesity (especially in the abdomen). Oral contraceptives are protective. After menopause, giving progesterone with estrogen protects against the development of uterine cancer. Uterine bleeding or spotting after menopause is a warning sign. Others include pelvic pain and pain with sexual intercourse and urination. If endometrial cancer is caught and treated early, survival rates are excellent.

2.3 Male Reproductive Cancers

Prostate Cancer

A man's prostate gland encircles the urethra just below the bladder. It makes fluids that nourish the sperm. After skin cancer, prostate cancer is the most commonly diagnosed cancer in men and the second leading cause of cancer deaths in men. The rate of diagnosis over a lifetime is just over 16 percent, or one in six men.[40] Most men with prostate cancer have a good prognosis for survival with adequate treatment. Overall, the risk of dying is about 3 percent. Some cases are, however, more aggressive. Black men, however, are more likely to be diagnosed when the cancer is more advanced and twice as likely to die of the disease than white men.

Other risks include family history, older age (it's rare before age 40), obesity, and higher consumption of meat and high-fat dairy products. Plant-based diets may decrease risk. Asian men have a much lower incidence of prostate cancer than Western men, which has been linked to a greater consumption of soy foods and green tea.[41],[42] Prostate cancer is more common in men living in higher latitudes, where the skin produces no vitamin D in response to UV radiation during the winter months.[43] Vitamin D insufficiency increases the risk of prostate cancer. One reason black men face a higher death rate may be because they are more at risk for vitamin D insufficiency than white men. Whether supplementation will lower the risk or aid treatment is under investigation.[44]

Until it spreads to other tissues, prostate cancer causes no symptoms unless it narrows the urethra (making urination more difficult) or releases blood into the urine.

Video Clip 16.1

Prostate Cancer

In this short video, Dr. Rajaratnam distinguishes prostate cancer from benign prostatic hyperplasia and explains how prostate cancer spreads.

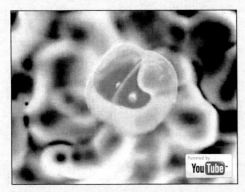

View the video online at: http://www.youtube.com/v/7YA1fumPaf0

Testicular Cancer

The testicles (also called testes) manufacture sperm and testosterone. Testicular cancer is the most common cancer in men between ages 15 and 39. However, this cancer can strike men of any age. While it's not a common cancer, the incidence has risen in the past 40 years. Scientists aren't sure why. Currently, 1 in 268 men develop testicular cancer during their lives. In 2013, an estimated 7,920 men will receive a diagnosis and 370 will die. Compared to white men, the condition is five times more common in black men and three times more common in Asian-American men. Fortunately, treatment is usually successful.

A key risk factor is having a history of one or two undescended testicles. (During fetal development, the testes start out in the abdominal cavity and, before birth, drop into the scrotal sacs.) Other risks include a personal or family history of cancer in the other testicle. Higher dietary consumption of red meat, fat, and milk and low intake of fiber, fruits, and vegetables have been linked to testicular cancer.[45] Entering puberty at a later age is associated with a lower risk.[46]

Signs of this cancer include enlargement of one testicle; a small, hard, painless lump; a feeling of heaviness in one testicle; and a dull ache in the groin. See the sidebar "Testicular Self-Exam" in Section 3. If testicular cancer is caught early, it can be cured with surgery to remove the cancerous testicle. For more aggressive tumors, chemotherapy or radiation therapy is usually recommended.

Bladder Cancer

The bladder is the reservoir for urine, storing it until you can conveniently find a restroom. The biggest risk for bladder cancer is smoking. Chemicals used as dyes (including dark hair dyes), in printing, and in the manufacture of leather, rubber, and paint can cause bladder cancer. Exposure to diesel fumes may put truck drivers at risk. Arsenic in drinking water and not drinking enough fluids also play a role. This cancer is more common in men than in women and in whites than in other races. If you notice a change in bladder habits (blood in the urine, burning with urination, and urinating more often and with a sense of urgency), contact your health care provider. Bladder infections and other benign conditions cause similar symptoms. Either way, diagnosis and treatment is in order.

Pancreatic Cancer

The pancreas is located behind the stomach. It makes the hormone insulin, which is secreted into the blood, and digestive enzymes, which are secreted into the small intestine. Pancreatic cancer is the fourth leading cause of cancer deaths and, because it's difficult to detect early, is one of the deadliest cancers. Risk factors include tobacco use, obesity, and chronic pancreatitis (long-term inflammation of the pancreas). Symptoms, which occur late in the disease, include jaundice (yellowing of the skin and eyes because of a buildup of bilirubin), back or abdominal pain, appetite loss, unintended weight loss, diabetes, and problems digesting foods, especially fatty foods.

Central Nervous System Tumors

These tumors involve the brain, spinal cord, and the membranes (meninges) encircling them. You often see the words "brain tumor" rather than "brain cancer" because some of the abnormal growths are benign rather than malignant. The tumors are named after the type of cell they arise from in the central nervous system.

Some of these tumors have a hereditary component, but most do not. Radiation exposure, usually from treating other cancers of the head or neck, represents a risk. As mentioned, the potential hazards of electromagnetic radiation, including cell phones, is still under investigation, as are chemicals used in the petrochemical industry.

Symptoms and signs, which depend on the size and location of the tumor, include new onset of headaches, seizures, problems speaking or thinking, personality changes, muscle weakness or paralysis, and loss of sensory perceptions such as vision or hearing.

No screening tests for central nervous system tumors exist. If suspicious symptoms or signs occur, imaging tests (brain scans) can reveal changes in the normal anatomy. Treatment depends on the characteristics of the tumor.

KEY TAKEAWAYS

- Skin cancer is by far the most common cancer. The three main types are basal cell carcinoma (the most common), squamous cell carcinoma, and melanoma (the most deadly).
- The most common cancer in women is breast cancer.
- The most common cancer in men is prostate cancer.
- The most common cancer in young men is testicular cancer.
- Lung cancer causes the most cancer-related deaths.
- For most cancers, signs and symptoms of the disease do not occur until the tumor is large enough to interfere with normal bodily functions or has spread to distant locations.

DISCUSSION QUESTIONS

1. What is the biggest risk factor for skin cancer?
2. Why does lifetime exposure to estrogen affect breast cancer and female reproductive cancers? What factors increase cumulative estrogen levels?
3. What are the risk factors for testicular cancer?
4. Go to the WebMD Cancer Risk Health Check at http://www.webmd.com/cancer/health-check-cancer-risk/default.htm. Follow all the steps. Watch and listen to videos about particular risks. Read "your health summary." Write down any cancers for which you're at above average risk and any risk factors you could change. Write down any questions you missed on the "test your knowledge" slide. Why was your answer wrong?

3. DETECTING, DIAGNOSING, AND TREATING CANCER

LEARNING OBJECTIVES

1. Identify key cancer screening tests.
2. Review diagnostic tools used to confirm the presence of cancer and stage its severity.

For most cancers, early detection and treatment is the ideal. That's because, with time, many cancers become bigger, more invasive, and more likely to metastasize. And the more the cancer has spread, the more difficult it is to eradicate. Diagnosis confirms positive screening tests, identifies the type of cancer, pinpoints the primary tumor, and assesses the stage of progression. Treatment methods attempt to remove cancerous cells and prevent *recurrences* (signs that the cancer has come back).

3.1 Screening Tests

The goal of routine screening tests is to catch cancer long before symptoms begin. Often, symptoms don't appear at all until the cancer has become large and has spread to distant tissues.

Screening tests need to have a good risk-to-benefit ratio. In other words, the potential physical or psychological harm of the test is low and the chances of ultimately reducing illness and death high. The test should be affordable (or at least covered by insurance) and readily accessible. The test should also be sensitive (not miss many cases of that cancer) and specific (not identify conditions other than that type of cancer). A false negative test means the lab reports that there isn't cancer when really there is. A false positive test means the report indicates a high likelihood of cancer when no cancer exists. No test is perfect. Because of perceived flaws, some tests have become controversial.

Unfortunately, fear represents a barrier to screening tests for cancer. Some people don't want to find out they have cancer. Plus some exams—fiber-optic exams of the intestinal tract, pelvic exams in women, digital rectal exams of the prostate for men—are more invasive. Nevertheless, for most cancers, early diagnosis and treatment can save lives. And treatment of cancer at early stages is less extensive.

Skin Cancer

You can screen yourself for this cancer by paying attention to changes in your scalp and skin, including your lips, ears, palms, soles, and under your nails. Your health practitioner should also inspect the skin all over your body during regular physical exams. He or she can create a "mole map" to help spot the development of new moles.

Signs of basal cell and squamous cell carcinoma are a new and persistent bump, crusty lesion, or sore that bleeds easily (and wasn't caused by trauma). Learn the pattern of freckles and moles. If a freckle or mole changes color, shape, or size, make an appointment to see your dermatologist (skin specialist) or family doctor. Most moles occur within the first 20 to 30 years of life. After that, new moles raise concerns about melanoma.

The acronym ABCDE provides a useful mnemonic for other warning signs of melanoma.

- **Asymmetry.** Compared to moles (which are benign), melanomas have irregular shapes.
- **Borders.** Moles have discrete edges. The edges of melanomas can be ragged or blurred.
- **Color.** Moles are usually a uniform color of brown. Melanomas can have red, pink, tan, blue, brown, and black coloration.
- **Diameter.** Larger size is more ominous. The ACS gives six millimeters (the diameter of a pencil eraser) as the threshold, noting melanomas sometimes are smaller. If you're suspicious, don't wait. Even small melanomas can metastasize.
- **Evolving.** A change in the shape, size, color, elevation (height and texture of the lesion) or new signs such as bleeding indicate danger.

Colon Cancer

An early sign of colon cancer is blood in the stool. Small amounts of blood aren't visible to the naked eye. For that reason, health practitioners use fecal occult blood or fecal immunochemical tests, which screen for any intestinal disorder that causes bleeding. The other test screening tests involve the use of a flexible tube that contains a video camera. *Sigmoidoscopy* examines the lower half of the colon. **Colonoscopy** examines the entire large bowel while the patient is sedated. Another option is *virtual colonoscopy*, which creates a two- or three-dimensional image from either computed tomography (CT), which uses X-rays, or magnetic resonance imaging (MRI), which uses a powerful magnet. For these procedures, patients need to fast and take laxatives to clear out the intestines beforehand.

While virtual colonoscopy is less invasive, sigmoidoscopy and colonoscopy allow the surgeon to remove precancerous lesions called polyps. A study found that examining the colon and removing precancerous lesions did, in fact, prevent colon cancer from occurring and reduced deaths from colon cancer.[47]

The ACS recommends a baseline colon examination at age 50, earlier if an individual is at higher risk. If the first test is normal, flexible sigmoidoscopy and virtual colonoscopy are repeated every 5

FIGURE 16.2

The ABCD system for recognizing melanoma. The right column contains photographs of normal moles. The left column illustrates, from top to bottom, asymmetry, irregular borders, unusual color variation, and enlarging diameter. The images don't capture the idea of changes in a lesion with time (and therefore lack the E for evolving).

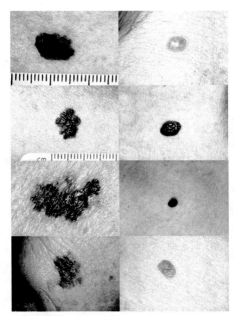

Source: Stevenfruitsmaak. 2008. Available at:
http://commons.wikimedia.org/wiki/
File:Melanoma_vs_normal
_mole_ABCD_rule_NCI_Visuals_Online.jpg.

colonoscopy

A visual examination of the colon (large bowel) with a flexible tube that contains a video camera.

years; colonoscopy is repeated at 10-year intervals. Tests for fecal blood occur with the annual physical exam.

Breast Cancer

Screening tests include a breast self-exam, clinical breast exam (done by a health practitioner), and mammography (a low-energy X-ray of the breasts) and other imaging tests. The use and timing of these tests have become controversial. Nevertheless, most experts agree that early detection improves survival and that the benefits increase with age, peaking during a woman's seventh decade.

For years, organizations such as the ACS have recommended annual screening with physical exams and **mammograms** beginning at age 40. In 2009, the US Preventive Services Task Force (USPSTF) issued the following recommendations: (1) Women without elevated risks should delay screening mammography until age 50; (2) if that baseline test is normal, screenings should only be repeated every two years until age 74.[48] The USPSTF argued that false positive tests (e.g., the mammogram shows an abnormality that is not cancer) lead to psychological harm and unnecessary testing, including biopsies. Furthermore, women over age 74 with positive tests may be subjected to treatment for a cancer that would not lead to serious symptoms or premature death. The agency also recommended against breast self-exam, noting that such exams don't prolong women's lives.

Not surprisingly, the USPSTF recommendation ignited a firestorm among the medical community. One, we lack better screening tests. Two, some studies have reaffirmed the value of mammography beginning at age 40. For instance, a 2011 Swedish study found that the benefit of mammography increased over time, with a 30 percent reduction in breast cancer mortality at the 15-year mark.[49]

The ACS continues to recommend mammograms and physical exams every one to two years beginning at age 40 and continuing as long as women are "in good health."[50] Women in their 20s and 30s are advised to have breast exams every three years. Women 20 and up should also do their own breast self-exams every month.

Women at high risk for cancer (close relative with breast cancer, carry the BRCA1 or BRCA2 gene mutation, personal history of breast cancer, and history of chest radiation therapy) are recommended to begin yearly screening at age 30 with both a magnetic resonance image (MRI) breast exam and a mammogram.

Genetic testing is recommended for certain populations, particularly Ashkenazi Jews, who are more likely to carry mutations of two genes related to breast and ovarian cancer: BRCA1 and BRCA2. Other groups have also been known to carry these mutations. The National Cancer Institute recommends women who descended from Ashkenazi Jews with any family history of breast or ovarian cancer to be tested. For women who are not of Ashkenazi Jewish descent, testing is recommended if they have a strong family history of breast and/or ovarian cancer or a blood relative known to carry either abnormal gene.[51]

This picture of a colon polyp was taken during a colonoscopy. Doctors usually remove the polyp and check for cancer cells in the tissue.

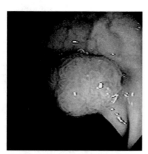

Source: Holland S. 2006. Available at: http://commons.wikimedia.org/wiki/File:Polyp.jpeg.

mammogram

An image of the breasts obtained by a low-dose X-ray technique called mammography.

Breast Self-Exam

Many doctors encourage women to examine their own breasts once a month. In that way, women become familiar with the normal appearance and texture of their breasts and can report changes to their primary care practitioners. A good time is after a menstrual period.

Start out by sitting or standing before a mirror with your hands on your hips. Check for a change in symmetry. It's normal for one breast to be a bit larger than the other. Raise your arms over your head and inspect your breasts again. If you see dimpling, puckering, or uneven texture or shape, consider them signs worth discussing with your doctor. Look and feel for any lumps in your armpits.

The next part is easiest to do while lying down. With your right hand behind your head, use the finger pads of your left hand to examine your right breast. Using small circular movements, start in the armpit and move up and down vertically until you reach the middle of your breastbone. Move with slow but firm pressure. Feel the hollow space above and below your collarbone. You're looking for new lumps. Gently squeeze the nipple. A tiny bit of clear discharge is normal; blood-tinged or yellowish discharge is not. Repeat on the other side.

Video Clip 16.2

How to Perform a Breast Self-Exam
A video featuring Laura Kruper, MD.

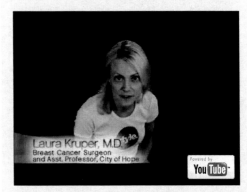

View the video online at: http://www.youtube.com/v/Ple5EJHmwqM

Cervical Cancer

The main screening tool is the Papanicolaou test (Pap test or Pap smear) plus or minus DNA tests for HPV strains associated with cervical cancer. These tests are done during a pelvic examination, ideally 10 to 20 days after the first day of the menstrual period. Cells gently scraped from the cervix are sent to the lab. The Pap test identifies precancerous and cancerous cells.

Women are usually screened at age 21. If the test is normal, it is repeated every three years. In the absence of significant risk factors, HPV testing is not added until a woman is 30 or older.[52] If the two tests are given together, repeat testing occurs at five-year intervals.

Testicular Cancer

This type of cancer is usually identified when a man or his doctor feels a lump on the testicle. In addition to routine physical exams, many health care practitioners recommend that teens and men get in the habit of examining their own testes once a month. If you're a guy, here's how.

Testicular Self-Exam

Stand in front of the mirror. A little asymmetry is normal. Often the right testicle is slightly larger than the left. You're looking for changes in color or size.

The next part is easier to do in a warm bath or shower because your scrotum will be relaxed, allowing better examination of the testicles. Soap helps your fingers to glide more easily. Using both hands, roll one testicle between your thumb and fingers with slight pressure. Feel for any lumps or variations in the contour along the front and sides of the testicle. Sometimes these bumps are described as a pea or grain of rice, which may be painless. While these lumps or swellings may not be cancer, they should be checked by your doctor as soon as possible. At the top and back of each testicle is the epididymis, a cord-like structure that transports the sperm. A lump there is usually a benign cyst, but should nonetheless be discussed with your physician.

Video Clip 16.3

How to Perform a Testicular Self-Exam
Phillip Alliotta, MD, explains how to do a testicular self-exam.

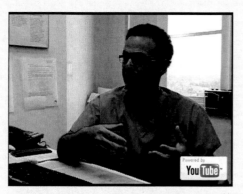

View the video online at: http://www.youtube.com/v/lYipPMweoPM

Prostate Cancer

Blood tests for prostate specific antigen (PSA), a protein unique to the prostate, are a widely used screening test. Other methods include the digital rectal exam (a gloved finger in the rectum feels the back contour of the prostate) and ultrasound exam.

Although the PSA test does detect prostate cancer before symptoms occurs, it has significant drawbacks.

In addition to cancer, other prostate conditions such as benign prostatic hyperplasia (enlargement), prostatitis (inflammation), and trauma increase PSA. In other words, an elevated PSA level isn't specific for prostate cancer. For that reason, positive tests sometimes generate needless anxiety and drive further testing with uncomfortable procedures like prostate biopsy. When prostate cancer is diagnosed, it's often slow growing and would not lead to serious problems or shorten a man's life. Large studies have failed to show that PSA screening saves lives.[53] ,[54] Treatment, on the other hand, risks surgical complications such as erectile dysfunction, urinary incontinence, and blood clots.

In 2011, the USPSTF recommended against routine PSA screening in men.[55] The rationale is that most cases don't occur until after age 50 and that most deaths don't occur until after age 75.[56] Also, the screening benefit for men over age 70 is zero; for men 50 to 59, the benefit is "small to none."

Other professional organizations disagree. The ACS recommends most men discuss prostate cancer screening with their doctors starting at age 50.[57] Black men (who are at higher risk) and men with a family history should meet with their doctors starting at age 45. The American Urological Association recommends men 40 years old and up begin screening on the grounds that prostate cancer doesn't cause symptoms until advanced stages when treatment success dwindles.[58]

Until more accurate screening tests become available, men need to make informed decisions with their doctors. New research suggests hope for an investigational urine test, which screens for markers of faulty genes present in over half of prostate cancers.[59]

Bladder Cancer

Urinalysis (examination of a urine specimen) can detect even microscopic amounts of blood. In addition to cancer, other conditions, particularly bladder infections, can also release blood. Cells in the urine can also be examined under the microscope. Newer tests are being developed to detect markers unique to bladder cancers. If cancer is suspected, cystoscopy and biopsy can confirm the diagnosis. The cystoscope is a thin tube with a video camera on one end that's inserted via the urethra.

3.2 Diagnosis

If screening tests indicate cancer, imaging studies include an ultrasound (the use of sound waves to visualize tissues), computed tomography (CT), or magnetic resonance imaging (MRI) to localize and determine the size and shape of the tumor(s). Physicians also use fiber-optic scopes (flexible tubes with an eye piece a one end and a lens at the other) to view the inside of hollow organs such as the gastrointestinal tract, urinary tract, and female reproductive tract.

The next step is usually **biopsy**, the removal of tissue. Samples of the tumor are usually taken with needles or scalpels. The tissue is then usually sent to a specialist called a *pathologist* to learn about the type and nature of the cancer.

For some cancers, the doctor may also sample tissue from nearby lymph nodes, to determine whether the cancer has already entered the lymph system. Other tests include examining tumor cells for particular markers. For instance, breast cancers cells that still have receptors (structures on the cell) that bind estrogen. In that case, drugs that block the receptors may decrease tumor growth. The data from the tests provides information on the size and location of the primary (original) tumor, the appearance of the cancer cells, involvement of lymph nodes, and evidence of metastasis. An **oncologist** (cancer specialist) then stages the cancer. **Staging** involves categorizing the cancer's severity from least to most advanced. It indicates the *prognosis* (the likely course of the illness) and the direction treatment should take. If the tumor is relatively small, localized (hasn't invaded neighboring tissues and lymph nodes), and shows no sign of metastasis, the prognosis is usually good.

3.3 Treatment

For slow-growing cancers, **watchful waiting** may be recommended. This strategy has become more common with prostate cancer, with sound results.[60] If biopsies and other tests indicate the cancer is not aggressive, a doctor may recommend periodic exams and/or repeat diagnostic testing to track the cancer's development. Aggressive treatment (with some combination of surgery, radiation, and medications to suppress male hormone production) is reserved for more advanced cancer, particularly in younger men.

For cancers that are more aggressive or that are otherwise likely to cause serious symptoms or shorten a person's life, the objective is to treat during the early stages. The goal of all treatment is to destroy cancer cells. Unfortunately, normal cells suffer too. Depending on the type and stage of the cancer, one or more treatments may be used. The three main treatment types are surgery, chemotherapy, and radiation therapy. The ultimate goal is putting the disease into long-term *remission*, a state in which no signs or symptoms of the cancer remain.

Surgery is often the first line of treatment. The lesion is removed by cutting it out (excision) or using extreme heat or extreme cold to destroy the abnormal tissue. Sometimes precancerous lesions can be eradicated, as is the case with suspicious-looking lesions on the skin, cervix, or in the colon. For cancers in their early stages, surgical excision may be all that's necessary. For others, radiation therapy and/or chemotherapy may precede or follow surgery, to increase the chances of destroying the cancer.

Radiation therapy uses high-energy (ionizing) radiation to shrink or eradicate cancers or to reduce symptoms caused by tumors. It can be used alone or in combination with surgery and/or chemotherapy. An external beam of radiation can be focused on a tumor. Radioactive material can also be implanted in or near the tumor. Sometimes radioactive agents are injected into the blood. For instance, radioactive iodine is given by injection. Because only the thyroid gland takes up iodine, cancer of that gland can be treated without widespread damage.

Side effects depend on the type of radiation therapy, dosage of radiation, and the location of the tumor. Some tissues are more sensitive than others. If the gonads (testes and ovaries) are exposed, infertility could result. Radiation to the intestinal tract can lead to bleeding and diarrhea. Skin can become inflamed. Injured tissue can form scar tissue. Radiation therapy early in life raises the risk of cancers in sensitive tissues that were exposed.

Chemotherapy ("chemo") involves the use of drugs to destroy the cancer cells, slow tumor growth, relieve symptoms caused by the tumor, or prevent invasion and metastasis. Often, the goal is to kill any cells surgery or radiation therapy didn't remove. It may also be used when surgery isn't feasible or to shrink a tumor before attacking it with surgery and radiation therapy. The drugs may be injected or swallowed. Doses are repeated daily, weekly, or monthly.

Many of these medicines target any rapidly dividing cell, which includes cancer cells, hair follicles, bone marrow, and those lining the intestinal tract. Side effects vary according to the medication and include discomfort at the injection site, nausea, vomiting, diarrhea, constipation, decreased appetite, muscle aches, hair loss, anemia, immune suppression, nerve tingling or numbness, and difficulty thinking and remembering. Some people have few side effects.

Hormone therapy is used in cancers such as prostate and breast cancer. Because testosterone fuels prostate cancer, drugs can be given to reduce blood levels of that hormone. Drugs can interfere with the production or estrogen and the ability of estrogen to stimulate breast cancer cells to divide.

Newer, more specific drugs are in various stages of development. For instance, some drugs can inhibit enzymes involved in cellular proliferation or stimulate those that cause cell death. Medications such as bevacizumab are antibodies against molecules that stimulate angiogenesis. Other new drugs inhibit molecular pathways involved in creating these new blood vessels. Either way, the goal is to cut off the tumor's blood supply, a strategy akin to laying siege to an enemy city.

biopsy

Removal of tissue for examination and analysis.

oncologist

A doctor specializing in cancer treatment.

staging

Determining the severity of the cancer.

radiation therapy

The use of high-energy radiation to damage cancer cells.

chemotherapy

The use of strong drugs to treat cancer.

Other immune-based treatments (*immunotherapy*) are being researched that would target cancer cells. Some carry chemotherapeutic drugs to the cancer cell. That means the chemo only kills the cancer cells and spares normal cells. For example, Herceptin (trastuzumab) contains antibodies to a breast cancer cells that carry a particular protein on their surfaces, thereby halting uncontrolled cell division. Immunotherapy could also be used to suppress processes that allow cancers to grow or to enhance the immune system tumor-fighting abilities. Custom-tailored antibodies could directly attack an individual's cancer cells.

Another experimental treatment is *gene therapy*, which would be of particular advantage for cancers caused by genetic defects. In this type of therapy, harmful genes could be silenced, protective genes could be turned on, and normal genes (delivered via microorganisms such as a harmless virus) could replace defective genes.

3.4 Living with Cancer

Having cancer is stressful for the individual and his or her close relatives and friends. People need to educate themselves about their treatment options, so they can make informed decisions with health care providers. There may be lots of tests, surgery, chemotherapy, radiation therapy, and follow-up appointments to check for recurrence. It's like running a marathon. All the elements vital for good health become even more important now: good nutrition, physical activity as much as possible, ample rest and sleep, the comfort of loved ones, and the sustenance of spiritual activities, whether they're religious or spending time watching the birds in your garden.

It helps to remain both hopeful and realistic. We've come a long way in treating cancer. Millions of cancer survivors can attest to that. Optimism, gratitude, and other positive traits buoy us up in troubled times. As with any chronic illness, people may bridle at becoming labeled—the leukemic or the breast or prostate cancer patient. Cancer should not eclipse an individual. Many people continue to work, raise families, create art, and compete athletically. For instance, hockey legend Mario Lemieux was diagnosed with Hodgkin's lymphoma. He survived the cancer and founded the Mario Lemieux foundation, which funds cancer research.[61]

Social support is tremendously important. In the mid-1980s, researchers demonstrated that women with breast cancer who perceived they had adequate social support survived significantly longer than those who didn't.[62] Many subsequent studies followed, though, once the word got out, it became difficult to find volunteers for the control group (no social support). Friends, family, and support groups of other cancer survivors all lighten the load. People with cancer who were previously unaccustomed to asking for help have a chance to learn to speak up and to receive assistance and encouragement. Those who care want to know how to assist, whether it's shopping, preparing meals, driving to appointments, giving a hug, listening, being the cheerleader, or delivering comic relief.

Sometimes the hardest thing is dealing with emotions. An overriding response to the word *cancer* is fear. It's a brutal reminder of the fact that we are all mortal. Many of us fear our death and the deaths of those we love. Upon hearing a cancer diagnosis, many people also become apprehensive about the treatment. People can become more upset about possibly losing their hair (even though many treatments don't cause hair loss) than about the cancer. In other words, the experience can be scary.

While cancer isn't a death sentence, news of a diagnosis causes many people to contemplate their mortality. In the late 1960s, psychiatrist Elisabeth Kübler-Ross, MD, described five emotional stages of grief many people pass through upon learning they have a life-altering or potentially life-threatening illness. Any life-altering event—a romantic breakup, receiving news that a loved one is seriously ill or injured, and so on—can trigger a similar sequence of emotions. In Kübler-Ross's work with dying patients, the pattern was often as follows:

1. **Denial.** "This isn't happening to me." "I am not ill." "I'm fine."
2. **Anger.** "Why did this happen to me? It's not fair. I didn't smoke. I ate vegetables." Blame comes in too. "I'm sick because this city is polluted, my boss stressed me out, and my mother fed me hotdogs."
3. **Bargaining.** "I just need some more time." "If I exercise every day, maybe nothing will happen." "If I do whatever the doctor says, could I just make it through till my grandchild is born?"
4. **Depression.** "Nothing matters anymore. What's the point in trying?"
5. **Acceptance.** This stage is where most of us would like to reach (and preferably long before we die), a place where we calmly, gracefully accept reality and make the best of every remaining moment. Often the dying person reaches this sweet surrender before his or her family members.

Surprisingly, many people are able to find the silver lining of a serious disease. A normal human response to any kind of malaise is to focus on what doesn't feel good. Unpleasant bodily sensations are designed to get our attention, to make us take care of ourselves. Once we've done what we need to do, we can shift our focus to all the body parts (and parts of our lives) that are functioning well. Doing so relieves distress. You can apply that principle to physical, emotional, social, financial, or spiritual afflictions. Illness causes some people to become more appreciative of all the good in their lives. They're grateful to have time to make wills, draw up advance directives (a written declaration of desires about medical treatment), make amends, right wrongs, forgive, and generally get their lives in order. Every moment becomes precious. People may transform their lives, and often the lives of those witnessing that metamorphosis.

On the other hand, there's no denying that aggressive cancers can cause pain and suffering. That's where **palliative care** comes in. Physicians, nurses, social workers, and other health specialists provide treatment aimed at relieving discomfort and distress. For patients nearing the end of life, **hospice care** shifts the goal from trying to cure the disease to improving quality of life, from extending life to creating a "good death." A team of specialists provides not just palliative care but multifaceted, compassionate support to patients and families.

palliative care

Health care aimed at reducing discomfort and distress.

hospice care

Compassionate end-of-life support to patients and their families.

KEY TAKEAWAYS

- Routine screening tests are designed to detect diseases at an early stage, often before symptoms begin.
- Sometimes authoritative organizations in the United States disagree about the timing or use of cancer screening tests. In that case, patients need to make informed decisions with their health care practitioners.
- For most cancers, early diagnosis and treatment improves the odds of survival.
- When a screening test is positive for cancer, diagnosis is confirmed with imaging tests, biopsies, and analysis of samples from the tumor.
- Diagnostic information allows oncologists to stage the tumor.
- Treatment varies depending on the type and stage of cancer. Common treatments include surgery, chemotherapy, and radiation therapy.
- A cancer diagnosis can trigger a complex sequence of emotions for the person with cancer and his or her loved ones. Social support is particularly important.
- Palliative care is used to decrease discomfort and increase quality of life. Hospice care provides compassionate end-of-life support to patients and their families.

DISCUSSION QUESTIONS

1. Which cancer screening tests should you get? How often should you get them? Of those tests, which have you actually had? Which have you missed? Do you plan to schedule an appointment with your student health center or family doctor?
2. What is the controversy surrounding breast self-exams and mammograms?
3. What are the weaknesses of the PSA test?
4. Have you ever had a life-altering event that caused you to experience Elisabeth Kübler-Ross's stages of grief? Describe the event and the emotions you had.

4. PREVENTING CANCER

LEARNING OBJECTIVE

1. **Learn how to prevent cancer by reducing or eliminate modifiable risk factors.**

Cancer is largely preventable. Because cancer takes 20 to 30 years to develop to an appreciable mass, the earlier prevention begins the better.

4.1   Reduce Known Risk Factors

Earlier in this chapter, we reviewed causes and risk factors for cancer. Your goal is to focus on reducing or eliminating the modifiable risks.

- **Stay away from tobacco smoke.** If you smoke, refer to Chapter 11 for resources for quitting.

- **Limit your alcohol intake.** According to the American Cancer Society (ACS), women should have no more than one drink a day and men should not exceed two. If you have a family history of breast cancer, you may choose not to drink at all. If you think you might have a problem with alcohol, contact your student health center or primary care doctor.

- **Protect your skin from ultraviolet radiation.** For practical tips, see "Making Sense of Sunscreens"

  One problem with avoiding the sun is that ultraviolet (UV) light stimulates vitamin D production in the skin. This vitamin seems to bolster immune system function and to protect people against cancer. Cancer develops more often in people living at higher latitudes, where winter sunlight is too weak to stimulate the skin's vitamin D production.[63] Low levels correlate with an increased risk of cancers of the colon, prostate, breast, and ovary.[64]

  However, it doesn't take long for your skin to produce plenty of vitamin D. If you're wearing a bathing suit, a single 20-minute exposure to summer sun produces 15,000 to 20,000 international units (IU) of vitamin D.[65] Compared to fair-skinned people, those with more skin pigmentation require relatively longer exposures to generate vitamin D.

  Alternatively, you can consider supplements. Only a few foods contain significant amounts of vitamin D: oily fish such as salmon and mackerel, egg yolks, liver, and fortified milk and orange juice. The Institute of Medicine (IOM) recommends 600 IU for people 1 to 70, and 800 IU for those older than 70.

- **Maintain a healthy weight.** As noted, being overweight and obese raise the risk of cancer. On the other hand, sustained weight loss can reverse the risk.[66],[67] See Chapter 10 for more information on weight management.

- **Be physically active.** Regular exercise helps maintain a healthy body weight, enhances antitumor immunity, and reduces the risk of some cancers.[68] In lab experiments, increased physical activity slows the growth of established tumors.[69] After a cancer diagnosis, moderate increases in physical activity reduce recurrence, improve function and quality of life, and increase survival.[70],[71],[72] The ACS recommends adults get at least 150 minutes of moderate-intensity exercise or 75 minutes of vigorous intensity exercise a week.

- **Eat a plant-based diet.** Compared to the American diet heavy in processed foods and meats, diets heavy in fruits and vegetables protect people against cancer.[73] Edible plants contain vitamins, minerals, fiber, healthy fats, and antioxidant and anti-inflammatory compounds. Some plant chemicals also promote a healthy immune system. Other plant chemicals are more directly anticancer.

  For example, people who follow a Mediterranean diet seem to have less cancer.[74] This diet is rich in a number of protective foods: vegetables, fruits, grains, legumes, and olive oil, as well as a moderate amount of red wine (which contains the anticancer chemical resveratrol).

- **Get enough sleep.** As mentioned, sleep deprivation and night-shift work raise cancer risks. You know you're sleeping enough if you awaken refreshed and feel alert all day. See Chapter 4 for tips about improving sleep habits.

- **Tame your stress level.** As noted in Chapter 3, the link between chronic stress and development of cancer is hard to pin down. Two things are clear. First, grinding stress suppresses the immune system, which you need to detect and kill cancer cells. Second, stressed-out people often turn to alcohol, tobacco, and junk food, which are all risk factors. Having cancer can be extremely stressful. Social support, relaxation methods, and other stress-relieving behaviors can improve outcomes and quality of life.[75]

- **Ditch plastic water bottles,** unless they promise that they're free of bisphenol A (BPA). Because BPA mimics estrogen, it's called an endocrine disruptor. Exposure early in life poses a risk for breast cancer and other ills.[76] Drink from steel, glass, or ceramic vessels. Store food in glass or ceramic containers.

- **Be wary of cosmetics.** Many chemicals pass readily through the skin (or, with inhalation, the lungs) to enter the blood. Dark hair dyes have been linked with some cancers. Many cosmetics contain phthalates, which disrupt natural hormones. Some nail polish and related products contain phthalates, formaldehyde, and solvents such as toluene and acetone.

- **Get vaccinated against the human papillomavirus (HPV).** The vaccines (Gardasil and Cervarix) target viral strains that most often cause cancer of the cervix, vagina, vulva (external female genitalia), anus, penis, mouth, and throat. HPV-related cancers of the mouth and throat in men and women have increased markedly over the past few years. Vaccines are also available against the hepatitis B virus, which can lead to liver cancer. These vaccines need to be given before exposure. See Chapter 13 for more information about immunizations.

Making Sense of Sunscreens

There's no doubt that ultraviolet radiation emitted from the sun, sunlamps, and tanning beds ages the skin and causes skin cancer. Proper use of sunscreen reduces the risk of sunburn, squamous cell carcinoma, and to a lesser extent, basal cell carcinoma.[77] However, sunscreens, particularly if they don't block UVA rays, do not appear to reduce the risk of melanoma and, may even increase the risk.[78] Sunscreens, especially those promising a high SPF (sun protection factor), provide a false sense of protection from UV light. People who apply them to prolong time outdoors may actually develop more sunburn.[79]

Until recently, sunscreens only needed to provide protection against UVB rays. The rules changed after recognizing that UVA also caused melanoma and other skin cancers. In 2011, the Food and Drug Administration released new label rules on sunscreens, saying they needed to offer at least an SPF of 15, with protection from both UVA and UVB rays, in order to make label claims about protecting against sunburn, premature skin aging, and cancer.

Some of the sunscreen terms deserve some explanation. SPF refers to the amount of UV radiation needed to produce sunburn on protected compared to unprotected skin. The SPF indicates UVB protection. The numbers are misleading. An SPF of 15 filters 94 percent of UVB radiation; and SPF of 30 filters only 3 percent more (97 percent).[80] That means, contrary to myth, you can't stay out in the sun twice as long with an SPF of 30. "Water resistant" means you can be in water 40 minutes before losing the sunscreen. "Very-water-resistant" products (formerly called "waterproof" or "sweatproof") allow for immersions twice that long.

Only a few sunscreen ingredients protect people against UVA: benzophenones (oxybenzone and sulisobenzone), avobenzone (Parsol 1789), ecamsule (Mexoryl), titanium dioxide, and zinc oxide. However even the most effective of these filters—that is, titanium dioxide—blocks only a quarter of UVA radiation.[81] Manufacturers often combine ingredients to improve coverage.

Zinc oxide and titanium dioxide, which are inert minerals, have the advantage of scattering and reflecting UVA and UVB radiation. Some people have aesthetic objections—the visible white smears on skin. More recent products use nano-sized (extremely small, also called micronized) particles, making them invisible on the skin. Micronized titanium dioxide does not completely protect people against UVA. Also, scientists now dispute whether nanoparticles enter skin cells and damage DNA.[82],[83]

Nonmineral agents are less visible but can cause skin allergic reactions. Some (benzophenone, oxybenzone, homosalate, 4-aminobenzoic acid or PABA, and others) may disrupt natural hormones. These chemicals are absorbed into the skin and enter the water supply when we shower and swim. The effect on humans and aquatic life isn't yet clear.[84] Aerosol sprays aren't recommended because of the risk of inhalation. For more information on sunscreen safety, check out the listing on the Environmental Working Group's Skin Deep at http://breakingnews.ewg.org/2012sunscreen.

In these two photographs, the man has sunscreen with an SPF of 50 on the left side of his face. The left photograph is taken in the visible light. The right photograph is taken under an ultraviolet lamp. In that image, the left side of his face appears darker because the sunscreen has absorbed the ultraviolet light waves.

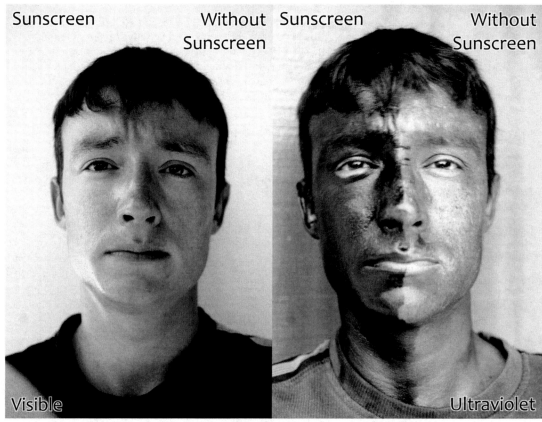

Source: Spigget. 2010. Available at: http://commons.wikimedia.org/wiki/File:UV_and_Vis_Sunscreen.jpg.

Sun Protection Tips

- When possible, avoid the intense midday sun (10 a.m. to 4 p.m.), particularly during summer months. Stay indoors, seek shade, or cover up. Remember that UVA penetrates clouds and glass.
- Cover up. Clothing and broad-brimmed hats are better than sunscreen at protecting your skin. The darker the color and the tighter the weave, the better the protection.
- Fifteen to 30 minutes before you go outdoors (or sit by a window), liberally apply sunscreen that promises UVA and UVB protection with an SPF of 30. One ounce (two tablespoons) usually covers exposed areas. Put on lip balm with sun protection. Reapply sunscreen and lip balm every 2 hours and after you come out of the water.
- Wear sunglasses to protect your eyes. (UV light can burn the eyes and increase the risk of squamous cell carcinoma on the eye's surface cataracts, a cloudiness of the eye's lens.[85])
- Do not use sunscreen to stay outside for prolonged periods. It's better to cover up with a hat and clothes and/or seek shelter. If you're outdoors a lot, consider investing in clothing that effectively blocks UV rays.
- Keep in mind that bright, reflective surfaces (white sand, snow, water, cement) intensify your UV exposure.
- If your skin begins to feel uncomfortable or turn pink, get out of the sun.
- Steer clear of tanning salons. If looking tanned is important to you, consider using a sunless tanning product. Also, keep in mind that a tan is a sign of skin damage, not glowing health.[86] One study found that 41 percent of indoor tanners met criteria for "tanning addictive disorder."[87] If you find you can't resist the urge to visit the tanning salon, contact your doctor.

4.2 Foods That Fight Cancer

In general, adopting a plant-based whole-foods diet and reducing "junk" food intake has several benefits. You're minimizing your exposure to potential carcinogens. Whether or not organically produced foods protect people against cancer isn't yet proven. Some chemicals used in the food industry may directly or indirectly increase cancer risk. Examples include pesticides, herbicides compounds in plastic packaging (bisphenol A [BPA], phthalates), growth hormones, and antibiotics. Foods can also be contaminated by heavy metals. If you're cash strapped, save your money for organic meats, because chemicals concentrate in animal fat. Pesticide and herbicide residues on fruits and vegetables are relatively low. Wash thoroughly before eating.

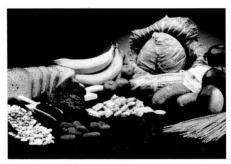

Source: National Cancer Institute. Available at:
http://commons.wikimedia.org/wiki/
File:Fruit,_Vegetables_and_Grain_NCI_Visuals_Online.jpg.

The ACS recommends you eat at least two-and-a-half cups of fruits and vegetables a day, choose whole grains over refined grains, and restrict your intake of meat and processed meat.

When you do eat animal flesh (fish, poultry, pork, or meat), cook with low heat—bake, braise, stew, or poach. Cooking meats at high temperatures by frying, broiling, or grilling can form the potentially carcinogenic substances heterocyclic amines and aromatic hydrocarbons. If you like to grill, reduce the time you subject meat to flames by first partially cooking in the oven or microwave, frequently turning the meat on the grill, and removing the charred portions before serving. High-temperature cooking of vegetables (especially potatoes) can generate the carcinogen acrylamide.[88]

The ACS also advises people to limit portion sizes. In animal studies, restricting calories (while maintaining nutrient intake) reduces cancer risk and generally increases longevity.[89],[90] While there's some evidence calorie restriction early in life can reduce breast cancer risk,[91] the degree of caloric restriction (e.g., a starvation diet) used in lab studies is unlikely to be attractive to most Americans. However, you may not have to go to extremes to see benefits.

Studying the impact of particular foods on cancer is complex. Most of the human studies are observational, meaning they provide evidence for *associations* between various diets and cancer but don't establish cause and effect. Some foods protect people against certain cancers and not others. Some help, but mainly if you consume them when you're young. One general rule is that research is more consistently positive for foods and whole herbs than for isolated phytochemicals (plant chemicals), vitamins, and minerals. In other words, good diet trumps supplements.

Some foods, spices, and herbs stand out as having anticancer ability. Most are rich sources of flavonoids and carotenoids (which reduce, among other functions, oxidation and inflammation—twin processes that promote cancer). Flavonoids belong to a broader chemical group called polyphenols, which provide multiple benefits for plants and those of us who eat them. Here's a partial list of promising foods and herbs:

- **Berries, cherries, and grapes.** The flavonoids that create those blue, red, and purple hues have antioxidant, anti-inflammatory, and anticancer cancer effects.[92],[93],[94] Berries, cherries, and grapes make great snack foods. Add them to smoothies. Top cereal, salads, and yogurt with berries.

- **Pomegranate** has shown promise as an anticancer agent.[95],[96] In men with prostate cancer, drinking eight ounces of pomegranate juice a day significantly slowed the rise in prostate specific antigen, a protein used to track benign and cancerous prostate conditions.[97] All parts of the pomegranate fruit—rind, pith, and juicy seeds—have valuable chemicals. Because commercial juices use the whole fruit, you can consume them all. You can snack on the seeds and add them to salads.

- **Cruciferous vegetables** include broccoli, cauliflower, cabbage, rapini, kale, collards, mustard greens, bok choy, arugula, watercress, and Brussels sprouts. They contain glucosinolates, which the body breaks down into anticancer substances. Animal and population studies link increased consumption of cruciferous vegetables with reduced cancer risk.[98],[99]

- **Orange fruits and vegetables** are rich in plant pigments called carotenoids, which protect people against a number of cancers.[100],[101] In America, tomatoes are a major source of dietary carotenoids such as lycopene. Regular consumption of tomatoes and tomato products has been linked with a reduced risk of prostate cancer[102],[103] and possibly breast cancer.[104],[105] Other foods rich in carotenoids include orange vegetables (carrots, pumpkin, sweet potatoes, winter squash), orange vegetables (cantaloupe, mangos, apricots, guava, goji berries), and dark-green leafy vegetables.

- **Whole grains.** Refined carbohydrates lead to spikes in blood sugar, insulin, and insulin-like growth factors, which can stimulate tumor growth.[106],[107] Whole (unprocessed) grains, legumes, and vegetables contain complex carbohydrates, which digest more slowly and contain fiber. Fiber-rich diets seem to protect people against colon cancer.[108]

- **Legumes** contain fiber and phytoestrogens (plant estrogens). Soybeans are a particularly rich source of phytoestrogens called isoflavones. Because they're weaker than human estrogen, they may lower the risk of estrogen-sensitive cancers. Population studies link higher consumption of soy foods with a reduced incidence of breast,[109] uterine,[110],[111] ovarian,[112],[113] prostate,[114] and colon cancer.[115] Consumption of soy decreases growth factors that increase breast cancer risk.[116] One concern has been whether isoflavones present a risk for breast cancer survivors. Reassuringly, a large study of Chinese and American women found that soy food consumption correlated with a reduced risk of recurrence.[117] While soy foods seem to be safe, some experts discourage against supplementing with soy protein or soy isoflavones.[118]

- **Seeds and nuts** contain vitamins, minerals, healthy fats, and fiber. Greater consumption correlates with a reduced risk of certain cancers, particularly colon cancer. Flaxseeds, sesame seeds, sunflower seeds, and pumpkin contain lignans, which our intestinal bacteria can convert into phytoestrogens.[119],[120] Flaxseeds, the richest source of lignans, inhibit the growth of breast,[121] colon,[122] and prostate cancer.[123]

- **Teas**, whether it's black, green, or oolong, all come from the same plant: *Camellia sinensis*. Population studies link higher tea consumption with a reduced risk of several cancers, including cancer of the bladder, esophagus, colon, pancreas, ovary, breast, and prostate. Green tea is particularly rich in a beneficial polyphenol called epigallocatechin gallate, which inhibits several steps of carcinogenesis and provokes cancer cell death.[124],[125] In general, drinking plenty of fluids like water reduces your risk of bladder cancer.

- **Curried foods** contain the spices turmeric and ginger. Both contain potent anti-inflammatory, antioxidant, and anticancer substances.[126] Curcumin, a chemical in turmeric, inhibits cancer cell growth and migration, blocks the creation of blood vessels to the cancer, and induces cancer cells to die.[127]

- **Garlic** enhances enzymes that detoxify carcinogens, quenches oxidation, inhibits proliferation of cancer cells, induces cancer cell death, and boosts immunity.[128] Populations who regularly eat it have a lower incidence of certain cancers. Because heat deactivates some of garlic's key ingredients, you can add raw, minced garlic to dressings, dips, soups, and sauces. Alternatively, you can crush the garlic, let it sit for 10 minutes (which allows time for critical enzymatic changes), and then add it to the pot after you've turned off the heat.[129]

- **Edible mushrooms** contain polysaccharides and other ingredients that enhance immunity and have anticancer properties.[130] Produce aisles often stock shiitake, maitake (hen of the woods), button mushrooms, portobello mushrooms, and oyster mushrooms—all of which taste delicious when lightly sautéed (plus or minus some garlic).

For additional information, check out this WebMD slides show on anticancer foods: http://www.webmd.com/cancer/ss/slideshow-cancer-fighting-foods.

KEY TAKEAWAYS

- One of the best things you can do to improve your health and avoid cancer is to stay away from tobacco products and smoke.

- Good nutrition is the cornerstone to good health. Cancer is less common among people who eat plant-based diets.

    - Preliminary scientific research suggests some edible plants have notable anticancer activity.

    - A simple way to incorporate healthful plant chemicals into your diet is to eat a variety of colorful fruits and vegetables.

- Other healthy lifestyle habits such as regular physical activity and sufficient sleep guard against cancer.

- The upsides of staying out of the sun are that your skin won't age as fast and is less likely to develop cancer. The downside is not receiving enough vitamin D.

DISCUSSION QUESTIONS

1. Find out the level of radiation in your area today. Go to the Environmental Protection Agency website, http://www.epa.gov/sunwise/uvindex.html. Write down the level. Read the recommendations for protecting yourself for each UV exposure category. What happens if you're on a bright, reflective surface such as white beach, snow, or water? What will you do to avoid excessive UV radiation today?

2. Why did sunscreens not require a UVA filter until recently?

3. Discuss how you could change your diet to incorporate foods thought to protect people against cancer. Be detailed. List the foods you ate at breakfast, lunch, and dinner. Next provide a menu for each meal that contains foods associated with a reduced cancer risk.

5. RECOMMENDED RESOURCES

5.1 Organizations and Websites

American Cancer Society. http://www.cancer.org.

American Institute for Cancer Research. http://www.aicr.org.

Harvard School of Public Health. http://www.diseaseriskindex.harvard.edu/update/hccpquiz.pl?lang=english&func=home&page=cancer_index.

International Agency for Research on Cancer, World Health Organization. http://www.iarc.fr.

National Cancer Institute, National Institutes of Health. http://www.cancer.gov.

ENDNOTES

1. Cancer facts and figures 2012. American Cancer Society. Available at: http://www.cancer.org/acs/groups/content/@epidemiologysurveilance/documents/document/acspc-031941.pdf. Accessed June 9, 2012.

2. Aggarwal BB, Danda D, Gupta S, Gehlot P. Models for prevention and treatment of cancer: problems vs promises. *Biochem Pharmacol*. 2009 Nov 1;78(9):1083–1094. Available at: http://www.ncbi.nlm.nih.gov/pmc/articles/PMC2748136/?tool=pubmed. Accessed June 9, 2012.

3. American Cancer Society guidelines on nutrition and physical activity for cancer prevention. American Cancer Society. Available at: http://www.cancer.org/acs/groups/cid/documents/webcontent/002577-pdf.pdf. Accessed June 17, 2012.

4. Cancer facts and figures for African Americans, 2011–2012. American Cancer Society. Available at: http://www.cancer.org/Research/CancerFactsFigures/CancerFactsFiguresforAfricanAmericans/cancer-facts-figures-af-am-2011-2012. Accessed June 22, 2012.

5. Cancer Research UK. Smoking and cancer: what's in a cigarette. Available at: http://info.cancerresearchuk.org/healthyliving/smokingandtobacco/whatsinacigarette/smoking-and-cancer-whats-in-a-cigarette. Accessed June 20, 2012.

6. Chen WY, Rosner B, Hankinson SE, Colditz GA, Willett WC. Moderate alcohol consumption during adult life, drinking patterns, and breast cancer risk. *JAMA*. 2011;306(17):1884–1890. doi:10.1001/jama.2011.1590.

7. Pan A, Sun Q, Bernstein AM, et al. Red meat consumption and mortality. *Archives of Intern Medicine*. 2012. doi:10.1001/archinternmed.2011.2287. Available at: http://www.archinternmed.com. Accessed June 19, 2012.

8. Davis S, Mirick DK. Circadian disruption, shift work and the risk of cancer: a summary of the evidence and studies in Seattle. *Cancer Causes Control*. 2006 May;17(4):539–545.

9. Hansen J, Lassen CF. Nested case-control study of night shift work and breast cancer risk among women in the Danish military. *Occup Environ Med*. 2012. doi:10.1136/oemed-2011-100240.

10. Sigurdardottir LG, Valdimarsdóttir U, Fall K, et al. Circadian disruption, sleep loss and prostate cancer risk: a systematic review of epidemiological studies. *Cancer Epidemiol Biomarkers Prev*. 2012 May 7 [Epub ahead of print]. doi:10.1158/1055-9965.EPI-12-0116.

11. Demark-Wahnefried W, Platz EA, Ligibel JA, et al. The role of obesity in cancer survival and recurrence. *Cancer Epidemiol Biomarkers Prev*. 2012 Jun 13 [Epub ahead of print]. doi:10.1158/1055-9965.EPI-12-0485.

12. Cooney KA, Gruber SB. Hyperglycemia, obesity, and cancer risks on the horizon. *JAMA*. 2005;293(2):235–236.

13. Wild SH. Diabetes, treatments for diabetes and their effect on cancer incidence and mortality: attempts to disentangle the web of associations. *Diabetologia*. 2011 Jul;54(7):1589–1592.

14. Jou PC, Feldman RJ. UV protection and sunscreens: what to tell patients. *Clev Clin J Med*. 2012;2–12;79(7):427–436. doi:10.3949/ccjm.79a.11110. Available at: http://www.ccjm.org/content/79/6/427.long. Accessed June 19, 2012.

15. Wischermann K, Popp S, Moshir S, et al. UVA radiation causes DNA strand breaks, chromosomal aberrations and tumorigenic transformation in HaCaT skin keratinocytes. *Oncogene*. 2008;17;27(31):4269–4280.

16. Godar DE, Landry RJ, Lucas AD. Increased UVA exposures and decreased cutaneous vitamin D(3) levels may be responsible for the increasing incidence of melanoma. *Med Hypotheses*. 2009;72(4):434–443.

17. Miller SA, Hamilton SL, Wester UG, Cyr WH. An analysis of UVA emissions from sunlamps and the potential importance for melanoma. *Photochem Photobiol*. 1998;68:63–70.

18. National Toxicology Program. Final report on carcinogens background document for styrene. *Report on Carcinogens Background Document*. 2008;(8–5978):i–398.

19. National Toxicology Program. Final report on carcinogens background document for formaldehyde. *Report on Carcinogens Background Document*. 2010;(10–5981):i–512.

20. Blair A, Freeman LB. Epidemiologic studies in agricultural populations: observations and future directions. *J Agromedicine*. 2009;14(2):125–131.

21. Wang HS, Sthiannopkao S, Du J, et al. Daily intake and human risk assessment of organochlorine pesticides (OCPs) based on Cambodian market basket data. *J Hazard Mater*. 2011 Sep 15;192(3):1441–1449.

22. Sappino AP, Buser R, Lesne L, et al. Aluminium chloride promotes anchorage-independent growth in human mammary epithelial cells. *J Appl Toxicol*. 2012 Mar;32(3):233–243. doi:10.1002/jat.1793.

23. National Cancer Institute at the National Institutes of Health. Antiperspirants/deodorants and breast cancer. Available at: http://www.cancer.gov/cancertopics/factsheet/Risk/AP-Deo. Accessed June 22, 2012.

24. Volkow ND, Tomasi D, Want G, et al. Effects of cell phone radiofrequency signal exposure on the brain glucose metabolism. *JAMA*. 2011;305:808–814, 828–829.

25. Larjavaara S, Schüz J, Swerdlow A, et al. Location of gliomas in relation to mobile telephone use: a case-case and case-specular analysis. *Am J Epidemiol*. 2011;174(1):2–11.

26. INTERPHONE Study Group. Brain tumour risk in relation to mobile telephone use: results of the INTERPHONE international case-control study. *Int J Epidemiol*. 2010 Jun;39(3):675–694.

27. World Health Organization. IARC classifies radiofrequency electromagnetic fields as possibly carcinogenic to humans. International Agency for Research on Cancer. Press Release No. 208. May 31, 2011. Available at: http://www.iarc.fr/en/media-centre/pr/2011/pdfs/pr208_E.pdf. Accessed June 21, 2012.

28. American Cancer Society. What are the key statistics about basal and squamous cell skin cancers? *Skin Cancer: Basal and Squamous Cell. Detailed Guide*. 2011. Available at: http://www.cancer.org/Cancer/SkinCancer-BasalandSquamousCell/DetailedGuide/skin-cancer-basal-and-squamous-cell-key-statistics. Accessed June 19, 2012.

29. American Cancer Society. What are the key statistics about melanoma? *Melanoma Skin Cancer. Detailed Guide*. 2011. Available at: http://www.cancer.org/Cancer/SkinCancer-Melanoma/DetailedGuide/melanoma-skin-cancer-key-statistics. Accessed June 19, 2012.

30. Kütting B, Drexler H. UV-induced skin cancer at workplace and evidence-based prevention. *Int Arch Occup Environ Health*. 2010 Dec;83(8):843–854.

31. Reed KB, Brewer JD, Lohse CM, et al. Increasing incidence of melanoma among young adults: an epidemiologic study in Olmsted County, Minnesota. *Mayo Clin Proc*. 2012. doi:10.1016/j.mayocp.2012.01.010.

32. Howlader N, Noone AM, Krapcho M, et al. (eds). *SEER Cancer Statistics Review, 1975–2009 (Vintage 2009 Populations)*. Bethesda, MD: National Cancer Institute; 2011. SEER Stat Fact Sheets: Colon and Rectum. Available at: http://seer.cancer.gov/statfacts/html/colorect.html. Accessed June 18, 2012.

33. Howlader N, Noone AM, Krapcho M, et al. (eds). *SEER Cancer Statistics Review, 1975–2009 (Vintage 2009 Populations)*. Bethesda, MD: National Cancer Institute. Based on November 2011 SEER data submission. SEER Stat Fact Sheets: Breast. Available at: http://seer.cancer.gov/statfacts/html/breast.html. Accessed June 18, 2012.

34. DQ® Cancer Information Summary. National Cancer Institute; Bethesda, MD. Breast Cancer Prevention (PDQ®)—Health Professional. Available at: http://www.cancer.gov/cancertopics/pdq/prevention/breast/healthprofessional. Updated April 30, 2009.

35. Schulz M, Hoffmann K, Weikert C, Nöthlings U, Schulze MB, Boeing H. Identification of a dietary pattern characterized by high-fat food choices associated with increased risk of breast cancer: the European Prospective Investigation into Cancer and Nutrition (EPIC)-Potsdam Study. *Br J Nutr*. 2008 Nov;100(5):942–946.

36. McCullough LE, Eng SM, Bradshaw PT, et al. Fat or fit: the joint effects of physical activity, weight gain, and body size on breast cancer risk. *Cancer*. 2012. doi:10.1002/cncr.27433.

37. What are the key statistics about breast cancer in men? Breast Cancer in Men. American Cancer Society. 2011. Available at: http://www.cancer.org/Cancer/BreastCancerinMen/DetailedGuide/breast-cancer-in-men-key-statistics. Accessed June 21, 2012.

38. Martin-Hirsch PL, Wood NJ. Cervical cancer. *Clin Evid*. 2011 Jul 27;2011. pii: 0818.

39. Rice LW. Hormone prevention strategies for breast, endometrial and ovarian cancers. *Gynecol Oncol*. 2010 Aug 1;118(2):202–207.

40. Howlader N, Noone AM, Krapcho M, et al. (eds). *SEER Cancer Statistics Review, 1975–2009 (Vintage 2009 Populations)*, National Cancer Institute. Bethesda, MD. November 2011. SEER Stat Fact Sheets: Prostate. Available at: http://seer.cancer.gov/statfacts/html/prost.html. Accessed June 18, 2012.

41. Kurahashi N, Iwasaki M, Sasazuki S, Otani T, Inoue M, Tsugane S; Japan Public Health Center-Based Prospective Study Group. Soy product and isoflavone consumption in relation to prostate cancer in Japanese men. *Cancer Epidemiol Biomarkers Prev*. 2007 Mar;16(3):538–545.

42. Kurahashi N, Sasazuki S, Iwasaki M, Inoue M, Tsugane S; JPHC Study Group. Green tea consumption and prostate cancer risk in Japanese men: a prospective study. *Am J Epidemiol*. 2008 Jan 1;167(1):71–77.

43. Schwartz GG, Hanchette CL. UV, latitude, and spatial trends in prostate cancer mortality: all sunlight is not the same (United States). *Cancer Causes Control*. 2006 Oct;17(8):1091–1101.

44. Schwartz GG. Vitamin D and intervention trials in prostate cancer: from theory to therapy. *Ann Epidemiol*. 2009 Feb;19(2):96–102.

45. SEER stat fact sheets: testis. Surveillance Epidemiology and End Results. National Cancer Institute. Available at: http://seer.cancer.gov/statfacts/html/testis.html. Accessed June 6, 2013.

46. Maule M, Malavassi JL, Richiardi L. Age at puberty and risk of testicular cancer: a meta-analysis. *Int J Androl*. 2012 Jun 19. doi:10.1111/j.1365-2605.2012.01286.x.

47. Schoen RE, Pinsky PF, Weissfeld JL, et al.; the PLCO Project Team. Colorectal-cancer incidence and mortality with screening flexible sigmoidoscopy. *N Engl J Med*. 2012;366:2345–2357.

48. Screening for Breast Cancer. US Preventive Services Task Force. November 2009. Available at: http://www.uspreventiveservicestaskforce.org/uspstf/uspsbrca.htm. Updated December 2009. Accessed June 18, 2012.

49. Tabár L, Vitak B, Chen TH, et al. Swedish two-county trial: impact of mammographic screening on breast cancer mortality during three decades. *Radiology*. 2011 Sep;260(3):658–663. doi:10.1148/radiol.11110469.

50. American Cancer Society recommendations for early breast cancer detection in women without breast symptoms. 2011. American Cancer Society. Available at: http://www.cancer.org/Cancer/BreastCancer/MoreInformation/BreastCancerEarlyDetection/breast-cancer-early-detection-acs-recs. Accessed June 18, 2012.

51. National Cancer Institute. BRCA1 and BRCA2: cancer risk and genetic testing. Available at: http://www.cancer.gov/cancertopics/factsheet/Risk/BRCA. Accessed June 18, 2012.

52. National Cancer Institute at the National Institutes of Health. Pap and HPV testing. Available at: http://www.cancer.gov/cancertopics/factsheet/detection/Pap-HPV-testing. Accessed June 25, 2012.

53. Andriole GL, Crawford ED, Grubb RL, et al.; PLCO Project Team. Prostate cancer screening in the randomized prostate, lung, colorectal, and ovarian cancer screening trial: mortality results after 13 years of follow-up. J Natl Cancer Inst. 2012.18;104(2):125–132.

54. Zhu X, van Leeuwen PJ, Bul M, et al. Disease-specific survival of men with prostate cancer detected during the screening interval: results of the European randomized study of screening for prostate cancer-Rotterdam after 11 years of follow-up. Eur Urol. 2011 Aug;60(2):330–336.

55. Screening for Prostate Cancer: US Preventive Services Task Force Recommendation Statement. Draft: Summary of Recommendation and Evidence. U.S. Preventive Services Task Force. November 2011. Available at: http://www.uspreventiveservicestaskforce.org/uspstf12/prostate/draftrecprostate.htm#ref1. Accessed June 18, 2012.

56. Howlader N, Noone AM, Krapcho M, et al. (eds). SEER Cancer Statistics Review, 1975–2009 (Vintage 2009 Populations). Bethesda, MD: National Cancer Institute; 2011. SEER Stat Fact Sheets: Colon and Rectum. Available at: http://seer.cancer.gov/statfacts/html/colorect.html. Accessed June 18, 2012.

57. American Cancer Society. American Cancer Society recommendations for prostate cancer early detection. Available at: http://www.auanet.org/content/media/psa09.pdf. Accessed June 18, 2012.

58. American Urological Association. Prostate-specific antigen best practice statement: 2009 update. Available at: http://www.auanet.org/content/media/psa09.pdf. Accessed June 18, 2012.

59. Tomlins SA, Aubin SM, Siddiqui J, et al. Urine TMPRSS2: ERG fusion transcript stratifies prostate cancer risk in men with elevated serum PSA. Sci Transl Med. 2011;3:94:ra72. doi:10.1126/scitranslmed.3001970 ra72.

60. Krakowsky Y, Loblaw A, Klotz L. Prostate cancer death of men treated with initial active surveillance: clinical and biochemical characteristics. J Urol. 2010 Jul;184(1):131–135.

61. Foundation history. Mario Lemieux Foundation. Available at: http://www.mariolemieux.org/about-us/foundation-history. Accessed March 12, 2013.

62. Morgenstern H, Gellert GA, Walter SD, Ostfeld AM, Siegel BS. The impact of a psychosocial support program on survival with breast cancer: the importance of selection bias in program evaluation. J Chronic Dis. 1984;37(4):273–282.

63. Lim HS, Roychoudhuri R, Peto J, et al. Cancer survival is dependent on season of diagnosis and sunlight exposure. Int J Cancer. 2006;119:1530–1536.

64. Bell DS. Protean manifestations of vitamin D deficiency, part 2: vitamin D deficiency and autoimmune disease. Medscape. South Med J. 2011 May;104(5):335–339. Available at: http://www.medscape.com/viewarticle/742625_2. Accessed August 11, 2011.

65. Thacher TD, Clarke BL. Vitamin D insufficiency. Mayo Clin Proc. 2011;86(1):50–60.

66. Linos E, Holmes MD, Willett WC. Diet and breast cancer. Curr Oncol Rep. 2007;9:31–41.

67. Eliassen AH, Colditz GA, Rosner B, et al. Adults weight change and the risk of postmenopausal breast cancer. JAMA. 2006;296:193–201.

68. Cust AE. Physical activity and gynecologic cancer prevention. Recent Results Cancer Res. 2011;186:159–185.

69. Jones LW, Viglianti BL, Tashjian JA, et al. Effect of aerobic exercise on tumor physiology in an animal model of human breast cancer. J Appl Physiol. 2010 Feb;108(2):343–348.

70. Irwin ML, Smith AW, McTiernan A, et al. Influence of pre- and postdiagnosis physical activity on mortality in breast cancer survivors: the health, eating, activity, and lifestyle study. J Clin Oncol. 2008 Aug 20;26(24):3958–3964.

71. Demark-Wahnefried W, Morey MC, Sloane R, et al. Reach out to enhance wellness home-based diet-exercise intervention promotes reproducible and sustainable long-term improvements in health behaviors, body weight, and physical functioning in improvements in health behaviors, body weight, and physical functioning in older, overweight/obese cancer survivors. J Clin Oncol. 2012 May 21 [Epub ahead of print].

72. Walsh NP, Gleeson M, Shephard RJ, et al. Position statement. Part one: immune function and exercise. Exerc Immunol Rev. 2011;17:6–63.

73. Boeing H, Bechthold A, Bub A, et al. Critical review: vegetables and fruit in the prevention of chronic diseases. Eur J Nutr. 2012 Jun 9 [Epub ahead of print].

74. Giacosa A, Barale R, Bavaresco L, et al. Cancer prevention in Europe: the Mediterranean diet as a protective choice. Eur J Cancer Prev. 2012 May 24 [Epub ahead of print].

75. Antoni MH. Psychosocial intervention effects on adaptation, disease course and biobehavioral processes in cancer. Brain Behav Immun. 2012 May 22 [Epub ahead of print].

76. Jenkins S, Betancourt AM, Wang J, Lamartiniere CA. Endocrine-active chemicals in mammary cancer causation and prevention. J Steroid Biochem Mol Biol. 2012 Apr;129(3–5):191–200.

77. Kütting B, Drexler H. UV-induced skin cancer at workplace and evidence-based prevention. Int Arch Occup Environ Health. 2010 Dec;83(8):843–854.

78. Gorham ED, Mohr SB, Garland CF, Chaplin G, Garland FC. Do sunscreens increase risk of melanoma in populations residing at higher latitudes? Ann Epidemiol. 2007 Dec;17(12):956–963.

79. Rodvall YE, Wahlgren CF, Ullén HT, Wiklund KE. Factors related to being sunburnt in 7-year-old children in Sweden. Eur J Cancer. 2010;46(3):566–572.

80. Jou PC, Feldman RJ. UV protection and sunscreens: what to tell patients. Clev Clin J Med. 2–12;79(7):427–436. doi:10.3949/ccjm.79a.11110. Available at: http://www.ccjm.org/content/79/6/427.long. Accessed June 19, 2012.

81. Couteau C, El-Boury S, Paparis E, Sébille-Rivain V, Coiffard LJ. In vitro UV-A protection factor (PFUVA) of organic and inorganic sunscreens. Pharm Dev Technol 2009;14(4):369–372.

82. Jaeger A, Weiss DG, Jonas L, Kriehuber R. Oxidative stress-induced cytotoxic and genotoxic effects of nano-sized titanium dioxide particles in human HaCaT keratinocytes. Toxicology. 2012 Jun 14;296(1–3):27–36.

83. Nohynek GJ, Dufour EK. Nano-sized cosmetic formulations or solid nanoparticles in sunscreens: a risk to human health? Arch Toxicol. 2012 Mar 31 [Epub ahead of print]. Abstract available at: http://www.ncbi.nlm.nih.gov/pubmed/22466067. Accessed June 19, 2012.

84. Krause M, Klit A, Blomberg Jensen M, et al. Sunscreens: are they beneficial for health? An overview of endocrine disrupting properties of UV-filters. Int J Androl. 2012 Jun;35(3):424–436. doi:10.1111/j.1365-2605.2012.01280.x.

85. Lucas RM. An epidemiological perspective of ultraviolet exposure—public health concerns. Eye Contact Lens. 2011 Jul;37(4):168–175.

86. Miyamura Y, Coelho SG, Wolber R, et al. Regulation of human skin pigmentation and responses to ultraviolet radiation. Pigment Cell Res. 2007;20:2–13.

87. Harrington CR, Beswick TC, Leitenberger J, Minhajuddin A, Jacobe HT, Adinoff B. Addictive-like behaviours to ultraviolet light among frequent indoor tanners. Clin Exp Dermatol. 2011 Jan;36(1):33–8. doi:10.1111/j.1365-2230.2010.03882.x.

88. Acrylamide in Food and Cancer Risk. National Cancer Institute. National Institutes of Health. 7/29/08. Available at: http://www.cancer.gov/cancertopics/factsheet/Risk/acrylamide-in-food. Accessed June 20, 2012.

89. Donaldson MS. Nutrition and cancer: a review of the evidence for an anticancer diet. Nutr J. 2004;3:19.

90. Elias SG, Peeters PH, Grobbee DE, van Noord PA. Transient caloric restriction and cancer risk (The Netherlands). Cancer Causes Control. 2007 Feb;18(1):1–5.

91. Michels KB, Ekbom A. Caloric restriction and incidence of breast cancer. JAMA. 2004 Mar 10;291(10):1226–1230.

92. Zafra-Stone S, Yasmin T, Bagchi M, et al. Berry anthocyanins as novel antioxidants in human health and disease prevention. Mol Nutr Food Res. 2007 Jun;51(6):675–683.

93. Neto CC. Cranberry and blueberry: evidence for protective effects against cancer and vascular diseases. Mol Nutr Food Res. 2007 Jun;51(6):652–664.

94. Do MH, Lee SS, Jung PJ, Lee MH. Intake of fruits, vegetables, and soy foods in relation to breast cancer risk in Korean women: a case-control study. Nutr Cancer. 2007;57(1):20–27.

95. Johanningsmeier SD, Harris GK. Pomegranate as a functional food and nutraceutical source. Annu Rev Food Sci Technol. 2011;2:181–201.

96. Adhami VM, Khan N, Mukhtar H. Cancer chemoprevention by pomegranate: laboratory and Clinical Evidence. Nutr Cancer. 2009;61(6):811–815.

97. Pantuck AJ, Zomorodian N, Belldegrun AS. Phase-II Study of pomegranate juice for men with prostate cancer and increasing PSA. Curr Urol Rep. 2006 Jan;7(1):7.

98. Johnson IT. Phytochemicals and cancer. Proc Nutr Soc 2007;66:207–217.

99. Talalay P, Fahey JW. Phytochemicals from cruciferous plants protect against cancer by modulating carcinogen metabolism. J Nutr. 2001 Nov;131(11 Suppl):3027S-33S.

100. Rao AV, Rao LG. Carotenoids and human health. Pharmacol Res. 2007 Mar;55(3):207–216.

101. Azqueta A, Collins AR. Carotenoids and DNA damage. Mutat Res. 2012 May 1;733(1–2):4–13.

102. Wei MY, Giovannucci EL. Lycopene, tomato products, and prostate cancer incidence: a review and reassessment in the PSA screening era. J Oncol. 2012;2012:271063:1–7.

103. Ellinger S, Ellinger J, Stehle P. Tomatoes, tomato products and lycopene in the prevention and treatment of prostate cancer: do we have the evidence from intervention studies? Curr Opin Clin Nutr Metab Care. 2006 Nov;9(6):722–727.

104. Do MH, Lee SS, Jung PJ, Lee MH. Intake of fruits, vegetables, and soy foods in relation to breast cancer risk in Korean women: a case-control study. Nutr Cancer. 2007;57(1):20–27.

105. Masala G, Assedi M, Bendinelli B, et al. Fruit and vegetables consumption and breast cancer risk: the EPIC Italy study. Breast Cancer Res Treat. 2012 Apr;132(3):1127–1136.

106. Jee SH, Ohrr H, Sull JW, et al. Fasting serum glucose level and cancer risk in Korean men and women. JAMA. 2005 Jan 12;293(2):194–202.

107. Pelucchi C, Bosetti C, Rossi M, Negri E, La Vecchia C. Selected aspects of Mediterranean diet and cancer risk. Nutr Cancer. 2009;61(6):756–766.

108. Kaczmarczyk MM, Miller MJ, Freund GG. The health benefits of dietary fiber: beyond the usual suspects of type 2 diabetes mellitus, cardiovascular disease and colon cancer. Metabolism. 2012 Mar 7 [Epub ahead of print].

109. Dong JY, Qin LQ. Soy isoflavones consumption and risk of breast cancer incidence or recurrence: a meta-analysis of prospective studies. Breast Cancer Res Treat. 2011 Jan;125(2):315–323.

110. Goodman MT, Wilkens LR, Hankin JH, et al. Association of soy and fiber consumption with the risk of endometrial cancer. Am J Epidemiol. 1997 Aug 15;146(4):294–306.

111. Ollberding NJ, Lim U, Wilkens LR, et al. Legume, soy, tofu, and isoflavone intake and endometrial cancer risk in postmenopausal women in the multiethnic cohort study. J Natl Cancer Inst. 2012 Jan 4;104(1):67–76.

112. Sakauchi F, Khan MM, Mori M, et al.; JACC Study Group. Dietary habits and risk of ovarian cancer death in a large-scale cohort study (JACC study) in Japan. *Nutr Cancer.* 2007;57(2):138–145.

113. Myung SK, Ju W, Choi HJ, Kim SC; Korean Meta-Analysis (KORMA) Study Group. Soy intake and risk of endocrine-related gynaecological cancer: a meta-analysis. *BJOG.* 2009 Dec;116(13):1697–1705.

114. Yan L, Spitznagel EL. Soy consumption and prostate cancer risk in men: a revisit of a meta-analysis. *Am J Clin Nutr.* 2009 Apr;89(4):1155–1163.

115. Yan L, Spitznagel EL, Bosland MC. Soy consumption and colorectal cancer risk in humans: a meta-analysis. *Cancer Epidemiol Biomarkers Prev.* 2010 Jan;19(1):148–158.

116. McLaughlin JM, Olivo-Marston S, Vitolins MZ, et al. Effects of tomato- and soy-rich diets on the IGF-I hormonal network: a crossover study of postmenopausal women at high risk for breast cancer. *Cancer Prev Res (Phila).* 2011 May;4(5):702–710.

117. Nechuta SJ, Caan BJ, Chen WY, et al. Soy food intake after diagnosis of breast cancer and survival: an in-depth analysis of combined evidence from cohort studies of US and Chinese women. *Am J Clin Nutr.* 2012 May 30 [Epub ahead of print].

118. Boyce J. Breast cancer. In: *Integrative Medicine*, David Rakel, Ed. Philadelphia, PA: Saunders/Elsevier; 2007:827.

119. Bergman Jungestrom M, Thompson LU, Dabrosin C. Flaxseed and its lignans inhibit estradiol-induced growth, angiogenesis, and secretion of vascular endothelial growth factor in human breast cancer xenografts in vivo. *Clin Cancer Res.* 2007 Feb 1;13(3):1061–1067.

120. Bergman Jungestrom M, Thompson LU, Dabrosin C. Flaxseed and its lignans inhibit estradiol-induced growth, angiogenesis, and secretion of vascular endothelial growth factor in human breast cancer xenografts in vivo. *Clin Cancer Res.* 2007 Feb 1;13(3):1061–1067.

121. Chen J, Power KA, Mann J, et al. Flaxseed alone or in combination with tamoxifen inhibits MCF-7 breast tumor growth in ovariectomized athymic mice with high circulating levels of estrogen. *Exp Biol Med (Maywood).* 2007 Sep;232(8):1071–1080.

122. Danbara N, Yuri T, Tsujita-Kyutoku M, et al. Enterolactone induces apoptosis and inhibits growth of Colo 201 human colon cancer cells both in vitro and in vivo. *Anticancer Res.* 2005 May–Jun;25(3B):2269–2276.

123. Demark-Wahnefried W, Polascik TJ, et al. Flaxseed supplementation (not dietary fat restriction) reduces prostate cancer proliferation rates in men presurgery. *Cancer Epidemiol Biomarkers Prev.* 2008 Dec;17(12):3577–3587.

124. Singh BN, Shankar S, Srivastava RK. Green tea catechin, epigallocatechin-3-gallate (EGCG): mechanisms, perspectives and clinical applications. *Biochem Pharmacol.* 2011 Dec 15;82(12):1807–1821.

125. Yang CS, Wang X. Green tea and cancer prevention. *Nutr Cancer.* 2010;62(7):931–937.

126. Pereira MM, Haniadka R, Chacko PP, Palatty PL, Baliga MS. Zingiber officinale Roscoe (ginger) as an adjuvant in cancer treatment: a review. *J BUON.* 2011 Jul–Sep;16(3):414–424.

127. Shankar S, Chen Q, Sarva K, et al. Curcumin enhances the apoptosis-inducing potential of TRAIL in prostate cancer cells: molecular mechanisms of apoptosis, migration and angiogenesis. *J Mol Signal.* 2007 Oct 4;2(1):10.

128. Cerella C, Dicato M, Jacob C, Diederich M. Chemical properties and mechanisms determining the anticancer action of garlic-derived organic sulfur compounds. *Anticancer Agents Med Chem.* 2011 Mar;11(3):267–271.

129. American Institute for Cancer Research. Cancer experts on garlic: chop, then stop. June 18, 2007. Available at: http://www.aicr.org/site/News2?abbr=pr_&page=NewsArticle&id=12154.

130. Xu T, Beelman RB, Lambert JD. The cancer preventive effects of edible mushrooms. *Anticancer Agents Med Chem.* 2012 May 2 [Epub ahead of print]. Available at: http://www.ncbi.nlm.nih.gov/pubmed/22583406. Accessed June 17, 2012.

CHAPTER 17
Environmental Health

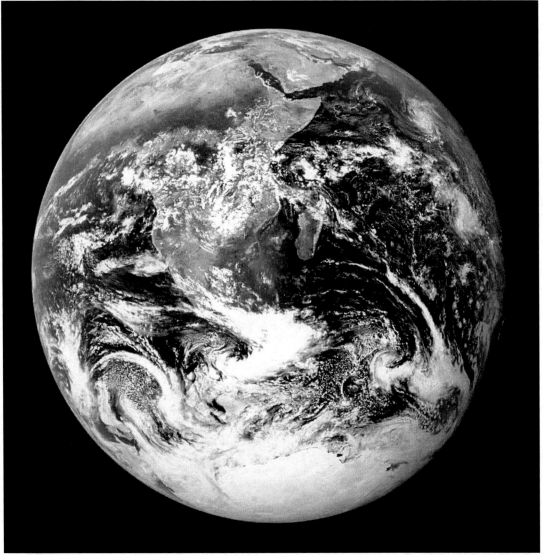

Source: Deglr6328. 2005. Adaptation of NASA. The blue marble. 1972. Available at: http://commons.wikimedia.org/wiki/File:The_Blue_Marble.jpg.

In many ways, environmental health is a fitting conclusion to this text. The subject has already come up repeatedly. In truth, your health is not just a personal issue. Beginning in Chapter 1, you learned that lifestyle and environmental factors have a much greater influence on your health and longevity than genetics. That theme recurred in all the chapters on major diseases (infectious diseases, diabetes, cardiovascular disease, and cancer). You learned how your social environment and the safety of your neighborhood influence health. Family planning, discussed in Chapter 7, has a profound effect on the environment—a concept we'll expand upon in this chapter. Chapter 8 examined the environmental impact of agriculture and individual food choices. In Chapter 13, you learned that your body forms an *ecosystem*, a complex system of interacting organisms and their physical environment. In this chapter, you'll learn how our behaviors impact broader ecosystems and how those ecosystems affect our health.

The global environment affects us all. The news media are full of ominous reports:

- 2012 Hottest Year on Record[1]

- Summer 2012 Brought Record-Breaking Melt to Greenland[2]

- Arctic Sea Ice Melts to Lowest Level on Record[3]

- Extreme Weather Linked to Global Warming[4]

- Hurricane Sandy Death Toll Climbs above 110[5]

- Typhoon Bopha Kills Hundreds in Philippines[6]

This chapter will explore the influence of the local and global environment on human health. It will also address the power of humans, collectively and individually, to affect the environment and the steps you can take now to improve planetary health.

In nature nothing exists alone.

- Rachel Carson, scientist, environmentalist, and author of Silent Spring

1. HUMANS AND THE ENVIRONMENT

LEARNING OBJECTIVES

1. Explain the reciprocal interaction between humans and the environment.
2. Define environmental health.
3. Discuss the relevance of population growth to environmental health.
4. Review common air and water pollutants and discuss ways to reduce your exposure.
5. Discuss the ways individuals can reduce solid waste.
6. Understand the impact of artificial lighting and noise on health.

environment

External surroundings, including living and nonliving things.

A reciprocal relationship exists between you and your **environment**, your external surroundings—both living and nonliving. Your actions can dramatically affect the health of the environment. Likewise, the environment profoundly affects your health. We can't live without oxygen, water, and soil rich enough to grow plants and graze animals. The earth provides a host of resources that we use for food, building materials, and the energy to light and heat our homes and power our machines.

The environment separates into two main components. The **natural environment** refers to areas and ecosystems that existed before human influence. The ever-growing human population affects that natural environment in many ways, from encroaching on wilderness areas and wildlife habitat to changing the chemistry of air and water. In contrast, the **built environment** refers to manmade structures such as buildings, parks, transportation systems, and energy networks.

Another categorical division is the local and the global environment. You fit into a local ecosystem that includes the built and natural environments. As you've learned in earlier chapters, a number of local environmental factors affect your health and well-being: social relationships; neighborhood safety; access to parks and recreation centers; and the quality of the food, water, soil, and air you breathe. You can even examine the environment you inhabit on a smaller scale—your living space. You can control some aspects of your personal environment, such as lighting, heating, sounds, smells, textures, and sights. You create positive environmental changes by putting a potted plant on the windowsill, hanging art on the walls, and playing peaceful music. Light a cigarette and you fill the air with toxic chemicals.

Our local environments contribute to the global environment, which affects us all. For example, air pollutants from Europe and Asia create a perceivable haze over the Arctic.[7] Our actions affect not only the health of people halfway across the globe but also the health of future generations.

As a species, humans have had an enormous impact on the planet. For centuries, we have controlled and exploited the natural world in order to grow crops, build cities, extract natural resources, manufacture goods, and live as safely and as comfortably as possible.

Yet *Homo sapiens* is one of many species occupying the earth. Our actions have altered multiple ecosystems, often in ways that ultimately harm us. For instance, we have cut and burned entire forests to create agricultural fields, pasture land, golf courses, and housing tracts.

Deforestation (loss of forest cover) has many adverse effects. Among their many functions, forests provide habitats for diverse species, filter the water (making it cleaner to drink), retain precipitation, stabilize the ground to prevent erosion, stabilize snow to inhibit avalanches, provide building materials and medicinal plants, offer shade and wind blocks, and take up atmospheric carbon dioxide. (Later, we'll discuss the role of carbon dioxide in global warming.) As one example of the impact on human health, removal of trees creates the right mix of sunlight, warmth, and puddles for mosquito breeding. In the Amazon, a 4 percent increase in deforestation led to a 50 percent rise in malaria.[8]

On a positive note, collective awareness about the relationship between our actions and human and planetary health has steadily climbed.

1.1   The Evolution of Environmentalism

While healers have long recognized that our environments affect our health, it took some time for society to recognize that human activities often degrade the natural environment, which, in turn, damages human health. The story begins with infectious microorganisms. Ancient physician Hippocrates broke ranks with contemporaries by proposing that environmental factors—as opposed to angry gods—caused illness. Much later, in the 1880s, scientists such as Robert Koch linked microbes to infectious illnesses.

Public health initiatives led to safe drinking water, sewage treatment, and the organized disposal of garbage, including hazardous wastes. Such programs to curb infectious diseases marked the beginning of **environmental health**, a discipline devoted to addressing the many external factors that can potentially affect health.[9] Initial efforts to prevent the spread of infectious disease expanded to the protection of air, water, and soil from physical, biological, and chemical pollutants and toxins.

The need to more broadly protect the environment arose with increasing migration from the countryside to cities. Denser populations intensified the challenge of providing clean water and sanitation. Rivers passing through cities became rank with sewage run-off. Smoke from wood and coal fires thickened the air with soot. Burning coal emitted sulfur dioxide and nitrogen oxides, both of which react with atmospheric water and other chemicals to form **acid rain**.[10] The acids fell to the ground as fog, mist, rain, and snow. They became incorporated into dust or smoke, settling onto soil, buildings, and plants and contributing to deforestation.

Efforts to regulate air pollution occurred as far back as 1306 in London.[11] Around 1760, the Industrial Revolution began in that city, increasing the release of pollutants into water and air. **Smog**, a combination of fog and chemical-laden smoke, blanketed the city. In December 1952, poor air quality led to 4,000 premature deaths, most of them due to respiratory and cardiovascular disease and most of them affecting the elderly.[12]

Industrialization radically increased use of **natural resources** such as water (used as a source of power), minerals (iron, asbestos, aluminum, stone, sand, lead, and mercury) and fossil fuels (coal, oil, and natural gas). **Fossil fuels** are those formed millions of years ago as prehistoric plants and animals became compressed under layers of earth. Because it takes so long to make them, fossil fuels are not renewable (easily replenished).

Furthermore, mining of minerals dramatically altered the landscape and introduced toxic industrial metals into the environment. Mercury, asbestos, and lead are prime examples. In 19th-century England, hats were made from felt (condensed wool), whose production involved mercury. *Mercury* damages the nervous system, including the brain—hence the expression "As mad as a hatter."[13] *Asbestos* fibers—used in insulation, drywall, concrete, bricks, and pipes—are easily inhaled, leading to lung cancer and other chronic chest diseases. *Lead*—used in metal alloys, bullets, batteries, ceramic glazes, cosmetics, and paint—damages many body systems, particularly the nervous system.

Industrialization did facilitate the growth of the middle class and a corresponding rise in living standards. However, increased prosperity correlates with increased consumption of goods, most of which use natural resources. Improvements in agriculture increased food production, which allowed the population to swell and further taxed natural resources.

In the mid-1900s, the Green Revolution radically increased food production through the use of mechanized farm equipment, improved crop varieties and irrigation techniques, pesticides (substances that destroy organisms such as insects, undesirable plants, and fungi), and synthetic fertilizer. Unfortunately, pesticides and fertilizers added to the pollution problem. For example, the pesticide DDT

deforestation

The removal of a forest or stand of trees.

environmental health

A discipline that addresses the many external factors that can potentially affect health.

acid rain

The deposition of atmospheric sulfur and nitric acids as precipitation or in dry form (smoke or dust).

smog

Fog thickened and darkened by air pollution.

fossil fuels

Energy resources derived from ancient plants and animals compressed in the ground for millions of years. They include oil (petroleum), natural gas, and coal.

effectively controlled crop insects, as well as malaria and typhus. However, it also caused cancer and killed marine organisms (crayfish, shrimp, fish).[14] Because it thinned eggshells, many bird species became unable to successfully reproduce.

In her 1962 book *Silent Spring* (which refers to a spring without birdsong), marine biologist Rachel Carson made the connection between this environmental devastation and DDT, as well as other pesticides. Her work inspired the environmental movement. She moved beyond **ecology** (the study of the relationship between organisms and their environment) and **conservationism** (the preservation of the natural environment) to **environmentalism**. Environmentalism extended beyond valuing the natural environment to regulating potential threats and disciplining polluters.

Environmental stewardship holds that humans have some obligation to preserve and protect natural settings. Motivations for doing so vary. Healthy ecosystems provide us with fertile agricultural soil, pollination (by insects and birds), and clean water and air.[15] In addition, nature has its own inherent worth, whether or not humans enjoy it or benefit from it. Proponents of that viewpoint believe we should protect plant and animal species, regardless of their apparent human value. Furthermore many people want future generations to inherit a world that retains some natural beauty and natural resources.

This evolution in attitudes has led to the creation of a number of nonprofit organizations and government agencies focused on the environment. In 1970, the US Environmental Protection Agency (EPA) was established.[16] The EPA's function is to research, monitor, set standards, and enforce regulations to protect the environment. April 22 of that same year marked the first Earth Day, a worldwide event intended to heighten awareness of environmental issues.[17]

Later in this chapter, we'll review the many ways of protecting the environment by conserving natural resources, reducing pollution and waste, improving energy efficiency, and developing "clean" energy resources.

FIGURE 17.1
London during the Great Smog of 1952

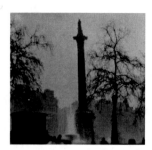

Source: Stobbs NT. Nelson's column in December. 1952. Available at: http://commons.wikimedia.org/wiki/File:Nelson%27s_Column_during_the_Great_Smog_of_1952.jpg.

Nature and Human Health

In addition to its intrinsic value, natural landscapes do us good. However, Americans have become indoor creatures. The trend toward dwindling outdoor time motivated journalist Richard Louv to write the 2005 book *Last Child in the Woods*, which became a *New York Times* best seller and received an Audubon Medal. In it, he describes the consequences of "nature-deficit disorder": diminished creativity, overweight and obesity, attention deficit disorder, and depression.

Sedentary, indoor lifestyles are linked to adult chronic ailments such as cardiovascular disease as well as chronic childhood conditions such as obesity, attention-deficit/hyperactivity disorder, asthma, diabetes, and vitamin D deficiency.[18]

Spending time outdoors encourages physical activity. A study in children found that physical activity rose by 20 to 27 minutes a week for each additional hour spent outside.[19] Furthermore, more outdoor time correlates with lower body weight and less television viewing.[20]

Natural settings help relax us, relieve stress, stimulate the senses, reduce mental fatigue after prolonged concentration, and improve attention.[21] People with access to green spaces are less likely to suffer from depression and anxiety.[22] They also live longer.[23]

Fortunately, a number of organizations are working to increase children's outdoor time.[24] Louv cofounded the Children and Nature Network (http://www.childrenandnature.org), which works with health care providers, researchers, educators, organizations, and individual to get kids outdoors. Adults haven't been left out of this movement. Doctors are starting to prescribe outdoor activity as a means to maintain health, prevent disease, and reduce the impact of chronic conditions.

1.2 Overpopulation: The Crux of the Problem

Overpopulation is the driving force behind environmental degradation. In the beginning, the human population grew at a slow rate. The hunter-gatherer lifestyle kept the population in check. In 1650, about half a billion humans walked the planet. Public health improvements, medical advances, and revolutions in agriculture and industry increased life expectancy. Between 1800 and 1930, the population doubled from 1 to 2 billion.[25] By 1975—a mere 15 years later—the population had again doubled.

In October 2011, world population passed the 7 billion mark[26] and continues to swell at a rate of 200,000 people each day.[27] By 2050, over 9 billion people may crowd the planet.[28] The most rapid development is concentrated in the poorest countries.

Population growth is a function of birth rates and death rates. If birth rates rise and/or death rates fall, the population grows. If both occur, there will be more people and they will live longer. Crowding leads to competition for land and water, typically at the expense of other species. Feeding and housing an increased population leads to deforestation and overfished rivers and oceans. Development pollutes air, water, and soil and consumes nonrenewable resources. Furthermore, overpopulation increases the risk of infectious diseases and deepens conditions of poverty and disadvantage.

In short, overpopulation stresses the planet. In most ecosystems, populations control themselves. When resources become overtaxed, species that depend on them die. Remove wolves and the deer population swells—until food shortages cause some animals to starve. Given that humans have the power to limit their fertility, we have other options than famine, thirst, and war to control our numbers.

Population growth depends on several factors:

1. **Childhood mortality.** In the developing world, parents often have more children, out of concern that some may die. The motivation is to have enough offspring to work fields and otherwise care for aging parents. Many children in these countries die before age five, mainly from infectious illnesses.[29] Improvements in sanitation and hygiene, access to medical care and vaccinations, and other factors have allowed more children to survive to adulthood. As child mortality rates decline, parents may choose to have smaller families.

2. **Education.** The most rapid population growth occurs in poor countries where largely uneducated girls marry and begin bearing children in adolescence.[30] Education increases a woman's social status and earning power, allowing her to postpone marriage and childbearing. Although better educated women tend to have fewer children, those children are more likely to survive because they're born into better socioeconomic conditions (less poverty, better hygiene, and increased medical care).[31]

3. **Access to contraceptives.** According to Save the Children, an organization dedicated to improving children's lives, "222 million women have an unmet need for family planning."[32] Many of these women live in poverty in the developing world. While the net effect is reduced fertility, contraceptive access has three effects on population. One, couples have fewer children. Two, more children survive when births are adequately spaced. Three, fewer women die as a result of pregnancy.[33] Meeting family planning needs lowers infant mortality an estimated 10 to 20 percent and maternal deaths by 35 percent.[34]

   Contraceptives shift population demographics from high birth rate and high death rates toward lower birth rates and death rates. The latter scenario leads to more stable and economically prosperous societies. Overall, quality of life improves.

As a solution to overpopulation, Stanford University professor and author of *The Population Bomb* Paul Ehrlich cofounded Zero Population Growth, now called the Population Connection. Sustainable population growth depends on voluntary family-planning programs. To hold the population steady, the average couple can have two children. For negative population growth, fertility rates need to decline further (assuming death rates stay constant).

Because fertility rates are highest in the developing world, organizations such as the United Nations Population Fund, the Population Connection, and Save the Children work to ensure that women everywhere have access to affordable birth control. Because of the link between human overpopulation and the extinction of other species, the Center for Biological Diversity created Endangered Species Condoms. To see their clever advertising, go to http://www.endangeredspeciescondoms.com.

The United Nations also recognizes that governments need to take action to improve education and women's rights.[35] Furthermore, international protocols can commit nations to stabilize population growth.

FIGURE 17.2 World Population Growth

This United States Census Bureau graph depicts world population from 1950 to 2050.

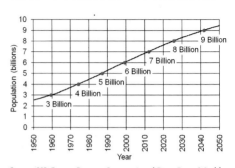

Source: US Census Bureau, International Data Base. World population: 1950–2050. 2012. Available at: http://www.census.gov/population/international/data/idb/worldpopgraph.php.

Progress has been made. According to the United Nations Population Fund, more than half of developing countries have adopted policies to curb fertility rates.[36] Since 1960, the global average birth rate has dropped from six children per woman to three.[37]

1.3 Water: A Critical Environmental Resource

FIGURE 17.3

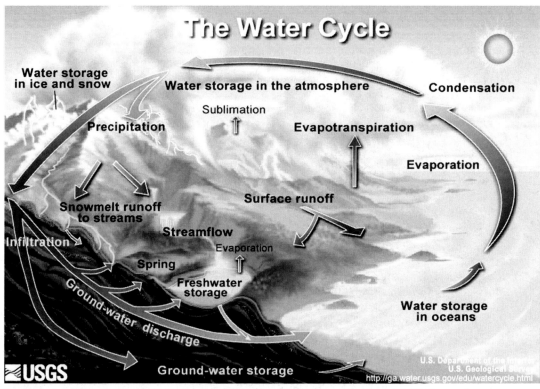

Source: John Evans/Howard Perlman/USGS. Water cycle. 2005. Available at: http://commons.wikimedia.org/wiki/File:Water_cycle.png.

All organisms require water. However, the distribution of water on earth is uneven, leaving some areas with precious little. Water covers 70 percent of the planet. The oceans hold about 97.5 percent of it, though it's too salty to drink. Another 2.4 percent lies on land. The remainder consists of atmospheric water vapor.[38] Some of the land water is stored in glaciers and ice caps. Only 1 percent of the earth's water is usable by humans, other animals, and plants.[39]

Water is constantly moving through the hydrologic (water) cycle. Surface water evaporates into the atmosphere. Cooling as it rises, water vapor condenses into clouds and eventually returns to the earth's surface as precipitation. From there, it may become **surface water** and be stored in streams, rivers, lakes, alpine snowpack and glaciers, oceans, manmade reservoirs, and wetlands (marshes, bogs, swamps). In temperate regions, snowpack and glaciers serve an important reservoir for freshwater, melting in the warmer months to feed streams and lakes.[40]

Precipitation may also penetrate deeper to become **groundwater**. Underground reservoirs called *aquifers* store groundwater. We tap into aquifers for household, agricultural, and other uses. Of the available freshwater, 99 percent is stored as groundwater.

Freshwater Shortages

According to the United Nations Environment Programme, 1.4 billion people live in river basins where water use has outstripped the rate of replenishment.[41] Regions already facing water scarcity include much of western North America, large regions of Africa, the Middle East, eastern Australia, South Asia, and the North China Plain—all areas dependent upon irrigated agriculture. Millions of the people affected are small farmers, who lack the means to move to moister climates.

Population growth and global warming will further strain this precious resource. Experts predict that by 2025, more than 2.8 million people living in 48 countries will face water stress or scarcity.[42] By 2050, that number could rise to 4 billion people (40 percent of the projected global population). Changes in temperature and precipitation as a result of global warming, as well as water pollution that impairs the use of water, are expected to worsen regional water shortages in many parts of the globe.

People in poorer nations bear the brunt of the scarcity of clean fresh water. According to the World Health Organization (WHO), 1.1 billion people in the developing world lack access to safe drinking water.[43] That's 3.5 times the population of the United States. A surprising amount of our drinkable water—42 percent of urban water in California—is used to irrigate lawns, parks, golf courses, and cemeteries. In Los Angeles, 70 percent of residential water went toward outdoor use—an amount that dropped after ordinances limiting lawn watering.[44]

The average American goes through 152 gallons a day. Ironically, daily per-person use in arid but emerald-lawned Phoenix in 2006 was more than 265 gallons. People in other developed countries get by with less. The average European manages on 53 to 80 gallons a day.[45] In contrast, in Mozambique, Africa, the average person has a mere 2.6 gallons a day—the amount that goes down the drain during a one-minute shower (with a low-flow showerhead) and one-hundredth of the per person daily use in Tucson.

Water Management and Conservation

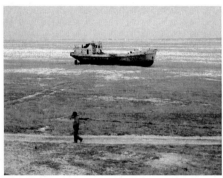

Ship lying aground in the former Aral Sea in Kazakhstan.

Scientists, conservationists, and city planners are searching for ways to cope with looming water shortages. In Australia, where much of the bone-dry continent has struggled with drought, the government has mandated restrictions on water use and has subsidized water tanks for homeowners to capture rainwater.

In addition, some Australian cities are spending billions of dollars on **desalination** plants, which remove salt from seawater to render it potable (safe to drink).[46] A plant recently began operations on the Thames River in London. Some US communities, particularly in arid southwest, are also considering desalination projects and the process has been used to improve the quality of Colorado River water delivered to Mexico.[47]

Opponents argue that the process is complicated, costly, harms marine ecosystems, and consumes energy, which further contributes to global warming and, hence, drought.[48] They prefer other measures, such as **water recycling**, which has a smaller economic and environmental impact. As described earlier, nature constantly recycles water. Humans have also long recycled water. For instance, water diverted from creeks and rivers to irrigate agricultural land eventually returns to surface and ground water systems. However, that water often has pesticides, synthetic fertilizers, and salts leached from the soil.

Source: Staecker. Orphaned ship in former Aral Sea. 2003.

Available at: http://commons.wikimedia.org/wiki/

File:Aralship2.jpg.

Increasingly, wastewater from municipal sewage systems has become a source of water. This reclaimed water can be used to irrigate crops and urban landscapes, flush toilets, and replenish groundwater aquifers. Industries can recycle and reuse water on site. Rapidly evolving treatment technology removes biological and chemical pollutants to make the water potable (safe to drink). Concerns remain about the ability to remove certain contaminants, such as pharmaceuticals.[49] While no health problems have been reported, public acceptance has lagged behind the technology.

A different form of recycling is capturing and reusing *gray water*—water used for bathing, showers, dishwashing, and clothes washing. This reclaimed water can irrigate outdoor areas. To protect plants, soap and other personal care products need to be nontoxic and low in sodium.[50]

The city of Tucson, Arizona, has adopted an ordinance requiring that new residential units be plumbed to divert gray water for irrigation.[51] Citizens can also receive tax credits for installing such systems.[52] The city estimates that water reclamation (recycling) saves more than six billion gallons of drinking water each year.[53]

Other states are taking steps to conserve freshwater. In 2012, the California state legislature passed a bill requiring municipal water suppliers to reduce use by 20 percent per person by 2020. Governments can accomplish their goals by restricting lawn watering, providing incentives for homeowners and farmers to install efficient irrigation systems, and motivating citizens to landscape with drought-tolerant plants.

Conservation works. Boston's efforts to conserve water (fix leaks in aging pipes, install low-flow shower heads and toilets) reduced water demands between 1980 and 2009 by a whopping 43 percent.[54]

Assess Yourself: How Can You Conserve Water?

If Europeans can maintain a high standard of living on half the water, we can surely follow suit. Because much municipal water goes to home use, citizens have the power to conserve this precious resource.

Examine the following list. Check off the things you're doing now. Resolve to adopt one new water-conserving habit. If you live in a dormitory, some goals may have to wait until you have your own place.

_____ I turn on the tap only when I really need water. I turn it off while I'm washing dishes, brushing my teeth, shaving, and soaping up in the shower (and I turn it on only to rinse).

_____ When hand-washing dishes, I fill a basin with soapy water and another with rinse water. In that way, I don't leave the tap running. (Note: Compared to hand washing, dishwashers use a lot less water.)

_____ I promptly repair leaky faucets.

_____ I shower rather than bathe.

_____ I take short (five minutes or less) showers.

_____ My showerhead is a low-flow fixture. (Before 1992, fixtures delivered 5.5 gallons a minute. The federal government has mandated that new fixtures can't exceed 2.5 gallons a minute.[55] To find out the rate of yours, time how many minutes it takes to fill a one-gallon bucket.)

_____ I have a low-flow toilet. (Toilets account for more than one-third of home water use.[56] Pre-1980 models use anywhere from 3.5 to 7 gallons per flush. Ultra low-flush toilets use 1.6 gallons per flush. To reduce the flow of your toilet without buying a new one, drop a few pebbles into an empty liter bottle, fill with water, and place in the toilet's tank.[57])

_____ I use a front-loading washing machine (which is water and energy efficient) and a water-efficient dishwasher.

_____ I wait to run the dishwasher and washing machine until I have a full load.

_____ I water houseplants with "gray water."

_____ When I landscape, I select plants resistant to drought. (That's important if you live in an arid region.)

_____ I make sure outdoor yard irrigation systems water efficiently (during cooler times of the day with no to little runoff on pavement).

_____ I take my car to a carwash rather than using a hose to wash it myself. (Going to the car wash uses less water. Municipal car washes are usually required to recycle water.)

_____ I eat foods that require less water to produce—more fruits and vegetables, less meat, dairy, and processed foods.

_____ I recycle paper, plastic, glass, and metal. (More water is used in creating these materials from their raw materials than from recycled products.)

1.4 Pollution: Problems and Solutions

pollution

The introduction into the environment of toxic substances (pollutants) that have adverse effects on living organisms and natural resources.

Pollution is defined as the introduction into the environment of substances with harmful effects. Physical, chemical, and biological alteration of air, water, and soil, including the introduction of toxic substances, can sicken us and other living creatures. Many of the pollutants discussed in this section are manmade.

Water Pollution

Degradation of water quality is a major concern worldwide. The pollution of freshwater sources and the oceans from the discharge of human, industrial, and agricultural waste has enormous implications for human health and the health of natural ecosystems. The absence of sanitation facilities results in the contamination of drinking water sources around the globe, particularly in Asia and Africa. Microbes in drinking water cause infectious diseases, mainly diarrheal illness, and represent the number one cause of death in children under five years old. According to the WHO, "More people die from unsafe water annually than from all forms of violence, including war."[58]

Freshwater fish and aquatic insects, plants, and animals are adversely affected by the discharge of pollutants, warmer water temperatures (often from power plants), and the destruction of wetlands that naturally filter out contaminants and provide important wildlife habitats. Loss of habitat and changes in the chemical and biological characteristics of rivers and streams can lead to reduction in species abundance and diversity.

Marine life has suffered too. Pollution, warmer water temperatures, and overfishing have stressed our oceans. Records tracking some 217 species of marine mammals, birds, reptiles, and fish show pronounced declines over the past four decades.[59] For a graphic created by the World Wildlife Federation, go to http://www.unep.org/dewa/vitalwater/article161.html.

In 1972, the United States enacted the Clean Water Act, which authorized the EPA to implement pollution controls. The result has been a significant improvement in the quality of surface water sources in the country. However, many challenges remain, including controlling chemicals from urban and agricultural storm water runoff and adequate regulation of surface and ground water pollution from oil and gas drilling.[60] A 2004 assessment of water quality by the states identified 44 percent of the assessed river and stream miles as being impaired, or not supporting one or more of their designated uses.[61]

Plastics and Human Health

Plastics are versatile, useful, pervasive, and, in many ways, unhealthy. On and around your own desk you may have multiple plastic-derived objects: insulation in the computer cables; CDs; the printer ink; the lenses of your glasses; and the casings of your phone, monitor, mouse, pens, and the keyboard under your fingertips. It's in containers that hold food, beverages, personal care products, and cleaning agents. It's in dental sealants, water pipes, toys, plastic cutlery, glue, clothes, and building materials.

Derived from natural gas and crude oil (petroleum), plastics are synthetic polymers (long chains of repeating units made from carbon, hydrogen, and other atoms). Each year, we produce more than 540 billion pounds worldwide—over 100 billion pounds in the United States alone.[62] More than 8 percent of the world's crude oil production goes into the production of plastics.[63] Disposable items account for a third of that volume. Thrown away, plastics endure a long time in the environment. Some industries have developed *biodegradable* (capable of decomposition) products derived from corn and other renewal resources.[64]

Certain types of plastic contain *endocrine disruptors*—substances that alter normal hormonal function. Two endocrine-disrupting chemicals in plastics have caught the attention of scientists and health advocates: bisphenol A (BPA) and phthalates. These chemicals are released from plastic into food, water, air, soil, and human bodies. In the human system—and nearly everyone has both chemicals in bodily fluids—they mimic the action of estrogen and interfere with the action of testosterone.

Exposure early in life may be particularly detrimental. A recent study showed that 93 percent of breastfed infants had BPA in their urine.[65] That means they were exposed via their mothers. Scientists have raised concerns that endocrine-disrupting chemicals affect the brain and behavior; hasten the onset of puberty; impair fertility; retard fetal growth; and raise the risk for obesity and breast, testicular, and prostate cancer.[66],[67],[68]

Here's how you can reduce your exposure harmful chemicals in plastics:

- Avoid these products:
    - plastic containers marked on the bottom with "7" or "PC" (for polycarbonate), which contain BPA
    - hard, clear plastic containers not labeled as BPA-free
    - plastic-wrapped foods such as deli meats and cheeses
- Look for canned foods that state they're BPA-free. (BPA is in the lining of tin cans.)
- Drink beverages in glass or steel containers.
- Store food in ceramic or glass containers.
- Microwave food in ceramic or glass containers, not plastic.
- Wash plastic beverage and food containers by hand in lukewarm water rather than in the dishwasher.
- Use wood rather than plastic cutting boards.
- Use plant-derived fragrances. Synthetic fragrances usually are phthalates.

If you have a baby, use glass bottles with nipples that don't contain phthalates. In 2012, the Food and Drug Administration banned BPA from baby bottles and "sippy cups," though it declined to ban the substance from food containers such as cans and water bottles.[69],[70] Don't accept hand-me-downs that may contain them. The same is true for toys marked with a "3" or "PVC," which stands for polyvinyl chloride.

For more ideas, check out "Eat like a Mennonite," a *New York Times* personal essay on avoiding BPA and phthalates (http://www.nytimes.com/2013/01/19/opinion/eat-like-a-mennonite.html?ref=opinion&_r=0).

Air Pollution

The atmosphere enveloping the earth is divided into five layers. This chapter will focus on the first two: the troposphere and the stratosphere. The troposphere begins at sea level and extends upward seven miles, becoming cooler and thinner in water vapor and life-sustaining gases as it rises. Only the bottom third—just over two miles—is breathable.[71] What we call "weather" occurs in the troposphere.

Parallel to the junction between the troposphere and the stratosphere are strong wind currents called *jet streams*. The predominant wind direction is west to east. The jet streams influence weather and airplane travel. The outer edge of the stratosphere contains ozone, a gas formed from the interaction of the sun's ultraviolet rays and oxygen. Stratospheric ozone shields life on earth's surface from the harmful effects of ultraviolet radiation. As we'll soon discuss, depletion of stratospheric ozone and excess tropospheric ozone damage health.

Sources of air pollutants are both natural and manmade. Natural causes include forest fires, volcanic eruptions, dust storms, decaying organic matter in swamps, fungal spores, and pollen blooms.[72] Most of the time, these natural air pollutants are minor in comparison to human-generated sources. All of our modes of transportation—train, car, truck, airplane—produce pollution from the combustion of fossil fuels. Power plants, industrial facilities, and modern agriculture also release particles and gases that are harmful to humans. Tobacco smoke and wood smoke from fireplaces pollute indoor and local outdoor air.

According to the WHO, indoor air pollution causes 2 million premature deaths a year; urban outdoor air pollution leads to 1.3 million deaths a year.[73] Respiratory illnesses account for many of these deaths.[74] Children, older adults, and people with lung disease are most vulnerable.

Air pollution is especially a problem in India and China, where rapid economic development has increased the use of fossil fuels such as coal for generating electricity, heating homes, and powering industrial plants.[75] Air pollution in one region can affect the entire planet because winds transport pollutants to distant locations.

In 1963, the US government enacted the Clean Air Act, which originally funded research into techniques for monitoring and controlling air pollution. Subsequent amendments strengthened the role of the EPA to monitor and enforce regulations on air pollutants. The EPA calculates outdoor air quality using the **Air Quality Index** (AQI) for the five major air pollutants: particulate matter, sulfur dioxide, nitrogen oxide, ozone, and carbon monoxide. The Clean Air Act regulates these pollutants, and the EPA establishes standards to protect public health. AQI values run from 0 to 500. The lower the number, the better the air quality.

TABLE 17.1 Air Quality Index (AQI)

Air quality index (AQI) range	Air quality condition	Color
0–50	Good	Green
51–100	Moderate	Yellow
101–150	Unhealthy for sensitive groups	Orange
151–200	Unhealthy	Red
201–300	Very unhealthy	Purple
301–500	Hazardous	Maroon
Note: The EPA divides AQI values into six categories, ranging from good to hazardous air quality. The category called "Unhealthy for Sensitive Groups" refers to children, older adults, and people with heart and lung disease.		

Source: AIRNow/Environmental Protection Agency. Air Quality Index (AQI): a guide to air quality and your health. 2011. Available at:

http://www.airnow.gov/index.cfm?action=aqibasics.aqi.

The Four Most Damaging Air Pollutants

Particulate matter is made of small particles suspended in the air in dry form or mixed with liquid droplets. Natural sources include dust, sea salt spray, smoke from wildfires, volcanic ash, pollen, fungal spores, and airborne bacteria and viruses. Manmade sources include aerosols and chemical fumes.

These fine particles make the air hazy, reducing visibility. They stain and corrode statues, monuments, and other structures. Wind carries suspended particles long distances. Eventually they settle to the ground, damaging plants and polluting soil and water.

The tiniest particles (those less than 10 microns in diameter) can be inhaled into the lungs to irritate the airways, leading to bronchitis, asthma attacks, decreased lung function, irregular heartbeat, and premature death.[76] Chronic exposure contributes to cardiovascular and respiratory diseases, including lung cancer.

Sulfur dioxide is a colorless gas that smells like a burnt match. In the presence of water vapor, it turns into a mist of sulfuric acid.[77] Manmade sources stem from the combustion of fossil fuels in power plants, iron and steel mills, pulp and paper mills, and petroleum refineries. Exposure irritates the eyes and inflames and narrows respiratory passages, triggering coughing and asthma symptoms. Sulfur dioxide can also react with other compounds to form small particles that can damage the lungs. When combined with water vapor, it forms sulfuric acid, leading to acid rain.

Nitrogen oxides are formed from nitrogen and oxygen. Nitrogen dioxide is the predominant chemical. This reddish-brown, strong-smelling gas arises from combusting fuels to generate power, heat homes, and run motorized vehicles. People who live or work near roadways are at particular risk for exposure. This gas inflames the eyes, nose, throat, and respiratory tract. Long-term exposure reduces lung function and triggers airway inflammation, especially in asthmatic children.[78] Like sulfur oxides, nitrogen oxides can become acidic components of particulate matter, thereby contributing to acid rain.

Ozone is an unstable molecule made of three oxygen atoms. This gas is colorless and odorless. In the troposphere, ozone results primarily from chemical reactions involving sunlight and gases generated by the burning of fossil fuels: nitrogen oxides, carbon monoxide, methane, and other hydrocarbons (compounds made of hydrogen and carbon).[79] Ground-level ozone levels tend to peak in cities on hot, sunny days. Ozone irritates respiratory linings, triggering asthma and causing sore throat, coughing, pain upon deep inhalation, and shortness of breath.[80] It also damages plants and reduces crop yields, further challenging the ability to feed the world's growing population.[81] Between the 1860s and the 2000s, ground-level ozone increased fourfold.

Stratospheric Ozone Depletion: The Ozone Hole

It's the worst of all possible combinations. Ozone levels have increased in the troposphere, where at ground level this gas causes serious health problems. In the stratosphere, where it shields us from ultraviolet light, ozone has been depleted. The main culprit is chlorofluorocarbons (CFCs), compounds made of carbon, chlorine, hydrogen, and fluorine. They were invented in the 1920s for use in propellants (including aerosol sprays), refrigerants, cleaning solvents, and foaming agents.[82] In the 1970s, scientists established a link between CFCs and ozone depletion. An expanding region of marked thinning over Antarctica was called the **ozone hole**. (A smaller ozone hole exists over the North Pole.) By 1984, about 40 percent of the stratospheric ozone had been lost.[83]

Consequences of depleted ozone stem from an increase in ultraviolet (UV) light reaching the ground and oceans. Scientists are concerned about damage to terrestrial plants and phytoplankton, which supports marine life.[84],[85] Excess UV radiation also decreases the productivity of terrestrial plants. In humans, increased exposure to UV rays suppresses immune function and heightens the risk of sunburn, skin cancer, and cataracts (vision-impairing cloudiness in the eye's lens). Because they live under the ozone hole, Australians have the highest rates of skin cancer.[86]

Beginning in the late 1980s, international protocols such as the Montreal Protocol were established to reduce and eventually ban the production of CFCs. Since then, stratospheric concentrations of ozone-depleting chemicals have steadily declined.

Indoor Air Pollution

In addition to air pollutants that enter buildings through doors and windows, other sources can pollute indoor air. Common examples include wood and coal-burning stoves, furnaces, lead, tobacco smoke, radon, mold spores, cleaning products, and off-gassing building materials.

The most prevalent indoor pollutant is **tobacco** smoke. It contains hundreds of toxic chemicals, including poisonous gases (carbon monoxide, hydrogen cyanide, ammonia, butane, toluene), carcinogens (formaldehyde, benzene, vinyl chloride), and toxic metals (arsenic, lead, and cadmium).[87]

Carbon monoxide is a colorless, odorless gas formed from incomplete combustion of natural gas, oil, coal, wood, tobacco, and other carbon-containing materials. Each molecule is made of one carbon and one oxygen atom (CO). (Carbon dioxide, on the other hand, contains two oxygen atoms.) Carbon monoxide binds tightly to hemoglobin, a protein in red blood cells that normally transports oxygen to tissues. The result is reduced oxygen delivery. Carbon monoxide poisoning causes headache, dizziness, fatigue, weakness, nausea, vomiting, and eventually death. The skin and mucous membranes redden.

Proper ventilation reduces exposure. Living spaces should have *carbon monoxide detectors* that set off an alarm when at critical levels. If yours goes off, go outside and breathe fresh air. Leave windows open until you can get a professional inspection. Never leave your car idling in a garage or other poorly ventilated space.

In addition to carbon monoxide, **formaldehyde** pollutes indoor air when released by materials such as carpets, particleboard, plywood, furniture, and adhesives. Workers in industries making these products are most at risk. Short-term effects include nausea; skin irritation; and burning of the eyes, nose, and throat. Long-term exposure has been associated with some types of cancer.[88]

Lead, a naturally occurring metal, can contaminate air as well as water and soil. Sources include plants that process ores and metals and make lead-acid batteries. In the past, motor vehicles fueled by leaded gasoline were a major source of atmospheric lead. Homes built before 1978 may have lead-based paint.[89] Over time, the paint chips away, turns to dust, and settles onto floors and outdoor soil.

Nonplastic plumbing installed before 1986 also contained lead. Corroded pipes then release lead. The EPA recommends that, if the tap hasn't been turned on for six hours or more, run the water until it becomes cold.[90] Because lead is used in ceramic glazes, imported pottery is another source. For

FIGURE 17.4 Antarctic Ozone Hole

Stratospheric ozone shields earth's inhabitants from the sun's ultraviolet light. Use of compounds called chlorofluorocarbons has thinned the ozone over the South Pole. Purple and blue colors represent areas of the least ozone.

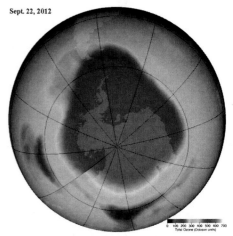

Sept. 22, 2012

Source: NASA. Antarctic ozone hole as at Sept. 22, 2012. 2012. Available at: http://commons.wikimedia.org/wiki/ File:2012_Antarctic_Ozone_Hole.jpg.

ozone hole

A region of marked thinning in stratospheric ozone.

more information on protecting yourself from lead, consult the EPA website (http://www.epa.gov/lead/parents.html#soil).

Lead enters the body when inhaled, ingested, or applied to the skin. It damages the nervous system, blood, kidneys, and other tissues.[91] Children are especially vulnerable to impaired brain development.[92] For that reason, use of lead in paint, in plumbing, in shotgun pellets (for hunting fowl), and as an additive to gasoline was eventually banned.

Radon is a naturally occurring odorless, colorless, tasteless, radioactive gas that comes from breakdown of uranium. Indoor radon ranks second to tobacco smoke as a cause for lung cancer and results in over 21,000 lung cancer deaths a year.[93] Sources include soil, rock, and, less often, well water. Radon in the ground under buildings or in building materials seeps into indoor air where it can be inhaled. People may also ingest it in contaminated water. The only way to determine whether this gas is in your home or workplace is to test the levels. You can find kits at hardware stores. Sealing cracks in foundations, basement floors, and walls can reduce radon. If it doesn't, ventilations systems may be needed.

Asbestos is another cancer-causing substance that can contaminate indoor air. This mineral fiber, which occurs naturally in rock and soil, has been used for insulation and as a fire retardant. It's found in products such as heat-resistant fabrics, building materials (shingles, vermiculite insulation, ceiling and floor tiles, walls and floors around wood-burning stoves, some cement products), and motor vehicle parts (breaks, transmission, clutch).[94] If asbestos was used in cement water mains, it can decay into drinking water.

When asbestos-containing products are disturbed (during installation or demolition), fibers can be released into the air. People who inhale the fibers may eventually develop lung cancer, mesothelioma (cancer of the lining of the chest organs), and asbestosis (a noncancerous, chronic lung disease). Despite the well-known risks, this material has not been banned in the United States.

If you suspect you have asbestos in your home, find out how to protect yourself on the EPA website (http://www.epa.gov/asbestos/protect-your-family.html).

What You Can Do to Reduce Air Pollution

Granted, a lot of air pollution comes from power plants and other industrial sources. But individual actions, such as driving automobiles and heating homes, also play a powerful role. Here's what you can do:

- Keep your car well-maintained and use it only when necessary.
- Avoid idling your car (unless you're waiting at a traffic light).
- Support the production of electricity that's not generated by coal-fired plants, which are a major source of air pollution. Some utilities offer programs in which ratepayers can elect to purchase energy from renewable sources.
- Test your home for radon. The EPA website has information about testing for radon and reducing home levels of this gas at http://www.epa.gov/radon/index.html.
- Don't smoke!
- Use water-based paints, stains, and paint strippers. Avoid those high in toxic volatile organic compounds ("VOCs"—toxic solvents that evaporate into the air).
- Use carpets and other building materials that are low in VOCs.
- Conserve energy. While the contribution from renewable sources is increasing, the United States still relies largely on fossil fuels for energy. So when you use electricity, you're contributing to the burning of fossil fuels.
- Consider the life-cycle energy cost of products that you buy, including processing, packaging, and transportation that consume energy and release pollutants.

Land Pollution and Solid Waste

Some pollutants are first introduced into the environment on the land. For instance, synthetic pesticides and fertilizers applied to crops also contaminate the soil. Precipitation carries those pollutants into surface and groundwater. Soil pollutants may also become incorporated into dust, which becomes airborne when blown by the wind. On the other hand, air pollutants from industries and vehicle exhaust eventually settle to the ground.

In addition, most of our **municipal solid waste** (trash) ends up in landfills. In a single year, Americans throw away about 250 million tons of trash.[95] Containers and packaging constitute one-third of solid waste.

Although we dump most of our trash in landfills, we're getting better at reducing that waste. Nearly 12 percent of solid waste is combusted for energy. About 34 percent is recycled or composted, a number that has crept steadily upward thanks to heightened public awareness, increased infrastructure, and a growing market demand for recycled materials.

Much household solid waste ends up in landfills, disposal sites where trash is buried between layers of dirt.

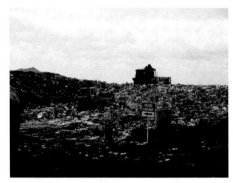

Source: Ashley Felton. Active tipping area of an operating landfill in Perth, Western Australia. 2006. Available at: http://commons.wikimedia.org/wiki/File:Landfill_face.JPG.

FIGURE 17.5 What Happens to the Stuff We Throw Away

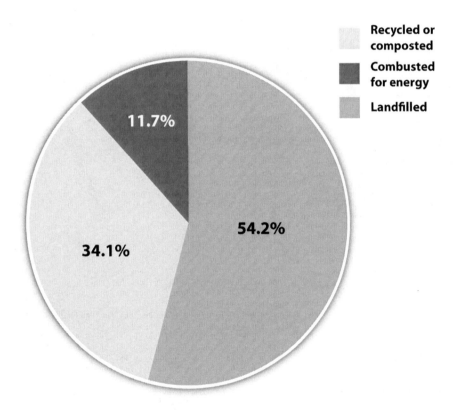

Source: Adapted from Environmental Protection Agency. What happens to the stuff we throw away. Recycling Basics. Available at: http://www2.epa.gov/recycle/recycling-basics.

The EPA defines recycling as "the recovery of useful materials, such as paper, glass, plastic, and metals, from the trash to use to make new products, reducing the amount of new raw materials needed."[96] Composting involves collecting organic waste (e.g., food scraps and yard clippings) and storing it under conditions that promote the breakdown of the material. Once the process is completed, compost can be used as a rich fertilizer.

Americans are best at recycling paper (a rate of 72 percent) and worst at recycling plastic containers and packaging (overall 13 percent).[97] About 35 percent of metals (aluminum, steel, and mixed metals) are recycled.

The benefits of recycling and composting are multiple and include the following:

- less waste taxing our landfill capacity
- conservation of the raw materials from which these products are composed

- reduced energy consumption and pollution involved in collecting and processing raw materials (A total of 85 million tons of solid waste recycled in 2010 reduced carbon dioxide emissions by 186 million metric tons, equivalent to removing 36 million cars from the road.[98] A 2009 mandatory recycling and composting ordinance in San Francisco led to a 12 percent reduction in the city's carbon emissions compared to 1990;[99] it plans to be a zero-waste city by 2020.)
- job creation in recycling and manufacturing industries[100]

Two other strategies help us conserve resources and protect the environment: **reduce** and **reuse**. A good way to minimize your environmental impact is to buy fewer goods. Consider sharing with friends and neighbors large items such as lawn mowers, power tools, clothes washers, and cars. Rent rather than buy infrequently used goods. Choose products with less packaging.

In addition to reducing your use of resources, you can reuse products already in circulation. Bring fabric bags to stores. Buy used goods. Donate items so others can reuse them. Repair items rather than tossing and replacing them. Build using refurbished materials. Buy products made from recycled materials, which supports the market for recycling.

Video Clip 17.1

Making Music on Recycled Materials

Landfill Harmonic is a 2014 documentary about Cateura, Paraguay, a town built on a landfill. To keep kids away from gangs and drugs, a school music program was started, using instruments made from recycled materials.

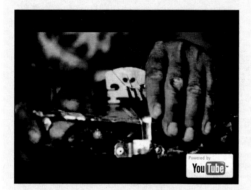

View the video online at: http://www.youtube.com/v/fXynrsrTKbl

Assess Yourself: Do You Reduce, Reuse, and Recycle?

Are you doing all you can to conserve valuable resources? Check off the things you're already doing and identify at least one new habit you could adopt.

_____ I buy goods that last.

_____ I buy reusable rather than disposable items (e.g., pens, razors, silverware, cups).

_____ I recycle aluminum, glass, plastic, paper, batteries, and electronic equipment.

_____ I carry beverages in reusable containers and bring my own cup to coffee shops.

_____ I bring reusable bags when shopping.

_____ I shop for minimally packaged products (or choose packaging made from recycled materials).

_____ I shop for products made from recycled materials.

_____ I repair items such as shoes, clothes, cars, and appliances so that they last longer.

_____ When possible, I buy durable goods that are gently used rather than new. (The manufacture of new goods consumes energy and water.)

_____ I donate my used books, clothing, furniture, and electronics.

_____ I buy rechargeable batteries for devices I use frequently.

_____ I compost organic matter—food waste, lawn clippings, leaves. (To learn how, go to http://howtocompost.org.)

In addition to the relatively nontoxic items we routinely toss, there are also **hazardous wastes**, those capable of harming humans and the environment. Household materials that qualify include batteries, motor oil, gasoline, antifreeze, paint, paint thinner and other solvents, and compact fluorescent bulbs (which save energy but contain small amounts of mercury). Some industrial materials are highly toxic, such as radioactive materials used in medicine and nuclear power plants.

One approach is to minimize your use of toxic products. For instance, you can buy paints lower in toxic chemicals and cleaning products made from biodegradable (decomposed by bacteria), nontoxic materials. You should also take batteries, electronic equipment, and other hazardous materials to collection centers for disposal. Do not dispose of hazardous wastes down the sink, into storm sewers, onto the ground, or in the trash. Doing so pollutes soil, water, and air. Your municipal recycling center can tell you where to take them. To find out more about recycling of nonhazardous and hazardous materials, consult Earth911.com or http://www.epa.gov/epawaste/basic-hazard.htm.

Light and Noise Pollution

The city lights, such as those in Spain and Portugal, can disrupt daily rhythms in humans and animals.

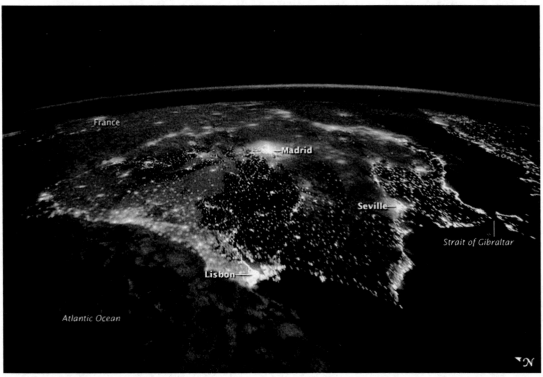

Source: NASA. Iberian Peninsula at night—NASA Earth Observatory. 2011. Available at: http://commons.wikimedia.org/wiki/

File:Iberian_Peninsula_at_Night_-_NASA_Earth_ Observatory.jpg.

When we talk about pollution, most people think of harsh chemicals. However, light and sound also have profound effects on living creatures.

Light pollution is excessive or intrusive amounts of light. Recall from Chapter 4 that darkness helps us sleep. Light, even small amounts emitted by electronic devices, inhibit the nighttime rise in melatonin, a hormone that regulates many cycles, including sleep. Breast cancer risk is higher among women who work nightshifts and live in communities where artificial lighting is bright enough to read outdoors at night. Urban lights also obscure our view of the night sky. Just think about how much better you see stars and planets when you're far from a city.[101]

Plants and animals are also affected by artificial light. It can hinder the normal adaptation of trees' and other plants' seasonal variations in natural light. In animals, artificial light can interfere with normal daily rhythms, nighttime navigation, breeding cycles, and foraging behaviors.[102]

Outside lights, especially those that point sideways and upward, are the main causes of light pollution.[103] A solution is to install lights that angle downward or that are activated by motion (turning on only as someone approaches your home).

Noise pollution involves the production of sounds loud enough to adversely affect the health of humans and other animals. If you live in an urban area (or even in a college dormitory), you understand that loud music, construction, honking cars, and sirens can be more than an annoyance. Loud noises disrupt sleep, fracture concentration, shatter peace of mind, generate stress (which is particularly hard on the cardiovascular system), and impair hearing.

A 2011 WHO report stated that environmental noise was second to air pollution in causing human disease, death, and disability.[104] Listening to MP3 players at high volumes has led to hearing loss in many teens and young adults. Earbud-style earphones increase the decibel (sound level) exposure. Fifteen percent of college graduates have hearing loss on par or worse than that of their parents.[105]

Many land animals use sound to communicate, navigate, and find food.[106] Our noise can disrupt these processes. The ocean has also become a noisy place due to underwater blasts, sonar and seismic surveys, shipping, and oil and gas industry activity. Marine mammals (whales, dolphins, and porpoises) that navigate and communicate using sound have been most adversely affected.[107]

Here's some sound advice: take care of your ears. Prolonged exposure to loud noises leads to tinnitus (ringing or buzzing in the ears) and permanent hearing loss. If you use a head set when listening to music and movies, use the kind that goes over your ears instead of earbuds. Keep the volume at a moderate level. Rather than turning up the tunes to drown out the noise around you, listen to lower-volume music with noise-canceling headphones. Wear ear protection (ear plugs, ear muffs, noise-reducing headset) when exposed to loud noises: attending loud concerts, riding or working on a motorcycle, or operating power equipment (chainsaw, jackhammer, lawnmower).

TABLE 17.2 How Loud Is Too Loud?

Decibels	Sound source
150	Firecracker
120	Ambulance siren
110	Chain saw, rock concert
105	Personal stereo system at maximum level
100	Wood shop, snowmobile
95	Motorcycle
90	Power mower
85	Heavy city traffic
60	Normal conversation
40	Refrigerator humming
30	Whispered voice
0	Threshold of normal hearing

Note: The National Institute on Deafness and Other Communication Disorders provides a scale of noise levels. Sound intensity is measured in decibels. Prolonged exposure to sounds at 85 decibels leads to hearing loss. Higher decibel levels more quickly damage hearing. Only one minute at 110 decibels can permanently impair hearing.

Source: National Institute on Deafness and Other Communication Disorders (NIDCD). How loud is too loud? Available at: http://www.nidcd.nih.gov/health/hearing/pages/ruler.aspx.

KEY TAKEAWAYS

- Environmental health began in an attempt to reduce exposure to infectious diseases. The field has since broadened to include all external factors (chemical, biological, and physical) that can potentially affect health.
- Industrialization and rapid population growth accelerated use of natural resources and the release of toxic compounds into the environment. Governments subsequently have enacted legislation to regulate pollution.
- Controlling population growth is critical to solving environmental problems.
- Freshwater is a limited resource. Looming water shortages make water conservation critical.
- Byproducts from burning fossil fuel are largely responsible for outdoor air pollution. Indoor air pollutants include tobacco smoke, chemicals in building materials, solvents, cleaning products, and radon.
- People can minimize solid waste production by buying fewer consumer goods, recycling, and reusing materials. Doing so also reduces pollution and consumption of natural resources.
- Light and noise pollution, though under-recognized, have a significant impact on health.

DISCUSSION QUESTIONS

1. Modern humans spend little time in natural environments. What does "being in nature" mean to you? How much time do you currently spend outside each week? Describe what you do. Do you ever go outside as a study break? If yes, how do you feel afterward? Is there a qualitative difference between being in an urban green space (a backyard or park) and a wilder natural setting (national park, wilderness area, ocean)?

2. Consider the concept of environmental stewardship. Some dismiss the concept as speciesist (discriminates based on species) or anthropocentric (assumes humans are the most important species). Others insist that we humans, who have so degraded the environment, have moral and ethical obligations to lessen the damage and protect nature.

   What do you think? What does environmental stewardship mean to you? Should we protect natural environments? For whom? Future generations of humans or all future life forms? Should we preserve species even if doing so might threaten human interests? (Examples include large predators.)

3. Go to this *National Geographic* website: http://environment.nationalgeographic.com/environment/ freshwater/water-footprint-calculator. Calculate your "water footprint." View the tips. What did you learn? Can you reduce your water use? How will you accomplish that goal? (Note: when you finish the calculation, click the link at the bottom that takes you to "Water Footprint Calculator Methodology and Tips.")

4. Go to the AIRNow website (http://airnow.gov). In the forecast tab, do you see any American cities with an air quality index worse than moderate? Click on the map over your region for more detailed information. How is your air quality today?

5. On the same EPA website, go to http://www.epa.gov/aircompare/index.htm. Click on "County Comparisons." Compare the county in which you live to another city you suspect might have worse air quality. How did your county stack up?

6. In addition to being a potent source of indoor air pollution, tobacco has other environment downsides. Go to this World Health Organization website: http://www.who.int/tobacco/research/economics/ rationale/environment/en/. Summarize what you learned about the environment degradation associated with growing and producing tobacco products.

2. CLIMATE CHANGE: CAUSES AND CONSEQUENCES

LEARNING OBJECTIVES

1. Explain the greenhouse effect.
2. Differentiate between renewable and nonrenewable energy resources.
3. Review the evidence for climate change and the consequences of global warming.
4. Examine ways groups and individuals can reduce greenhouse gas emissions.

FIGURE 17.6 How the Earth's Greenhouse Effect Works

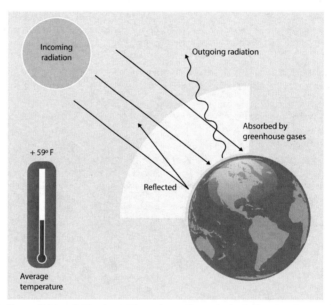

*Source: Adapted from NOAA; Conway T, Belnay L. How the earth's greenhouse effect works. Available at: http://www.esrl.noaa.gov/gsd/outreach/
education/climgraph/CG_Figure_16.gif.html.*

Life as we know it depends on the temperature of the land, air, and oceans. Temperature variations affect the range of plants and animals. They also shape weather patterns. The source of warmth is the sun. After it penetrates the atmosphere, some of the sun's energy is absorbed by the earth and some is radiated back into space.

Greenhouse gases are gases that absorb heat energy in the atmosphere. Without them, the earth would be a frozen, inhospitable place. Prime examples include carbon dioxide, methane, and water vapor, which trap heat much as the glass does in a manmade greenhouse. The atmospheric concentration of these gases changes the temperature of the planet through a complex mechanism known as the **greenhouse effect**.

A net increase in these gases enhances the greenhouse effect. The end result is **global warming**, a term describing the increase in the earth's temperature. The other term for this phenomenon is *climate change*. (*Climate* refers to average weather patterns over a long period of time.)

The Intergovernmental Panel on Climate Change (IPCC), created by the United Nations Environment Programme to assess climate change,[108] has issued reports confirming the evidence of global warming and attributing it to human activities.[109] Those activities include fossil fuel combustion, which releases greenhouse gases into the atmosphere, as well as deforestation, which reduces the ability of the planet to absorb **carbon dioxide** (CO_2). While a few skeptics remain, a 2009 survey found that 97 percent of climate scientists thought that human activities had contributed to steadily rising global temperatures.[110]

Carbon dioxide is the greenhouse gas that contributes to most of the enhanced greenhouse effect. Historically, carbon dioxide levels were fairly stable (barring the occasional volcano). Then came the Industrial Revolution, after which carbon dioxide levels have risen from 285 to more than 400 parts per million.[111] ,[112] (Scientists measure these gases in the atmosphere. To determine levels in earlier periods, they assay carbon contained in tree rings and in bubbles trapped in ice cores.)

greenhouse gases

Gases that absorb heat energy in the atmosphere. These include carbon dioxide, methane, and water vapor.

greenhouse effect

The phenomenon whereby atmospheric gases such as water vapor, carbon dioxide, and methane trap solar radiation and consequently warm the earth's surface.

global warming

Increase in the earth's temperature.

Carbon dioxide is a part of a complex process called the **carbon cycle**. All life forms derive from carbon. Our bodies, our food, our clothes, and many of our building materials are carbon based. The carbon cycle describes how carbon moves from one "reservoir" to another. The main reservoirs of carbon are living land organisms, fossil fuels, the oceans, and the atmosphere. Some reservoirs release carbon into the atmosphere; others act as carbon sinks, removing carbon dioxide from the atmosphere.

carbon cycle

A combination of processes by which carbon-containing compounds move between different reservoirs—the atmosphere, oceans, and living organisms.

FIGURE 17.7 The Carbon Cycle

This image shows the movement of carbon between land, atmosphere, and oceans. Yellow and red numbers reflect the contribution from natural fluxes and human activity, respectively, in gigatons of carbon per year. A balance between carbon storage and carbon release into the atmosphere holds temperatures fairly steady.

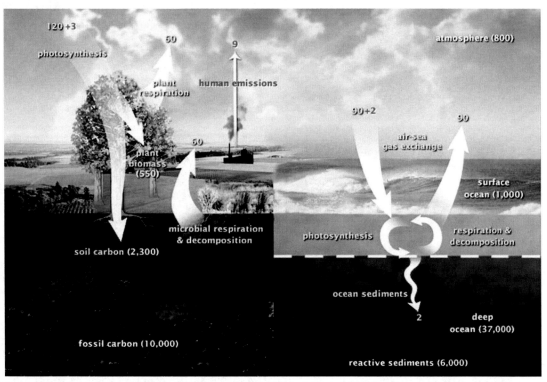

Source: US Department of Energy, Biological and Environmental Research Information System. Climate placemat: energy-climate nexus. 2008. Available at: http://commons.wikimedia.org/wiki/File:Carbon_cycle.jpg.

All organisms act as both sources and sinks for carbon. While living, plants, animals, and microorganisms tie up carbon in their cells. All organisms also break down carbon-based nutrients to create energy. This process, called *cellular respiration*, releases carbon dioxide. Every time you exhale, carbon dioxide leaves your body. Decomposition and combustion of organic matter also release carbon dioxide. Since the Industrial Revolution, humans have generated a steadily increasing amount of atmospheric carbon dioxide from burning fossil fuels.

Through *photosynthesis*, plants, ocean-dwelling plankton, algae, and some bacteria harness light energy to convert water and carbon dioxide into carbohydrates and oxygen. Fast-growing trees are especially good at removing atmospheric carbon dioxide. Undisturbed biomass (e.g., old-growth forests), soil, and sediments layering the ocean floor *sequester* carbon, meaning they act as long-term reservoirs for carbon. Clear-cutting or burning a forest leads to a net increase in atmospheric carbon because an important carbon sink is lost and the stored carbon is released.

FIGURE 17.8 Photosynthesis and Carbon Capture

Plants take in water and atmospheric carbon dioxide and, using energy from sunlight, create carbohydrates and oxygen, which is released into the air. The net effect is that atmospheric carbon is removed and captured in the plant until the plant decomposes or burns.

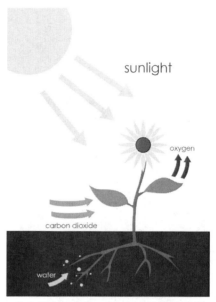

Source: At09kg. The scientific process of photosynthesis. 2011. Available at: http://commons.wikimedia.org/wiki/File:Photosynthesis.gif.

A longer-term cycle deposits atmospheric carbon in rocks such as limestone and releases it when volcanoes erupt.[113] Carbon-containing rocks that undergo millions of years of heat and pressure eventually become shale. In the same way, pressurized organic material (dead plants and animals) becomes crude oil and natural gas. All are reservoirs of sequestered carbon. Additionally, the ocean absorbs carbon dioxide, which dissolves and is eventually released again as a gas.

For hundreds of thousands of years, the carbon cycle remained fairly steady. A massive phytoplankton bloom might remove extra carbon. The occasional volcanic eruption released large amounts carbon dioxide. Climate varied with such fluctuations in carbon dioxide levels; the temperature rose and fell in tandem with levels of carbon dioxide.

Humans have altered the carbon cycle through activities such as removing forests and burning wood and fossil fuels—processes that increase atmospheric carbon dioxide. Records show that, since the Industrial Revolution, carbon dioxide levels have risen rapidly—and so have average global temperatures. In fact, climate change is accelerating.

In addition to carbon dioxide, other important greenhouse gases include water vapor, methane, nitrous oxide, and sulfur hexafluoride. **Water vapor**, the most abundant of the greenhouse gases, is simply aerosolized water. Scientists are more concerned with the other gases because human activities are largely responsible for their increase, which means we have some ability to control their levels.

Methane, like carbon dioxide, is a colorless, odorless gas. The main constituent of natural gas, methane can be combusted. Because decomposition of organic plant and animal matter releases methane, swamps, marshes, and oceans are sources. Ruminants (hoofed, cud-chewing animals such cattle, sheep, goats, bison, deer, and elk) release methane from their intestinal tracts. Humans liberate this gas through mining for fossil fuels and transporting natural gas.[114] As a greenhouse gas, methane is more than 20 times more powerful than carbon dioxide.

Nitrous oxide is colorless and nonflammable. Oceans and rainforests release it. Human sources include the use of fertilizers, the burning of fossil fuels, nylon production, and automobile catalytic converters.[115]

Sulfur hexafluoride is an extremely strong greenhouse gas and one that persists in the atmosphere for more than a thousand years.[116] Electric power plants are the main source.

2.1 Energy Production and Greenhouse Gases

FIGURE 17.9 Greenhouse Gases and Global Temperatures Rise in Tandem

This graph shows actual global temperature averages over a decade and predicted temperatures based on factors such as greenhouse gases, manmade sulfate emissions, solar variability, and changes in ozone levels. The gray bands indicate normal temperature variability. As you can see, global temperatures and greenhouse gases have risen in parallel.

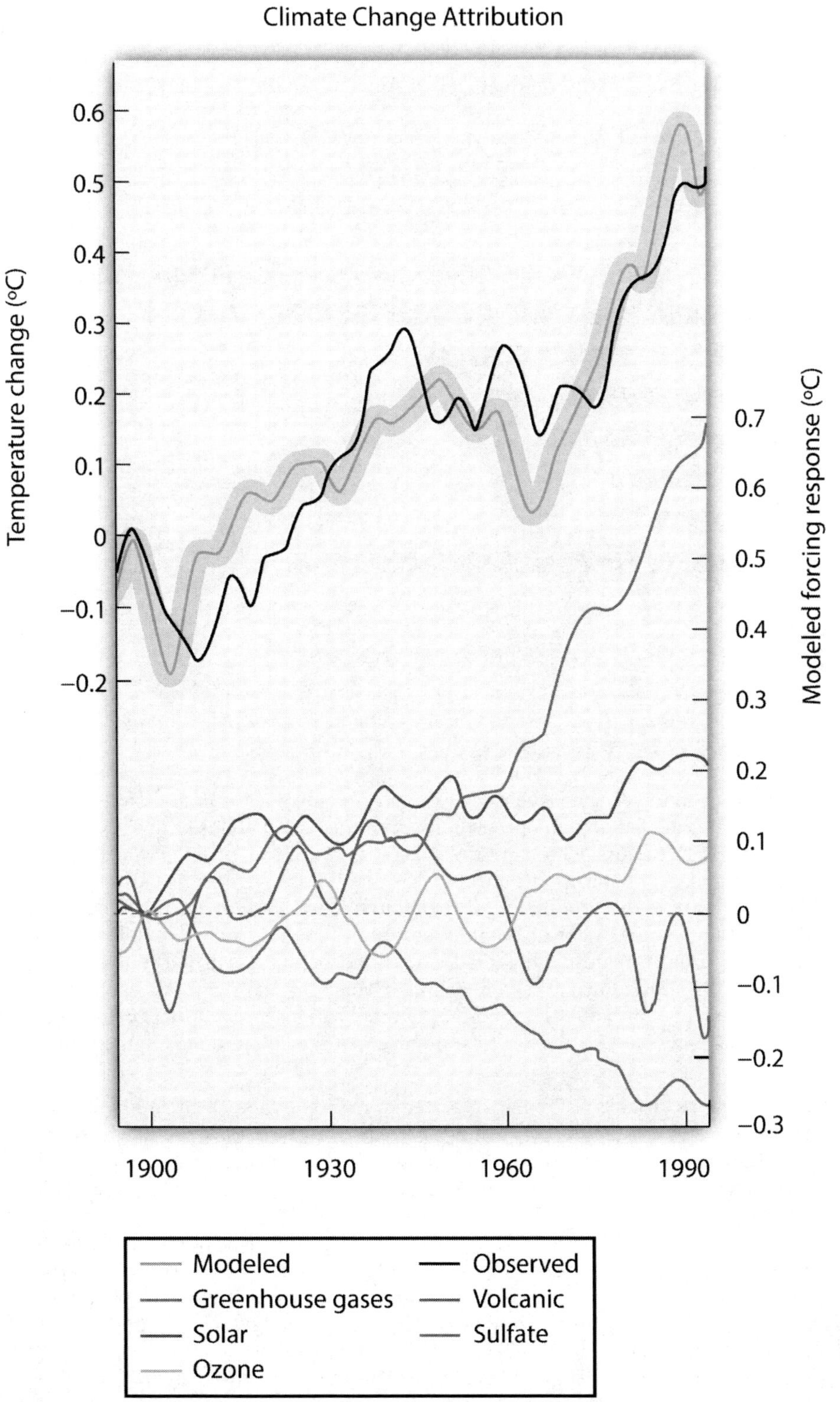

Climate Change Attribution

Source: Adapted from Rohde RA. Climate change attribution. 2006. Data source: Meehl GA, Washington WM, Ammann CM, Arblaster JM, Wigley TML, Tebaldi C. Combinations of natural and anthropogenic forcings in twentieth-century climate. J Clim. 2004;17:3721–3727. Available at: http://commons.wikimedia.org./wiki/File:Climate_Change_Attribution.png.

nonrenewable energy resources

Energy resources that natural processes either don't replace or do so over a long period of time.

Energy resources are either nonrenewable or renewable. **Nonrenewable energy resources** are those natural sources of energy that either aren't replenished or do so very slowly. Examples include fossil fuels (coal, oil, and gas) and nuclear power.

Most of the world relies on combustion of wood and **fossil fuels** for energy. *Combustion* is a chemical reaction wherein atmospheric oxygen reacts with carbon and hydrogen in fuel, creating carbon dioxide, water vapor, and energy in the form of heat and light. In addition to releasing greenhouse gases, fossil fuel combustion produces many of the air pollutants discussed earlier.

The term *carbon footprint* refers to the amount of greenhouse gases, particularly carbon dioxide, that a person, group, or product emits. Due to our appetite for fossil fuels, the United States is the biggest producer of greenhouse gases. While Americans represent 5 percent of the world's population, we emit 25 percent of the carbon dioxide. Compared to global per capita averages, each American emits four times more carbon dioxide—a total of 21 tons a year.[117] Europeans, despite their high standard of living, produce half the carbon dioxide that Americans do.

FIGURE 17.10 Energy-Related Carbon Dioxide Emissions by Country

This bar graph shows contributions for the countries that emitted the most carbon dioxide between 1890 and 2007. Richer countries consume more energy resources. Notice which country comes out on top.

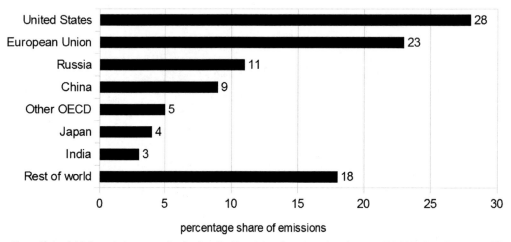

Source: EnescotShare of global cumulative energy-related carbon dioxide emissions for major emitters between 1890–2007. 2012. Data source: IEA. World Energy Outlook 2009. Paris, France: International Energy Agency (IEA); 2009:180. Available at: http://commons.wikimedia.org/wiki/ File:Share_of_global_cumulative_energy-related_carbon_dioxide_emissions_for_major_emitters_between_1890-2007.png.

Nuclear energy is also used to generate electricity. The process involves atomic fission (the splitting of atoms), which sparks a heat-releasing chain reaction. Uranium is usually used in these reactions. Fission takes place in nuclear reactors, which are designed with a number of safety mechanisms to keep the reaction from getting out of control. The advantage is that it doesn't generate carbon emissions.

The main disadvantage is the production of toxic radioactive waste material. A permanent solution to the problem of radioactive waste disposal has not been found. Moreover, while modern nuclear plants are designed to protect against radiation leaks, those measures can fail. For example, after a tsunami hit Japan in 2011, a meltdown at the Fukushima Daiichi nuclear plant released radioactive materials into the environment. This and other nuclear plant failures have cast doubt on the safety of nuclear power facilities, causing several countries to announce that they plan to reduce their use of nuclear power.[118]

renewable energy resources

Energy resources that natural processes readily replace.

Renewable energy resources are readily replaced in nature. Examples include solar, wind, wave, and geothermal power. Because they don't produce greenhouse gases, they provide a solution to climate change. Furthermore, these resources are *sustainable*, meaning they allow people to maintain a good-quality standard of living without compromising the health and energy needs of future generations.

Solar power utilizes light or heat energy from sunlight. Solar thermal (heat) technologies take advantage of the sun's warmth. A simple example is using the sun's energy to warm water for household use. More complicated technology concentrates solar energy to create steam, which operates a turbine. Solar energy can also be converted directly into electricity using *photovoltaic cells*. In this case, sunlight striking photosensitive materials produces an electric current.

Wind power indirectly stems from solar energy. When the sun heats the earth's surface and the oceans irregularly, cooler air (which is heavier) displaces warmer air, resulting in global and regional wind currents. Sailors have long harnessed the wind for transportation; farmers developed windmills to pump water and grind grain. Modern-day wind turbines are used to generate electricity.

Like wind, moving **water** is a type of kinetic energy made possible by the sun. For centuries, humans used running water to turn wheels to grind grain, lift water onto fields, and do other work. More recently, *hydroelectric power* plants used the energy of water running down rivers or released from dams to turn turbines that generate electricity. The energy of waves can be used in a similar fashion. In addition, the gravitational pull of the moon creates a steady source of *tidal energy* that can be harnessed to generate electricity.

Geothermal power makes use of the warmer temperatures in the earth's core. Rather than generating heat, the earth's heat is moved. Warm air and water can be used to regulate heat in buildings. In some areas, geothermal energy is relatively close to the surface, making it accessible to produce steam to run a turbine.

Plants store the sun's energy as chemical energy (carbohydrates). Living and recently living plants form **biomass**, which can serve as a source of energy (*biofuel*). Woody plants (trees), plants high in sugar (corn), grasses, agricultural waste, and household garbage can all serve as biofuel. As long as the plant grows relatively quickly and is sustainably harvested, biomass counts as a renewal source of energy.

However, biomass combustion does release greenhouse gases and particulate matter. Furthermore, the net energy efficiency of biomass can be reduced if the crops are grown with synthetic fertilizers and planted, harvested, and transported using fuel-burning machines.[119]

 Video Clip 17.2

Global Warming 101

This 2007 National Geographic video explains the basics of global warming, its causes, and its consequences. Note that, since this video was made, average temperatures have climbed further.

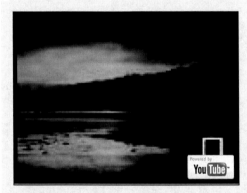

View the video online at: http://www.youtube.com/v/oJAbATJCugs
Source: National Geographic.

2.2 Consequences of Climate Change

An obvious result of climate change is **higher average temperatures**. In early 2013, the National Oceanic and Atmospheric Administration (NOAA) reported that 2012 was the hottest year on record for the United States.[120] Widespread summer heat and drought followed by a mild winter raised the national average temperature to 55.3°F—a full degree warmer than the previous record for 1998 and 3.2 degrees above the average for the entire 20th century. While short-term weather variations are normal, global climate change underlies this marked and consistent alteration.

Predicting how high temperatures will rise is difficult. The IPCC estimates that global temperatures will have risen between 3.2 and 7.1°F between the preindustrial era and the end of this century.[121] The exact amount of warming depends largely upon the extent to which we continue to burn fossil fuels.

The IPCC has documented increased air temperatures, especially in northern latitudes; decreases in snow and ice; and rising sea levels.[122] As of early 2013, 2012 is the hottest year on record in the contiguous United States.[123] The year's average temperature was 55.3°F (a full degree above the last record set in 1998.) During that summer, scorching heat and drought gripped two-thirds of the country.

FIGURE 17.11 Projected Temperature Increases

The National Oceanic and Atmospheric Administration used data to graph projected increases in global temperature rises based on three scenarios for greenhouse gas emissions. The lowest (blue) would lead to a 2°C increase by 2100. Higher (green) emissions would raise the temperature 3°C. The highest would ratchet up global averages by 4°C. (Each degree Celsius is 1.8 degrees in Fahrenheit.)

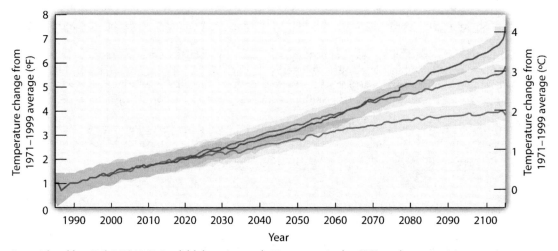

Source: Adapted from Hnilo J; NOAA. Projected global warming over the 21st century using three SRES greenhouse gas emissions scenarios.

ClimateWatch Magazine. 2010. Available at: http://commons.wikimedia.org/wiki/

File:Projected_global_warming_over_the_21st_century_using_three_SRES_greenhouse_gas_emissions_scenarios._Data_from_CMIP3_282007%29.png.

Hot, dry weather creates tinder for **wildfires**. In the United States in the summer of 2012, wildfires scorched nearly 10 million acres.[124] ,[125] Produce prices soared. As grasslands parched and the cost of hay and grain soared, ranchers were forced to cull their herds.

Another consequence of climate change is more **extreme, unpredictable weather**: more hurricanes, tornados, storms, heat waves, and cold spells. Some areas will experience more heat waves and drought; other regions will see more precipitation and storms. While most of the United States baked during 2012, Alaska experienced record cold. Winter storms battered the Pacific Northwest. Hurricane Sandy ravaged coastal areas from the Caribbean to New England; Typhoon Bopha hit the Philippines.

Extreme weather patterns are continuing. In the Southern Hemisphere in 2013, Australia and Tasmania suffered record-breaking heat, drought, and widespread fires.[126] Meanwhile, north of the equator, Eastern Russia froze, China endured the coldest winter in 30 years, and floods inundated the Middle East and the United Kingdom.[127]

Warmer temperatures means more polar ice melts in summer. In the summer of 2012, the rate of loss of Arctic sea ice was 50 percent higher than expected.[128] Increased melting glaciers and polar ice increases sea levels. Because water expands as it warms, warmer oceans also increase sea levels.

Video Clip 17.3

Retreating Alaskan Glacier
This time-lapsed video documents the retreat of the Mendenhall glacier in Alaska. Note that since this video was uploaded in 2009, the rate of glacier loss has accelerated.

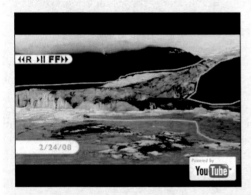

View the video online at: http://www.youtube.com/v/6dFbuaz130c
Source: Extremeicesurvey.org.

Since the early 1990s, scientists have recorded an average annual **rise in sea level** of 0.14 inches (3.5 millimeters).[129] The pace has been accelerating. By the end of the century, scientists expect sea level to rise between 2.5 to 6.5 feet (0.8 to 2 meters). More dire predictions call for a 23-foot rise, which would submerge some coastal cities. The result is loss of coastal wetlands and mangroves, contamination of aquifers and agricultural land, larger storm surges, and massive damage to property from coastal flooding.

Water shortages are another problem. A shift in rainfall patterns will increase regional aridity. Declining winter snowfall and earlier spring thaws diminish the mountain snowpack. Since 1970, Northern Hemisphere snow cover has steadily declined.[130] Reduced snowpack and earlier spring runoff means that, during the summer months, less water is available to sustain rivers and streams. Diminished irrigation water lowers agricultural yields.

In addition, higher temperatures increase surface evaporation and transpiration (the water absorbed by plants and evaporated into the atmosphere). Consequently, water shortages will become widespread in areas such as the southwestern United States.[131] By 2050, the retreat of Himalayan glaciers is estimated to endanger the food security of 70 million people.[132]

Temperatures in *permafrost* (ground that remains frozen all year) have steadily risen. Animals and plants adapted to the permafrost have lost habitats. In parts of Alaska, highways, airstrips, and buildings have begun to crack and crumble where the ground now thaws in summer.[133]

Unfortunately, loss of snow and ice amplifies global warming. For one, snow and ice reflect sunlight back into space, which minimizes the absorption of heat by the planet. Particulate matter from dust storms, fires, and urban pollution can travel thousands of miles on wind currents and settle on snowfields, darkening them and causing them to absorb more of the sun's energy. The heat increases melting. Bare ground and unfrozen oceans absorb even more energy. And so, a vicious cycle ensues.

Climate change will **disrupt ecosystems** and push many species toward extinction unless they can adapt or migrate. The timing for seasonal events has altered. Trees and plants flower and leaf earlier in the spring, disrupting the timing of their availability to species that depend on them. Migration patterns for animals shift. Rising sea levels have jeopardized animals such as sea turtles that breed on low-lying beaches and waterfowl that rely on marshes. Warming waterways and oceans disrupt riparian (river) and marine life.

Some animal species can move to find more suitable habitats—the major exceptions being polar animals such as penguins and polar bears who have simply run out of icy habitats and others whose habitat has been constrained by human settlements. Since plants don't migrate easily, many species may become extinct before they can adapt. Pests such as the pine beetle have infested and heat-stressed trees, blighting landscapes and creating dry tinder for forest fires.

The **impacts on human populations** are multiple, and low-income populations will be most vulnerable. The rise of the oceans presents one of the most serious threats to human societies from climate change. Millions of people living in areas subject to inundation and cyclical **flooding** will be displaced. This will exacerbate population pressures in other parts of the world, with the attendant issues of political instability, food insecurity, and disease.

The increase in extreme weather events and long-term changes in precipitation patterns will also affect public health, with risks ranging from localized storm damage to **drought** and flooding that render land unsuitable for agriculture. Crop failures and loss of pastureland spawn food insecurity and outright **famine**. Compounding the problem is the decline in seafood due to overfishing and ocean warming, pollution, and acidification (from increased uptake of carbon dioxide). Malnutrition increases susceptibility to infections and other illnesses. A loss of biodiversity resulting from the impairment of habitat for susceptible species will have long-term implications for the development of new food sources and medicines.

A warmer world means more **heat-related illness** and death, particularly in the elderly and in those with underlying heart and lung diseases.[134] The earlier onset of spring and higher carbon dioxide levels (which will stimulate the growth of plants such as ragweed) increase pollen counts, aggravating respiratory allergies and asthma.[135] On a brighter note, milder winters may decrease deaths from heart attacks an stroke.[136]

Infectious diseases will likely increase. Flooding can contaminate water with microbes, leading to diarrheal illnesses such as cholera and typhoid. Flooding and excessive precipitation from storms allow disease-causing fungi to proliferate. Water scarcity results in poorer sanitation and hygiene.[137]

Infectious diseases previously limited to the tropics have already spread into northern latitudes. For example, the mosquito-borne West Nile virus, in more severe forms, adversely affects the nervous system. The virus, which is common in Africa, West Asia, and the Middle East, was first detected in the United States in 1999. In 2012, there was a record of 5,387 cases in people from 48 states.[138] Dengue fever, another mosquito-borne infectious disease, has also spread.[139] Disease-carrying ticks have migrated northward. However, regions that become drier could see reduced mosquito survival and a consequent decrease in mosquito-borne infections.

 Video Clip 17.4

Climate Change Is Not a Partisan Issue
Unfortunately, global warming has become a polarizing political issue. However, the response to global warming, a scientifically proven phenomenon, requires bipartisan cooperation. Watch "It's Time to Find Common Ground," a speed-drawn video featuring the opinions of two scientists, one a Republican, the other a Democrat.

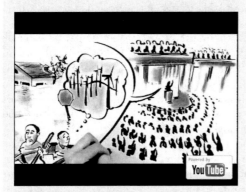

View the video online at: http://www.youtube.com/v/TLg3B1Vi3Xl
Source: Union of Concerned Scientists.

2.3 Responding to Climate Change

Carbon dioxide persists for a very long time in the atmosphere—an average of 200 to 300 years.[140] That means we can't halt, much less reverse, global warming in our lifetimes. However, we can immediately take action to mitigate the long-term impacts on future generations. The solution is a dramatic reduction in greenhouse gas emissions. In addition, we must prepare and adapt to climate change.

We've already seen that positive changes are possible. For a few years, beginning in 2008, the economic crisis reduced the world's carbon dioxide emissions by cutting consumption of electricity, oil, and gas.[141] Scientists and climate activists viewed this small decline in greenhouse gas emissions as an opportunity to change policies on carbon emissions and alter the course of global warming. After all, climate change will prove much more costly than an economic recession. Unfortunately, the economic crisis has made it more difficult for governments to adopt sustainable energy policies.

In 2009, the leaders of the world's 8 major economic powers adopted a goal to limit global warming to 2°C (about 3.6°F).[142] However, negotiations under the United Nations Framework Convention on Climate Change have not resulted in the formal commitments needed to achieve this goal, and the window of opportunity is fast closing.[143] According to the International Energy Agency's (IEA) 2012 report, *World Energy Outlook*, carbon dioxide emissions then rebounded to record highs, oil imports rose, American oil and gas production increased, gas prices declined, and energy efficiency worsened.[144]

Large-Scale Solutions

While individual efforts to reduce carbon emissions are vital, large-scale changes in government policy and international cooperation are also required to effect meaningful reductions in atmospheric carbon. To varying degrees, governments around the globe have taken measures to promote greater energy efficiency, reduce use of fossil fuels, and support sustainable energy development. Some efforts are also being made, in many cases with the support of nongovernmental organizations, to curb deforestation by preserving forests and planting more trees.

International treaties have attempted to reduce greenhouse gas emissions. The Kyoto Protocol to the United Nations Framework Convention on Climate Change sets binding targets for industrialized countries to reduce greenhouse emissions. As of 2011, 191 parties had signed it.[145] While the United States' representative to the convention signed the protocol, Congress has not ratified it. Objections to ratification include the fact that developing countries were excluded from the agreement. A 2012 amendment to the Kyoto Protocol established new commitments for carbon reductions.[146]

Although the United States is not participating in the Kyoto Protocol, the government has taken some steps to reduce greenhouse gas emissions. The Clean Air Act requires the US Environmental Protection Agency (EPA) to protect the public from harmful air pollutants. Furthermore, the US Supreme Court has determined that the EPA has the power to regulate greenhouse gas emissions.[147] Although the EPA found that such emissions endanger both public health and public welfare and has the power to set standards for major sources, implementation of solutions is difficult and faces significant opposition.[148]

Around the globe, however, there is evidence of success. According to the IEA, China aims to reduce energy intensity 16 percent by 2015.[149] Likewise, Japan plans to cut its electricity use 20 percent by 2030. The European Union (EU) agreed to cut energy demands by 20 percent by 2020.

A number of countries, such as those belonging to the European Union, have adopted a **cap-and-trade** system. This market approach sets prices on pollutants—in this case, carbon dioxide emissions. The cap, or limit set by the government, is allocated to industries as permits (carbon credits). Industries that need to increase their emissions above this cap can only do so by buying carbon credits from another company. They may also offset their emissions by investing in clean energy development and in forest preservation. Over time, the emissions allowances would be steadily reduced. In the United States, carbon markets have been established on a regional basis.[150]

Another strategy is **carbon capture and storage**. As the name suggests, industries such as power plants that generate a lot of carbon dioxide capture it, compress the gas to a liquid, transport it via pipelines, and store it in geological formations underground. Although the technology could reduce carbon dioxide emissions, more energy is required to capture and compress the gas. Another concern is that carbon dioxide will leak out again. On the positive side, this technology, which is yet to be widely available, could provide a means to reduce carbon dioxide emissions during the decades required to make the transition from fossil fuels to renewable energy resources.

At home and abroad, economic stimulus packages have, to a small degree, promoted development of clean, **sustainable energy**. Continued subsidies are needed to expand renewable energy resources—a critical step in restricting greenhouse gas emissions. According to the IEA, hydroelectric power generation has steadily increased, and wind and solar technologies have grown, though not fast enough to keep pace with fossil fuel use.[151]

Ideally, renewables would account for two-thirds of electricity generation by 2035. (Currently, fossil fuels provide 80 percent of the world's energy needs.) To meet that goal, policy makers will need to do more to support businesses that develop and use sustainable energy sources. As the technology advances, the costs to renewables will fall. Also, as the cost of carbon emissions (and the cost of fossil fuels) rises, incentives to use renewables will mount.

Improving **motor vehicle efficiency** is also an important step toward controlling emissions. In the United States, passenger vehicles contribute a quarter of our yearly energy-related carbon dioxide emissions.[152] The United States has committed to improve fuel efficiency of cars to 35.5 miles per gallon and light-duty vehicles to 39 miles per gallon. Subsidizing the development of fuel-efficient cars and providing monetary incentives for buying them speeds their adoption.

Hybrid vehicles have secured a greater share of the domestic and foreign car markets. They combine a fuel-based power system with an energy storage system that can be recharged by braking energy and the gas engine. This system significantly improves fuel efficiency.

Electric cars are powered solely by electric motors. These vehicles need to be plugged periodically into an electricity source to recharge the batteries. While the electric cars emit no greenhouse gases, they do rely on electricity, most of which is currently generated by fossil fuel combustion. However, electric cars do nonetheless reduce carbon emissions.[153] And in theory, increased generation of electricity using nuclear power and renewable energy resources would further reduce these vehicles' environmental impact. Carports with in-roof solar panels have already been developed to recharge electric vehicles.[154]

FIGURE 17.12 Electric Car Charging in Amsterdam

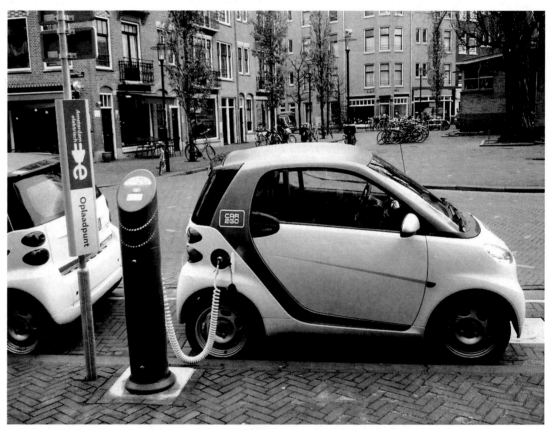

Source: Hirlimann L. Electric car charging Amsterdam. 2011. Available at: http://commons.wikimedia.org/wiki/

File:Electric_car_charging_Amsterdam.jpg.

The biggest challenge to curbing climate change is the increase in global population, most of which is occurring in Asia and Africa. Heavily populated China and India are developing at a rapid pace—a pursuit that devours energy resources. Growing populations, combined with increases in the standard of living, result in a rapid increase in energy use. The IEA estimates that 1.3 billion people currently lack electricity.[155] In these countries, much of the new electricity generation is based on coal-fired power plants, which are significant emitters of greenhouse gases. The goal is to shift energy use away from fossil fuels, especially coal, and toward renewable resources.

Cities Going Green

Denver Bike Sharing

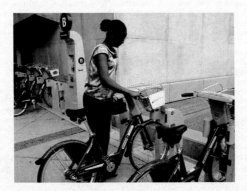

© Denver Bike Sharing

Cities can support greener transportation methods. They can increase access to public transportation, adding bus lines, trains, and subways. (Raising parking fees indirectly promotes carpooling and mass transit.) Cities can create bike lanes to improve cyclists' safety.

Car-sharing programs have become popular in large cities. Compared to car rentals, car sharing is designed for people who make short intercity trips. Members can go online to locate the nearest available car, reserve it, and then unlock it with a membership card. Membership fees and hourly rates cover gas, maintenance, and insurance. You can go to CarSharing.net to learn more and find out car sharing is available where you live.

Bike-sharing programs, which began in Europe, have spread all over the world. At the end of 2012, 497 cities around the globe operate bike-share programs. In the United States, 29 cities from Irvine, California, to Washington, DC, have bike-share program, with an additional 27 in the planning stages.[156]

Typically, stations are set up near public transportation stops and other important venues (e.g., business and retail districts, college campuses). Reasonably priced memberships allow users undock a bike, ride to a short distance to their destination, and then redock. The results have been impressive.

Denver Bike Sharing serves as a shining example. Between the program's start in 2010 and the end of 2012, users collectively pedaled 1,051,006 miles, reduced carbon emissions by 1,477,396 pounds, spared 75,109 gallons of gasoline, and saved $1,279,407 in parking costs and $259,126 at the gas pump. Riders also burned 31,530,189 million calories and lost an estimated 9,008 pounds[157] Members also reported subjective improvements in fitness and mood.

2.4   What You Can Do

Many people feel helpless against a problem as massive as climate change. However, individuals can collectively make a huge impact, both by reducing their own carbon footprint and acting as models for others. Simple lifestyle modifications reduce your carbon footprint <u>can</u> save you money.

There are other benefits. Air and water quality improve. If you commute on foot or bicycle, you're getting exercise, improving your health, and possibly losing weight. You may engage more with your community and reduce the need for expensive new roads and highways.

Here are simple things you can do:

- Change your transportation mode. Take public transit (bus, train, ferry). Walk or cycle. Buy a fuel-efficient car, which can double your gas mileage.

- Within reason, use human power rather than machine power. When cleaning a hard floor, sweep rather than vacuum. Use a rake rather than a leaf blower, a push mower rather than a gas-powered lawn mower, a snow shovel rather than a snow blower.

- Replace incandescent light bulbs with compact fluorescent bulbs or light-emitting diode (LED) bulbs. Switching from incandescent to compact fluorescent light bulbs could lower electricity costs about $150 a year.[158] LED bulbs save even more.

- Turn off lights and electronics when not in use. It only takes a second. Leaving printers, monitors, computers on gobbles energy. According to the Union of Concerned Scientists, a laser printer left on can waste $130 in energy costs annually. Appliances with LED lights such as toasters consume energy when plugged in, even if not in use.

- Wash your clothes in cold water. They'll get just as clean and last longer. (Compared to cold-water wash, a hot water cycle creates five times the emissions.[159]) Whenever possible, air dry clothes rather than tossing them into the dryer.

- Adjust the thermostat (and your layers of clothing) so that you rely less on heating and air conditioning.

- Insulate attics and hot water heaters. Use double-paned windows. Weather stripping on doors keeps out drafts.

- Let your hair air dry for a while before finishing it off with the blow dryer (or skip the blow dryer).

- Buy locally made products.

- Avoid unnecessary packaging. Bring your own bags to stores. Buy items, including foods, that haven't been boxed and bagged.

- Drink tap water. Sip from a reusable container (glass, ceramic, or steel). Ask for water without ice at restaurants. It takes energy to make ice and to keep it frozen—more still if it's transported. Plus, room temperature water is better for your digestion.

- Recycle, reuse, and generally reduce consumerism. Each store item requires energy—to make it, package it, transport it to store and home, and, if it's perishable, keep it at the right temperature. Question your motives. Do you need it or do you want it?

- If you're in the market for a new car, buy the most fuel-efficient model you can. If you're not, keep your car in good working order (tire pressure, regular oil changes, and tune-ups). Drive at a steady, moderate speed (rather than speeding up to stop signs and traffic lights.) You'll get better gas mileage.

- Plant a tree. In addition to capturing carbon dioxide and releasing oxygen, trees provide shade. Depending on where they're planted, they can reduce costs of cooling homes and cars. Deciduous trees shade homes in summer but let in warming sunlight in winter.

- Vote to support candidates with a strong environmental track records. Find out whether they support renewable energy resources. Ask how they plan to curb global warming.

- Donate to organizations that help protect the planet.

Making Green Food Choices

Agriculture consumes water and oil (to grow, package, chill, and transport food); plastic, paper, and metals (for packaging); and chemicals (pesticides, herbicides, antibiotics, preservatives). Your food choices impact the environment. Here are some things you can do to be healthier and greener.

- Eat low on the food chain. That means consuming more grains, vegetables, and fruits and less meat. Factory farming pollutes air and ground water. Chemical contaminants concentrate in the fat of animals (and end up inside of you, the consumer). Cattle and other ruminants release the greenhouse gas methane. Forests may be cleared for grazing land. A parcel of arable land devoted to raising edible plants feeds more people than the same parcel devoted to raising livestock. (In areas where the land is already open and not amenable to agriculture, it makes perfect sense to run cattle, sheep, and goats.)

- Buy locally produced foods. In that way, you reduce the fossil fuels consumed in shipping and transportation. There may be exceptions to that rule. For instance, some fruits and vegetables require fewer resources to produce in a warmer climate, even when you factor in the cost of getting it to your door.

- Buy foods in season. Those fresh strawberries at the supermarket in January traveled a long, fuel-intensive distance.

- Support small, organic farmers. By definition, they don't use synthetic fertilizers, pesticides, genetically modified seeds, nontherapeutic antibiotics, and growth hormones. Their agricultural practices are generally more sustainable. Animals usually receive more humane treatment at small farms. And the sewage from these farms is much less than from factory farms.

- Cut down on packaged foods and beverages. Lots of energy is consumed in the materials and manufacturing. Some plastics leach chemicals into foods and beverages. Single-serving packages are particularly wasteful. It's better to buy a bigger container.

- Buy sustainable seafood. Many species have been overfished. You can find a pocket guide to ocean-friendly seafood at the Monterey Bay Aquarium website (http://www.montereybayaquarium.org/cr/cr_seafoodwatch/download.aspx).

- Compost table scraps. Doing so enriches soil and reduces the load heading to the landfill.

KEY TAKEAWAYS

- Industrialization has increased use of energy resources, mainly nonrenewable resources such as fossil fuels.
- Combustion of fossil fuels emits greenhouse gases, magnifying the greenhouse effect.
- A steady climb in levels of greenhouse gases has warmed the planet.
- Global warming has multiple consequences:
  - warmer average temperatures on land and in the oceans
  - loss of snow and ice
  - severe and widespread droughts in certain areas
  - rising sea levels and coastal flooding
  - altered weather patterns with more extreme weather events
  - loss of habitat for humans and other living organisms
  - an increase in illnesses such as heat stress, asthma, allergies, and infectious diseases
- Solutions to climate change pivot on efforts to reduce greenhouse gas emissions.
  - Large-scale programs enacted by international bodies and national, state, and local governments are essential.
  - Changes in the habits of individuals can have profound effects on the environment.

DISCUSSION QUESTIONS

1. Pick one renewable energy resource. Using the Internet, search for the pros and cons of that energy resource. For example, here's a website on the pros and cons of solar power: http://www.clean-energy-ideas.com/articles/pros_and_cons_of_solar_energy.html. Make a list and add your own thoughts about this method's feasibility.

2. Go to the webpage for the Union of Concerned Scientists book *Cooler Smarter: Practical Steps for Low-Carbon Living* (http://coolersmarter.org), click on the interactive web tool, and fill out the questionnaire. Make note of recommendations and tips. Now write at least three ways you can reduce your carbon footprint. What barriers might prevent you from making those changes?

3. If you drive, you've probably noticed that gas prices rose during the last several years. Gas has always been more expensive in Europe. Higher gas prices cause people to drive less, or at least purchase fuel-efficient cars. Some experts think we should keep gas prices high, or perhaps raise them. After all, crude oil is not limitless. What do you think? Do you see any downsides? Which groups might be hurt the most?

3. RECOMMENDED RESOURCES

3.1 Books

Diamond J. *Collapse: How Societies Choose to Fail or Succeed*. New York, NY: Penguin Books; 2005.

Friedman S. *Hot, Flat, and Crowded: Why We Need a Green Revolution—and How It Can Renew America*. New York, NY: Farrar, Straus and Giroux; 2008.

Kolbert E. *Field Notes from a Catastrophe: Man, Nature, and Climate Change*. New York, NY: Bloomsbury USA; 2006.

Union of Concerned Scientists. *Cooler, Smarter: Practical Steps for Low-Carbon Living*. Washington, DC: Island Press; 2012.

3.2 Organizations and Websites

Center for Biological Diversity. http://www.biologicaldiversity.org.

Environment and Human Health, Inc. http://www.ehhi.org.

Environmental Defense Fund. http://www.edf.org.

Environmental Protection Agency. http://www.epa.gov.

Extreme Ice Survey. http://extremeicesurvey.org.

Intergovernmental Panel on Climate Change. http://www.ipcc.ch.

National Geographic. http://environment.nationalgeographic.com/environment/global-warming.

National Oceanic and Atmospheric Administration. http://www.noaa.gov.

Natural Resources Defense Council. http://www.nrdc.org.

The Nature Conservancy. http://www.nature.org.

One Health Initiative. http://www.onehealthinitiative.com.

Population Connection. http://www.populationconnection.org.

Population Matters. http://www.populationmatters.org.

Sierra Club. http://www.sierraclub.org.

United Nations Environment Programme. http://www.unep.org.

United States Global Change Research Program. http://www.globalchange.gov.

USGS Water Science School. http://ga.water.usgs.gov/edu.

World Health Organization: Environmental Health. http://www.who.int/topics/environmental_health/en.

3.3 Videos

Global Warming, What You Need to Know (2012). Discovery Channel. 1 hour, 27 minutes. http://www.youtube.com/watch?v=xcVwLrAavyA.

James Balog: Time-Lapse Proof of Extreme Ice Loss (2009). In 2007, Balog founded Extreme Ice Survey, a long-term photography project that has documented the retreat of multiple glaciers in the Northern Hemisphere. In this 2009 TED talk, he discusses climate change and narrates time-lapse photographs documenting the retreat of major glaciers. http://www.youtube.com/watch?v=bAbDDA3otfc.

ENDNOTES

1. The making of the hottest year on record: USA temperature update. *ClimateWatch Magazine*. National Oceanic and Atmospheric Administration. Available at: http://www.climatewatch.noaa.gov/video/2012/ the-making-of-the-hottest-year-on-record-usa-temperature-update. Accessed December 16, 2012.

2. Scott M. Summer 2012 brought record-breaking melt to Greenland. National Snow and Ice Data Center. December 5, 2012. Available at: http://www.climatewatch.noaa.gov/article/2012/ summer-2012-brought-record-breaking-melt-to-greenland. Accessed December 16, 2012.

3. Zabarenko D. Arctic Sea ice melts to lowest level on record. Reuters. September 19, 2012. Available at: http://www.reuters.com/article/2012/09/19/ arctic-ice-idUSL1E8KJB5F20120919. Accessed December 16, 2012.

4. Extreme weather linked to global warming, Nobel Prize-winning scientist says. *Science Daily*. August 20, 2012. Available at: http://www.sciencedaily.com/releases/ 2012/08/120820114041.htm. Accessed December 16, 2012.

5. Serna J. Hurricane Sandy death toll climbs above 110, N.Y. hardest hit. *Los Angeles Times*. November 3, 2012. Available at: http://articles.latimes.com/2012/nov/03/ nation/la-na-nn-hurricane-sandy-deaths-climb-20121103. Accessed December 16, 2012.

6. Whaley F. Philippines Struggles to Reach Typhoon's Victims. *New York Times*. December 5, 2012. Available at: http://www.nytimes.com/2012/12/06/world/asia/ typhoon-said-to-have-killed-hundreds-in-philippines.html. Accessed December 16, 2012.

7. Law KS, Stohl KS. Arctic air pollution: origin and impacts. *Science*. 2007;315(5818):1537–1540. doi:10.1126/science.1137695.

8. Robbins J. The ecology of disease. Sunday Review. *New York Times*. July 14, 2012. Available at: http://www.nytimes.com/2012/07/15/sunday-review/ the-ecology-of-disease.html?pagewanted=all&_r=0. Accessed December 20, 2012.

9. Environmental health. World Health Organization. Available at: http://www.who.int/ topics/environmental_health/en. Accessed December 20, 2012.

10. What is acid rain? US Environmental Protection Agency. Available at: http://www.epa.gov/acidrain/what/index.html. Accessed December 21, 2012.

11. What is the history of air pollution in London? King's College London. Available at: http://www.londonair.org.uk/LondonAir/guide/LondonHistory.aspx. Accessed December 20, 2012.

12. Livingstone K. 50 years on: the struggle for air quality since the great smog of December 1952. Greater London Authority. December 2002. Available at: http://legacy.london.gov.uk/mayor/environment/air_quality/docs/50_years_on.pdf. Accessed December 20, 2012.

13. As mad as a hatter. The Phrase Finder. Available at: http://www.phrases.org.uk/ meanings/mad-as-a-hatter.html. Accessed December 20, 2012.

14. Rahman MM. Insecticide substitutes for DDT to control mosquitoes may be causes of several diseases. *Environ Sci Pollut Res Int*. 2012 Sep 6 [Epub ahead of print]. http://www.ncbi.nlm.nih.gov/pubmed/22956113. Accessed March 5, 2013.

15. Ecosystems services. Ecosystems Research. Environmental Protection Agency. Available at: http://www.epa.gov/research/ecoscience/eco-services.htm. Accessed March 5, 2013.

16. Origins of the EPA. United States Environmental Protection Agency. Available at: http://www2.epa.gov/aboutepa/origins-epa. Accessed June 6, 2013.

17. Origins of the EPA. Originally published in *The Guardian*, Spring 1992. EPA Historical Publication-1. United States Environmental Protection Agency. Available at: http://www2.epa.gov/aboutepa/guardian-origins-epa. Accessed December 22, 2012.

18. Perrin JM, Bloom SR, Gortmaker SL. The increase of childhood chronic conditions in the United States. *JAMA*. 2007;297:2755–2759.

19. Cleland V, Crawford D, Baur LA, Hume C, Timperio A, Salmon J. A prospective examination of children's time spent outdoors, objectively measured physical activity and overweight. *Int J Obes*. 2008 Nov;32(11):1685–1693.

20. Kimbro RT, Brooks-Gunn J, McLanahan S. Young children in urban areas: links among neighborhood characteristics, weight status, outdoor play, and television watching. *Soc Sci Med*. 2011 Mar;72(5):668–676.

21. McCurdy LE, Winterbottom KE, Mehta SS, Roberts JR. Using nature and outdoor activity to improve children's health. *Curr Probl Pediatr Adolesc Health Care*. 2010;5:102–117.

22. Maas J, Verheij RA, de Vries S, Spreeuwenberg P, Schellevis FG, Groenewegen PP. Morbidity is related to a green living environment. *J Epidemiol Community Health*. 2009 Dec;63(12):967–973.

23. Mitchell R, Popham F. Effect of exposure to natural environment on health inequalities: an observational population study. *Lancet*. 2008;372:1655–1660.

24. Davison KK, Edmunds LS, Wyker BA, Young LM, Sarfoh VS, Sekhobo JP. Feasibility of increasing childhood outdoor play and decreasing television viewing through a family-based intervention in WIC, New York State, 2007–2008. *Prev Chronic Dis*. 2011 May;8(3):A54. Available at: http://www.ncbi.nlm.nih.gov/pmc/articles/PMC3103559/ ?tool=pubmed. Accessed July 28, 2011.

25. Human population: a key factor in species extinction. Center for Biological Diversity. Available at: http://www.biologicaldiversity.org/campaigns/overpopulation/ index.html. Accessed January 6, 2013.

26. As global population nears 7 billion, UN capitalizes on new opportunities. UNEP News Centre. United Nations Environment Programme. September 14, 2011. Available at: http://www.unep.org/newscentre/ default.aspx?DocumentID=2653&ArticleID=8866. Accessed December 26, 2012.

27. Population growth rate. DEPweb. The World Bank Group. Available at: http://www.worldbank.org/depweb/english/modules/social/pgr/index.html. Accessed December 26, 2012.

28. *Science* magazine podcast on food insecurity. Transcript, February 12, 2010. Available at: http://www.sciencemag.org/content/suppl/2010/02/11/327.5967.837-b.DC1/ SciencePodcast_100212.pdf. Accessed November 1, 2012.

29. Black RE, Cousens S, Johnson HL, Lawn JE. Global, regional, and national causes of child mortality: a systematic analysis. *Lancet*. 2010;375:1969–1987. doi:10.1016/S0140-6736(10)60549-1.

30. Coleman I. Why the global effort for access to contraception is so important. *The Atlantic Monthly*. July 12, 2012. Available at: http://www.theatlantic.com/international/ archive/2012/07/why-the-global-effort-for-access-to-contraception-is-so-important/ 259729. Accessed January 5, 2013.

31. Rawe K, with Dunford A, Steward J, Espey, Stoeckel J. Every woman's right: how family planning saves children's lives. Save the Children. 2012. Available at: http://www.savethechildren.org/atf/cf/ %7B9def2ebe-10ae-432c-9bd0-df91d2eba74a%7D/ EVERY_WOMANS_RIGHT_REPORT_JUNE_2012.PDF. Accessed January 5, 2013.

32. Rawe K, with Dunford A, Steward J, Espey, Stoeckel J. Every woman's right: how family planning saves children's lives. Save the Children. 2012. Available at: http://www.savethechildren.org/atf/cf/ %7B9def2ebe-10ae-432c-9bd0-df91d2eba74a%7D/ EVERY_WOMANS_RIGHT_REPORT_JUNE_2012.PDF. Accessed January 5, 2013.

33. Ahmed S, Li A, Liu L, Tsui AO. Maternal deaths averted by contraceptive use: an analysis of 172 countries. *Lancet*. 2012;380(9837):111–125. doi:10.1016/ S0140-6736(12)60478-4.

34. Coleman I, Lemmon GT. Family planning and U.S. foreign policy. Council on Foreign Relations Press. 2011. Available at: http://www.cfr.org/women/ family-planning-us-foreign-policy/p24683. Accessed January 5, 2013.

35. McDougall R. Too many people: Earth's population problem. Optimum Population/ Population Matters. 2010. Available at: http://www.populationmatters.org/ wp-content/uploads/population_problem.pdf. Accessed January 6, 2013.

36. Population growth and poverty: what are the connections. International Conference on Population and Development. Available at: http://www.unfpa.org/conversations/ factsheets/popgrowth_poverty_eng.pdf. Accessed January 6, 2013.

37. Coleman I, Lemmon GT. Family planning and U.S. foreign policy. Council on Foreign Relations Press. 2011. Available at: http://www.cfr.org/women/ family-planning-us-foreign-policy/p24683. Accessed January 5, 2013.

38. The earth's water budget. WW2010 Project. Department of Atmospheric Sciences, University of Illinois at Urbana-Champaign. Available at: http://ww2010.atmos.uiuc.edu/(Gh)/guides/mtr/hyd/bdgt.rxml. Accessed December 24, 2012.

39. Where is earth's water located? The USGS Water Science School. United States Geological Survey. Available at: http://ga.water.usgs.gov/edu/earthwherewater.html. Accessed December 24, 2012.

40. The water cycle: water science for schools. United States Geological Survey. Available at: http://ga.water.usgs.gov/edu/watercyclesummarytext.html. Accessed December 24, 2012.

41. Water scarcity index. *Vital Water Graphics: An Overview of the State of the World's Fresh and Marine Waters*. 2nd ed. United Nations Environment Programme. 2008. Available at: http://www.unep.org/dewa/vitalwater/article77.html. Accessed December 26, 2012.

42. Increased global water stress. *Vital Water Graphics: An Overview of the State of the World's Fresh and Marine Waters*. 2nd ed. United Nations Environment Programme. 2008. Available at: http://www.unep.org/dewa/vitalwater/article141.html. Accessed January 4, 2013.

43. Health through safe drinking water and basic sanitation. World Health Organization. Available at: http://www.who.int/water_sanitation_health/mdg1/en/index.html. Accessed December 20, 2012.

44. Wulff DL. Water conservation, recycling and California's future. *Bilingual Weekly*. January 26, 2012. Available at: http://bwnews.us/2012/01/26/ what-happened-to-water-conservation. Accessed January 8, 2013.

45. Beyond scarcity: power, poverty, and the global water crisis. *Human Development Report 2006*. New York, NY: Palgrave Macmillan; 2006. Available at: http://hdr.undp.org/ en/media/HDR06-complete.pdf. Accessed January 8, 2013.

46. Onishi N. Arid Australia sips seawater, but at a cost. *New York Times*. July 10, 2010. Available at: http://www.nytimes.com/2010/07/11/world/asia/11water.html?_r=0. Accessed January 8, 2013.

47. Reclamation: managing water in the west. Colorado River Basin Water Supply and Demand Study. US Department of the Interior. Bureau of Reclamation. December 2012. Available at: http://www.usbr.gov/lc/region/programs/crbstudy/finalreport/ Study%20Report/StudyReport_FINAL_Dec2012.pdf. Accessed March 5, 2013.

48. Desalination: An ocean of problems. Food and Water Watch. February 3, 2009. Available at: http://www.foodandwaterwatch.org/reports/ desalination-an-ocean-of-problems. Accessed January 8, 2013.

49. Ginebreda A, Muñoz I, de Alda ML, Brix R, López-Doval J, Barceló D. Environmental risk assessment of pharmaceuticals in rivers: relationships between hazard indexes and aquatic macroinvertebrate diversity indexes in the Llobregat River (NE Spain). *Environ Int*. 2010 Feb;36(2):153–162. doi:10.1016/j.envint.2009.10.003. Accessed March 5, 2013.

50. Water recycling and reuse: the environmental benefits. United States Environmental Protection Agency. Available at: http://www.epa.gov/region9/water/recycling. Accessed January 8, 2013.

51. Water recycling and reuse: the environmental benefits. United States Environmental Protection Agency. Available at: http://www.epa.gov/region9/water/recycling. Accessed January 8, 2013.

52. Arizona state tax credit for gray water. City of Tucson, Arizona. Available at: http://cms3.tucsonaz.gov/water/aztaxcredit. Accessed January 8, 2013.

53. Reclaimed water. City of Tucson, Arizona. Available at: http://cms3.tucsonaz.gov/water/reclaimed. Accessed January 8, 2013.

54. Postel S. Lessons from the field: Boston conservation. *Natl Geogr Mag*. Available at: http://environment.nationalgeographic.com/environment/freshwater/lessons-boston-conservation. Accessed January 8, 2013.

55. Install low-flow fixtures. Energy.gov. Available at: http://energy.gov/energysaver/articles/reduce-hot-water-use-energy-savings. Accessed January 17, 2013.

56. Facts about ultra low flush toilets. Massachusetts Water Resources Authority. Available at: http://www.mwra.com/publications/ulftoilets.pdf. Accessed January 17, 2013.

57. Do one thing, save 10 gallons of water a day. *The Daily Green*. Available at: http://www.thedailygreen.com/going-green/tips/brick-in-toilet. Accessed January 19, 2013.

58. Water quality facts and statistics. World Water Day 2010: Clean Water for a Healthy World. UN Water. Available at: http://www.unwater.org/wwd10/downloads/WWD2010_Facts_web.pdf. Accessed March 5, 2013.

59. Planet index 2007 for marine species population. *Vital Water Graphics: An Overview of the State of the World's Fresh and Marine Waters*. 2nd ed. United Nations Environment Programme. 2008. Accessed December 26, 2012. Available at: http://www.unep.org/dewa/vitalwater/article161.html.

60. German B. Report: EPA struggling to keep pace with "fracking" boom. The Hill. October 9, 2012. Available at: http://thehill.com/blogs/e2-wire/e2-wire/261033-report-epa-struggling-to-keep-pace-with-fracking-boom#ixzz2JE0PDOAc. Accessed March 5, 2013.

61. National water quality inventory: report to congress, 2004 reporting cycle: findings. United States Environmental Protection Agency. Available at: http://water.epa.gov/lawsregs/guidance/cwa/305b/upload/2009_05_20_305b_report_report2004pt3.pdf. Accessed March 5, 2013.

62. Trafton A. One word: bioplastics. MIT News. Massachusetts Institute of Technology. November 17, 2009. Available at: http://web.mit.edu/newsoffice/2009/bioplastics.html. Accessed January 2, 2013.

63. Thompson RC, Moore CJ, vom Saal FS, Swan SH. Plastics, the environment and human health: current consensus and future trends. *Philos Trans R Soc Lond B Biol Sci*. 2009;364:2153–2166.

64. Trafton A. One word: bioplastics. MIT News. Massachusetts Institute of Technology. November 17, 2009. Available at: http://web.mit.edu/newsoffice/2009/bioplastics.html. Accessed January 2, 2013.

65. Mendonca K, Hauser R, Calafat AM, Arbuckle TE, Duty SM. Bisphenol A concentrations in maternal breast milk and infant urine. *Int Arch Occup Environ Health*. 2012 Dec 5 [Epub ahead of print]. Available at: http://www.ncbi.nlm.nih.gov/pubmed/23212895. Accessed January 2, 2013.

66. Wargo J. *Plastics That May Be Harmful to Children and Reproductive Health*. North Haven, CT: Environment & Human Health; 2008. Available at: http://www.ehhi.org/reports/plastics/ehhi_plastics_report_2008.pdf. Accessed January 2, 2013.

67. Halden RU. Plastics and health risks. *Annu Rev Public Health*. 2010;31:179–194. doi:10.1146/annurev.publhealth.012809.103714.

68. Snijder CA, Heederi D, Pierik FH, et al. Fetal growth and prenatal exposure to bisphenol A: the generation R study. *Environ Health Perspect*. 2013. doi:10.1289/ehp.1205296. Available at: http://ehp.niehs.nih.gov/2013/01/1205296. Accessed January 9, 2013.

69. Tavernise S. FDA makes it official: BPA can't be used in baby bottles and cups. *New York Times*. July 17, 2012. Available at: http://www.nytimes.com/2012/07/18/science/fda-bans-bpa-from-baby-bottles-and-sippy-cups.html?_r=0. Accessed January 2, 2013.

70. Flore K. FDA rejects BPA ban. MedPage Today. March 30, 2012. Available at: http://www.medpagetoday.com/PublicHealthPolicy/PublicHealth/31953?utm_content=&utm_medium=email&utm_campaign=DailyHeadlines&utm_source=WC&eun=g236011d0r&userid=236011&email=lwhite27@mscd.edu&mu_id=5231323. Accessed January 13, 2013.

71. Tomlinson S. The layers of the atmosphere: atmospheric structure and composition. About.com Weather. Available at: http://weather.about.com/od/weathertutorials/a/atmoslayers.htm. Accessed December 29, 2012.

72. Sources of pollutants in the ambient air. Air Pollution Control Orientation Course. US Environmental Protection Agency. Available at: http://www.epa.gov/apti/course422/ap3.html. Accessed December 29, 2012.

73. Air quality and health. Fact sheet no. 313. World Health Organization. Available at: http://www.who.int/mediacentre/factsheets/fs313/en/index.html. Accessed December 30, 2012.

74. Fang Y, Naik V, Horowitz LW, Mauzerall DL. Air pollution and associated human mortality: the role of air pollutant emissions, climate change and methane concentration increases during the industrial period. *Atmos Chem Phys Discuss*. 2012;12:22713–22756. Available at: http://www.atmos-chem-phys-discuss.net/12/22713/2012/acpd-12-22713-2012.pdf. Accessed December 30, 2012.

75. Coal in China: consumption, production, mining and liquification. Facts and Details. Available at: http://factsanddetails.com/china.php?itemid=322. Accessed March 5, 2013.

76. Particulate matter. Health. United States Environmental Protection Agency. Available at: http://www.epa.gov/airquality/particlepollution/health.html. Accessed December 30, 2012.

77. Air quality: air quality pollutants. The Weather Network. Available at: http://www.theweathernetwork.com/airquality/airpollutants. Accessed December 30, 2012.

78. Air quality and health. Fact sheet no. 313. World Health Organization. Available at: http://www.who.int/mediacentre/factsheets/fs313/en/index.html. Accessed December 30, 2012.

79. How is ozone formed in the atmosphere? 20 Questions: 2010 Update. Earth System Research Laboratory. National Oceanic & Atmospheric Administration. US Department of Commerce. Available at: http://www.esrl.noaa.gov/csd/assessments/ozone/2010/twentyquestions/Q2.pdf. Accessed December 29, 2012.

80. Ground-level ozone. Health Effects. United States Environmental Protection Agency. Available at: http://www.epa.gov/glo/health.html. Accessed December 30, 2012.

81. Avnery S, Mauzerall DL, Liu J, Horowitz LW. Global crop yield reductions due to surface ozone exposure: year 2000 crop production losses and economic damage. *Atmos Environ*. 2011;45:2284–2296.

82. What are chlorofluorocarbons (CFCs)? A hole in the ozone. Upper Midwest Aerospace Consortium. Available at: http://www.umac.org/ocp/WhatareChlorofluorocarbonsCFCs/info.html. Accessed December 31, 2012.

83. Is the ozone layer diminishing? A hole in the ozone. Upper Midwest Aerospace Consortium. Available at: http://www.umac.org/ocp/IstheOzoneLayerDiminishing/info.html. Accessed December 31, 2012.

84. Environmental effects of ozone depletion and its interactions with climated change: 2010 assessment. United Nations Environment Programme. Available at: http://ozone.unep.org/Assessment_Panels/EEAP/eeap-report2010.pdf. Accessed December 31, 2012.

85. Ozone hole consequences. The Ozone Hole. Available at: http://www.theozonehole.com/consequences.htm. Accessed December 31, 2012.

86. Australian skin cancer. The Ozone Hole. Available at: http://www.theozonehole.com/consequences.htm. Accessed December 31, 2012.

87. Chemicals in tobacco smoke. Centers for Disease Control and Prevention. Available at: http://www.cdc.gov/tobacco/data_statistics/sgr/2010/consumer_booklet/chemicals_smoke/index.htm. Accessed December 31, 2012.

88. Formaldehyde and cancer risk. National Cancer Institute. Available at: http://www.cancer.gov/cancertopics/factsheet/Risk/formaldehyde. Accessed December 31, 2012.

89. Real estate disclosure: lead. United States Environmental Protection Agency. Available at: http://www.epa.gov/lead/property.html. Accessed December 30, 2012.

90. Lead: protect your family. United States Environmental Protection Agency. Available at: http://www.epa.gov/lead/parents.html#testdw. Accessed December 30, 2012.

91. Lead poisoning. Mayo Clinic. Available at: http://www.mayoclinic.com/health/lead-poisoning/FL00068. Accessed December 20, 2012.

92. About lead poisoning. Kids Health. American Academy of Pediatrics. Available at: http://kidshealth.org/parent/medical/brain/lead_poisoning.html. Accessed December 20, 2012.

93. Health risks: radon. US Environmental Protection Agency. Available at: http://www.epa.gov/radon/healthrisks.html. Accessed January 4, 2013.

94. Learn about asbestos. US Environmental Protection Agency. Available at: http://www.epa.gov/asbestos/learn-about-asbestos.html#asbestos. Accessed January 4, 2013.

95. Municipal solid waste generation, recycling, and disposal in the United States: facts and figures for 2010. US Environmental Protection Agency. Available at: http://www.epa.gov/epawaste/nonhaz/municipal/pubs/msw_2010_rev_factsheet.pdf. Accessed January 2, 2013.

96. Municipal solid waste. Wastes: Non-Hazardous Waste. US Environmental Protection Agency. Available at: http://www.epa.gov/epawaste/nonhaz/municipal/index.htm. Accessed January 2, 2013.

97. Municipal solid waste generation, recycling, and disposal in the United States: facts and figures for 2010. US Environmental Protection Agency. Available at: http://www.epa.gov/epawaste/nonhaz/municipal/pubs/msw_2010_rev_factsheet.pdf. Accessed January 2, 2013.

98. Municipal solid waste generation, recycling, and disposal in the United States: facts and figures for 2010. US Environmental Protection Agency. Available at: http://www.epa.gov/epawaste/nonhaz/municipal/pubs/msw_2010_rev_factsheet.pdf. Accessed January 2, 2013.

99. Lydon T. For climate's sake, finish your veggies. *High Country News*. March 13, 2013. Available at: http://www.hcn.org/wotr/for-climates-sake-finish-your-veggies. Accessed June 6, 2013.

100. Recycling basics. US Environmental Protection Agency. Available at: http://epa.gov/recycle/recycle.html. Accessed January 2, 2013.

101. Chepesiuk R. Missing the dark: health effects of light pollution. *Environ Health Perspect*. 2009 January;117(1):A20–A27. Available at: http://www.ncbi.nlm.nih.gov/pmc/articles/pmc2627884. Accessed January 13, 2013.

102. Chepesiuk R. Missing the dark: health effects of light pollution. *Environ Health Perspect*. 2009 January;117(1):A20–A27. Available at: http://www.ncbi.nlm.nih.gov/pmc/articles/pmc2627884. Accessed January 13, 2013.

103. Lenahan M. What is light pollution? Green Living. *Natl Geogr Mag*. Available at: http://greenliving.nationalgeographic.com/light-pollution-2221.html. Accessed January 12, 2013.

104. Noise pollution a critical public health problem, new WHO report says. European Public Health Alliance. July 27, 2011. Available at: http://www.epha.org/spip.php?article4501. Accessed January 12, 2013.

105. Fausti SA, Wilmington DJ, Helt PV, Helt WJ, Konrad-Martin D. Hearing health and care: the need for improved hearing loss prevention and hearing conservation practices. *J Rehabil Res Dev*. 2005;42(4 Suppl 2):45–62. Available at: http://www.rehab.research.va.gov/jour/05/42/4suppl2/fausti.html. Accessed January 13, 2013.

106. Noise effect on wildlife. Federal Highway Administration. US Department of Transportation. Available at: http://www.fhwa.dot.gov/environment/noise/noise_effect_on_wildlife. Accessed January 13, 2013.

107. O'Carroll E. Noise pollution threatening marine life. *Christ Sci Monitor*. December 5, 2008. Available at: http://www.csmonitor.com/Environment/Bright-Green/2008/1205/noise-pollution-threatening-marine-life. Accessed January 12, 2013.

108. Climate change and global warming. Global Issues. Updated December 2, 2012. Available at: http://www.globalissues.org/issue/178/climate-change-and-global-warming. Accessed December 28, 2012.

109. Roach J. Global warming "very likely" caused by humans, world climate experts say. *Natl Geogr News*. February 2, 2007. Available at: http://news.nationalgeographic.com/news/2007/02/070202-global-warming.html. Accessed December 28, 2012.

110. Doran PT, Zimmerman MK. Examining the scientific consensus on climate change. *EOS*. 2009;90(3):22–23. doi:10.1029/2009EO030002. Available at: http://tigger.uic.edu/%7Epdoran/012009_Doran_final.pdf. Accessed March 5, 2013.

111. Carbon cycling and sequestration integrative biology and science through systems science. Report from the March 2008 workshop. US Department of Energy. Office of Science. Office of Biological and Environmental Research. Available at: http://genomicscience.energy.gov/carboncycle/report/CarbonCycle012609LRnocover.pdf. Accessed December 28, 2012.

112. Mastersky R; Nature magazine. Global CO2 levels approach worrisome milestone. *Sci Am*. May 1, 2013. Available at: http://www.scientificamerican.com/article.cfm?id=global-co2-levels-approach-worrisome-milestone. Accessed June 6, 2013.

113. The slow carbon cycle. Earth Observatory. NASA. Available at: http://earthobservatory.nasa.gov/Features/CarbonCycle/page2.php. Accessed January 9, 2013.

114. Basics of the carbon cycle and the greenhouse effect. Earth System Research Laboratory. National Oceanic & Atmospheric Administration. US Department of Commerce. Available at: http://www.esrl.noaa.gov/gmd/outreach/carbon_toolkit/basics.html. Accessed December 29, 2012.

115. Basics of the carbon cycle and the greenhouse effect. Earth System Research Laboratory. National Oceanic & Atmospheric Administration. US Department of Commerce. Available at: http://www.esrl.noaa.gov/gmd/outreach/carbon_toolkit/basics.html. Accessed December 29, 2012.

116. Basics of the carbon cycle and the greenhouse effect. Earth System Research Laboratory. National Oceanic & Atmospheric Administration. US Department of Commerce. Available at: http://www.esrl.noaa.gov/gmd/outreach/carbon_toolkit/basics.html. Accessed December 29, 2012.

117. Shulman S. Smarter ways to keep the planet cool. Catalyst: Union of Concerned Scientists. Spring 2012. Available at: http://www.ucsusa.org/publications/catalyst/sp12-cooler-smarter.html. Accessed January 10, 2013.

118. World energy outlook 2012: executive summary. International Energy Agency. Available at: http://iea.org/publications/freepublications/publication/English.pdf. Accessed January 9, 2013.

119. Energy crops. Biomass Energy Centre. Available at: http://www.biomassenergycentre.org.uk/portal/page?_pageid=75,17301&_dad=portal&_schema=PORTAL. Accessed December 24, 2012.

120. Eilperin J. 2012 hottest year on record in contiguous U.S., NOAA says. *Washington Post*. January 8, 2013. Available at: http://www.washingtonpost.com/national/health-science/2012-hottest-year-on-record-in-continental-us-noaa-says/2013/01/08/5c9dc1ae-55d9-11e2-8b9e-dd8773594efc_story.html. Accessed January 9, 2013.

121. Roach J. Global warming "very likely" caused by humans, world climate experts say. *Natl Geogr News*. February 2, 2007. Available at: http://news.nationalgeographic.com/news/2007/02/070202-global-warming.html. Accessed December 28, 2012.

122. Climate change 2007: synthesis report. IPCC Fourth Assessment Report: Climate Change 2007. Intergovernment Panel on Climate Change. Available at: http://www.ipcc.ch/publications_and_data/ar4/syr/en/mains1.html#1-1. Accessed December 29, 2012.

123. Extreme events of 2012. *Climate Watch Magazine*. National Oceanic and Atmospheric Administration. January 9, 2013. Available at: http://www.climatewatch.noaa.gov/video/2013/extreme-events-of-2012. Accessed January 14, 2013.

124. Hottest month ever recorded. *Climate Watch Magazine*. National Oceanic and Atmospheric Administration. August 8, 2012. Available at: http://www.climatewatch.noaa.gov/image/2012/july-2012-hottest-month-on-record. Accessed August 13, 2012.

125. Fires burn through some states' budgets. *Denver Post*. August 23, 2012:5A.

126. Siegel M. Record heat fuels widespread fires in Australia. *New York Times*. January 9, 2013. Available at: http://www.nytimes.com/2013/01/10/world/asia/record-heat-fuels-widespread-fires-in-australia.html. Accessed January 10, 2013.

127. Lyall S. Heat, flood or icy cold, extreme weather rages worldwide. *New York Times*. January 10, 2013. Available at: http://www.nytimes.com/2013/01/11/science/earth/extreme-weather-grows-in-frequency-and-intensity-around-world.html?ref=earth. Accessed January 12, 2013.

128. McKie R. Rate of arctic summer sea ice loss is 50 percent higher than expected. *The Observer*. August 11, 2012. Available at: http://www.guardian.co.uk/environment/2012/aug/11/arctic-sea-ice-vanishing. Accessed January 12, 2013.

129. Sea level rise. *National Geographic*. Available at: http://ocean.nationalgeographic.com/ocean/critical-issues-sea-level-rise. Accessed January 14, 2013.

130. Future climate change: increasing greenhouse gas concentrations will have many effects. Available at: http://www.epa.gov/climatechange/science/future.html. Accessed January 14, 2013.

131. Reclamation: managing water in the west. Colorado River Basin Water Supply and Demand Study. US Department of the Interior. Bureau of Reclamation. December 2012. Available at: http://www.usbr.gov/lc/region/programs/crbstudy/finalreport/Study%20Report/StudyReport_FINAL_Dec2012.pdf. Accessed March 5, 2013.

132. Measuring glacier change in the Himalayas. Global Environmental Alert Service. United Nations Environment Programme. Available at: http://na.unep.net/geas/getUNEPPageWithArticleIDScript.php?article_id=91. Accessed December 24, 2012.

133. Goddard Space Flight Center. Melting permafrost causes erosion. NASA. USGS. Available at: http://landsat.gsfc.nasa.gov/pdf_archive/cape_halkett_4web.pdf. Accessed January 12, 2013.

134. Neale T. Global warming: more killer heat waves? *MedPage Today*. May 23, 2012. Available at: http://www.medpagetoday.com/PublicHealthPolicy/EnvironmentalHealth/32887. Accessed January 14, 2013.

135. Epstein PR. Climate change and human health. *N Engl J Med*. 2005;353:1433–1436. doi:10.1056/NEJMp058079. Accessed January 12, 2013.

136. McMichael AJ. Globalization, climate change, and human health. *N Engl J Med*. 2013;368(14):1335–1343.

137. Shuman EK. Global climate change and infectious diseases. *N Engl J Med*. 2010;362:1061–1063. doi:10.1056/NEJMp0912931. Accessed January 12, 2013.

138. 2012 West Nile virus update: December 11. Centers for Disease Control and Prevention. Available at: http://www.cdc.gov/ncidod/dvbid/westnile/index.htm. Accessed January 12, 2013.

139. Cooney CM. Climate change and infectious disease: is the future here? *Environ Health Perspect*. 2011;119(9):a394–a397. Available at: http://www.ncbi.nlrn.nih.gov/pmc/articles/PMC3230419. Accessed January 12, 2013.

140. Cook DR. Carbon dioxide duration in the atmosphere. NEWTON: Ask A Scientist! Available at: http://www.newton.dep.anl.gov/askasci/wea00/wea00296.htm. Accessed January 12, 2013.

141. World energy outlook 2009. International Energy Agency. Available at: http://www.worldenergyoutlook.org/media/weowebsite/2009/WEO2009.pdf. Accessed January 9, 2013.

142. G8 leaders agree to global warming goals. United Nations Environment Programme. July 9, 2009. Available at: http://www.unep.org/Documents.Multilingual/Default.asp?DocumentID=593&ArticleID=6245&l=en. Accessed March 5, 2013.

143. Global warming & climate change. *New York Times*. Available at: http://topics.nytimes.com/top/news/science/topics/globalwarming/index.html. Updated January 8, 2013. Accessed March 5, 2013.

144. World energy outlook 2012: in-depth study on energy-efficiency. Overview. International Energy Agency. Available at: http://www.iea.org/media/workshops/2012/energyefficiencyfinance/1aBirol.pdf. Accessed January 9, 2013.

145. Status of ratification of the Kyoto Protocol. United Nations Framework Convention on Climate Change. Available at: http://unfccc.int/kyoto_protocol/status_of_ratification/items/2613.php. Accessed January 12, 2013.

146. Doha Amendment. United Nations Framework Convention on Climate Change. Available at: http://unfccc.int/kyoto_protocol/doha_amendment/items/7362.php. Accessed March 5, 2013.

147. *Massachusetts v. Environmental Protection Agency*, 549 US 497 (2007). Available at: http://www.law.cornell.edu/supct/html/05-1120.ZS.html.

148. Steps the EPA must take to reduce global warming emissions. Union of Concerned Scientists. Available at: http://www.ucsusa.org/global_warming/solutions/big_picture_solutions/steps-the-epa-must-take-to-reduce-global-warming-emissions.html. Accessed January 12, 2013.

149. World energy outlook 2012: in-depth study on energy-efficiency. Overview. International Energy Agency. Available at: http://www.iea.org/media/workshops/2012/energyefficiencyfinance/1aBirol.pdf. Accessed January 9, 2013.

150. Regional Greenhouse Gas Initiative. Available at: http://www.rggi.org. Accessed March 5, 2013.

151. World energy outlook 2012: executive summary. International Energy Agency. Available at: http://iea.org/publications/freepublications/publication/English.pdf. Accessed January 9, 2013.

152. Vehicle solutions. Union of Concerned Scientists. Available at: http://www.ucsusa.org/global_warming/solutions/vehicle_solutions. Accessed January 12, 2013.

153. Gribben C. Debunking the myth of EVs and smokestacks. Electric Vehicle Association of Great Washington, DC. Available at: http://evadc.org/wp-content/uploads/2012/07/pwrplnt.pdf. Accessed January 12, 2013.

154. Breyer A. Solar car ports: the new rising stars. *Solar Novus*. August 27, 2012. Available at: http://www.solarnovus.com/index.php?option=com_content&view=article&id=5551:solar-car-ports-the-new-rising-stars&catid=38:application-tech-features&Itemid=246. Accessed January 12, 2013.

155. World energy outlook 2012: executive summary. International Energy Agency. Available at: http://iea.org/publications/freepublications/publication/English.pdf. Accessed January 9, 2013.

156. Meddin R. World bike-sharing map. Bike Share Philadelphia & the Bike-Sharing Blog. Available at: http://bike-sharing.blogspot.com. E-mail communication, January 24, 2013.

157. Duvall A, Burnap P, e-mail communication, January 21, 2013.

158. Shulman S. Smarter ways to keep the planet cool. Catalyst: Union of Concerned Scientists. Spring 2012. Available at: http://www.ucsusa.org/publications/catalyst/sp12-cooler-smarter.html. Accessed January 10, 2013.

159. Shulman S. Smarter ways to keep the planet cool. Catalyst: Union of Concerned Scientists. Spring 2012. Available at: http://www.ucsusa.org/publications/catalyst/sp12-cooler-smarter.html. Accessed January 10, 2013.

Index